VISION AND AGING
GENERAL AND CLINICAL PERSPECTIVES

VISION AND AGING

GENERAL AND CLINICAL PERSPECTIVES

EDITED BY ALFRED A. ROSENBLOOM, JR.
AND MEREDITH W. MORGAN

Professional Press Books
Fairchild Publications
New York

Dedicated with love to our wives, Sarah and Ida,
and to our children

Table of Contents

Contents

Contents

Foreword

The publication of *Vision and Aging: General and Clinical Perspectives* is indeed welcome. The growing sophistication and complexity of the field of aging has many facets. For example, there is the recognition of the heterogeneity of the aged population and the proper emphasis on successful aging as a state of potential health and growth. There is also the demographic imperative. Moreover, there have been many professional advances: indeed, the research literature on aging has more than doubled in the past two decades. All these factors underscore the need for practitioners to review and expand their knowledge of the field of vision and aging.

This book not only deals with the identification, assessment, and correction of visual disabilities that occur in the older adult; it also places the technical issues of visual function in the aged within a psychological and social context. The impressive group of contributing authors is drawn from the fields of psychology, sociology, gerontology, education, optometry, and medicine. The authors provide the essential scope and depth of knowledge that sharpens this text's focus on a holistic perspective of viewing patients as unique and diverse individuals. The editors, Meredith W. Morgan and Alfred A. Rosenbloom, Jr., should be congratulated for their monumental effort and the unique and valuable contribution they have made to optometric gerontology.

James E. Birren, Ph.D.

Dean, Ethel Percy Andrus Gerontology Center
University of Southern California
Los Angeles

Preface

The purpose of this book is to bring into focus the vast variety of concepts concerning vision and aging. By so doing, vision care practitioners will be able to relate these concepts to the larger goal of providing vision care as a part of comprehensive health service to older persons. In various respects this text is an updating and expansion of optometry's first and only volume on aging—*Vision of the Aging Patient,* edited by Monroe J. Hirsch and Ralph E. Wick. Over 25 years have passed since its publication; moreover, it has been out of print for at least a decade. In the meantime, the number of aging individuals both healthy and unhealthy, vigorous and infirm has increased dramatically so that today every eighth person in the United States is over 65 years of age. Nearly every individual in this diverse group needs optometric care. Optometrists must be prepared to offer this needed care as informed and sympathetic health care practitioners.

Several guiding principles which serve as a framework for this text deserve comment. Aging is *not* a disease—even though there are physiological, psychological, sociological and visual changes with time. Diversity rather than homogeneity becomes the norm with increasing age. Physiological indicators, for example, show a greater range of differences in persons over 65 than in any other age group. As a consequence, norms as performance guidelines cannot be accurately established with any certainty.

Chronological age is a convenient but imprecise indicator of physical, mental and emotional status. For general reference and purposes of discussion only, the editors have defined the aged as being at least 65 years of age. Persons in the age bracket 65 to 74 are sometimes referred to as the *young-old* in contrast to persons in the age range from 75 to 84 who are referred to as the *old.* Those persons over 85 are referred to as the *old-old* and they are more likely to have some significant health care problems due to degenerative or disease conditions.

Because of the unique characteristics of aging, its diversity and complexity, this book is necessarily the work of many individuals. Each of the 27 contributors has undertaken to discuss the aspect of vision and aging with which he or she is most conversant. These authors include optometrists, physicians, psychologists, sociologists and other health professionals. Many participating authors are also educator-scientists who have made important contributions to the advancement of knowledge through research and teaching.

This text is not intended to be a specific topic text, such as refraction techniques and analyses, disease recognition and/or treatment. For example, the chapter on disease and pathology does not include illustrations of the conditions discussed since these are available in many specific texts as identified in the chapter's reference list. This particular chapter is, however, as others, an overview of those specific ocular conditions which are most prevalent in the elderly and which should be kept in mind when serving an older population. This text, then, is directed to the complex vision care of a specific category of patients.

The editors were guided by the overriding goal of imparting knowledge and understanding fundamental to comprehensive and primary vision care of elderly persons rather than imparting skill in testing methodology. In the selection of topics to be discussed and the type of information to be provided, the editors had in mind a primary readership of vision care colleagues, both practitioners and students. What would these readers want and need to know? How much prior knowledge could be assumed? The editors have, for example, assumed that the reader already has skill and knowledge in the various techniques of routine vision and eye examination procedures.

Limitations of space prohibited the inclusion of everything we wished to include; consequently, some topics have been treated only briefly or omitted entirely. So, too, many authors and colleagues who have made important contributions to the field of vision and aging are missing from this book. In some instances, the editors have recognized some of these important contributors through appropriate bibliographic references.

In order to provide the older patient with comprehensive primary care, the optometrist must be aware of not only the ocular and vision conditions of the elderly patient but also must be knowledgeable about those services within the community which improve the quality of life for elderly persons.

The collaborating authors have not met to discuss their special contributions. In a larger sense the prevailing theme of aging is the single concept to which each author adds a unique contribution. The necessary unity in planning and presentation has been the task of the editors. Having read and re-read the various chapters, the editors feel particular pride in and appreciation for the writers who so generously and painstakingly have given of themselves by sharing with us their knowledge and by helping us to understand and appreciate the concepts that each has discussed.

The editors also wish to acknowledge the valued editorial assistance of the copy editor, Mary C. Berry. She provided valuable assistance with details of the editorial process and with the solution of problems of contemporary English usage and style.

Science, it has been said, lives in the details which are universally valid. *Vision and Aging: General and Clinical Perspectives* is not a text whose only purpose is recounting past and present knowledge. Rather its overriding intent is to bring into perspective the continuing quest of practitioners and scientists seeking a more perfect understanding not only of patient care but also of other human services for all aging individuals. The editors hope that every reader of this book may someday find the material personally beneficial.

Meredith W. Morgan
Alfred A. Rosenbloom, Jr.

Introduction

A characteristic of mature industrialized societies is increased average longevity and increased average age of the population. The United States is now becoming such a society and will reach a steady state around 2030, when the distribution of the population by age will be rectangular; there will be equal proportions of people under age 19 and over age 55, as well as a substantial percentage over 75 (and even 85) years of age. With increased expectations of living into old age and with the anticipation of approaching the biologically determined upper limit of the human life-span (estimated at 110 to 120 years), the prevalence of age-related disorders will increase. Indeed, a byproduct of increased average longevity is an increased probability that a given individual will survive to the age of risk of certain diseases prevalent in both old age and, increasingly, old-old age.

Visual disorders are high on the list of such diseases, and impaired vision is one of the most common and disabling conditions of old age. Geriatricians and laypeople alike are increasingly concerned with issues of the quality—more than simply the quantity—of life as old age is achieved. To paraphrase John F. Kennedy, it is more the life in the years than simply the years of life that we must sustain as the population ages progessively. In this regard, no function appears more important than the retention of vision—not only for the maintenance of independence and function, but also for the fullest enjoyment of life.

The frontiers of knowledge relating to the aging process are also being extended through an intensified research effort. This effort has a dual purpose: (1) to understand the aging process ("primary aging") stripped of the associated time-determined concomitants of aging that, through interventions both prior to and during old age, may be retarded or prevented altogether ("secondary aging"); and (2) to determine the means whereby the disabilities associated with aging might be alleviated through treatment.

In both regards *Vision and Aging: General and Clinical Perspectives* is of major interest. It is becoming increasingly apparent that much of what we have accepted as inevitable in aging may indeed not be so. A fuller understanding of the nutritional, behavioral, and environmental determinants of time-related disease emphasizes that function can be preserved into very old age at levels not significantly less than those of middle age and young adulthood. For example, if atherosclerosis can be prevented, cardiovascular function can be maintained into the eighth and ninth decades. The same may prove to be true for the visual disorders of old age; cataract, glaucoma, and macular degeneration may possibly be preventable or even able to be delayed further through appropriate preventive strategies. At the same time, improved surgical, medical, and prosthetic treatment of the disorders highly prevalent in old age may preserve function and retard progression and disability. Finally, geriatric practitioners are becoming increasingly aware of the inextricable interrelationships among the biological, psychological, and social determinants of function and the quality of life in old age. The integration of information about, and sensitivity to, all three spheres of human feelings and endeavor mark the effective geriatric practitioner. Equally important is an awareness that attitudes that preserve the dignity and self-respect of aging patients, although important in caring for patients of all ages, are central to the appropriate care of elderly people.

Increased awareness of the emotional and physical needs of the growing proportion of elderly people, the changing patterns of normal versus abnormal aging in our maturing society, and the sophistication of scientific advances require widespread dissemination of the principles and practice of gerontology among health professionals. *Vision and Aging: General and Clinical Perspectives* is a text that practitioners addressing the visual needs of an aging population will find indispensable. The scope and depth of this text and the wide range of expertise characteristic of its contributors make this volume a significant contribution to the field of gerontology.

William R. Hazzard, M.D.

David J. Carver Professor of Medicine
Director, Center on Aging
Johns Hopkins Medical Institutions
Baltimore

VISION
AND
AGING
GENERAL AND
CLINICAL
PERSPECTIVES

Chapter 1

A Functional Perspective on Aging

Eleanor E. Faye and Robert Rosenberg

The Meaning of Aging

Conventional wisdom advises us that as we age, some of our parts wear out and die. Aging and the diseases that frequently accompany it are realities that everyone faces—some with good fortune, a benign course, and relative wellness, and others with pain, loneliness, disability, and poverty. In fact, older people do not specifically think of themselves as old unless an illness or disability requires an involuntary change in behavior. An individual may suddenly feel old when no longer able to walk as fast, do as much without tiring, or remember as keenly; another individual who is forced to retire at age 65 may suddenly feel old.

Getting old occurs in relation to the ability to function. We are all aging, but not necessarily aged. The active elderly seem to function much as they always have. Others are well but physically inactive. Still others are ill but controlled on medications, or physically ill but mentally alert. Finally, there are those who are not mentally alert or who are too frail to care for themselves. In any case, it is the individual behavior, as well as the organ or tissue state, that determines the diagnosis and course of treatment for the older patient.

Vision and Aging

The aging person who is experiencing visual impairment is facing an involuntary modification of behavior. Added to the problems of personal adjustment is the need to keep in touch with reality and the environment through normal sensory input, but a diminution of sensory input from the eyes or ears interferes with that vital connection. The vision care practitioner's role includes recognition of changes in an aging person's behavior that signal a visual or other sensory deficiency indicating a need for appropriate intervention (either treatment or referral).

What is good eye and vision care for the aging patient? Eye care should be consistent and ongoing, particularly for older people. They need continuity of care from a practitioner who knows them, understands how to evaluate their symptoms, and is interested in helping them retain their visual connections. The clinician must control personal bias toward aging, evaluate what stage the eye has reached, and determine what functional level the patient is capable of attaining. At the same time the clinician must be aware of the level of performance of the other body systems and their interaction with visual performance by taking an adequate medical history (including drugs, dosages, and side effects), visual history, nutritional history, and social history.

The psychological aspects of aging should interest the practitioner who cares for aging persons. The evaluation of vision should also take into consideration age-related responses to all psychophysical measures of function: foveal acuity with high-contrast acuity symbols, ambient acuity with visual field tests, contrast sensitivity, color vision, binocular function, and dark adaptation.

The percentage of vision disorders increases with age, so inevitably more older patients' evaluations result in a determination of low vision. After state-of-the-art medical and surgical treatment has been completed, a clinician should be able to initiate whatever visual rehabilitation is indicated. Although no blanket statements can be made about prescribing or advising rehabilitative care for an older person, the care given by the clinician depends on the progression of the disorder and the patient's expectations, objectives, and ability to learn new techniques and carry them out after a period of adjustment and learning.

Low-vision aids represent a means of sensory augmentation by which the visually impaired person seeks to put residual sight to use. Some forms of magnifying devices have been available for more than half a century, but they often have been overlooked as an integral part of eye and vision care by ophthalmologists and optometrists. Fortunately, practitioner experience and consumer demand have escalated at the same time. Not only have technological advances been made in the sophistication of low-vision aids, but the practitioner also has become aware of the complexity of prescribing successfully. Adapting to sensory augmentation is not a simple adjustment. Although clinicians and older people both recognize the advantage of some forms of sensory augmentation, the successful use of either an optical or hearing aid requires skill, patience, and an awareness of differences in patient's patterns of coping with impairment and disability.

For referral for multiple services to help integrate activities for older patients, the practitioner should be aware of local agencies for the aging, for rehabilitation, and for the visually impaired. For the clinician who wishes to offer a full range of eye and vision care, this book brings together thoughts of experts in the clinical aspects of vision and aging. It is hoped that by reading their contributions, clinicians will see the value of becoming actively involved in geriatric care, whether professionally in practice, in community centers through lecturing or screening programs, or merely by visiting institutionalized elderly people as an interested member of the community.

In the traditional world of health care, "cure," in the sense of restoring normal organ function, is the ultimate goal, and the success or failure of diagnosis and treatment is usually measured in those terms. In vision care, these same criteria are accepted in assessing visual health; in addition, however, performance tests are important in determining the success of treatment. In vision care, age alone is not a good predictor of individual performance or behavior. Performance relates less to the apparent organ lesions than to anatomic, physiological, and psychological factors, all dynamic functions that make up processes whose rates of change—usually expressed as population means related to popula-

tion age—often defy accurate measurement.

Individual Differences

To understand the relationship between population means, population age, and individual performance, it is helpful to visualize a population as a parade marching down a boulevard. As we observe the parade, we can predict only where the crowd will be at a given time. We cannot know in advance if one or more marchers will drop out, drop back, or run ahead of the rest. In other words, knowing the performance means of a population as a function of age is of interest, but it does not predict individual performance in geriatric care; only individual assessment discloses an individual's position in the age group "parade."

Because of the large individual differences observed in the older population, conventional wisdom would advise us not to divide people into chronological age groups as if they were separate species. We grow up, mature, and grow old at different rates, so there are no valid norms by which to declare what stage anyone has achieved. Instead, we observe that there are greater differences among older individuals than among younger people. The hallmark of good geriatric care is individual assessment, comprehensive evaluation, and goal setting based on individual wants and needs.

Suggested Readings

Butler, R. N., and M. I. Lewis. *Aging and Mental Health.* 2d ed. St. Louis: Mosby, 1977.

Faye, E. E., et al. *Clinical Low Vision.* 2d ed. Boston: Little, Brown, 1984.

Greenberg, D., and L. Branch. A Review of Methodologic Issues Concerning Incidence and Prevalence Data of Visual Deterioration in Elders. In *Aging and Human Visual Function*, eds. R. Sekuler, I. Kline, and K. Dismukes. New York: Alan R. Liss, 1982, pp. 279–296.

Hussian, R. A. *Geriatric Psychology: A Behavioral Perspective.* New York: Van Nostrand Reinhold, 1981.

Sekuler, R.; I. Kline; and K. Dismukes, *Aging and Human Visual Function.* New York: Alan R. Liss, 1982.

Snow, C. P. "The Price of Our Success," *New York State Journal of Medicine*, November 1964, pp. 2811–2815.

Chapter 2

The Maturing of the United States

Daniel F. Detzner

Everyone wants to live a long and healthy life, but it seems that no one wants to grow old. This paradox is most visible when one of the 15,000 people in the United States who annually turns 100 celebrates a centenary. Newspaper, magazine, and television reporters inquire about health, exercise, diet, and the secrets of living a long life. We marvel at their stamina, listen to their advice, and hope for similar good fortune. In the same media there are advertisements for cosmetic products promising an end to gray hair, wrinkles, age spots, and other signs of growing older. Although long life is valued, there are strong tendencies to fear the aging process and to negatively stereotype older people. These contradictions have roots deeply embedded in Western tradition and the U.S. experience. To understand why longevity is prized while the process leading toward it—and the people who achieve it—is not, it is necessary to trace the origins of U.S. values associated with aging. These values explain the complex and ambiguous attitudes that people in the United States have about growing old and being old.

Since the vast majority of people reading these words will live to an advanced age themselves, it is important to understand the social context within which those lives will be lived. The world of the future will be significantly older than the world of today. During the next several decades, our lives, work, family, friends, and neighborhoods will be dramatically altered by the rapid aging of the U.S. population. Because so many people will live longer lives, the strain on the national budget, the health care professions, and other major institutions will increase geometrically. Increasingly, the taxpayers, clients, and patients of tomorrow will be classified as "older people," and so will we. If we are to understand

the significance of these changes and their multiple effects on our lives, we must begin by examining the deeply ambiguous origins of U.S. values.

Paradox of Aging

In a market economy, the physical needs of society for food, shelter, and clothing are primary concerns. After those needs are served, entrepreneurs seek out the more elusive psychological and social needs of people and develop products that promise to fulfill them (Hughs 1971, Chap. 1). Marketing strategists design advertising campaigns to highlight the unique attributes of their products, and with careful analysis, the deeply rooted human needs for which these products are created becomes clear. For example, a 1923 popular magazine advertisement for a hair product, Kolor-Bak, illustrates how the underlying fear of aging can be effectively used to create and sell a product. The advertisement boldly states the following:

GRAY HAIR! SHE WAS HORRIFIED.

A woman gazes into her mirror with dismay. Gray streaks mar the beauty of her hair. "Is my youthful appearance going? Am I to look old?" Later she sees in the mirror an amazing change. The original color has returned. She is young again. A clean, colorless liquid has brought a wonderful and gratifying transformation.

Thousands of similar messages are repeated every day for a multitude of products, all designed to help consumers overcome the physical changes associated with growing older. Gray hair, wrinkles, and bifocal glasses are portrayed as stigmatic symbols of physical decline to be avoided at any cost (Goffman 1963, Chap.1;

Ward 1977). A multibillion dollar cosmetics industry promises to assist millions who feel a psychological and social need to avoid the negative label of "old." For the most part, the mass media have ignored the complex realities of late life, choosing instead to negatively stereotype the elderly as sick, silly, senile, and sitting in the rocking chair waiting for the end (Aronhoff 1974; Martel 1968).

Advertisements for products promising lasting youthfulness reflect and reinforce the contradictory messages about aging that have been passed down to us through Western culture. One part of this message can be traced back more than two millenia to the classical Greek concept of ideal forms. In the *Republic,* Plato argues that the human mind envisions idealized images of the proper structure for government, architecture, and human life. These abstract forms may be impossible to achieve; however, they provide a utopian model through which imperfect mortals may view their lives and creative efforts. In this notion we find the source of Western culture's idealization of youth, and it is here that the antipathy for all things old can be traced. Evidence for the idealization of the youthful body can be found throughout classical art and literature. Classical Greece viewed the youthful years with envy, because the young were seen as strong, heroic, beautiful, and without limits. In contrast, the very old were looked on with distaste, because they were weak, physically declining, and close to the limits of human life. To die young in the full bloom of youthful vitality, was considered heroic by the ancient Greeks, whereas old age was considered a sad misfortune (Durant 1966, Chap. 13). For more than 2,000 years, westerners have returned to ancient Greek sources for inspiration; this continuing influence helped create a youth cult that shapes modern values about all stages of the life cycle.

The origins of the youth cult and the consequent devaluation of old age may be even more deeply embedded in human history than this brief review of Greek thought suggests. A desire to avoid the limitations of the body and a dream of immortality seem to be universal attributes of human nature. Legends about a magical fountain of youth appear throughout world history in many different cultures separated by space and time. The persistence of this legend from ancient times into the modern era is additional evidence of the enduring human desire to avoid

the effects of aging and the ultimate finality of death. By recognizing the continuing influence of ancient legends and classical ideals, we can begin to understand the modern attraction of cosmetic products that help disguise normal processes of aging.

A more positive message about late life can be traced to ancient Hebrew sources in the Middle East. The basic text for this alternative vision is the Old Testament, where advanced age brings status and prestige. The very old were seen as blessed persons whose lives had been spared by Yahweh as an example of virtue rewarded. In this religious tradition, the wicked die young, and the rare older person exaggerates his or her age to add weight to opinions. The life cycle is portrayed as cyclical, with each stage having its own intrinsic value, responsibilities, and purpose. In their final years, the old have significant social roles, such as wise person, prophet, teacher, and priest. Even though the old are valued because of their knowledge and virtue, they also may be resented by impatient youth, because they have the authority to uphold age-old cultural traditions. Despite this fact, elders have an important place in ancient Hebrew tradition that continues to influence Western thought. The influence of this positive message, however, is closely intertwined with the negative messages coming from classical Greece. These two roots form the basis for the contradictory feelings about old age that are so prevalent in the modern era (Slater 1963).

The value any culture or historical period places on old age goes beyond a secular idealization of youth or sacred respect for longevity. In his classic anthropological study of 71 cultures, Simmons suggests that age status is primarily related to the wealth and technological development of a society (Cowgill 1974; Simmons 1945). Old people who no longer can be productive may be cast aside by undeveloped societies with scarce resources. A subsistence economy cannot tolerate the dependent status of the sick, crippled, and old. In contrast, technologically developed societies often have the resources to create dependency in these groups by policies such as mandatory retirement and sophisticated medical techniques, which extend life beyond natural expectations. It has become apparent in some advanced societies, particularly the United States, that increased longevity and nonproductivity may be too expensive for even the wealthiest of nations. This reality may create intergenerational tensions as higher taxes on the shrinking younger generation pay for entitlement programs for an expanding older population. Further strains will occur in technologically developed societies as the middle-aged and elderly realize that their knowledge and skills are rapidly dated in the postindustrial information age (Toffler 1970). Modern societies demand the new knowledge and creative energy of the young while devaluing the potential contributions of the old (Kidder 1981). The elderly's loss of social and economic status must be considered one of the most significant costs of modernization.

Simmons's pioneering research sparked a debate among anthropologists and gerontologists concerning the effects of modernization on the status of the elderly. This debate and the contradictory messages passed down to us from ancient times demonstrate that old age is more than a socially defined period of time toward the end of life. It has a larger symbolic meaning that grows out of its complex relationship with the economic and cultural values of a society and their roots in the human psyche.

Quest for the Fountain of Youth

These complex messages and symbolic meanings about old age were brought to the New World with the first exploratory voyages. A few years after Columbus's discovery, a 39-year-old Spanish nobleman named Ponce de León began a search for the legendary fountain of youth along the coast of Florida. He had heard tales of a magic spring with rejuvenating waters from the Carib Indians (who populated the Caribbean islands that stretch from Florida to South America). These stories were so similar to European legends that he decided to organize a major search in the newly discovered land. After eight unsuccessful months of testing every stream, river, and inlet along the Florida peninsula, Ponce de León returned home just in time to celebrate his 40th birthday (Morison 1974, 502–531).

Ponce de León's attempt to escape from the limits of age was unsuccessful, but this fact did not deter millions of young and middle-aged Europeans from following in his footsteps during the next 400 years. His quest is symbolic of the romantic dreams that post-Renaissance Europeans hoped to make real in the New World. Although few expected to find a fountain of youth, there was a strong desire to escape from

the layers of authority and centuries of tradition imposed on them by elders. Among lower-class and peasant youth, there was a widespread ambition to flee from the economic and religious boundaries of the Old World. Personal ambition was fueled with energy produced by the Renaissance, Reformation, and French Revolution, while economic interests and natural curiosity fostered the Age of Discovery. These social, economic and technological upheavals provided millions of young people with their first opportunity to escape (Elliot 1970, 54–78).

To the young immigrants who flocked to U.S. shores, the New World represented a rebirth, a fresh start, and a second chance to develop as individuals unencumbered by the traditional limits of family, state, and religious authority. The New World they sought had no past, no geographical boundaries, and no elderly authority figures who bound them to grim duty. In the absence of these traditional restrictions, the New World immigrant could hope for a rejuvenation into the individualistic self-made man that has become the archetypal hero of U.S. life and literature (Chase 1957; Lewis 1955).

For more than three centuries, millions of young Europeans pursued their dreams by leaving behind their parents, grandparents, and places of birth to seek their fortune on the boundless U.S. frontier. A steady stream of young people settling the new nation kept the median age of the population under 23 years of age until the early years of the 20th century (*Historical Statistics* 1960, ser. A, 22, 83, 84, and 86). In a recurring pattern of epic proportions, the new immigrants followed Horace Greeley's advice to "Go West Young Man." Clearly, the new nation and the western frontier was a place for the young (Smith 1950). Few older persons were willing to subject themselves to the difficulties of passage from Europe, and even fewer were willing to leave their ancestral homes for the uncertainty of life in the United States (*Historical Statistics* 1960, ser. A, 86–94). To the aged, the Old World offered security and a sense of place that would be impossible to find in the rapid change of life on the North American continent.

Despite their desire to escape from Old World boundaries, the new North Americans transplanted many European values to the New World. The Greek idealization of youth was apparent from the early years, and so was the influence of Judeo-Christian values. Although their authority may have been resented by the younger generation, the rare people who lived to an advanced age in the New World were more often than not respected (Achenbaum 1978; Fisher 1977). The strength of family ties and economic necessity required that the young and middle-aged pay attention to the advice of their elders. Because families were relatively large, integration of older family members was not a major problem. A slower paced, seasonal, farm life enabled most older persons to continue their productive years until death. Retirement was unknown until well into the 20th century. As a result, the elderly were not defined as a personal, family, or social problem for most of U.S. history (Handlin and Handlin 1971).

Although the small number of elderly persons who lived in the early United States were able to command respect, this does not mean that old age was valued. Even in the New World the old embodied the authority, tradition, and limits from which the young sought escape. Characteristics traditionally associated with youth, such as strength, vitality, energy, progress and optimism, were those needed to settle and develop the new land. Consequently, the newly developing culture elevated youth to a place of eminence not seen in the Western world since classical Greek times.

Growing Old in Public

By the middle of the 20th century, the dominance of the Greek ideal was most readily visible in the media of mass communication. It was here that fear of aging and dreams of longevity could be viewed on a daily basis, and it was here that paradoxical images of old age were instantaneously projected to millions. Like Plato's conception of ideal forms, the modern notion of "image" helps explain the negative stereotyping of the aged. According to Kenneth Boulding (1956), *images* are culturally based, individually shaped mental pictures of the world that are mirrorlike reflections of basic values, beliefs, and attitudes. Images can be romantic, idealized abstractions about a stage of life or inaccurate, misinformed stereotypes about a diverse group of individuals. Similar subjective images that are widely shared eventually become a "public" image that is recorded in the popular culture of the period. When they are repeated often enough by powerful image purveyors like television and mass circulation magazines, these images can take on a life of their own. Public images not only reflect widespread beliefs and opinions; they also subtly socialize the young into the dominant culture's way of viewing the world.

Negative Images

The public image of old age in the last half of the 20th century is complex, ambiguous, and largely negative. The roots of this image can be seen in Thomas Cole's 19th century paintings entitled "The Voyage of Life." In this series of four paintings, "Childhood" and "Youth" are portrayed in light, sunny, and optimistic tones, whereas "Adulthood" and "Old Age" are filled with dark, foreboding, and ominous clouds looming overhead (Kasson 1975).

When any group of people is asked what the dominant image of old age is in the modern United States, the answers are reminiscent of Cole's paintings. Old age is filled with sickness, senility, loneliness, and fear. Images of physical decline, dependency, and death cloud the future. "Dirty old man" and "little old lady" are well-known public images that unconsciously reflect the negative and simplistic notions of many about a large and highly diverse segment of the population. Mental pictures of a leering older man and a frail older woman restrict the elderly to a narrow range of acceptable behaviors based on the assumption of poor mental or physical health. The image of "sickness" seems to predominate in many popular magazines and advertising campaigns. Old age is portrayed as a time of sadness and loss or silliness and dementia. This image assumes that older people are incompetent, confused, or childlike. The image of older person as sickly relegates the more than 25,000,000 people now over 65 years of age to the rocking chair, the hospital, and the nursing home. Like other negative images, this stereotype has little basis in the realities of health and daily life for the vast majority of older people (National Center for Health Statistics 1971).

The sickness image has its parallel in advertising campaigns that encourage denial or stigmatization of the normal aging processes. Cosmetic manufacturers use youth, as well as the qualities associated with youthfulness, to encourage middle-aged consumers to purchase their wares. The physical changes that normally occur with increased years are portrayed as negative examples of what will happen if the unwary fail to use the product. Large cosmetic companies, such as the Olay Company, have used women's fear of looking older as their major advertising theme for many years. Because of the success of these kinds of advertisements, motivational analysts have begun to use the promise of eternal youthfulness to advertise products that range from dish soap to film processing.

In recent years the fear of aging and the cult of youth have spawned some bizarre services by medical practitioners who advertise lasting youth and life extension for those who can afford it. For large sums, the wealthy can purchase medical procedures such as deep facial peels, dermabrasion, plastic surgery, and hair transplants to conceal wrinkled skin and receding hairlines. At some clinics, placental extracts and lamb embryos are injected into older men and women in hopes of rejuvenation. Examples like this indicate how deeply rooted is the fear of age and how far individuals are willing to go in their quest for eternal youth (McGrady 1968).

Cosmetic advertisements are easily recognized examples that illustrate negative public images in the popular media; however, they are not the only examples. Recent studies by gerontologists indicate that the emphasis on the negative also can be found in children's books, prime time television, films, magazine cartoons, and poetry (Ansello 1976; Aronhoff 1974; Smith 1979; Sohngen and Smith 1978; Wolfenstein and Leites 1950). They reveal how widespread the tendency to emphasize the negative has become and how all aspects of modern culture have been affected. To what extent these negative images reflect or shape U.S. attitudes is difficult to measure; however, a public opinion survey sponsored by the National Council on Aging reveals an astonishingly broad range of negative opinion about older people by the younger and middle generations (Harris and Associates 1975). When such a negative portrait of late life is projected by all forms of media and apparently believed by such a wide range of people, it is not surprising that few people over 65 years of age are willing to identify themselves as "old" (Tuckman and Lorge 1957).

At the deepest personal level distaste for old age is linked to fear of death. In his Pulitzer Prize–winning book, *The Denial of Death*, Ernest Becker (1973) argues forcefully that man's heroic self-image causes a repression of the very idea of death. Because older people are chronologically closer to death, they are stigmatized and segregated by society in order to maintain the illusion of immortality. Death denial is much easier in the 20th century than it was in the past, because death has become remote from daily life. High infant mortality, epidemics, and shorter life spans made death and dying a commonly accepted occurrence only a few decades ago. Today, however, death has become insulated, isolated, and sterilized in formalized institutions such as hospitals, churches, and mortuaries (Sudnow 1967). The most common reaction of hospital patients when told they are terminally ill is outright denial (Kubler-Ross 1969). The extremes of denial are exhibited by members of the Cryonic Society of America, who carry out their fantasies of immortality by having their bodies frozen at death to await the discovery of a cure for their fatal disease and a method for reincarnation (Ettinger 1964).

Positive Images

Although the dominant public image of old age appears to be negative, the popular media always have portrayed some positive images. A 1868 Currier and Ives print illustrates a 19th century example. In this popular print, an older couple sits contentedly by the fireside while a beloved granddaughter sits at the knee of grandfather. The grandmother is knitting nearby while awaiting the arrival of her granddaughter's parents. The title of this romantic family-oriented portrait is "Old Age–The Season of Rest." This early example of a satisfying old age has been echoed more frequently during the last few decades. Older people now are portrayed more frequently in creative, educational, life-enhancing, and hopeful ways by the media. Growing older is shown as a natural and inevitable process that is not always filled with sickness, loneliness, or despair. The advertising industry appears to be catching up with the demographic realities of U.S. life; older people now more frequently are shown as warm and kindly figures whose years of experience have prepared them to speak wisely about a consumer product (Brown 1974).

Although the number of positive images remains relatively small, these images nevertheless present an alternative to the rather bleak picture that has prevailed. Occasionally, more realistic portraits of the later years are presented in the media as sketches or short biographies of older people whose activities are presented as "news" because they do not fit the negative stereotypes. Popular magazine and television stories about people in their 90s and 100s who enjoy good health and mental alertness high-light the admiration we continue to have for lon-gevity. Older people with unusual or unexpected activities are occasionally portrayed as eccentric examples of the possibilities of late life. Stories about seventy-year-old marathon runners, mountain-climbing octogenarians, and yoga-performing women in their 90s are life-enhancing images that are meant to inspire and give hope. The potential of old age is illustrated by articles and stories about accomplished artists like Miró, Picasso, Casals, and others, who did not reach their creative peaks until well past their 65th birthdays.

A few of these positive role models whose activities receive continuing media attention become larger-than-life symbols or public images of productive old age. Their lives demonstrate by example that the later years need not be a season of rest, disengagement, or decline. One of the most interesting examples is a man who came to national attention during the early years of the Great Depression. In 1933 Francis Townsend was a 66-year-old retired physician who developed a plan for national economic recovery and income security of the elderly. Although the Townsend Plan has serious eco-nomic flaws, Townsend's idea nevertheless initiated a national debate on the responsibili-ties of government to its senior citizens that con-tinues today. Townsend's leadership brought together hundreds of thousands of older people into a well-organized movement that ultimately pressured President Roosevelt to establish the commission that recommended congressional approval of the Social Security Act. The Town-send Movement was the first nationwide effort to organize older people into a coherent interest group to lobby on their own behalf (Holtzman 1963). Townsend became a repository of hope for millions of older people who were severely affected by unemployment and the absence of a national income maintenance program. As a nationally recognized figure, Townsend projected a public image of an intelligent, angry, and ener-getic older man who had decided to fight for the rights of his peers. Current national leaders like Maggie Kuhn of the Grey Panthers and Con-gressman Claude Pepper of the House Rules Committee are continuing the tradition and public image established by Townsend more than 50 years ago.

As Townsend's image faded in the 1940s, an older woman from upstate New York came into the national spotlight. Anna Mary Robertson Moses, affectionately known to millions as Grandma Moses, first came to national attention in 1940, when her paintings were shown at the Galerie St. Etienne in New York City. Although she never had formal training, Grandma Moses's romantic paintings of her 19th century child-hood evoked nostalgic emotions in the thousands of persons who flocked to her exhibits (Kallir 1946). Between 1940 and 1946 her "primitive" paintings were displayed at 37 galleries across the United States and Europe. The instant fame she received in her 70s and 80s goes beyond the clarity of her work or the nostalgic longing for a simpler past. She became the topic of innumer-able high school essays and a kind of national grandmother figure at a time when the world was once again torn by war. In addition to teaching an appreciation for U.S. rural history, Grandma Moses exemplified the creative poten-tial of the later years. She lived for 26 years after her 65th birthday and did not even begin to paint seriously until her late 70s. Although she experi-enced many of the same losses of other older woman—including the death of her husband, declining income, and physical frailty—she con-tinued to grow, create, and contribute to the lives of all she touched. Her life and public image demonstrated that older people need not be con-tent with the rocking chair or the nursing home.

Grandma Moses and Francis Townsend are only two examples of older people whose activi-ties were spotlighted as alternative public images of healthy, energetic, and creative old age. There are, of course, millions of ordinary individuals who grow old in interesting and crea-tive ways but never are noticed by the national media. These people serve as dynamic examples and positive models to their family, friends, and neighbors. Occasionally, the national media will focus on a group of these ordinary older people who are engaged in activities usually considered beyond the interests or capabilities of the elderly. One example is the worldwide attention given to an unusual softball team in St. Petersburg, Florida. The Three-Quarter Century Softball Club is composed of men 75 years of age and older who play a regular schedule of seven-inning games against high school and women's teams (Bakewell 1974). These men, some of whom are well into their 80s and 90s, have been proving for more than a half-century that good health, exercise, and team sports are not the exclusive domain of the young.

Another group that presents an alternative public image of openness and experimentation in late life is the Senior Actualization and Growth Experience (SAGE). Founded in the early 1970s by Gay Luce and Eugenia Gerrard, SAGE was designed to provide personal growth experiences for both healthy and ill senior citizens living in the San Francisco Bay area. Using ancient and modern relaxation techniques such as massage, biofeedback, meditation, and tai chi, hundreds of older people have learned how to relax their bodies and enhance their personal energy (Fauman 1976). Although the SAGE project was relatively small, it attracted national attention in the gerontological network and funding by the National Institute of Mental Health. The project provides hope to elderly people seeking new areas of strength to compensate for the losses that naturally accompany the last stage of life, and it is still another illustration of the inadequacy of the predominately negative images.

Maturation Process

These individuals and groups exemplify creative efforts by older people to improve their quality of life. Coincidentally, their lives and activities improve the public image of old age and help negate commonly accepted stereotypes. Despite the national attention these positive examples have received, the vast majority of younger and middle-aged people in the United States continues to see the elderly in negative, stereotypical, and inaccurate ways. For example, only 5 percent of a national opinion sample thought older people were sexually active; only 19 percent considered the elderly to be open-minded and adaptable; and less than one-third thought they were bright and alert (L. Harris and Associates 1975). The survey reveals a widespread lack of knowledge about elementary aspects of growing older and stereotypical images of the aged. Because of this widespread ignorance and negative image, most people over 65 prefer not to be identified as "old"; however, older people's attitudes about themselves and their peers are quite different from those of the younger generations. In a speech before the annual meeting of the National Council on Aging, Louis Harris interpreted his survey's message from the elderly to the rest of the nation:

Look, you are drowning us with pity and your bad conscience has convinced us that the plight and

lot of older people is well nigh hopeless. Well, we want to tell you that we are in much better fettle, in much better command of our competence and capabilities, and much more willing to bear our share of societal responsibilities than you even imagined (Harris 1974).

Apparently, this message has not yet filtered down to the general population. People continue to be inundated by public images flashed at them on television screens or billboards. Whether these images are positive or negative, they cannot substitute for a thorough understanding of the physical, psychological, and social changes that occur with normal aging. To overcome the cultural influences of the ancient Greeks, the powerful influence of the modern media, and our own fears and idiosyncratic notions about late life, it is necessary to develop a deeper understanding of the diversity and potential of people who are old.

Undoubtedly, this understanding and attitude change will take time to come about in the years ahead, even though the number and diversity of the older population will continue to grow at dramatic rates. Educators only recently have begun to develop a K–12 curriculum on the multiple processes of aging (Jacobs 1974). Although gerontology courses and programs have grown rapidly in undergraduate and graduate departments during the last decade, they affect a small percentage of the population (Association of Gerontology in Higher Education 1981). In the health professions, the debate continues over whether geriatrics should be a specialty, be integrated into the traditional curriculum, or be ignored altogether (Goldman 1974). Even though health care professionals interact with older patients more than any other age group, relatively few have studied the complex and interrelated processes of physical development through the life span in an integrated curriculum (Freeman 1971). The results of this disinterest in the elderly are predictable. One study revealed that the primary diagnosis for people admitted to a nursing home was inaccurate for 64 percent of the patients; secondary diagnosis was either not made or inaccurate for 84 percent of the aged patients (Miller and Elliot 1976). Because these problems are beginning to be addressed, future health care professionals will be far more knowledgeable about the elderly than those today; however, it will be many years before the effects of their training become widespread.

During the last three decades, a large gerontological research literature has been published as professional associations and journals attempted to keep pace with the explosion of knowledge in the field. Although a great deal still is unknown, significant cross-sectional data, longitudinal studies, and cross-cultural research have been completed. Despite the dissemination of this new knowledge in courses, journals, and popular books, the average person today probably knows less about older people than did those who lived at the turn of the century. This may be true because of the modern tendency for all age groups to live, work and recreate in age-segregated environments (Townsend 1970). There are national political pressures to segregate the aged, because federally funded programs and services are usually more cost effective if offered in an age-segregated setting (Estes 1979). Across the United States there are thousands of long-term care facilities, high-rise apartment complexes, senior centers, and congregate dining sites that bring people of the same age together. Evidence suggests that informal helping networks develop in these segregated environments, but the cost to other generations may be very high (Hochschild 1973). When the old are separated from the young and middle-aged, the younger people lose the opportunity to learn about late life in the old-fashioned way—by observing and participating in its joys and sorrows.

Implications for the Health Care Professional

Without an opportunity for regular contact with a broad range of older people, the tendency for the young and middle-aged to be subconsciously influenced by the negative public images surely must increase. Health care professionals and others who work directly with the elderly may find it even more difficult to develop a positive outlook, because the elderly who most frequently seek their services do, in fact, fit many of the stereotypes generalized to the entire older population. Typically, people who need health care or social services are experiencing physical decline, mental confusion, social disengagement, or economic problems. Healthy, well-adjusted, middle-class retirees who experience their final years as a time of release, relaxation, and reflection rarely need the services of a clinic or social worker. As a result, those professionals who have a significant effect on the lives of many older

people may have the greatest tendency to view them in negative ways. Their negative attitudes and low expectations are likely to be subtly transmitted to their patients and clients, resulting in a diminished quality of care. The health care professional who truly believes that older people should not expect to see, hear, walk, or think very well in their later years will pass on these attitudes to their patients, who certainly will fulfill those prophecies without adequate health care (Krause 1977).

To overcome these tendencies it is necessary to view the elderly in a very different way. It is important not to define them in strictly physical terms, since physical loss and decline are human realities, and if they are emphasized, inevitably they lead to negative stereotyping. Instead of defining older people in terms of their diseases, deficiencies, and disabilities, we must begin to view them in terms of their experience, perspective and potential. Accomplishing this alternative viewpoint requires a suspension of judgment or instant classification when encountering older people for the first time. Chronological age or physical status must be temporarily ignored to enable us to see the elderly as full persons with a long and varied past. The process for uncovering this past was first discussed by Robert Butler (1963), former director of the National Institute of Aging, more than 20 years ago.

According to Butler, older people have a natural tendency to reminisce and reflect on their earlier years. Although the desire to review life experiences exists at all ages, it appears to grow more intense in the later years and during periods of major life changes and transition (Lewis 1971; McMahon and Rhudick 1964). Although life review can take place in the recesses of individuals' own minds, it is more valuable when shared with others, because it enables the older people to pass on their experiences and enables the listeners to see the individuals as full persons.

Life review can be therapeutic for the elderly; however, we do not need to be therapists to engage older people in life review conversations (Liton and Olstein 1969). Active listening skills, a sincere interest, and a few questions are all that usually are necessary to bring forth a flood of memories and a storehouse of insights. Life reviews can take the form of structured interviews that are written down in a coherent life history, but more frequently they are casual remarks that are integrated into daily conversations. The interested listener can turn these informal comments into life history questions as a way of getting to know the individual in a deeper, more meaningful way.

Listening to the life stories of older people can be beneficial to almost anyone; however, this process may be particularly valuable for health care professionals and others in frequent contact with the elderly. Instead of seeing someone as a frail, poor, and lonely older woman with multiple health problems, it may be possible to see her as a full human being with a fascinating life history. By using life review as a communication technique, the skilled practitioner can better understand the problems, needs and coping abilities of patients and clients. Life review is also a way to diminish the influence of media stereotypes while creating more positive personal images of the later years. It can help diminish natural generational differences and the multiple effects of age segregation. Finally, life review can help individuals understand their own aging process and the value of long life.

While explaining his conception of ideal forms, Socrates told the story of a man who was chained to the wall of a cave for his entire life. Because he could not turn around to see the actual people walking past the mouth of the cave, his reality was based on the dark shadows that flitted past his limited vision. When the chains were broken, the man turned around and was amazed to see distinct silhouettes of people walking past the mouth of the cave and was certain that he had finally seen reality in its truest form. After he struggled out of the cave into bright sunlight, he was once again surprised to learn that the shadows and images that he had thought real were merely reflections of the true human form. After living in society for a time, the man began to realize how imperfect these human creatures were, and he began to wonder whether they were merely shadowy reflections of an ideal human form that only could be imagined by ordinary mortals.

Like the man in the cave, many of us believe that the realities of old age are the shadowy images we see directly in front of us. Although it is true that late life is filled with significant losses and major transitions, it is also true that only in old age can we achieve a full sense of accomplishment, completion, and self-actualization. It is obvious that health declines with advanced age and that ultimately we all perish, but we do not always realize that the intellect, personality, and spirit can continue to grow until the last moments of life. Even though we know that the body is frail and ultimately finite, we also know that the aging process occurs at widely variable rates, and with proper exercise, nutrition and health care the inevitable decline can be delayed until the very end.

It is possible to overcome the shadowy pictures and dark images of old age that have been shaped by the culture and projected by the mass media. To break the chains that bind us and the fears that blind us, we must struggle past the cultural values associated with youthfulness and the stigmatic notions associated with old age. Using life review as an everyday technique to understand the realities of the life span is one helpful technique. We should not expect to find, however, that everyone over 65 will be like Francis Townsend or Grandma Moses, or that all elderly people are capable of softball at 70, tai chi at 80, and wisdom at 90. We should find that all people grow old in their own individual ways and that as people age they become well-defined and different from their peers. Although gerontologists can make generalizations about older people, the reality is that all people's aging experiences are highly personal and uniquely their own. Like the man in the cave, we can strive to understand these complex realities, but we are similarly doomed to fail. By inquiring into the lives of those we meet and work with, it is possible to gain a few insights and a more clear vision of what lies over the horizon.

References

Achenbaum, W. *Old Age in the New Land,* Baltimore: Johns Hopkins, 1978.

Ansello, E. "Ageism in Picture Books: How Older People Are Stereotyped." *Interracial Books for Children* 7 (1976): 4–6.

Aronhoff, C. "Old Age in Prime Time." *Journal of Communication* 2 (1974): 86–87.

Association for Gerontology in Higher Education. *National Directory of Educational Programs in Gerontology.* Washington D.C.: Association for Gerontology in Higher Education, 1981.

Bakewell, G. *The History of the Kids and Kubs Three-Quarter Century Softball Club.* St. Petersburg, Fla.: Three-Quarter Century Softball Club, 1974.

Becker, E. *The Denial of Death,* New York: Free Press: 1973.

Boulding, K. *The Image,* Ann Arbor: University of Michigan Press, 1956.

Brown, L. "Commercials on TV Now Put Age before Beauty." *Minneapolis Tribune,* August 25, 1974, 8D.

Butler, R. "The Life Review: An Interpretation of Reminiscence in the Aged." *Psychiatry,* 26 (February 1963): 65–76.

Chase, R. *The American Novel and Its Tradition*, Doubleday, Garden City, N.Y.: 1957.

Cowgill, D. "The Aging of Populations and Societies." *Annals of the American Academy of Political and Social Science* 415 (1974): 1–18.

Durant, W. *Life in Ancient Greece*. New York: Simon and Schuster, 1966.

Elliott, J. *The Old World and the New (1492–1650)*. London: Cambridge University Press, 1970.

Estes, C. *The Aging Enterprise*. San Francisco: Jossey-Bass, 1979.

Ettinger, R. *The Prospect of Immortality*. Garden City, N.Y.: Doubleday, 1964.

Fauman, R. *New Image of Age*. Washington, D.C.: National Institute of Mental Health, 1976 (Videotape).

Fisher, D. *Growing Old in America*. New York: Oxford University Press, 1977.

Freeman, J. "Medical Ethics in Geriatrics." In *Research and Training in Gerontology*. Washington D.C.: U.S. Government Printing Office, 1971.

Goffman, I. *Stigma: Notes on the Management of Spoiled Identity*. Englewood Cliffs, N.J.: Prentice-Hall, 1963.

Goldman, R. "Geriatrics as a Specialty; Problems and Prospects." *Gerontologist* 14 (December 1974): 468–471.

Handlin, O, and M. Handlin *Facing Life: Youth and Family Life in American History*. Boston: Little, Brown, 1971.

Harris, L. "Who the Senior Citizens Really Are." Speech to the annual meeting of the National Council on Aging, Detroit, October 2, 1974.

L. Harris and Associates. *The Myth and Reality of Aging in America*. Washington, D.C.: National Council on Aging, 1975.

Historical Statistics of the United States: Colonial Times to the Present. Washington, D.C.: U.S. Government Printing Office, 1960.

Hochschild, A. *The Unexpected Community*. Englewood Cliffs, N.J.: Prentice-Hall, 1973.

Holtzman, A. *The Townsend Movement: A Political Study*. New York: Bookman Associates, 1963.

Hughs, G. *Attitude Measurement of Marketing Strategy*. Glenview, Ill.: Scott, Foresman, 1971.

Jacobs, H. "Education for Aging in the Elementary and Secondary School System." In *Learning for Aging*, eds. S. Grabowski and D. Mason, Washington, D.C.: Adult Education Association, 1974.

Kallir, O. *Grandma Moses: American Primitive*. Garden City, N.J.: Doubleday, 1946.

Kasson, J. "The Voyage of Life: Thomas Cole and the Romantic Disillusionment." *American Quarterly* 27 (1975): 42–56.

Kidder, T. *The Soul of a New Machine*. Boston: Little, Brown, 1981.

Krause, E. *Power and Illness*, New York: Elsevier, 1977.

Kubler-Ross, E. *On Death and Dying*, New York: Macmillan, 1969.

Lewis, C. "Reminiscing and Self-Concept in Old Age." *Journal of Gerontology* 26 (April 1971): 240–243.

Lewis, R. *The American Adam: Tragedy and Tradition in the Nineteenth Century*. Chicago: University of Chicago Press, 1955.

Liton, J., and S. Olstein. "Therapeutic Aspects of Reminiscence." *Social Casework* 5 (May 1969): 263–268.

Martel, M. "Age-sex Roles in American Magazine Fiction (1890–1955)." In *Middle Age and Aging*. ed. B. Neugarten.

Chicago: University of Chicago Press, 1968.

McGrady, P. *The Youth Doctors*. New York: Coward, 1968.

McMahon, A. and P. Rhudick. "Reminiscing: Adaptational Significance in the Aged." *Archives of General Psychiatry* 10 (March 1964): 292–298.

Miller, M. and D. Elliot. "Errors and Omissions in Diagnostic Records on Admission of Patients to a Nursing Home." *Journal of the American Geriatrics Society* 24 (March 1976): 108–116.

Morison, S. *The European Discovery of America: The Southern Voyagers, (1492–1616)*. New York: Oxford University Press, 1974.

National Center for Health Statistics, *Health in the Later Years: Data from the National Center for Health Statistics*. Washington, D.C.: U.S. Government Printing Office, 1971.

Simmons, L. *The Role of the Aged in Primitive Society*, New Haven, Conn.: Yale University Press, 1945.

Slater, P. "Cultural Attitudes toward the Aged." *Geriatrics* 18 (1963): 308–314.

Smith, H. *Virgin Land: The American West as Symbol and Myth*, Cambridge, Mass.: Harvard University Press, 1950.

Smith, M. "The Portrayal of Elders in Magazine Cartoons." *Gerontologist*. 19 (1979): 408–412.

Sohngen, M. and R. Smith, "Images of Old Age in Poetry." *Gerontologist* 18 (1978): 181–186.

Sudnow, D. *Passing On: The Social Organization of Dying*. Englewood Cliffs, N.J.: Prentice-Hall, 1967.

Toffler, A. *Future Shock*. New York: Random House, 1970.

Townsend, C. *Old Age: The Last Segregation*. New York: Grossman, 1970.

Tuckman, J. and I. Lorge, "Self Classification as Old or Not Old." *Geriatrics* 12 (1957): 661–671.

Ward, R. "The Impact of Subjective Age and Stigma on Older Persons," *Journal of Gerontology*. 32 (1977): 227–232.

Wolfenstein, M. and N. Leites, *Movies: A Psychological Study*. Glencoe, Ill.: Free Press, 1950.

Chapter 3

Themes and Variations: Social Aspects of Aging

Karen Altergott
C. Edwin Vaughn

Each older person is unique. From birth and childhood background through the environments, activities, and associations of many years of adulthood, experience embellishes the uniqueness of each biography. Each story can be told in all its detail, although there are common themes from one to another. This chapter will examine themes and variations of the aging experience in modern society. Similarities in the process of aging are generated by physiological and psychological processes, as is seen in other chapters. Common themes or similarities also are generated by people's living within the same culture and society, being a member of a human population with particular characteristics, and sharing a historical era. In contrast, variations on these themes are introduced by people's holding different social positions within society based on social class, ethnic background, and gender, as well as experiencing different conditions and opportunities. The patterns that can be discovered provide an understanding and background for practical action, although in clinical practice and daily life, individual uniqueness is never to be neglected.

Case Studies

A comparison of two older individuals illustrates the variety in old age and the challenge of identifying themes. Mr. Vaughan celebrated his 93rd birthday at a large family picnic held on his front lawn. His four children (ranging in age from 49 to 72), grandchildren, great-grandchildren, and even a few great-great-grandchildren were present. The elder Vaughan was the center of attention and a lively participant in the event. He was much admired and appreciated by those

present. Mr. Vaughan still lives in the house that he helped build in 1911. His first wife died more than 20 years ago, and he remarried when he was in his late 70s. His second wife now keeps house for them, and he continues to do his chores on his farm. Through subsistence farming and a minimal retirement pension from Social Security, Mr. Vaughan is able, from his own perspective, to do reasonably well. He is in good health. At age 90 he finally agreed to get a hearing aid, which he admits "makes things sound better." In his early 90s his vision had deteriorated to the point where traditional bifocals did not provide adequate correction. Until this was correctly diagnosed as a vision problem, friends and relatives began to fear he was becoming senile. Mr. Vaughan is highly respected in his community and receives frequent visits. He enjoys life but also is looking forward to "seeing his maker."

Mrs. Sanfield's husband died when she was 50. For several years she continued to live in the family home and kept in close touch with her two daughters. However, she complained of being lonely and bored. When she was 60 years old, her doctor advised her to quit driving the car because of her vision impairment; this greatly limited her mobility. Over a period of a few years several of her lifelong friends died, and her three grandchildren moved away. With increasing deterioration in her health and strength, she required additional assistance in housekeeping, grocery shopping, and transportation. Her two daughters tried to help, but since both were working full-time, they had limited time and energy to give. The daughters became increasingly concerned about the amount of alcohol their mother drank, which they associated with mild bouts of depression. Mrs. Stanfield began to lose weight and experienced multiple minor health problems. Her doctor suggested that she soon would require additional care. After talking it over, the daughters agreed that their mother would move in with the younger daughter. However, the presence of the older woman brought strain into this daughter's marriage and career. While expressing concern, this daughter felt she could not continue to deal with this responsibility in her home. Without talking to their mother, the daughters made arrangements to place her in a nursing home. Mrs. Stanfield saw this action as abandonment and greatly resented the idea. When the daughters made their weekly visits, their mother complained about the treatment and expressed a wish to get back into her own home. As the months went by, the frequency of her daughters' visits decreased. Three years later Mrs. Stanfield died in the nursing home at the age of 71.

What did Mr. Vaughan and Mrs. Stanfield share? Both experienced the social aging process, lived as members of the aging population, shared a particular historical era, and faced a society with certain practices and policies toward older people. They faced similar cultural attitudes and expectations toward aging. The nature of their aging varied because of their class and ethnic backgrounds, family and community context, gender, health, goals, and personal style. Together, social context and individual characteristics shape the aging experience and the conditions of late life. Since it is difficult to see the themes when we are confronted with such diversity, we will begin by describing the social theories regarding the common experiences in aging.

Themes of Aging in a Social Context

Theories: Emphasizing Different Themes

Theories provide an understanding and explanations for why people age as they do. Biological theories explain the changes of physical function and death; psychological theories explain cognitive (or intellectual) and affective (or emotional) changes; and social theories explain changing social positions, roles, and activities of people. The sociology of aging developed around disengagement and activity theories. Each seemed to emphasize different themes.

Disengagement Theory. Disengagement theory (Cumming 1975; Cumming and Henry 1961) posits that as people age, they tend to become increasingly ready to withdraw from diverse social activities and involvements and to focus dwindling energies on private activities. Likewise, as people age, social expectations regarding what they should or must do for others and for themselves diminish. Less and less involvement is demanded of the aging individual, and at a certain point, the individual is "released" from social obligations. This condition could be a burden or a pleasure, depending on the congruence with individual readiness to withdraw. The lack of rehabilitative services for newly blind older people may reflect an assumption that they are both ready to withdraw and be free of social obligations. The fact that most older people, including the visually impaired, do not fit the disengagement model is one reason this theory has been challenged.

Activity Theory. Activity theorists were unwilling to grant that withdrawal and declining involvement are intrinsic to the social aging experience. In fact, they suggested that maintaining roles and activity is the only way to experience a satisfactory old age. If people experience role loss — and therefore less activity — they also lose role support, suffer diminished self-esteem, and have lower life satisfaction. The way to avoid this downward trend in social involvement and satisfaction is to replace lost roles with new roles and activities (Lemon, Bengtson, and Peterson 1972). These activities, however, must be meaningful to the individual. Meaningless activities sometimes imposed on older people by well-intentioned practitioners are not likely to produce satisfaction. Although it is an appealing theory, activity theory does not explain how some people can reduce roles and activities and still be quite satisfied in old age.

Continuity Theory. According to continuity theory, individuals maintain the same style of coping with life as they age, but the events and challenges to be coped with vary. Hence, those who coped with loss by withdrawal and resignation early in life also would disengage in the face of loss in late life. People who coped with loss by actively and successfully replacing lost activities early in life would attempt the same in late life, when losses are more common. Continuity theory posits a continuity of personal style in the face of changed opportunities and barriers. It helps explain the differences among older people. However, what explains the changing opportunties and barriers older people face?

Exchange Theory. First applied to old age by Dowd (1975), exchange theory suggests that older people have fewer valued social resources to exchange and therefore have less influence on others in social interaction. They face fewer opportunities to act and interact, because their participation is not highly valued. Sometimes barriers result in social exclusion. Whether these barriers are physical (such as overly bright lights, glaring floors, or glass walls in public places), normative (such as exclusion from paid work on the basis of age), or informal (such as a preference to work with, treat, or associate with younger people), the result is the same: older people lose power and opportunities. They eventually must comply with whatever others around them demand and learn to live with the limits placed upon them. Exchange theory explains the disadvantaged position older people have in societies and in relationships with others, including professionals.

Subculture of Aging Theory. Rose (1965) suggests that older people may congregate and develop a somewhat separate value system in part to avoid the powerlessness and low status imposed on them by their position in the larger U.S. society. On the one hand, contact with other older people, common interests and experiences, residential segregation, social welfare programs based on age, and the ability of older people to define themselves as a group enhance the aged subculture. On the other hand, contact with offspring, age integration, continued employment, and shared values and beliefs with younger people can reduce the salience of an aged subculture. Subculture of aging theory helps explain the emergence of age-segregated residences but also suggests that value differences and segregation may lead to conflict between young and old.

Role Theories. Role theories of aging developed early. The term *roleless roles* was applied to older people by Burgess (1950) to indicate the lack of expectations for older people. Rosow (1974) further developed a theory of role loss to explain how older people come to this roleless fate. He

suggests that, in addition to role loss through death or social distance, expectations for action could gradually dwindle. For example, less and less advice or assistance is expected of an aging father, and older people may be assigned vacuous roles (those that no one considers important or useful).

According to role theory, loss depends on the type of society in which an older individual lives, since the roles that are available to different age groups vary (Cowgill and Holmes 1972). Few older people are actually roleless; they have social relationships, activities, and abilities. However, in interaction with strangers and with professionals, these roles may be invisible. Too few expectations may be placed on older people. Their role competence may be underestimated. This is detrimental to the social integration and well-being of the aged.

Age Stratification Theories. One theoretical framework that may help integrate the many competing theories is age stratification (Riley, Johnson, and Foner 1972). This framework recognizes that in all societies, people are differentiated on the basis of age, and some roles are available or unavailable to an individual as a result of age. Individuals under the age of 14 are rarely allowed to marry. Older women like Mrs. Stanfield may lack partners and social approval or face economic loss if they remarry (for example, through a reduction of Social Security benefits). Whenever age-based laws, expectations, or opportunities exist, they influence the individual's experiences.

The age stratification framework also recognizes the many processes involved in aging. As time passes, individuals age, society changes, and new people reach old age. Since each aggregate of people born at about the same time (for example, those born in the 1930s) has a historically unique situation, each of these cohorts experiences youth, middle age, and old age in a somewhat different manner. Social aging is complex, and many processes must be taken into account. Many research findings published before 1970 may be misleading, because researchers made simple comparisons of young, middle-aged, and older people without recognizing the impact of cohort membership and historical context (Schaie 1970).

Finally, this theory suggests that older people cannot be understood without examining people of all ages in the society. It suggests that we compare the social condition of the aged and of the young, the relationships among age groups, and the distribution of roles and resources across the age strata rather than just describe the conditions, relationships, and resources of those who are currently old.

Social theories, then, are developed around common themes of aging–involvement and withdrawal, power and dependence, opportunities and behavior, individual and social changes–and a good theory would explain both the common experiences and the variations in the experience of social aging. The common experiences of old age are shaped by the *number of older people* in a population, the *cultural meanings* of age, and the *societal arrangements* for old age. By describing these general characteristics of an aging society, we set the stage for understanding today's (and tomorrow's) aging individual.

Numbers: Demography of Age

The absolute and relative size of the older segment of the population is consequential for aging individuals. The aged, whether a relatively large segment of the population or not, are recognized as a separate segment in all known societies (Cowgill 1974)–even in societies with life expectancies of 50 years or less. Older people always constitute a minority in a society (Cowgill 1974). If that minority is small (for example, if 3 percent of the population is over the age of 65), older individuals may feel isolated, deviant, and out of date even while being esteemed for their rarity (Fischer 1975). If that minority is large (for example, in 1980 11 percent of the U.S. population was over the age of 65 and some European societies have even higher percentages, U.S. Bureau of the Census 1980), older individuals may feel a sense of community and political influence. At the same time, there may be too few geriatric health practitioners to meet the needs of the millions over the age of 75. Difficulties in paying for health and personal services also may exist.

The proportion of older people relative to other age cohorts in every modern society is rising. To some extent this is due to increases in longevity. At birth in 1930, a white female in the United States could expect to live to be 64; a white male, 60; and a black male or female, 49. Infant mortality and deaths during youth and adulthood kept life expectancy low. In contrast, life expec-

tancy at birth for those born in 1980 is 78 for a white female, 71 for a white male, 74 for a black female, and 65 for a black male. Each individual born today has a better chance of surviving to old age than an individual born 50 years ago. This is more because of improved nutrition, public health measures, and less dangerous and deadly occupations than because of the conquest of diseases.

However, the most dramatic cause for the recent increase in the proportion of older people in Western societies is the decreased birth rate. With fewer children entering society, the proportion of the population over the age of 65 increases (without, of course, increasing the number of older people). Demographers have shown, for example, that if birth rates remain low, the proportion of older people in the U.S. population could increase to more than 20 percent. However, if the birth rate increases, the percentage of older people could remain about the same, but the U.S. population would double (U.S. Bureau of the Census 1980).

The gender composition of the older population also has consequences for the individual and society. Almost all older populations have more females than males (Cowgill 1974). Although there are slightly more males than females at the time of conception, males die at a more rapid rate throughout the life cycle. Social causes such as war and higher-pressure lifestyles for some men, as well as the fact that women appear to have better overall health, produce an abundance of females over males (see Table 3–1). In the United States among persons over 70 years of age, women outlive men an average of 8 years. Most societies have a higher proportion of widows than widowers among their populations.

Table 3–1
Number of Men per 100 Women in Late Life

Age	Number of Men
55–64	88
65–74	76
75–84	66
85 +	44

Source: Current Population Reports, Series P. 25, No. T40. Washington, D.C.: U.S. Government Printing Office, 1980.

The demographic trends also include, however, an increased number of adult years in the married state. Contemporary marriages are much less likely to end by death before old age (Uhlenberg 1980) than were marriages in the early 1900s. The trend toward early childbearing and small families also has changed the experience of older married life, since children reach adulthood while their parents are still middle aged. Older couples can expect to have many years alone together after the departure of adult offspring and prior to the death of either spouse for the first time in human history. The emergence of this "postparental" stage of marriage is a striking change in U.S. family life.

The demography of aging has changed dramatically. More people are reaching old age, and there is a relatively high proportion of older people in our society. What does it mean to live in an "aging society"? The cultural meaning of reaching old age is the next theme to be considered.

Culture: Meanings of Age

Each of the demographic trends previously described relies on chronology—the calculation of time. Using chronological age is a cultural invention; many societies do not even use chronological numbers to mark periods in the life cycle. In addition to marking the number of years since birth, chronological age identifies individuals in another way: all people the same age were born at the same historical era. The Great Depression cohort, for example, shares a great deal because of this common historical location. The "baby boom" cohort in the United States (those born from 1946 to 1965) will share many experiences because of the relatively large size of the group entering society and the historical events the members of this aggregate share.

In the U.S. past, retirement was linked to ability to perform job-related tasks, not to a particular age (Fischer 1975). This ability-related criteria is referred to as *functional age.* Chronological age does not give us perfect insight into functional age, and declines in function should not be taken for granted as an unavoidable part of aging. Mr. Vaughan, described in the first case study, is in his 90s and is still doing many of the things he did at age 50. A successful interior decorator returned to school at age 55 and is, at 69, having a successful career as an assistant professor of psychiatry. A factory worker, lungs damaged by the industrial environment, gratefully takes early retirement at 63. In terms of functional age, who is the youngest?

Functional age often can be modified through medical intervention, such as correcting sensory loss or treating reversible conditions; through training, such as mobility instruction for the visually impaired; through services, such as home nursing care; or through coping strategies of the individual, such as obtaining Talking Books to stay well informed about current events in spite of vision loss.

Age also indicates the proportion of the expected lifetime a person has lived. At age 33, a person can be reasonably sure that more than one-third of life has past. At 71, a person may balance past and future and be aware that most of his or her time has past, leading perhaps to resolution and integration of life in a process of review (Butler 1982). In terms of probable nearness to death, a 55-year-old man is "older than" a 55-year-old woman because of differences in longevity. Stopping smoking may improve health and reduce nearness to death.

Social age is somewhat more complex than chronological or functional age, because it depends on what people perceive and define as youthful. To dress youthfully may change a person's self-identity and social identity. Eye tucks and eye surgery may be equally effective in making a person seem youthful. Conversely, spectacles and hearing aids become outward symbols of age and are sometimes hidden or avoided by the consumer because of a negative social connotation.

The socially defined meanings of age are so pervasive in our society that they have given rise to distinct notions of age-appropriate behavior—expectations that the young have for the old and expectations that the old frequently adopt for themselves (McTavish 1971; Neugarten, Moore, and Lowe 1968). Older people in our culture attract attention if they violate these expectations by having sexual interests, having plastic surgery to enhance appearance, remarrying after the death of a spouse, or remaining successful in business in later years. Being a successful or busy older physician, lawyer, community leader, volunteer, businessperson, or mechanic is an exception rather than what people expect of older people. Imagery commonly communicated through the mass media favors youth; these images include physical vitality, athletic interests, efficiency, new ideas, and current fashions. These are not expected of the elderly. Many older individuals respond to pervasive attitudes about being old by adopting negative images and attitudes about their own situation as elderly people.

The negative imagery common in our society about being old has given additional impetus to stereotypical ideas about older people. Much of this negative imagery results from our assuming that being old is somehow a "problem." Research frequently focuses on the multiple illnesses, physical decline, or other assumed negative attributes of older people rather than on the way they transcend their minor to severe impairments. This stereotyped negative thinking is frequently labeled agism, which is similar to racism, sexism, and other forms of prejudice in our society (Levin and Levin 1980).

Negative age stereotypes encourage older people to play a role that includes being asexual, intellectually rigid, unproductive, ineffective, and disengaged. Older people are encouraged by stereotypes of old age to stay out of the way, be invisible, and yet enjoy the "golden years" and "be happy" (Levin and Levin 1980).

Health care practitioners, of course, are influenced by the various meanings of age in their culture. Frequently they share negative stereotypes about the elderly, and their attention is focused on the young. Of particular concern is access to optimal vision care. Fifty percent of blindness is preventable; thus, older people, friends, relatives, and professionals should not assume that vision loss and blindness is simply a part of aging. This thinking in terms of agist stereotypes denies older people access to diagnosis and treatment for visual impairments, which in turn produces dependency and decline (Vaughan 1984). Eye and vision care are equally important for people of all ages. Programs to prevent blindness and to encourage elderly people to seek means of maximizing their vision deserve more attention. As this group increases in size and ability to purchase services, more attention is likely to center on its needs.

Society: Structures of Age
Older people living in modern industrial countries such as the United States, Great Britain, and Japan are influenced by general conditions in the wider society. According to the comparative studies of Cowgill and Holmes (1972), the status of older people is higher in societies where they are able to perform useful and valuable functions and where the extended form of the family serves as a functional household unit. These conditions are not present, in general, in North American or Western European societies.

The difficulties of older people in terms of housing and health care seem to increase as they make up a larger portion of the population. Rapid social changes, new technologies, an altered occupational system, geographical mobility, urbanization, and the changing family structure also affect older people. Loss of socially valued positions in the work place, community, and home become frequent experiences. At the personal level this may result in increased economic dependency because of separation from regular employment, subordinate relations to one's grown children and to social workers or other professionals, the loss of a major focus of activity and self-identity, the loss of an independent household either for economic or health reasons, increased involvement in age-segregated groups and organizations, and dependency on others for transportation and other personal needs.

The social and economic policies in modern societies play a major role in shaping the degree of dependence or independence of older individuals. In preliterate cultures, status depended upon serving functional roles in private groups; in complex postindustrial societies, however, status depends on a person's position in both private and public spheres. Table 3–2 lists some of the private and public advantages and disadvantages of the aged in modern times. The position of the aged in society depends a great deal on forces outside the individual's control, as can be seen in this list. These societal conditions produce common themes in the experiences of old age. The consequences of these conditions are a major topic of study in the field of social gerontology, or the sociology of aging (Binstock and Shanas 1976).

The demographic, cultural, and societal conditions described so far are shared by all older people in our society. These social forces create similarities in the experience of aging and operate outside any individual's control. In addition to the common themes that result from sharing a society and a historical context, aging is a differentiated experience as well. To complicate our understanding of older people, we turn to some of the variations on the theme.

Variations: Many Ways of Growing Old
All older people in U.S. society are affected by the same demographic, cultural, and social

Table 3-2
Advantages and Disadvantages of Old Age in Modern Society

The Aged in Public Life

Advantages

- Older people are overrepresented among politicians.

- Older people are well represented among the voting public (but diverse enough to be divided—the old are not a voting block).

- Self-aware groups represent the interests of the aged; these include professionals in the "aging enterprise" (Estes 1979) and the aged themselves.

- Explicit policy transfers income and benefits and improves the condition of most of the aged.

Disadvantages

- Older people are separated by policy and practice from employment opportunities.

- The health needs of the aging population exceed the health care system's capacity, and some needs (such as treatment for chronic conditions) are not well incorporated into the health care system.

- Older people are dependent on income transfer policies that are not uniformly favorable.

The Aged in Private Life

Advantages

- More generations survive at one time, and more of one's peers reach old age.

- The husband-wife relationship is more likely than ever to endure (even considering the divorce rate), because there are fewer premature deaths.

- Technology allows contact and visiting across the miles (for example, air travel and the telephone).

Disadvantages

- One-fifth of older U.S. citizens have no surviving children. Mobility scatters families, and divorce separates and complicates kin relations.

- Remarriage is difficult for women because of the demographic imbalance.

- Mobility continues to disperse family members.

realities previously discussed, but there are certain variations in the experience of aging. It is common in popular and professional publications to write of all people over 65 as being the same. No matter how much they have in common, however, there is also a great diversity among people aged 65 and older.

Old Is Old Is Old?

It is important, for example, to recognize differences among the "young-old," "old," and "old-old." The basic distinction between these categories is based on the differential functional status among people in each decade of late life. Of the 25.5 million older people in the United States, 61 percent are 65 to 74 years old, 30 percent are 75 to 84 years old, and almost 9 percent are 85 or older ("Every Ninth American" 1982). That 2.2 million people in U.S. society are over the age of 85 is truly a societal accomplishment, but it also produces societal responsibility.

The daily lives and the functional abilities of the various age groups among the aged depend a great deal on the policies and practices in a society. For example, relatively few people over the age of 85 work for pay. Pensions for this group are rare and are diminished to almost nothing by inflation even if they are received. The quality of life of those 85 and over depends on personal, familial, and societal provisions for the life-style associated with very old age.

People 75 to 84 are likely to begin to experience some of the more serious decrements associated with old age, since the probability of disability, illness, and social losses increases around age 75. The conditions and quality of life for this age group are no less determined by social practice and societal policy. Are preventive and curative health programs and supportive services available? Can individuals requiring medical care afford the services? Or are people forced into premature institutionalization and dependency by a narrow vision of what a community member must be able to do for himself or herself?

Finally, the youngest group of the aged—those 65 to 74—may be the most comfortable in terms of health, personal condition, and societal position (although many exceptions exist). These are the aged with fewer debilitating conditions, better economic provisions, and usually a richer set of associates and activities. Therefore, whether or not younger adults recognize the difference between a 58-, 67-, 76-, or 85-year-old, those who serve the needs of older people and those with a more sophisticated view of the aging population recognize that these individuals tend to be very different.

Ethnicity and Race

Whether a person is a white, black, Native American, Hispanic, or Asian American transforms the aging experience. Among whites the ethnic roots traced further elaborate the differences. Elderly Jewish, Italian, Irish, German, and other immigrant groups embellish the theme of aging in many ways. The diversity of ethnic strands woven into this aging subculture transforms and complicates it (Myerhoff 1978). Immigration from Europe in the past and from Central and South America and Asia in the present have affected our image of aging. Twenty years ago the image of *grandmother* was more frequently blurred with images of the "old country" than it is today (Cain 1967).

When ethnicity combines with race, as among blacks in the United States, the variations in patterns of aging become even more complex.

Some have argued that in our industrial society, being old and being a member of a minority group constitutes double jeopardy. Not only do blacks suffer the effects of living in a racially discriminatory society their whole lives; they also suffer steeper declines in status, health, and income in old age (Dowd and Bengtson 1978). However, minority elderly were found to be similar to the white elderly in terms of life satisfaction and frequency of social contact. In fact, elderly Mexican Americans and blacks had a higher level of primary group interaction with children and grandchildren than was characteristic of the white group studied (Dowd and Bengtson 1978). This family involvement may well be the most important legacy elders receive from their ethnic heritage.

Societal forces of discrimination lead to greater poverty and poorer health; a higher proportion of elderly blacks than elderly whites live in old age poverty. Social support systems within the black community draw on the resources of younger generations. The black aged are more likely to continue a process of exchange and contact with relatives and others, perhaps because of continued low access to social programs and benefits.

Economics and Economic Sufficiency

Whether wealthy or poor, people age. Economic resources, prestige, and power are three dimensions along which people differ, and each influences the experience of aging. There is greater economic variation among the aged than among other adults.

Older individuals are both wealthy (many U.S. millionaires are over the age of 65) and poor (5.4 million older U.S. citizens had incomes below the poverty level of $4,896 per year for couples and $3,895 per year for individuals in 1978) (Soldo 1980). The wealthy clearly have positions, histories, and resources that allow them greater control over some aspects of their own late lives than do middle-income or poor older people.

Many older U.S. citizens experience poverty for the first time in old age. An elderly widow may lose her husband's pension at the same time as she loses her lifelong companion. Many working people never receive the pension they expected. Private pension reform legislation has changed, but not eliminated, the risks faced by the individual hoping to receive a pension. Even if pensions are received, most pensions are not inflationproof. At 3 percent inflation, each $100 of a pension at age 60 would be reduced to $55 at age 80. At 10 percent inflation, each $100 of a pension would be worth only $15 after 20 years. Savings, it seems, provide protection in old age only for those with high earnings throughout adulthood. Furthermore, many U.S. citizens face major expenses before retirement, such as college for their offspring and help for elderly parents. A "life cycle squeeze" exists for the middle aged, the patron generation in the middle that helps both younger and older generations (Hill 1970; Oppenheimer 1974). Also, many deplete their savings during periods of disability and unemployment before retirement. The economic shortfall in late life may lead to the neglect of preventive health care, especially since much of this type of care is not reimbursed by Medicare. This especially affects vision, hearing, foot, and dental care.

U.S. public policies of income transfer are discussed in Chapter 6. Government sources such as Social Security are the only source of income for half of all married couples and two-thirds of nonmarried individuals in old age. Blacks, the very old, and women receive substantially less than white men, an inequality that produces extreme poverty for many.

Because of relatively high rates of home ownership among the aged, the decrease in expenditures that may accompany the economic independence of children and retirement, and the existing (although incomplete) income transfer and medical benefits programs, older people in the United States tend to say that their income is adequate, even though it may be objectively low (Schultz 1976). However, according to a national pool, 24 percent of older U.S. citizens find the high cost of living their greatest problem; 41 percent say that a lack of money is a somewhat serious or very serious problem for them (Louis Harris and Associates 1975).

Gender
Much of the literature on the aged ignores the differences in the experience of aging for men and women. Women and men face different opportunities in most societies throughout life. Roles, relationships, and resources are different for men and women in U.S. society. Social themes of aging, therefore, are substantially modified by gender.

Women live longer than men, are more likely to spend part of old age living alone, and are more likely to experience poverty. These objec-

tive conditions influence many other aspects of the aging experience.

Most older men have wives; their wives are their principle confidants, companions, and helpers. Women who are married also spend a great deal of time with their husbands, receive help from them, and have them as confidants. However, older women also are likely to have other friends and confidants, as well as to maintain kin relationships to a greater degree than are older men (Lowenthal and Haven 1968). This perhaps eases the transition to widowhood for women, whereas the experience of being widowed for a man is perhaps more isolating (Berardo 1970).

When men and women face health problems in old age, they may cope in very different ways. Women may rely on relatives more. Men may become more dependent on a spouse or if unmarried, may become isolated or less able to care for themselves adaquately.

Marital and Parental Status
Not all adults in U.S. society marry, and some married people divorce or are widowed. Not all adults become parents, and some people outlive some or all of their offspring. Variations in life experiences during early life lead to variations in the family status of older adults. Shanas et al. (1968) found that four-fifths of the U.S. elderly had at least one surviving child. For most of these elderly parents, one child lived within an hour's drive. An interesting development in modern society is that many generations coexist. Four- and five-generation families can become more common. Thus, even though the number of children in each generation may be small, an elderly person could have many descendents. The number of surviving kin—siblings as well as offspring—influences the lives of older people. Ranging from no surviving relatives to a virtual clan, kin structure affects the aging experience.

Of the men in 1980 who were 65 years of age and older, 75 percent lived with their spouse, 17 percent lived alone or with a nonrelative, and 7 percent lived with another relative. Of the women in the same age category in 1980, 38 percent lived with a spouse, 43 percent alone or with a nonrelative, and 19 percent lived with a relative ("Every Ninth American" 1982). Older people who return to living alone after being married are much less positive about their daily lives than are either those never married or the currently married (Gubrium 1974).

According to many researchers, relationships between older parents and their mature adult children who have left home are usually supportive and involve much mutual contact (Shanas 1979). Next to a spouse, a child is the most likely source of assistance. These close family members may be important to the health care practitioner as well, since they can frequently facilitate (or interfere with) treatment programs.

There is evidence that today's grandparenting has lost some of its emotional and experiential salience. Grandparents have fewer grandchildren than in previous generations. People become grandparents at earlier ages and often are involved in work or a busy social life. With the lengthening of life and the telescoping of generations, many people, by retirement age, are great-grandparents.

Today four out of ten people aged 65 and older report that they have great-grandchildren. These great-grandparenting roles are even more tentative than are the roles in grandparenting. Contacts may become limited to family reunions and major ceremonial events such as funerals, marriages, and graduations.

In summary, most older people have contact and exchange support with some family members. The relationship of older adults to their children, grandchildren, and great-grandchildren is variable, depending on ages, family size, emotional closeness, and physical proximity. Some elderly people reach old age with few or no surviving kin. Family structure is one of the great differentiators in old age.

Health and Mobility

Increased longevity in our society is accompanied by an increase in the probability of experiencing health problems in later years. Much of the money spent on health care in the United States is spent by the elderly, yet few physicians specialize in geriatric medicine. Overmedication is a commonly reported problem. "Senility" and other symptoms associated with mental health problems have, in many clinical cases, been reversed or eliminated when medications were reduced or changed. Overmedication can occur at any age, but people of advanced age apparently have less tolerance for most forms of medication—ranging from over-the-counter to prescription drugs. Some conditions cannot be reversed. Only careful diagnosis of the source and nature of older people's health problems can determine whether a condition is reversible or not.

Vision problems for the aged provide examples of both correctable and irreversible conditions. Blindness is greatly feared by people of advanced years, and older people do experience increased problems with vision. Either because of lack of knowledge or resources, however, many vision problems that develop in later life are untreated or undertreated. Low-vision aids and rehabilitation services are underutilized by older persons. This underutilization and the concomitant limits on mobility and social participation can be counteracted by public education and professional awareness.

What are the current facts regarding vision and aging? Age is the best predictor of blindness and visual impairment (Padula 1982). Approximately 1.4 million people in the United States have severe visual impairments (the inability to read normal newspaper print with conventional glasses), and 500,000 individuals are legally blind. The estimated prevalence of legal blindness among individuals over age 65 is approximately 230,000, and according to 1977 figures, there are nearly one million people over age 65 with severe visual impairment (Padula 1982).

"What are the conditions which produce vision loss in late life? Among persons 65 and older, macular degeneration is responsible for 60 percent of legal blindness. Cataracts and glaucoma are eight times more prevalent in older persons and retinal disorders are six times more common in this same population. Macular degeneration, cataracts, glaucoma, diabetic retinopathy, and optic nerve atrophy are the major diseases affecting older person's eyes" (Vaughan 1984, 3). Prevention and treatment methods are improving rapidly. Access to care and the rapidly growing need are problems however. The "'projection for the year 2,000 is that there will be between 272,000 and 376,000 elderly individuals who are legally blind and 1,760,000 with severe visual impairments" (Padula 1983, 315). This projection is probably conservative, because it does not take into account the disproportionate growth in the number of people of advanced age (over 75 or 85 years).

Whether people maintain physical and mental health into their 90s or suffer irreversible decrements at age 60 leads to great variation in the aging experience. Even if limiting health conditions exist, however, an individual may have enough help to overcome these limits. Health concerns are a problem not only for the aged individual, but also for society. Policy debate revolves around the rising costs of Medicare and Medicaid in the United States and health care throughout the world. There is increasing awareness that institutional care for the elderly is not only usually less desired by the older people themselves, but is also the most costly form of providing health care.

This concern has given rise to a rapidly growing sector of care for the elderly; in-home care services, which range from chore and homemaking services to health-related services provided by visiting nurses and other related professionals. In-home services enable older individuals to maintain themselves in their preferred environments while providing the requisite care at a cost much lower than that of institutional care. In-home care services work well only when a comprehensive health care system is in place; the entire array of health services must be available. Some people require nursing home care; others need comprehensive health services in the home, whereas still others require only minimal services to maintain themselves in their home environment. Much of the anxiety that older people experience about their health problems will be reduced when people have confidence in the availability of a comprehensive health care system.

Public policy is only now being considered relative to blindness in late life. One survey recently completed demonstrated that nearly ten percent of the in-home services provided in Michigan in a recent year were associated with blindness as a major cause of dependency. Some have argued that if only one-third of the public money spent on providing maintenance services were spent on rehabilitation services, older blind people could learn to do many things for themselves at far less public expense. Furthermore, increased self-esteem comes from mastering one's mobility, housekeeping, and other problems rather than from being taken care of by others at public expense.

Methodological issues abound in both medical and functional definitions of blindness and varying degrees of vision loss (Greenburg and Branch 1982). A relevent and useful definition in terms of service delivery and efforts to improve vision follows: any change in vision that interferes with the processing of information and requires that a person manage ordinary tasks in new or more complicated ways. The provision of care to those experiencing varying degrees of vision loss should include education, emotional support, accurate diagnosis and correction where possible, appropriate aids and appliances, and rehabilitative services.

Conclusion

Older individuals experience a wide variety of situations. It is difficult to generalize about all aged people—young-old and old-old, black and white, rich and poor, male and female, married and single, socially integrated and isolated, healthy and limited by health conditions. Theories of social aging help us understand the experiences and important aspects of old age.

The age structure of modern populations indicates the historically unique situation we face: more people survive to old age than ever before. This will affect both our culture and our social structure. The culture shapes the image we have of aging and old age. Although slightly negative in tone today, the image of old age may change if people increasingly become old without becoming ill, poor, and isolated. The structures of our society—families, work organizations, service organizations, and communities—and the policies of our government constitute and modify the life conditions older people face. Variations in the aging experience based on age, gender, ethnicity, race, class, health, and family status exist.

The vision care professional who recognizes the aging experience of older people in general and the variations among older patients can help improve the quality of life for older citizens. Almost everyone will experience some vision loss with advanced age. Severe pronounced sensory loss potentially impairs our ability to participate fully in our social environment. Biologists' and psychologists' contributions to knowledge regarding vision, technological efforts to improve vision, and the impaired individual's coping strategies cannot succeed if we ignore the social context in which older people live. Economic deprivation, social isolation, geographic isolation, and ignorance are but a few of the conditions preventing many older people from receiving professional help in obtaining improved vision or rehabilitative services. Education, vision correction, and the prevention of blindness will be enhanced insofar as the social context of aging populations is incorporated into public policy and service delivery efforts.

References

Berardo, F. M. "Survivorship and Social Isolation: The Case of the Aged Widower." *Family Coordinator* 19 (1970): 11–25.

Binstock, R., and E. Shanas. *The Handbook of Aging and the Social Sciences.* New York: Van Nostrand, 1976.

Burgess, E. "Personal and Social Adjustments in Old Age." In *The Aged and Society,,* ed. Milton Derber. Champaign, Ill.: Industrial Relations Reserve Association, 1950.

Butler, R. *Aging and Mental Health.* St. Louis: Mosby, 1982.

Cain, L. "Age and Generational Phenomena: The New Old People in Contemporary America." *Gerontologist* 7 (1967): 83–92.

Cowgill, D. "The Aging of Populations and Societies." *The Annals of the American Academy of Political and Social Science* 415 (1974): 1–18.

Cowgill, D. O., and L. D. Holmes. *Aging and Modernization.* New York: Appleton-Century-Crofts, 1972.

Cumming, E. "Engagement with an Old Theory." *International Journal of Aging and Human Development* 6 (1975): 187–191.

Cumming, E., and E. Henry. *Growing Old: The Process of Disengagement.* New York: Basic, 1961.

Dowd, J. J. "Aging as Exchange: A Preface to Theory." *Journal of Gerontology* 30 (1975): 584–594.

Dowd, J. J., and V. Bengtson, "Aging in Minority Populations: An Examination of the Double Jeopardy Hypothesis." *Journal of Gerontology* 33 (1978): 427–436.

Estes, C. L. *The Aging Enterprise.* San Francisco: Jossey-Bass, 1979.

"Every Ninth American." *Congressional Record.* Washington, D.C., 1982.

Fischer, D. H. *Aging in America.* New York: Oxford University Press, 1975.

Greenburg, D. A., and L. G. Branch. "Review of Methodological Issues Concerning Incidence and Prevalence Data of Visual Deterioration in Elders." In *Aging and Human Visual Functions.* Modern Aging Research, Vol. 2, eds. R. Sekuler, R. D. Kline, and K. Dismukes. New York: Alan R. Liss, 1982, pp. 279–296.

Gubrium, J. "Marital Desolation and the Evaluation of Everyday Life in Old Age." *Journal of Marriage and the Family* 35 (1974): 107–113.

Hill, R. *Family Development in Three Generations.* Cambridge, Mass.: Schenkman, 1970.

Lemon, B.; B. Bengtson; and J. Peterson. "An Exploration of the Activity Theory of Aging: Activity Types and Life Satisfaction among In-Movers to a Retirement Community." *Journal of Gerontology* 27 (1972): 511–523.

Levin L., and W. Levin. *Agism: Prejudice and Discrimination against The Elderly.* Belmont, Calif.: Wadsworth Publishing, 1980.

Lopata, H. "Support Systems of Elderly Urbanites: Chicago of the 1970s." *Gerontologist* 15 (1975): 35–41.

Louis Harris and Associates. *The Myth and Reality of Aging in America.* Washington, D.C.: National Council on the Aging, 1975.

Lowenthal, M. F., and C. Haven. "Interaction and Adaptation: Intimacy as a Critical Variable." *American Sociological Review* 33 (1968): 20–30.

McTavish, D. "Perceptions of Old People: A Review of Research Methodologies and Findings." *The Gerontologist* 11 (1971): 90–102.

Michigan Commission for the Blind. *Services for the Elderly Blind in Michigan: The Senior Blind Program and Related Issues.* Unpublished manuscript, Lansing: Michigan Department of Labor, 1983.

Myerhoff, B. *Number Our Days.* New York: Dutton, 1978.

Neugarten, B.; J. Moore and J. Lowe. "Age Norms, Age Constraints, and Adult Socialization." In *Middle Age and Aging.* ed. B. Neugarten. Chicago: University of Chicago Press, 1968, pp. 22–28.

Oppenheimer, V. K. "The Life Cycle Squeeze: The Interaction of Men's Occupational and Family Life Cycles." *Demography* 11 (1974): 227–245.

Padula, W. V. "Low Vision Related to Function and Service Delivery." In *Aging and Human Visual Functions.* Modern Aging Research, Vol. 2, eds R. Sekuler, R. D. Kline, and K. Dismukes. New York: Alan R. Liss, 1982, pp. 315–322.

Riley, M. W.; M. Johnson; and A. Foner, *Aged and Society: A Sociology of Age Stratification.* Vol. 3. New York: Basic, 1972.

Rose, A. "The Subculture of the Aging: A Framework for Research in Social Gerontology." In *Older People and Their Social Words.* eds. A. M. Rose and W. Peterson, Philadelphia: Davis Co., 1965.

Rose, A. M., and W. Peterson. *Older People and Their Social Worlds.* Philadelphia: Davis, 1965.

Rosow, I. *Socialization to Old Age.* Berkeley: University of California Press, 1974.

Schaie, K. W. "A Reinterpretation of Age-related Changes in the Cognitive Structure and Functioning." In *Theory and Research in Life-span Development Psychology,* eds. L. R. Goulet and P. B. Baltes. New York: Academic Press, 1970.

Schultz, J. *Economics of Aging.* Belmont, Calif.: Wadsworth Publishing, 1976.

Sekuler, R.; D. Kline; and K. Dismukes. *Aging and Human Visual Function,* Modern Aging Research, Vol. 2. New York: Alan R. Liss, 1982.

Shanas, E. "Social Myths Hypothesis: The Case of the Family Relations of Old People." *Gerontologist* 19 (1979): 3–9.

Shanas, E.; P. Townsend; D. Wedderburn; H. Friis; P. Milhoj; and J. Stenhouwer. *Old People in Three Industrial Countries.* New York: Atherton Press, 1968.

Soldo, B. "America's Elderly in the 1980s." *Population Bulletin* 35, no. 4 (1980).

Uhlenberg, P. "Death and the Family." *Journal of Family History* 5 (1980): 313–320.

U.S. Bureau of the Census, U.S. Department of Commerce. *Current Population Series,* P25, No. 704, Washington, D.C.: U.S. Government Printing Office, 1980.

Vaughn, C. E., "Blindness Prevention among the Elderly." Columbia: University of Missouri, Center for the Study of Aging, 1984.

Chapter 4

Age-Related Disorders: Physiological and Pathological

Derek M. Prinsley

During the 20th century, and particularly in its later decades, there has been an almost worldwide improvement in life span expectancy. There have always been some survivors into very old age, and highly respected individuals they were. The Bible gave the human life span as three score years and ten: in those days and until very recently, only relatively few reached 70 years. Now, for the first time in history, most people are going to reach maturity and beyond.

It is difficult to pinpoint the beginning of the process of aging in the human being; it goes on for many years, however, and during that period, changes take place in body structures in response to normal aging, injury, or disease. A new field of knowledge is accumulating about aging—gerontology—and a new discipline of care for elderly people is gradually spreading, making modern medical and social treatment available to people of all ages.

Demographic Considerations

Expectations of life at birth in a developed country such as Australia or the United States is 70.3 years for men and 75.2 years for women. Life expectancy in less-developed countries is much shorter, mainly because of high infant mortality. In East Timor men live for 42.9 years and women, 44.8 years. In Bangladesh expectation is 48 years for both men and women.

The reasons for the difference between developed and developing countries are mainly environmental, but major advances in therapeutics have conquered many of the fatal diseases that were so prevalent, particularly among children. Better obstetric and neonatal care has greatly lowered neonatal mortality. Infectious diseases of childhood used to be potential killers when complicated by respiratory infections.

Diphtheria and scarlet fever patients once required extensive wards in hospitals for infectious diseases. Tuberculosis, while still a menace, is no longer a widespread and often lethal condition in adolescents. Serious disease in middle age is more responsive to treatment, and disorders of the past such as diabetes and pernicious anemia are now fully controllable. Improved survival in infancy, adolescence, and maturity has resulted in many more people's reaching old age. The remaining causes of mortality for adults in Western society are mainly related to accidents, stress, pollution, and overindulgence.

In the developing world, advances in medicine, nutrition, and environmental safety still must develop further before life expectancy at birth approaches figures resembling those for the Western world. Death rates among children are still high, especially because of bowel infections related to poor water supply and poor sanitation. Life-saving drugs are in short supply and not available in rural areas. Nutrition is often poor, and medical help is rarely available. Nevertheless, even under such ill-favored conditions, survivors from childhood will reach maturity. It is clear already that much larger numbers of old people can be seen, even in countries with high infant mortality.

If people can survive to maturity, life expectancy from then on does not differ greatly throughout the world. In Australia a man aged 65 can expect to live a further 13.6 years and a woman 15.5 years. U.S. data show average life expectancy at age 65 to be 15 years (13 years for men and 17 years for women). As a result of this sex difference in life expectancy, which begins at birth, there are 143 older women per 100 older men, and the disparity continues to grow with age (U.S. Department of Health, Education, and Welfare 1975). In East Timor a man will survive a further 10.2 years after age 65 and a woman, 11.1 years; in Bangladesh, 10.8 years and 11.5 years for men and women, respectively.

Demography, the statistical study of life in human communities, shows that the growth of numbers of aged people, although widespread, is not uniform. Some parts of the world now have reached the maximum point of the bulge in numbers of old people and can anticipate a gradual reduction coinciding with a reduced birth rate.

In some countries in western Europe, the retired population has reached 16 percent of the total. In Britain in 1900, 5 percent of the population was over the age of retirement. In 1974 the figure had reached 16.4 percent. In Australia the retired population is still only 10 percent and will continue slowly rising over the next 20 years. Countries that accepted a large immigration of population shortly after World War II face a quite sudden bulge in the near future. Most immigrants were fit young adults who are now aging and countries such as Canada and Australia will be faced with the need for additional services to provide for their old new citizens.

Population pyramids in the past showed steady attrition for total numbers because of disease. Survivors reaching old age were relatively few. Modern population pyramids are more rectangular or box shaped, with greater numbers reaching 70 years, great numbers therefore reaching 80, and more survivors even to age 90. All creatures have a programmed life span. Elephants reach 60 years; horses, 30 years; and rats and mice, only 3 years. If all went well and disease and stress were eliminated, the life span of a human being would probably be 90 years. People would wake up on their 90th birthday, have a good breakfast, and quietly cease to live! Unfortunately, few people will have that happy ending. These days humans can expect to reach their 80s.

A number of isolated communities in the world are reputedly astonishingly long lived. Two well-described populations—in the high Andes and in the Caucasus region of the Soviet Union—certainly can demonstrate large numbers of very old people, many over the age of 100. It is claimed that a healthy, active life, eating simple food, and avoiding stresses of city conditions promote the long survival of these people, and these factors may be part of the explanation. Much more likely, however, is genetic makeup. Isolated populations intermarry, and when long life is part of the genetic make up, children of such marriages will be equally long lived. The old adage is true: if people want a long life, they must choose their parents carefully.

Physiological and Pathological Causes of Changes with Aging

There are three phases of mammalian life. First, in the embryonic phase, the individual is totally dependent on maternal support. The second period is healthy adult life, when the creature is in equilibrium with the environment by maintaining all body functions and has the capacity to repair injury or damage. The third phase, senescence, is prolonged in humans. In most animals this phase is short after the reproductive period is over. Senescence in humans is a period when maintenance and repair of tissues gradually becomes less effective, organ functions deteriorate and cells die and are not replaced. However, age-related changes do not occur simultaneously in all organs or tissues. In addition, these changes may not be significant and may affect only limited areas.

Changes in the body with increasing age are the result of two processes: physiological and pathological. Physiological age changes are inevitable and are unlikely to be treatable. Time-related involutional changes cannot as yet be prevented, although some effects can be ameliorated (for example, by fitting hearing aids and spectacles). Skin wrinkles and loss of hair have less effective forms of treatment. Pathological changes are the result of wear and tear, stress, and disease. Degenerative arthritis of weight-bearing joints is not normal aging but the result of damage. Maturity-onset diabetes is all too often the result of overeating and lack of normal exercise. Many of the pathological processes that cause aging effects are amenable to treatment, and improvement in life style is probable even if complete cure is less common. Aging and disease are not synonymous, although it must be admitted that advanced age does bring an increased occurrence of illness. Older people consult their physicians on an average of four times per year; young people, about once every fourth year.

To accept the limitations of aging without question is therefore quite incorrect. To regard a patient's advanced chronological age as a reason for therapeutic inactivity is equally fallacious. All health care disciplines concerned with elderly patients emphasize recognizing treatability, defining those failings that are physiological and need to be considered in any therapeutic program, and identifying those changes that are due to potentially reversible pathological processes. To be able to manage this differentiation successfully, the practitioner must have a basic understanding of aging processes and changes in competence of organs with advancing years.

Cell Changes

There are two types of cell populations in the body and a matrix of supportive or connective tissue. The first group consists of cells that are capable of mitosis and that continue to reproduce themselves throughout life. The skin, the liver, the endothelial lining of blood vessels, and the epithelial layer of the cornea are constantly able to repair damage and reproduce by mitosis. These cells are therefore much younger than the whole organism. Nevertheless, the capacity to reproduce falls off in old age. Fibroblasts taken from a young adult and grown under laboratory conditions are capable of reproduction some 50 times, whereas fibroblasts that are apparently similar in structure taken from an aged adult are capable of reproduction only about 5 times— the Hayflick (1965) phenomenon.

The second cell population is more specialized and not capable of reproduction. These are the fixed postmitotic cells, which are the same age as the whole human being. Nerve cells and muscle cells are not replaced after loss. Function of the fixed postmitotic cells tends to deteriorate slowly, and there is also a slow reduction in the numbers of these cells. The conduction capacity of aged neurons is slowed, and total numbers are diminished. The slowed reaction time of the elderly and the reduced capacity for new learning illustrate the aging processes in the central nervous system. In the eye the choriocapillaris vessels become attenuated. The endothelial cells lose their nuclei and are replaced with hyaline tissue. This is a prelude to disciform macular degeneration.

Other Causes of Changes in Aging

The supportive connective tissue normally is supple, strong, and elastic. With aging, however, changes occur in the molecular structure of collagen; cross-linking of macromolecules results in hardening, rigidity, and loss of elasticity of connective tissue. The hardening of the connective

tissue that makes up the medial layer of an artery is evident when the radial pulse is palpated. When the artery of a young adult is compressed under the finger, there seems to be no substance to feel. The sensation under the finger when the artery of an aged person is compressed is that of a piece of string.

The significance of loss of elasticity is seen in the steady rise of systolic blood pressure with aging, a physiological response to push adequate amounts of blood through a rigid and possibly narrowed artery instead of through an elastic tube that stretches to accommodate the bolus of blood expelled by each ventricular systole. There are many practical issues in measuring blood pressure in older people. The thickness of the artery wall may lead to a fallaciously high reading. The interpretation of diastolic pressure depends upon identifying the end point on auscultation of the disappearance of the sound. Single estimations of blood pressure levels are equally unreliable as a valid measure. The determination of an abnormality of blood pressure in older people therefore requires repeated and painstaking observations.

Every species appears to have a biological clock that influences the onset of puberty, cessation of reproductive capacity, and duration of life. Attempts to extend the life span indefinitely are therefore doomed to fail, but an extension of healthy life to the preordained termination point is possible and should be the aim of all therapeutic effort. Attempts to retard the aging process and maintain good health require some background relating to the causes of aging. All living creatures have two fundamental capacities: to reproduce themselves exactly and to take in food substances and turn them into energy. Errors in these mechanisms are considered to be responsible for some changes in aging.

The deoxyribonucleic acid (DNA) molecule contains the code for protein synthesis. With increasing age, DNA errors accumulate; with repeated reproduction, chromosomal abnormalities appear. Faulty protein production results, with cell abnormality. Errors may accumulate at the stage of transfer of information from the DNA molecule by messenger ribonucleic acid (mRNA) (Orgel 1963).

Energy is produced from food intake through the action of enzymes (protein substances that catalyze specific biochemical reactions). Enzyme activity in old age decreases; as a result, the capacity to convert sources of energy from the environment and use them decreases.

There is increasing interest in faults in the immune defense mechanisms of the body as a cause of aging. A reduced defense capacity results in a higher incidence of infections in old age. Viruses that have been present in the body for many years may become virulent when immunity is reduced. The virus of herpes zoster (shingles) can be present for many years before an overt attack of shingles is seen in old age, usually when other disease processes wear down the body's defenses. Other failures of the immune defense mechanism are seen when the body makes mistakes in identifying its own cells. Antibodies then develop and a number of identified autoimmune diseases can result. Thyroid antibodies result in thyroid depression and myxedema. Antibodies to parietal cells of the stomach result in a form of macrocytic anemia. Other antibodies remain to be discovered, including a possibility of an antibrain antibody.

Adverse environmental conditions accelerate aging. Poverty, poor housing, repeated illness, and malnutrition are clearly involved. Malnutrition in the form of undernutrition and overnutrition appear to have an equally adverse effect on humans. Underfed rats live longer than rats fed *ad libitum,* because arterial degeneration and renal failure does not occur (Everitt 1982). The little old lady so often described in anecdotes is probably old because she is little. It is certainly unusual to see a nonagenarian who is not very thin. (See the section on "Nutrition" later in the chapter.)

Effects of Aging

Whereas the causes of aging are still theoretical, the tissue changes have been firmly established, and the effects of tissue changes can be found in all body structures. Aging processes proceed at a variable rate. Joints may fail in an intellectually well preserved individual, or the brain may fail when other bodily systems are still in good order. Visible effects of aging are obvious in most individuals, including changes in the skin, hair, posture, and ability to move, and even the ability to think and learn quickly. The skin becomes wrinkled, inelastic, and thin; the disappearance of subcutaneous fat and the loss of much of its protective function results in persisting purple patches of discoloration in exposed areas from bruising caused by trivial injuries. The skin is dry because of a relative absence of sweat glands and deterioration of autonomic

functions, which then fail to stimulate sweating in hot conditions in the remaining sweat glands.

Changes in the eyes and visual function are dealt with in detail in other chapters. Inner ear function is involved with both hearing and sensation of position in space. Deteriorating semicircular canal function in old age often means that elderly people become very dependent on vision to orient their head position. Poor vision and darkness increase the risk of loss of balance and falls. A deterioration of hearing may not be perceived when conversation takes place on a one-to-one basis in quiet surroundings. However, most elderly people have marked difficulty in hearing in noisy surroundings.

The appreciation of food and enjoyment of meals is limited by deterioration in nasal mucosa function. The tongue is only responsible for limited taste sensation, which does not change greatly; however, the sense of smell is the main organ used to savor food. Thus overseasoning food and adding excessive quantities of salt and strongly flavored condiments is common when the sense of smell has deteriorated, and excess salt is not desirable at any age. An absence of teeth, which now is becoming less common, leads to an inadequate diet and, frequently, indigestion. Better conservative dentistry and the addition of flouride to water supplies is having an effect; many older people have their own teeth and consequently expect and need dental care.

Reduced Mobility

One of the major problems in old age is reduced mobility. The aging of collagen and loss of elasticity of connective tissue result in stiffer joints, and the loss of muscle tone reduces strength. Poor balance from neurological deterioration and degeneration of joint surfaces combine to make ambulation slow and unsteady. The hardness and strength of bones depends on mineral content. Lack of activity is one of the prime reasons for reduced calcium content in the bones, which results in osteoporosis. Women are particularly liable to loss of bone minerals and resulting osteoporosis. Immediately after menopause there is a heavy loss of calcium that is never made up. Regrettably, there is still no effective treatment of osteoporosis, but additional calcium at menopause is advisable.

The etiology of osteoporosis is uncertain. Reduced physical activity certainly leads to a diminution of bone mineral. It is thought that many patients with osteoporosis had only a small bone mass before mineral loss took place. The role of calcium intake – particularly in the form of dairy foods – in the prevention of osteoporosis is still unclear. One thing is certain: additional calcium in the diet can do no harm. A significant proportion of patients with osteoporosis also have low vitamin D levels, and supplementation with vitamin D for a short period may be necessary.

There are four common types of disabling fractures: fracture of the neck of the femur, fracture of the surgical neck of the humerus, Colles' fracture of the wrist, and fracture of the upper or lower table of thoracic and lumbar vertebrae. Fractured neck of the femur is a major cause of prolonged and expensive hospitalization, with much subsequent permanent invalidism and significant mortality.

Changes in Respiratory and Cardiac Systems

The respiratory reserve in old age is reduced by increased stiffness of the lungs that is due to age changes in elastic tissues and reduced mobility of the thorax. Pathological changes are caused by pollution (industrial or vegetable in origin) and repeated infections. The result is always shortness of breath on exertion.

Cardiac output and competence are affected mainly by changes in coronary arteries and increased peripheral resistance in systemic vessels caused by increasing rigidity in vessel walls. Mention has been made of the physiological increase in systolic pressure commonly found in response to increased peripheral resistance. Prolonged and considerable elevation of blood pressure eventually leads to myocardial failure that primarily affects the left ventricle. Considerable judgment consequently is necessary before introducing drugs to lower blood pressure when there has been a necessary rise in systolic pressure to maintain perfusion.

Coronary arteries carry blood flow that readily can be increased when greater cardiac output in exertion requires increased blood supply to cardiac muscle. Increasing rigidity of coronary artery walls limits the capacity to increase flow. The integrity of the endothelial lining of the arteries depends on the ability for repair. In old age, faults in endothelium destroy smoothness; the resulting deposition of platelets is followed by organization of clots and narrowing of the lumen. The deposition of atheromas in the wall

of the artery may further narrow the lumen. A consequence of narrowed, rigid coronary arteries is inadequate blood flow with resulting crushing cardiac pain on exertion (angina of effort) relieved by stopping exertion. A sudden obstruction by a clot in a coronary artery (coronary thrombosis) causes similar crushing pain that persists.

Equally common and much less dramatic is the gradual occlusion of small branches of coronary arteries over the course of years, usually without any dramatic symptom at the time. The result of chronic ischemia of cardiac muscle is the slow replacement of muscle by fibrous tissue and gradually decreasing competence of cardiac function, which eventually leads to congestive cardiac failure. Ischemic heart disease following this sequence of events is by far the most common cause of chronic congestive heart failure in old age.

Pathological Changes in the Skull

The many syndromes produced by obstruction of various parts of the arterial tree within the skull can be covered only partially in this chapter. Computerized tomography (CT) scanning has helped localize precisely lesions within the brain. Intellectual changes produced by localized lesions in the brain are not as obvious as motor, sensory, or visual disturbances, but they have some quite characteristic features. For example, frontal lobe lesions may not affect memory, but they lead to indifference and a lack of inhibition in social behavior and continence. There is a marked deterioration in intellectual functions and response.

Syndromes resulting from focal lesions in the temporal lobe of the dominant hemisphere cause speech disturbance, difficulty in word finding, and some inability to understand speech. Left temporal lobe lesions affect verbal memory, writing ability, and numerical calculation; right temporal lobe lesions affect visual memory, reading and learning. A temporal lobe lesion is often associated with a contralateral upper quadrant hemianopia.

Focal lesions in the parietal lobes cause visuospatial disorganization, particularly in three-dimensional situations. There is neglect of the opposite side of the body more commonly with right parietal lobe lesions. Parietal lobe lesions big enough to involve the visual pathways cause a contralateral lower quadrant hemianopia. If it is situated posteriorly, there may be visual agnosia. Anterior parietal lobe lesions may cause focal sensory seizures, whereas posterior lesions may cause unformed visual seizures (Marsden 1978).

Better localization of the lesions causing strokes has improved understanding of rehabilitation possibilities. A thrombosis in the area of the internal capsule is the equivalent of the main cable of a telephone network being cut. The result is extensive motor paralysis of the opposite side of the body, with little or no intellectual upset. A thrombosis nearer to the cortex of the cerebral hemisphere produces a much more limited paralysis of the contralateral limbs but always intellectual impairment. The rehabilitation of cortical strokes is consequently more difficult to achieve because of intellectual difficulties, although the degree of paralysis may be much less than in capsular strokes.

Migraine, a disorder with recurring, intense, and often unilateral headaches, is a lifelong problem that may persist into old age. Spasm of cerebral blood vessels followed by dilatation results in headache and nausea. Visual disturbances accompany the phase of spasm when the basilar artery system is involved. When the carotid system is involved, dilatation may cause intense frontal headache, sometimes with pain in the eye or face. At the beginning of the attack, before the headache develops, there may be various types of visual phenomena. Bright spots and colors, hemianopia, shimmering vision to one side, rings of light that open out into a series of angles, and linear bright colors called *fortification spectra* may last for several minutes before fading and development of headache. The personality types subject to migraine tend to calm down in later years and migraine attacks become less frequent. Uncorrected anomalies of vision may cause attacks and require correction. Awareness of the multiplicity of visual disturbances preceding the headache should help the practitioner make accurate diagnoses.

The neurons making up the brain belong to the fixed postmitotic population. Cells lost in this system are lost forever. It is not certain at what age people reach their peak; however, it would probably be true to say that after age 30, the pinnacle of brain function has been passed, and intellectual brilliance depends much more on experience to produce correct responses. The elderly individual is left with somewhat reduced capacity to learn new facts quickly and to adapt to new conditions. Thus, instructions given to elderly patients always should be repeated until the person concerned is able to repeat the instructions accurately and with understanding.

With advancing old age there is a slow loss of nerve cells in the brain, with typical findings upon pathological examination. When there is excessive loss of nerve cells, intellectual function deteriorates and dementia results. This condition is called Senile Dementia of the Alzheimer Type (SDAT). Although there are several causes of dementia, such as cerebral thrombosis or tumor, it is clear that the majority of people with dementia in old age are suffering from SDAT, or Alzheimer's disease, as it is now commonly referred to in the United States.

The cause of excessive loss of brain cells is not known, but with increasing numbers of people surviving into old age, there are more cases of this distressing condition in the community. The gradual decline into dementia may occur in people who are otherwise physically well, although frequently there are other major physical disabilities accompanying the demented state. Although the statistics are somewhat imprecise, it is thought that approximately five percent of the population over the age of 65 suffers from Alzheimer's disease, and over the age of 80, possibly 20 percent are affected to a greater or lesser extent.

Other Nervous System Changes
The neurons of the peripheral nervous system also consist of postmitotic cells. With the slow loss of cells and deterioration of cell function, nerve impulses in general tend to be somewhat slower in the elderly. Proprioceptive function tends to deteriorate; when added to poor vision and deteriorating balance, this makes the already poor stability of elderly people even worse.

Function of the autonomic nervous system also may deteriorate. One of the more important effects of the decline of the autonomic function is failure of the blood pressure to correct itself on a change of posture. Blood pressure normally falls when the body is in a reclining position for a long time. A healthy adult, on standing upright, undergoes immediate correction of blood pressure and cerebral blood flow is maintained. In the elderly, autonomic response is delayed; on standing up, many elderly people have a postural drop of systolic blood pressure that may produce dizziness and, in extreme cases, may cause a fall. Another effect of autonomic deterioration is a decline in bowel motility. Constipation is almost universal among the elderly. Lack of bulk in the diet, reduced fluid intake, and lack of mobility add to constipation.

The capacity to adjust to changes in environmental temperature deteriorates with age. Shivering (the mechanism for warming the body in cold conditions) does not occur in older people. Sweat evaporation (the normal method of cooling) is also defective because of deteriorated autonomic function and fewer sweat glands in the skin of older people.

Endocrine System Failure

Two endocrine system failures in old age are of extreme importance, as their diagnosis and appropriate treatment are truly effective. Diabetes of maturity onset is caused by inadequate secretion of insulin by the beta cells in the pancreas. The result is decreased tolerance of carbohydrates, especially simple sugars, with resulting rise in blood sugar levels, thirst, polyuria, and glucose in the urine. The patients are usually overweight. Vascular complications of diabetes occur, and slow degeneration takes place in arteries and nerve tissue.

Control of maturity-onset diabetes can be achieved by control of carbohydrate intake, weight reduction, and increased exercise in most cases. Oral hypoglycemic agents stimulate the flagging beta cells to produce more insulin, and those not controlled by dietary restriction then can be controlled. Insulin is only required in this group to cover an emergency such as acute illness or a surgical procedure. It is advisable to use only short-acting hypoglycemic agents in the sulfonylurea group if oral treatment is required. The action of long-acting hypoglycemic drugs may persist overnight and cause faintness the following morning from hypoglycemia with marked postural hypotension on getting out of bed; this could set the stage for a fall.

A smaller number of diabetics of the juvenile-onset type who always need insulin are now reaching old age. Well-controlled diabetics are said to avoid many of the vascular complications of diabetes and those who have had a successful lifetime of insulin treatment have had to be well controlled. There is an increased incidence of cataracts and retinal deterioration in diabetics.

The second endocrine failure is myxedema that is due to lack of thyroxin secretion. Practitioners may mistake the insidious onset of this condition for aging unless they are aware of the syndrome. There is a gradual slowing of all bodily function. Slow pulse; slow, deep, husky speech; slow thought; increasing deafness; thinning of hair; increasing obesity; dryness of the skin; and constipation all can be attributed to age. The total picture is nevertheless typical, and once suggested is instantly recognizable. Any member of the caring professions is entitled to make the diagnosis on simple clinical observation, which can be readily confirmed biochemically and successfully cured by replacement therapy.

Problems in Drug Administration

Nephrons, the individual filters in the kidney, decrease in number in old age; the capacity of the distal tubules to reabsorb fluid also deteriorates. Old age thus is accompanied by increased frequency of micturition. Reduced renal capacity to excrete toxic substances is of great significance when medication is administered. Drugs are excreted by the kidneys after metabolism in the liver or excreted unchanged by the kidneys. Kidney deterioration thus can lead to toxic drug levels when normal doses have been administered.

Further problems are created after drugs have been administered by changes in volume of distribution of drugs. Fat-soluble drugs tend to be stored in the increased fatty tissue of the elderly; this is particularly important with many hypnotic drugs, which thereby may have marked hangover effects lasting for days. Decreased serum protein levels lead to reduced protein binding of drugs and consequently, increased levels of active drug in the serum. Reduced body fluid and reduced protein binding of drugs in the circulation lead to higher drug levels and possible toxic effects. Metabolism of drugs (the breaking down of drugs, particularly in the liver) is reduced, and the capacity of the kidneys to excrete drugs or their metabolites is reduced. Consequently, all drug doses for older patients must be modified to a lower level to allow for the changes in drug metabolism and excretion.

Diagnosis and the Older Patient

Treatment of disease can proceed only if an accurate diagnosis has been achieved. Medical conditions associated with eye disorders are mainly connected with arterial conditions; infections; endocrine disorders; immune disorders; neurology, rheumatology, and dermatology. Nevertheless, in old age the most common disorders are of the heart, lung, and intestines, as well as cancer.

Diagnosis must be made after an accurate and full history and a physical examination. Getting an accurate and full history from an elderly patient is frequently a work of art. A full examination is time consuming, allowing for dressing and undressing. The whole procedure nevertheless is both worthwhile and essential. Further investigation of elderly patients, if still necessary, calls for some balance to avoid the pitfalls either of inadequacy or overinvestigation, which may be unpleasant for the patient. Most elderly patients have several well-authenticated diagnoses at the same time. Multiple pathology is common; however, only one condition is the cause of the immediate disabling problem, and therapeutic efforts should be concentrated on the problem, not the whole range of possible treatment of coincident disorders. Investigation should be selective and carried out only to discover conditions that can be treated (Prinsley 1981).

Urine should be examined routinely for sugar, protein, and bile. Anemia in old age is frequently unsuspected, and a routine full blood examination is essential. Hematology results can be interpreted in the elderly in exactly the same way as in other age groups and follow-up investigation proceeded with, when indicated, to complete the diagnosis. An erythrocyte sedimentation rate (ESR) above 40 mm in 1 hour should alert the clinician to the possibility of polymyalgia and myeloma. Polymyalgia and its association with arteritis is very significant, as retinal artery occlusion is a complication.

Biochemical investigations should be interpreted with awareness that the normal range may be broadened. Results can be upset by dehydration, use of diuretics, or circulatory disturbances. Impaired glucose tolerance is common, but abnormal blood sugar levels should be regarded as significant only if the patient has been on a normal diet and has been taking normal exercise before the investigation. Serum protein, mineral, and vitamin investigations may give evidence of malnutrition, and dietary iron deficiency is common.

Nutrition

Recent observations of nutritional status in institutionalized older people have drawn attention to the likelihood of malnutrition in the midst of plentiful food supplies (Flint 1981). Heat-labile and water-soluble vitamins are easily destroyed in large-scale catering. Folate deficiency is common when green vegetables are overcooked and kept hot for hours before serving. (This subject is considered further in Chapter 7.) There is clear evidence that education about proper nutrition is still necessary. Dietary requirements in old age are little different from those of any other age. A mixed diet with adequate fiber and protein, as well as a shift from simple sugars to vegetable types of carbohydrate, should be provided. Recommendations for the control of obesity and continued adequate exercise are good advice.

Community Care

The life style of the elderly always has been related to the community's attitudes toward its older members. Western society has tended to become less well oriented toward, less respectful of, and certainly less inclined to continue the tradition of the extended family. Although the golden age of several generations all living together in one house may have had its problems if it ever existed, the modern nuclear family leaves its elderly members to fend for themselves in many cases. Older people living with a family are protected, and competent older couples also manage well when income, housing, and health are adequate. There is a vast difference between living with family and living alone when the frailties of old age become a burden.

Increasing frailty with advancing years inevitably causes problems, even when health is otherwise good. Age-related changes include diminishing physical strength and dexterity, which makes ordinary activities of daily living increasingly difficult, from housekeeping to any normal social life. Lack of motivation, lack of fresh sensory input, poor concentration, and decreased capacity for sustained effort reduce activity. Lack of transportation, lack of finances, and unsuitable housing are frequent additional burdens.

The recognition of unfavorable factors has led to the construction of a scale of deprivation. The group at the top of the scale, who are particularly at risk, consists of people over 80 years old, living alone, who have recently been hospitalized themselves or recently bereaved. Other important factors in the scale of deprivation are poor mobility, failing brain function (which is often not realized), a disorganized life style after retirement, and poor housing. Retirement migration is not always the happiest way of life when family, familiar surroundings, and organized support services have been left behind.

History of Care for the Elderly

Support services to assist elderly people have a long history. Planning was first mentioned at the jubilee of King Amenophis III in 1375 BC. King David, 3,000 years ago, was recommended treatment with a fair virgin. Hippocrates, 2,400 years ago, recommended exercise and a spare diet. In less ancient times, the churches were involved in providing accommodation for the homeless and dependent. In Europe many of these splendid "hospitals," now hundreds of years old, are still in use and are architectural treasures. In Britain the Poor Relief Acts of 1601 made local parishes responsible for those who could not help themselves. The Poor Laws were superseded by Boards of Guardians in 1834. The awful old institutions known as workhouses followed. More enlightened welfare arrangements did not begin until 1929 with the abolition of the Poor Laws. Following the 1948 Health Acts, centrally funded, specially built welfare homes for the frail aged were created. In Australia somewhat similar arrangements were made, with the construction of Benevolent Homes for those of all ages left destitute in the early days of colonization. Many of these establishments have now become modern geriatric centers, with very different aims of rehabilitation and return to the community, rather than long-term, almost custodial, care.

The development of support services in the community has been relatively late. In Western countries the pattern is variable in quality, quantity, and content. Making sensible use of support services requires knowledge of local arrangements.

Support Systems

In addition to the scale of deprivation, there is a scale of supports for the elderly, with the most important elements at the top of the scale. At the very top of the scale for those elderly who cannot live independently is living with family—either the spouse or younger members. If that is not possible, a caring family member who visits every day comes next. The importance of the good neighbor is not in giving physical assistance, but in helping with simple tasks outside the house such as shopping and in observing if there is trouble. A doctor and nurse who will visit and someone who will provide transportation come high on the list. A house that is con-

veniently located and manageable and adequate income support come before organized community services. At-home help or a paid or subsidized housekeeping service can assist in domestic maintenance. A service that delivers meals provides a balanced diet for those too feeble or lacking in motivation to prepare meals for themselves. Mobility aids and gadgets within the house to make life easier and safer are provided by a variety of agencies.

Backing up community support services are various forms of sheltered housing and accommodation. Small groups of houses and apartments for the elderly give mutual support. Retirement villages seem to provide a satisfactory and happy life style for those who make that choice. Independence is largely maintained, and catering and house maintenance arrangements are the residents' responsibilites. For those who can no longer manage such day-to-day activities, a more sheltered existence in hostel-type accommodations insures that a roof and meals are provided. This saves the older person who is merely frail from having to live with sick people, which is the case when nursing homes are the only alternative to struggling and failing in the community.

The emphasis now is certainly away from institutions, but survival in the community frequently depends on organized support services if family support is not available. Institution and community are not interchangeable, but admission to an institution may be the result of lack of even minimal community support services. The development of community services depends not only on available finances and personnel, but also on legislation and location. Some city provisions would be inappropriate in rural areas. Manageable small population groups and a wealth of volunteer effort facilitate services in rural areas that could not be contemplated in a city. Complex financial structures in most countries create difficulties in paying for special housing, hostels, transportation, pensions and allowances, personal services, aids and appliances, assistance to volunteer groups, supporting payment for private accommodation, and the like (Prinsley 1982). Cost-consciousness includes much more than the price of medical investigation, treatment, and spectacles.

Mention has been made of domiciliary nursing services, housekeeping services, and services that bring food to people's homes. Such services are well developed. Paramedical practitioners have a major role to play in many countries, but as yet they have scarcely impinged on community care. The training of occupational therapists and physiotherapists includes an increasing commitment to care of the elderly. A visiting physiotherapist has a role more as educator for members of the household to continue simple remedial exercises than as therapist. The occupational therapist can assess a house and the hazards likely to trouble a patient with any disability. Suitably minor modifications can be made, danger points removed, and appropriate appliances and aids provided.

Centers for the display of aids and appliances of all kinds, including visual aids, are now to be found in major centers in western countries. The Disabled Living Foundation in London was the prototype of these valuable resources, which can demonstrate aids for all types of disability and give advice and instruction about suitable appliances. Personal alarm systems are now available in various forms. A simple button device worn on a cord around the neck, when pressed, can activate a permanently staffed control center through a monitor attached to the house telephone. Thus, an elderly person living alone can feel secure, especially if disabled by mobility problems or poor vision.

Various forms of day care and day clubs are valuable for social contact, observation, and provision of services such as hairdressing, bathing, and podiatry, as well as a meal at midday. Social contact is of particular value for those living alone, and for those who live in a strained domestic situation. More formal day hospitals, where rehabilitation treatment and medical and nursing care are provided, also give social contact. Day care and day hospitals together prevent social and medical breakdown and are steadily increasing in numbers as their value in maintaining life in the community is appreciated.

Further ideas of accommodation for elderly people have continued to evolve. Hostels for the frail have been constructed by voluntary effort, religious groups, and local and regional authorities. The United States has been in the forefront in constructing multilevel complexes for the aged that incorporate self-care units or apartments, hostels for the frail, and nursing home accommodation for those in need for total care. In Australia religious groups have followed this pattern successfully, and an occasional development of this type now exists in Great Britain.

Complexes with such a wide range of facilities for support and care are expensive to staff, especially when rehabilitation facilities are added. Admission to the system at whichever level is appropriate at the time when help is necessary avoids the dreadful concept of steady deterioration through self-care apartment to hostel to nursing home bed, until departure in a box.

Supportive family attitudes to aged parents may make such arrangements appear quite appropriate. However, those offering advice must consider ethnic diversity of views about aged relatives. The idea of a grandparent being removed from the family home would fill some families with shame and horror, and others with welcome relief. A sensitive social worker is clearly part of any team involved in the care of elderly patients. Family background, resources, and attitudes need to be known when caring plans are being made.

Concepts of health care of the elderly must incorporate a group with a range of skills. Geriatric medicine always involves a team, and all the members of the team—physicians, nurses, paramedical personnel, social workers, and the family— are involved. The physician has the responsibility of seeing that the usual medical principles are applied, making a proper diagnosis, and providing necessary treatment. The other members of the team have equally important roles. Chronological age should not be a limiting factor; improved quality of life is the aim, and this may be achieved by any members or all of the team. Nevertheless, some degenerative diseases are a challenge to the best efforts and progress in spite of treatment. There is still no reason to stop trying to help the person maintain quality of life.

Medical and caring techniques to manage such growing commitments are developing with increasing sophistication. The specialty of geriatric medicine is attracting lively minds and skilled practitioners who accept the challenge. Geriatric medicine is not included in health education—still with inadequate time devoted to it but, it is hoped, with increasing impact and improving attitudes in the next generation of health care practitioners.

Older people have to cope with many problems. Physical weakness leads to reduced mobility. Arthritis, strokes, Parkinson's disease, heart failure, and chronic lung disorders are common and disabling. Psychological problems include loss of role, bereavement, family neglect or rejection, reduced income, depression, and the generally poor attitudes of society toward the elderly. The environment presents a hostile front, with traffic hazards, difficult access to public buildings, and fear of crime.

Role of the Optometrist

Although optometrists may be faced with difficult problems in their own field, they must keep in mind all the additional difficulties that may be part of the lives of many elderly patients. The etiology of disease is multifactorial for many older people, yet they present with only one illness or problem. Sorting out the whole patient may be a formidable task, but it is all too frequently necessary when simple questioning reveals that the illness brought to the practitioner is only the tip of an iceberg of social, financial, psychological, and environmental difficulties. A society may be judged by the way it cares for its aged citizens.

The clock cannot run forever, but, it is hoped, can be kept running smoothly: "Senescence, like Mount Everest, challenges our ingenuity by the fact that it is there, and focusing our attention on it is unlikely to be fruitless" (Comfort 1979, 331). This is a worthy sentiment to encourage optometrists to focus their attention on worthy recipients of their skills.

References

Comfort, A. *The Biology of Senescence.* 3rd ed. London: Churchill-Livingstone, 1979.

Everitt, A. V. "Nutritional and Hypothalamic Influence in Aging." In *Nutritional Approaches to Aging Research,* ed. G. B. Moment. Boca Raton, Fla.: CRC Press, 1982, pp. 245–256.

Flint, D. M. "The Elderly." In *Food and Nutrition in Australia,* ed. M. Wahlqvist. North Ryde, Australia: Cassell Australia, 1981, pp. 362–367.

Hayflick, L. " The Limited In Vitro Life of Human Diploid Cell Strains." *Experimental Cell Research* 37 (1965): 614–636.

Marsden, C. D. "The Diagnosis of Dementia." In *Studies in Geriatric Psychiatry,* eds. A. D. Isaacs and F. Post. Chichester, England: Wiley, 1978, pp. 94–118.

Orgel, L. E. " The Maintenance of the Accuracy of Protein Synthesis and Its Relevance to Aging." *Proceedings of the National Academy of Sciences of the United States of America* 49 (1963): 517–521.

Prinsley, D. M. "Investigating the Elderly Patient." *Medical Journal of Australia* 2 (July 25, 1981): 25–26.

Prinsley, D. M. "The Provision of Community Services for the Elderly." In *Recent Advances in Geriatric Medicine,* No. 2, ed. B. Isaacs. London: Churchill-Livingstone, 1982, pp. 241–257.

U.S. Department of Health , Education and Welfare. National Clearinghouse on Aging. *Facts about Older Americans: 1975.* Washington D.C.: U.S. Government Printing Office, 1975.

Chapter 5

Psychology of Aging

Susan Bettis

Aging is characterized by a progressive decrease in the intensity of the adaptive process. The limitation of the adaptive capacities of an aging organism promotes the development of pathology in old age as well as the possibility of an easier disruption of regulatory mechanisms. (Frolkis 1977, 177)

Aging is measured biologically, psychologically, and sociologically (Birren 1959). All three of these factors influence the amount of success an organism experiences in the adaptational process. This chapter will begin by sharing some current information from the areas of neurological psychology, cognitive/perceptual psychology, and social psychology to show the multiple influences affecting the adapting aging individual. The first section examines normative psychological processes. The chapter continues by considering a small sample of the non-normative life events faced by many elderly people. A final section on individual differences concludes the chapter. A complete review of the psychology of aging is well beyond the scope of this chapter.

We are all aging and likely to become old. Each of us—professional, student, adult, child, and older patient—is at some stage of the aging process. It is therefore to our mutual advantage to recognize one another's age-related expectations, resources, and adaptive styles.

Normative Psychology of Aging

Neuropsychological Changes in Aging

The human brain and central nervous system is a miracle of complexity. As the human's communications center, it collects and processes internal and external information, allowing adaptation to the environment. On a hot day our body tells our brain that it is overly warm. Searching the environment, we find the direct sunlight to be too penetrating and move to the shade. Although this example may seem overly simple, the results of not moving into a cooler space could be heat stroke and death. By moving to the shade, we adapt and survive.

Any major loss of sensory function such as vision or hearing necessitates major compensations on the part of the organism to continue successful interaction with the immediate world. As we age, not only are we faced with sensory decline, but meeting the challange to adapt also becomes increasingly difficult.

Anatomic Changes in the Aging Brain. The neuron is the basic building block of the brain and central nervous system. Neurons carry messages to the body like a telephone carries information from one terminal to another. Humans have billions of nerve cells at birth, but aging results in the progressive death of these cells over the life span (Bondareff 1977; Brody 1955, 1973, 1980). However, humans still have a tremendous number of these nonreplaceable cells at their disposal. A common, although not universal, structural change in the aging brain, then is atrophy and neuronal death. Brain atrophy is found alarmingly often in old men (Bondareff 1977), but little correlation between degree of cell loss and ability to function has been determined (Brody 1980).

A second common change in the structure of the brain results from the development of structures called *neurofibrillary tangles*. These tangles, which may be likened to neuronal "spaghetti," are made up of clumps of nonfunctioning neurons. Described as "a thickening and twisting of neurofibrillary networks within the cytoplasm" (Brody 1980), these masses develop in most elderly brains and are seen in major proportion in dementia patients (see the discussion later in the chapter).

A third change in the structure of the aging brain is the development of *senile plaques*. These plaques, consisting of pieces of broken neurons, tend to congregate at the synaptic gap between neurons. The number of these plaques is quite small in normally functioning elderly people, but plaques are numerous in people with Alzheimer's disease (Tomlinson and Henderson 1976).

Finally, alterations in the chemical structure of neurons is the most commonly occurring change in the brain. Lipofuscin begins to collect in the cells of many of the body's organ systems, including the brain. By age 90, certain neurons in the central nervous system are made up of 75 percent lipofuscin (Strehler 1977). It could be assumed that this build-up would interfere with cell metabolism, but the role of lipofuscin in decreased functioning is not known.

The total functional cost of these changes to the normally aging individual is not yet fully understood. The range of individual differences in cognition, an area of the brain particularly affected, may prevent the development of an effective predictive model of aging and functional loss.

Physiological Changes in the Aging Brain. The chemical "messengers" that communicate from one nerve cell to the next are called *neurotransmitters*. The study of these chemicals is one of the most exciting and rapidly growing areas in psychology. Around 30 of these chemicals have been identified to date, each with a different function. Neurotransmitters regulate all our cognitive and emotive behaviors, including memory, pain, and mood. Their role in mental illness, substance abuse, obesity, and even senility is in the initial phase of exploration. One of the fascinating aspects of these substances is that an excess can cause one set of problems, whereas deficit amounts result in something very different. For example, an excess of one neurotransmitter, dopamine, is suspected as being involved in schizophrenia. When dopamine deficits occur, however, Parkinson's disease results.

Dopamine regulates motor behavior, which explains the difficulty with walking seen in people with Parkinson's disease. Dopamine is a monoamine. Two other monoamines (catecholamines) are serotonin and norepinephrine. Serotonin regulates the sleep-wakefulness cycles by stimulating the onset of sleep as well as eating, and it is involved in psychological depression. Norepinenphrine regulates waking, memory, and eating and is also suspected as serving an antidepressant role. Monoamine oxidase (MAO) is an enzyme that metabolizes the catecholamines or monoamines (Cooper, Bloom, and Roth 1982). MAO levels increase with age. It is possible to associate this change with a depressive state accompanying old age (Samorajski and Hartford 1980). This may also explain in part the sleep problems common in older people (see the discussion later in the chapter).

As yet, only a few clinical applications for neurotransmitter research exist. One example is the replacement of dopamine in parkinsonism patients with drugs like L-dopa. We cannot help but speculate that an adjustment in serotonin and norepinephrine through drugs such as amoxapine, which work on both these catecholamines, might also be helpful in Parkinson's disease. If one member of this neurotransmitter family is being affected (dopamine), then we could speculate that others are also in need of adjustment. This could be very helpful in alleviating associated sleep problems.

This concept is worthy of discussion for two reasons. First, many of the behaviors that are idiosyncratic to older populations are the result of physiological changes in the brain—a natural part of aging. Second, when these changes exceed the normal range, a pathological condition results just as surely as if the person had had a stroke or head trauma from a car accident; they are just not visible. Some neurotransmitter manipulations exist, such as using dopamine to treat Parkinson's disease, but basically we are at the beginning phases of a new science. As study on brain structure and process continues, many more secrets of aging will be discovered.

Thus, as we add to length of life, it is exciting to consider how much neurological research may add quality to these added years. Psychological depression can be treated and memory and learning, enhanced. One of the objects of research is to develop nondrug interventions that will modify these processes. An example is the use of running and other aerobic exercises to increase both norepinephrine and endorphine levels, thus elevating mood and, in some individuals, producing the "runner's high." We must more fully understand the physiological determinants of behavior before we can understand the sociophysical components.

The effects of the anatomic and physiological changes in the elderly range from a simple slowing of reaction time all the way to vegetative states seen in the final stages of Alzheimer's disease. Many of the daily complaints we hear from the elderly, including forgetfulness, low mood, difficulties in falling and staying asleep, and increased sensitivity to pain (to mention but a few), are the results of these changes. What may seem like a bid for attention is usually a reaction to some very real physical experiences.

Cognitive and Perceptual Changes in Aging

The cognitive functions including memory, learning, and problem solving have been the subject of much study. Despite this considerable effort, debates concerning age-related loss versus the maintenance of adult intellectual competency are not uncommon. Baltes and Schaie (1974, 1976) have championed the belief that a "general and universal decline in intellectual performance" is a myth and is not supported by data. The opposing viewpoint, represented by Horn and Donaldson (1976, 715), states that "it is premature to argue that existing results indicate the myth of intellectual decline."

As the debate continues, a working definition of intelligence and a more valid delineation of its components may result. "Intelligence is usually defined as the ability to learn and/or manipulate symbols. Intelligence is an inference from competence demonstrated in several situations, but competence may involve more than simply intelligence; motivation, and personal styles may be involved as well" (Schaie and Geiwitz 1982, 201). This debate seems necessary to answer questions concerning intelligence at any age. In the meantime, research results do exist that clarify some of the critical changes in learning style that occur with age.

Memory. There are three stages in human memory. *Acquisition,* or short-term memory, is the process of recording a stimuli for a few seconds. The information when encoded, goes into *storage,* or long-term memory. *Retrieval* occurs when information is recalled into active thought. One of the commonly held myths is that as we age, short-term memory skills are lost but long-term memory stays intact even in individuals with organic brain syndromes. Closer examination, however, reveals that what appears to be good memory for historic events is really nothing more than anecdotal memory or memory for a few events from a person's childhood that are repeated regardless of stimuli (Craik 1977).

Intelligence and Learning Ability. Adaptation to loss of cognitive capacity and functional ability depends on the following (Ebersole and Hess 1981, 474–475)·
1. Previous IQ (people with higher IQs retain function better).
2. Preexisting personality factors (basic needs and expectations, defense mechanisms, coping capacity, tolerance for anxiety, emotional status, and attitude).
3. Relationship network (number, type, and stability).
4. Prevailing attitudes toward aging.
5. Environmental supports and resources.

The most outstanding psychological features of aging are the impairment of *short term memory* and the *lengthening of response time.* Both factors contribute to lower scores of the elderly on standard tests of "intelligence." Many studies show that the measured intelligence of older people is typically underestimated. Measured declines usually involve speed of response. Age decrements are negligible on tests that depend on vocabulary, general information, and well-practiced activities. Sensory deprivation–the result of hearing and visual impairment–may impair intellectual responses.

Some elderly people suffer from mild, non-progressive memory impairment. Memory of recent events is more affected than remote or long-term memory. With increases in age, the retention of things heard is superior to that of things seen. Short-term memory is 5 to 30 seconds; recent memory is 1 hour to several days.

Learning may not be as difficult as we might assume for the elderly. Two factors are important: the type of material to be learned and the time alloted for its retention. Two types of intelligence or learning styles exist (Willis, Blieszner, and Baltes 1981). *Fluid intelligence*–the learning style of the young–is the ability to learn new material without an existing structure on which to "hang" the new stimuli. We are born without much exposure to the world; everything is new, and learning must happen in an experiential void. As we reach our adult years, our experience forms a number of structures or outlines in which to fit new information. Thus, new stimuli that relate to previous learning will be more easily retained.

The second factor that influences learning in the elderly is time. The longer the exposure to the new stimuli, the greater the chance of memory storage. Indeed, one study indicates that when older people are exposed to a stimulus for at least 12 seconds, they have higher recall rates than people in their 20s (Adamowicz 1976). When all time pressures are taken off the older individual, there is no significant difference in problem-solving ability between age groups. Time pressure may produce an arousal level in the elderly that interferes with performance. This is the result of trying to cope with the lengthening reaction time between stimulus and response. (Most adolescents and young adults probably have been frustrated by being behind an older automobile driver or older shopper in line.) This slowness in reaction time is often mistaken for the loss of intelligence, but it is simply an elongation in the time necessary to process information and to retrieve content from long-term memory. When coupled with short-term memory loss and perceptual decline, however, it can make dealing with the elderly a frustrating experience.

The idea that intelligence radically deteriorates with age is simply wrong. When the same age group is measured radically at a number of points in time and compared with itself (longitudinal research), individual IQs remain about the same or show very little decline. Only when illness intervenes does ability decline. Indeed, when a sudden loss in cognitive function occurs, it often signals that death is imminent (the "terminal drop" phenomenon) (Botwinick 1977).

Implications for the optometrist attempting to work with the older patient are many. It is necessary to go slowly. Relating new material to the past experience of the elderly will aid in learning. When a rapid decline in intellectual function is noted, referral to a medical specialist is advised. "Just growing old" is not a sufficient explanation for this rapid loss. Above all, optometrists must monitor their stereotypes and assumptions about the learning capacities of elderly patients. Realizing that the different age groups' learning styles are unique and not necessarily deficient may prevent condescension from the professional and embarrassment on the part of the older patient.

Perception. Multiple interactive perceptual changes occur with aging. Presbycusis and other types of hearing loss are common (Corso 1977). Hearing loss can begin in the early 30s for men and the late 30s for women (Schaie 1982). Hearing decline is nearly universal for people in their 70s, but the degree of loss varies from individual to individual. Our bones become porous, and the ear canal loses its abililty to carry sound. Loss of teeth causes the jawbone to deteriorate, eliminating another means of carrying vibratory information. Arthritic changes in the joints affect the inner ear as the malleus, incus, and stapes lose their vibratory capacity. The tympanic membrane also changes in its vibratory characteristics, which changes the nature of sound. Neuronal loss occurs in the inner ear. The sum total of these changes is the loss of audition, and it can be one of the most devastating occurrences in later life. Social isolation may result. The inability to hear and carry on a converation causes the hearing handicapped and others to withdraw from each other as discourse becomes strained. Threats to personal safety can occur when the environment cannot be monitored. Paranoia, a common mental disorder, can result from hearing decline (see the discussion on paranoid behavior later in the chapter).

Taste sensitivity also diminishes (Schiffman 1979). Although this may not seem as devastating as visual or auditory losses, nutritional deficits may result when food no longer is appealing. A decrease in the number of taste buds begins in women in the early 40s and in men some ten years later. Of the four primary taste sensations (salt, sweet, sour, and bitter), salty tastes seem most vulnerable to age-related changes (Schiffman, Orlandi, and Erickson 1979). This may lead to oversalting, a dangerous habit. Decrement in sweet and sour sensitivity follow and are almost as common as salt sensitivity decrement.

The sense of smell, through which we glean much pleasure, is also a warning system for toxic substances in the environment. Odor sensitivity seems relatively stable over the life span (Engen 1977). Given that olfaction takes up more area in the brain than any other sensory system, it may be the least vulnerable to neuronal death.

Touch has several dimensions. The ability of the skin to judge temperature does not seem to decrease significantly with age (Kenshalo 1977). Other touch-related activities, such as pain detection, vibratory detection, and pressure sensitivity, have proved difficult to investigate and have produced conflicting results.

Thus, perceptual responses decline in old age. For some people, the sensory response decline is almost insignificant. For vision and hearing, however, significant losses may occur. Such losses proceed gradually, and people adapt to them until their effects become cumulative and occasionally incapacitating.

There is a strong relationship between cognition, perception, and consciousness; they work together for adaptive purposes. Decrements in one area can limit the functions of another. Studies have shown that when individuals are placed in stimulus-free environments for any period of time, hallucinations and states much like psychosis ensue, and paranoia may result (Diamond 1978; Heron 1957). Any sensory decline increases the elderly person's vulnerability to stimulus deprivation. Efforts must be made to avoid a world composed exclusively of one room in a nursing home or a person's own home, no matter how extensive the individual's health problems.

On the other end of the continuum is sensory overload—having more stimuli to cope with than the sensory mechanisms of the body can effectively process. We may be more susceptible to stimulus overload as we age (Watson 1978). Attending to a stimulus is made difficult, if not impossible, when stimuli from the background intervene. For example, an elderly woman in a noisy airline terminal who is attempting to reroute her airplane flight may literally be unable to function in that complex, demanding, fast-moving environment.

As we age, optimal stimulus levels may be required for us to function. The interaction between cognition, perception, and consciousness is synergistic. All three functions equal more than the sum of each single function. Interestingly, sleep pattern highlight this interaction.

The topic of sleep-related problems frequently arises in conversations between older people (Gurland 1976). The fact that sleep aids are the over-the-counter medication most frequently purchased by the elderly is a testament to the amount of frustration experienced. As we age, our sleep patterns change. It takes longer for us to fall asleep, and we awaken more often during night. Fifty percent of older people complain of insomnia (Feinberg and Carlson 1968). This con-

stant regaining of consciousness prevents the elderly from entering deep sleep cycles (Stages 3 and 4), in which refreshing and resorative sleep occurs. When the flow in and out of these stages is interrupted, people experience fatigue during the waking hours.

Whereas Stage 3 and 4 sleep are marked by slow brain wave activities, rapid eye movement (REM) or dream, sleep produces brain wave patterns that are often more vigorous than those of waking states. REM sleep has a critical, though little understood, function. People deprived of dream activity become irritable and are unable to solve problems. When allowed to dream after deprivation, people spend most of their time in REM activity, as though to catch up. The relationship between cognition and consciousness is marked, since there is a positive correlation between REM activity and cognitive function (Prinz, Marsh, and Thompson 1974). People affected by organic brain syndromes dream less and less as their dementia worsens. By the latter stages of this disease, no REM activity can be measured.

Implications. Optometrists have an important role in the maintenance of perceptual and cognitive functioning. First, the importance of maintaining optimal visual functioning throughout life is obvious. Furthermore, given the synergistic nature of cognition and perception, enhancement of one skill area or sensory system will enhance others. Similarly, deprivation must be prevented to promote optimal psychological functioning.

Sociopsychological Factors in Aging
What motivates older people? What goals do they share with their peers? What values do they have in common?

Health has become a national obsession in our society, and a high priority of older people is health maintenance. Unfortunately, many negative side effects result. Older people tend to self-diagnose and self-treat rather than seek help from a trained professional. When the multiple losses in aging are considered, this tendency should not be surprising. Examples of this decline and typical attempts at self-help are many. As people age, their energy decreases. Many older people use thyroid medication to fight depression. Metabolic decreases mean lower caloric need; the appetite decreases at the same time as the body's need for food decreases.

A side-effect of this is a change in bowel habits that leads many older persons to assume they are constipated. As a result, laxative abuse is common and addictive. As has been mentioned, sleep patterns change, and over-the-counter sleep aids are purchased despite their negative side-effects.

This compulsion to self-treat includes vision care. As close-up work becomes more difficult, if not impossible, a trip to the corner druggist's eyeglass display may be substituted for adequate vision care. Glaucoma is not considered, examination for cataracts is not sought, and correction for failing distance vision and binocular function often are ignored. When over-the-counter eyeglasses do not work, older people may experience a sense of decline and helplessness concerning their visual condition.

Vision care practitioners need to be aware of older people's preference (and economic incentives) for self-help. Of course, motivation toward health maintenance is both positive and negative. At its best, it can motivate older patients to seek aid and keep them receptive to it.

A second prime motivator for older people is the impetus to meet social needs. Relationship patterns have varied greatly over the past hundred years. Most presently elderly people grew up in rural settings where social contacts were taken for granted. It was not uncommon to know everyone in town, to marry the girl or boy next door, and to remain in one's home town for a lifetime. These expectations are no longer valid. Urbanization and mobility cause many neighbors to live like strangers. For older people this can present problems for two reasons. First, as we age we frequently face the loss of a loved one. Half of all women are widowed by the age of 60. This leaves them vulnerable to isolation that many do not succeed in combating. Second, elderly people may share certain biases and physical limitations that may preclude their actively seeking replacement of lost relationships.

One of the most prevalent debates in gerontology has been between theorists who believe that older people disengage from their social surroundings at the same time as society disengages from them (Cumming and Henry 1961) and those who believe that when disengagement does occur, it is not normal and natural but is rather a sign of depression and resignation:

Older people are the same as middle age people with essentially the same psychological and social needs. In this view the decreased social interaction that characterizes old age results by the withdrawal by society from the aging person, and the decrease in interaction proceeds against the desires of most aging men and women. The older person who ages optimally is the person who stays active and who manages to resist the shrinkage of his social world. He maintains the activities of middle age as long as possible and then finds substitutes for those activities he is forced to relinquish. (Havinghurst, Neugarten, and Tobin 1968, 173)

Striking up a conversation with strangers or detaining optometrists with personal chatter long after the vision examination has ended are manifestations of this need to make interpersonal contact.

It has been commonly known that life transitions and high stress have the least negative effect on the person with a full and well-balanced set of relationships. Furthermore, women have been shown to be people oriented throughout life, whereas men are less so in their career development years. As men age, however, there is a tendency for friends and family to take on increased importance. This is heightened when loss of resources forces the older individual to ask for help with activities of daily living. Since dependence is a dreaded fear for many, a small amount of assistance with one or two activities of daily living may prevent a total collapse of health maintenance.

The wish to remain independent is a third motivator in the lives of the elderly. The stereotype of the lonely oldster waiting for an invitation from an adult son or daughter to come live with him or her rarely exists in real life. To maintain one's own life style and decision-making freedom is important at any age. For the older person faced for the first time with threats to self-definition, this freedom may be even more precious.

As human beings we are all "wired" to strive for competence. This is the basis of human motivation. Like younger people, older people strive to remain healthy and independent and to have fulfilling interpersonal relationships. Again, elderly people must stay as functional as possible to fulfill their potential. Any professional faced with meeting the needs of older people must consider that the treatment of choice is the treatment that will give them the greatest amount of self-determination and mastery of their environment. Without these, depression is likely to result. The fact that white males over 70 have the highest rate of suicide in our society is a testament to the seriousness of this problem.

Nonnormative Psychology of Aging

Nonnormative development in aging involves decline, loss, and pathology. Nonnormative aging can be due to many causes. This section will discuss only the more common problems. Psychological depression and learned helplessness are two of these. Paranoia is more common among older people than in younger populations (Eisdorfer 1980). Finally, this section will cover the organic brain syndromes and aphasias, the relatively mysterious diseases that strike millions of people in the United States.

Learned Helplessness and Depression

To understand depression in older people, we must understand the concept of learned helplessness. Seligman (1975) assigned dogs in the laboratory to one of two experimental conditions. Both groups of dogs received electric shock, but when these shocks were neither predictable nor controllable, the animals would do nothing to avoid the shock, even though escape was possible. These animals were said to be in a state of learned helplessness, which is considered to be a type of psychological depression. Gerontologists have found that this laboratory-induced depression resembles a condition with which many elderly are faced. Unable to predict or control the blows that life delivers, the relationship between cause and effect breaks down, and depression sets in (Arling, Parham, and Teitelman 1978; Neiderehe 1977).

Just how prevalent depression is among the elderly is not known. Using one criterion for incidence, some feel it is very common (Pfeiffer and Busse 1973); others using another set of criteria feel that the rate may be no higher than for other age groups (Zemore and Eames 1979). The gerontology literature, however, assumes frequent occurrence of depression. Even if the incidence of depression is no higher than for younger groups, the fact that the elderly have diminished resources with which to combat depression makes it a topic worth discussing. So also does the fact that depression is assumed to occur so widely among older people.

Symptoms of depression include apathy and flat affect, sleep disturbances, changes in eating habits, fatigue, decision-making difficulties, con-stipation, disinterest in sex, and psychosomatic complaints such as headaches and stomach problems. The difficulty in measuring depression in the elderly stems from the fact that many of the normal aspects of aging resemble depressive symptoms. As we age, our range of response diminishes; our sleep patterns change; food becomes less interesting; we experience more tiredness; our interest in sex, although by no means nonexistent, is less than in our younger years. Bowel habits change and mimic constipation. We become less sure of our decision-making abilities and may become less inclined to take risks. This problem is exacerbated by the fact that older people do not use the word *depression* to describe themselves. For them, depression is synonymous with mental illness. They insist that they are not mentally ill—they may feel low or blue, but not depressed.

How can we diagnose depression? Reactive, or situationally caused, depression (as opposed to chronic, or long-term, depression) will be discussed here. First, sudden change of behavior or life-style should be monitored. Second, when a majority of the symptoms of depression exist and seem much greater than what might be attributable to normal aging, suspicion of depression may be warranted. Finally, when life seems to be a constant and intense daily battle with non-organically caused aches and pains, depression may be the explanation.

When depression is diagnosed and treatment sought, the prognosis is usually good, particularly when a strong support system (family and friends) and the following exist: "first onset of symptoms prior to the age of seventy; recovery from previous depressions; introversion; multiple interests; severe symptomology; confusion or irrationality; and emotionality" (Gerner 1979, 121). To be effective, treatment may include chemotherapy, cognitive therapy, behavior modification, or a combination of these.

The use of antidepressants has proved successful with the elderly, but these drugs must be used very cautiously, as they have a much greater impact on the elderly. Doses of one-third to one-half those prescribed for younger people are usually mandatory to avoid toxicity (often signaled by a ringing in the ears). Although chemotherapy is not always the treatment of choice, it may be used when psychotherapy is neither available nor desirable or it can be used in conjunction with psychotherapy.

Depressed people commonly engage in negative talk about themselves, including negative evaluations of themselves, their environments, and their futures; examples are "I am not as good as I once was," "Nothing will ever be as good as it used to be," and "Things are going to continue to get worse." Cognitive therapy (Beck 1976) counters this talk with a more accurate assessment of the person in his or her situation. A second treatment for depression, then, is cognitive therapy.

Depressed people fail to engage in events that are pleasant and rewarding (Lewinsohn and MacPhillamy 1974). Behavior therapy works at getting the depressed person to engage in rewarding activities. By engaging in pleasant events, depression subsides. Research suggests that using behavior therapy and cognitive therapy concurrently is the treatment of choice for many older depressed people (Zarit 1980).

A second major mental health problem common in older populations is paranoia, typified by suspiciousness, hypervigilance, and oversensitivity. It is often seen in nursing home residents and individuals in the beginning phases of organic brain syndromes. Paranoia may result from one or a combination of three factors or from none of these factors. The first is sensory deprivation (Cooper, Garside, and Kay, 1974). When auditory loss prevents an older woman, for example, from hearing a conversation between two people standing nearby, she may assume they are whispering and are talking about her. She then becomes certain that a scheme is being developed against her. Second, paranoia may result when decision-making powers are usurped from the elderly person—for example, when an older man is moved without warning, or when his house is sold without his consent. Finally, memory loss will heighten this problem dramatically. When the nursing home resident forgets that she sent her favorite dress to the dry cleaners, upon being unable to find it she will assume that it was stolen and accuse the next person with whom she comes in contact.

Paranoid behavior can take many forms. As the elderly become concerned about being victimized, many complaints may surface. Worry about being overcharged for vision care or being given the wrong prescription is a form of paranoia. The best way to cope with this is to prevent it in the first place by giving as much initial information as possible—even more than might seem necessary without talking down to the older person. Any method to increase the reception of information will help counteract paranoia. This may be facilitated either by correcting as much as possible for sensory decline so the person can receive environmental cues, by increasing the amount of information available, or both. The more accurately a person reads his or her environment, the less paranoia will result. It should be remembered, however, that when paranoia and more advanced stages of organic brain syndromes exist, nothing may be helpful. (Although the disorder may not be reversible, management is possible and may provide some symptom relief.)

The average age of onset for most serious forms of mental illness is usually no later than early middle age (Hendricks and Hendricks 1981). Older people who are schizophrenic, for example, have been so most of their adult lives. Paraphrenia, or what is thought to be a late-onset schizophrenia (Kay 1972), is usually not an emotional illness but some form of organic brain syndrome or aphasia (Fish 1960). Nonpsychotic forms of psychopathology in the aged are not uncommon. Estimates of their incidence range from 10 to 15 percent to as high as 60 percent, depending on the source (Blazer 1980; Hendricks and Hendricks 1981). By far the largest contributor to emotional and behavioral problems in the elderly is organic brain syndromes.

Organic Brain Syndromes

Although not exclusively a problem of the elderly, the organic brain syndromes are primarily associated with advancing age. Numerous disorders fall under this category, but this chapter will cover only three, focusing on those that are most disruptive to the individual.

Acute organic brain syndrome is commonly called *delirium*. This short-term problem with a rapid onset is basically the result of toxicity. Toxicity may result from failure of the body systems to provide nutrition and oxygen to the brain while filtering out toxins or from external sources such as drugs, alcohol, or natural gas leaks. Delirium produces a great fluctuation in symptoms. Diagnostic criteria include reduced awareness of the environment and an inability to sustain attention. There are perceptual disturbances, such as misinterpretations, illusions, and hallucinations. At times the person's speech is incoherent, the sleep-wake cycle becomes disturbed, and the person often becomes hyperactive. Often there is memory impairment and disorientation. (American Psychiatric Association 1980). Just how prevalent this reversible organic brain syndrome is would be impossible to ascertain, as there are hundreds of possible causes for delirium. Any time a sudden dramatic loss of cognition and attention is seen, immediate medical referral should be obtained to help prevent the acute dementia from becoming chronic.

Chronic organic mental disorders are not reversible. The two primary types are multi-infarct dementia and Alzheimer's disease. *Multi-infarct* comes from a Latin work meaning "many small holes." Multi-infarct dementia results from small strokes in the brain that cause impaired functioning. Its onset is comparatively sudden, and the loss is stepwise. A stroke or series of strokes starts the initial loss. The person then stabilizes at a certain level of functioning until the next cardiovascular event. At this time, further cognitive and behavioral loss occurs.

This disorder, which constitutes 10 percent of all dementia cases, results in part from high blood pressure. Thus, treatment for hypertension can go a long way toward preventing further loss. Although the damage from multi-infarct is not reversible, it is possible to arrest the development of further decline. This is not true, however, of chronic organic brain syndromes of the Alzheimer's type.

The term *senility* usually refers to Alzheimer's disease, or primary degenerative dementia. The onset of Alzheimer's disease, unlike multi-infarct dementia, is slow and insidious. The first symptom commonly is memory loss, and the loss is progressive. Impairment in abstract thinking and judgment, confusion, and unpredictable behavioral patterns are all common symptoms. The person in the final stages of this disorder is in a completely vegetative state.

Eisdorfer (1981, cited in Rathbone-McCuan and Hashimi 1982, 280) has listed five phases that the person with Alzheimer's disease and the family go through:

Phase one consists of questioning and suspicion that something is going wrong with the family member. Something is different and something is wrong, but no one seems to know exactly what is happening.

Phase two involves the search for medical information. Often a crisis event can trigger entry into phase two. The victim may go out for a walk and be unable to find his or her way home. A series of small car accidents may ensue that are untypical for this person. Or the ability to cook new recipes may suddenly diminish from the repertoire of the older woman.

Phase three includes the period of extended care giving. The individual is usually living within the community but is faced with increasing dependency on the people around him or her. Towards the end of this phase other alternatives will be considered.

Phase four includes the period of transition from living at home to institutional placement. This is a very difficult period for the family and for the victim if any awareness of this transfer is there.

By phase five the patient is shifted from marginal abilities to function into a complete vegetative state. Death will probably follow within a matter of months, although sometimes the victims can live for years in this state.

The cause of Alzheimer's disease is yet to be established. Theories abound, but most of them would best be filed in the mythology of the subject. A cure or even the ability to arrest the loss does not now exist. This dementia, which accounts for 60 percent of all dementias, leaves victims with no real recourse except physical care and daily maintenance.

The elderly are often stereotyped as senile, suffering from confusion and forgetfulness. However, the idea that aging is synonymous with senility could not be farther from the truth. In actuality, only a very small percentage of the older population is cognitively impaired. Even those in their 80s and 90s have a dementia rate of only 11 percent.

Some people feel the real sufferers of organic brain syndrome are the family members trying to care for their declining loved ones in their homes. For the families of persons with organic brain syndromes, life can become a very tedious, limiting experience. As people with these syndromes deteriorate, more and more functions decline. Memory declines first; then they become unable to function on a daily basis, such as to prepare meals and do housekeeping. Bowel and bladder control problems follow. Eventually, complete nonfunction may occur.

Through the progression of this decline, decision-making points arise for the family, causing much distress. The hardest decision concerns when and if to institutionalize. For some people a nursing home placement creates a great deal of guilt; they feel they should have continued to nurse the person at home (for example, if only they were stronger, did not have to go to work, or were less fatigued). Those who are forced to place a frail family member in a nursing home must be given all the support and validation possible. Research has demonstrated that older family members are rarely "dumped."

In the early phases of organic mental disorders, the greatest frustration to the family and victim results from the difficulty in diagnosis; the only sure way to make a diagnosis is through autopsy. Even the computerized axial tomography (CAT) scan, for all of its sophistication, cannot give enough information to make a certain assessment. To add to this, in 17 percent of all organic brain syndromes, Alzheimer's syndrome and multi-infarct dementia exist concurrently. Depression, even when strictly psychological, can in its extreme form mimic organic brain syndromes. This area is one of the great medical frontiers in which pioneering efforts are being made. Given the degree of tragedy that involved individuals experience, we can only hope that a major breakthrough occurs soon.

In summary, dementia involves trauma to the brain and central nervous system that results in a loss of function. The chronic disorders are the most serious form of dementia. Of these, multi-infarct dementia is the more treatable of the two most common forms. The most prevalent form (Alzheimer's disease) is the most serious and least treatable of the chronic forms of dementia.

The Aphasias

Because of their significant effects on communication options for use in the clinical setting, the aphasias also merit attention here. Aphasia, although not officially an organic brain syndrome, is the impairment or loss of speech that is due to brain damage, usually from a cardiovascular accident to the left side of the brain (language function for most people is located in the left hemisphere). When damage occurs, aphasia results; the type depends on the extent and location of the damage. Broca's aphasia, or anterior aphasia, is the most treatable. The person with Broca's aphasia is fully aware and cognitively functional but cannot find the words to speak. Called tip-of-the-tongue aphasia, the person stutters and searches for the word he or she wants.

Wernicke's aphasia, or posterior aphasia, is less reversible. Most victims recover very little

skill as compared with those with Broca's aphasia. This problem, functionally the reverse of Broca's aphasia, occurs when the person maintains a perfectly normal speech pattern (in terms of cadence) but makes absolutely no sense; words spoken are complete nonsense.

A second problem that can result from cardiovascular accident that could present a problem to the unaware optometrist results from the inability of the person to recognize or cope with the half of their body that is controlled by the impaired hemisphere. Denial of the existence of a hand, a foot, or half the face is common. Those with a stroke in the right hemisphere may refuse to eat food on the left side of their plate, shave the left side of their face, or dress the left side of their body. Giving an eye examination to someone who denies the existence of one of their eyes may be frustrating. Remember that this person is not trying to be contrary but rather has yet to reassimilate full body awareness. Visual assessment may have to wait until this happens if denial is total and unyielding.

Individual Differences in Aging

At birth we share more characteristics than we do at any other point in human development. From that moment on, we become more individualistic and increasingly unique. Aging means becoming more and more idiosyncratic; we become less like others and more like ourselves. Individual personality traits become accentuated. But what does this say about human change?

The great debate in human development concerns change versus nonchange in the lives of individuals. Do we make major changes in our interests, values, or interpersonal styles as we age? Or has the die been cast by our early 20s (Costa, McCrae, and Arenberg 1980; Woodruff and Birren 1972)? At this point most researchers feel that personality is stable over the adult and aging periods of our lives. However, we cannot underestimate the effects of crisis events, such as job loss, widowhood, or illness. Little research exists in this area, but it is likely that major personality changes in middle and later life are preceded by a major event or loss. Although these transitions account for adjustment in life-style, in the majority of cases the changes are limited to certain parameters. One analogy that may be helpful in understanding this is to think of a person's personality over a life span as being like a rock pile. The shape of the pile of rocks can take on numerous variations, but the building blocks of the pile—the rocks themselves—stay the same. This autonomy may be critical for good adjustment to old age.

Adjustment to old age is also determined by people's attitudes toward their life and toward the aging process. Individuals with a positive attitude toward aging and their own lives will make the best adjustment. A study of Bourque and Back (1970) has shown that such individuals rate their own lives as being significantly better than the lives of their peers. This finding has been repeatedly obtained among people in their later years. We might suspect, therefore, that older people are generally optimistic and that this orientation affects overall life satisfaction. As resources diminish, however, and as physical abilities decline, it is not uncommon for older people to become unsure of themselves and their ability to operate. Professionals trying to serve older people and meet their health care needs must remember that certain adjustments in examination techniques and procedures are helpful in working with such individuals.

Implications for
Optometric Practitioners

What does this mean for the optometrist dealing with an 87- or 73-year-old patient? First, maintaining competence in visual functioning is important for all age groups, but perhaps especially for the elderly. Since sensory decline for older people occurs in all five senses, the loss of one sense will not be offset by growing acuity in another. Thus, every possible step should be taken to promote optimum visual function.

Once an intervention has been devised, it must be used properly. This may require more effort than with the young. If there is any doubt at all that the person will be able to accurately utilize the intervention, writing down all instructions for future reference is appropriate. A follow-up telephone call after a few weeks is also helpful. When vision care is being provided, all instructions should be shared with the care provider so that this person can also monitor visual treatment. When auditory decline also exists, it is wise to ask the older person in a noncondescending manner to repeat instructions just given.

It is important to remove all competing stimuli during the examination. For example, the optometrist who normally plays the radio while working or has an office off a very busy hallway should quiet the room for the time the older person is there.

In conclusion, the following will facilitate working with older adults:
1. Speak loudly, slowly, and at low pitches.
2. Take social needs into account; allow time for digression.
3. Reduce interference from others, telephone calls, background noise, and glare.
4. Minimize time pressures.
5. Cover major concepts, not scattered facts.
6. Whenever possible, help the patient relate new material to past learning.
7. Be willing to repeat instructions and explanations.
8. Communicate by involving as many sensory systems as possible.

The optometrist is in a unique role when it comes to providing the elderly with access to the elements that make life a rich and positive experience. To maintain optimal visual performance is to maintain patient independence and self-determination. Time, patience, and effective communication skills may mean the difference between a self-sufficient lifestyle or one of increasing depression and dependence on others. The rewards for the involved optometrist are many.

References

Adamowicz, J. K. "Visual Short-Term Memory and Aging." *Journal of Gerontology* 31 (1976): 39–46.

American Psychiatric Association. *Diagnostic and Statistical Manual of Mental Disorders.* Washington, D.C.: American Psychiatric Association, 1980.

Arling, G.; I. A. Parham; and J. Teitelman. "Learned Helplessness and Social Exchange: Covergence and Application of Theories." Paper presented at the 31st annual scientific meeting of the Gerontological Society, Dallas, November 1978.

Baltes, P. B., and K. W. Schaie. "Aging and I.Q.: The Myth of the Twilight Years." *Psychology Today* 7 (1974): 35–40.

Baltes, P. B., and K. W. Schaie. "On the Plasticity of Intelligence in Adulthood and Old Age: Where Horn and Donaldson Fail." *American Psychologist* 31 (1976): 720–725.

Beck, A. T. *Cognitive Therapy and the Emotional Disorders.* New York: International Universities Press, 1976.

Birren, J. E. "Principles of Research on Aging." *Handbook of Aging and the Individual: Psychological and Biological Aspects,* ed. J. E. Birren. Chicago: University of Chicago Press, 1959.

Blazer, D. "The Epidemiology of Mental Illness in Later Life." In *Handbook of Geriatric Psychiatry,* eds. E. W. Busse and D. G. Blazer. New York: Van Nostrand Reinhold, 1980, pp. 249–272.

Bondareff, W. The Neural Basis of Aging. In *Handbook of the Psychology of Aging*, eds. J. E. Birren and K. W. Shaie. New York: Van Nostrand Reinhold, 1977, pp. 157–176.

Botwinick, J. "Intellectual Abilities." In *Handbook of the Psychology of Aging*, eds. J.E. Birren and K. W. Shaie. New York: Van Nostrand Reinhold, 1977, pp. 580–605.

Bourque, L. B., and K. W. Back. "Life Graphs: Aging and Cohort Effects." *Journal of Gerontology* 25 (1970): 249–255.

Brody, H. "Organization of the Cerebral Cortex; 3. A Study of Aging in the Human Cerebral Cortex." *Journal of Comparative Neurology* 102 (1955): 511–556.

Brody, H. Aging of the Vertebrate Brain. In *Development and Aging in the Nervous system*, ed. M. Rockstein. New York: Academic Press, 1973, pp. 121–133.

Brody, H. Neuroanatomy and Neuropathology of Aging. In *Handbook of Geriatric Psychiatry*, eds. E. W. Busse and D. G. Blazer. New York: Van Nostrand Reinhold. 1980, pp. 28–45.

Cooper, A. F.; R. F. Garside; and D. W. K. Kay. "A Comparison of Deaf and Nondeaf Patients with Paranoid and Affective Psychoses." *British Journal of Psychiatry* 129 (1974): 532–538.

Cooper, J. R.; F. E. Bloom; and R. H. Roth. *The Biochemical Basis of Neuropharmacology.* 4th ed. New York: Oxford University Press, 1982.

Corso, J. F. "Auditory Perception and Communication." In *Handbook of the Psychology of Aging*, eds. J. E. Birren and K. W. Schiae. New York: Van Nostrand Reinhold, 1977, pp. 535–553.

Costa, P. T.; R. R. McCrae; and D. Arenberg. "Enduring Dispositions in Adult Males." *Journal of Personality and Social Psychology* 38 (1980): 793–800.

Craik, F. I. "Age Differences in Human Memory." In *Handbook of the Psychology of Aging*, eds. J. E. Birren and K. W. Schiae. New York: Van Nostrand Reinhold. 1977, pp. 384–420.

Cumming, E., and W. Henry. *Growing Old: The Process of Disengagement.* New York: Basic, 1961.

Diamond, M. C., "The Aging Brain: Some Enlightening and Optomistic Results." *Scientific American* 65 (1978): 66–71.

Ebersole, P., and P. Hess. *Toward Healthy Aging.* St. Louis: Mosby, 1981.

Eisdorfer, C. "Paranoia and Schizophrenic Disorders in Later Life." In *Handbook of Geriatric Psychiatry*, eds. E. W. Busse and D. G. Blazer. New York: Van Nostrand Reinhold, 1980, pp. 324–337.

Engen, T. Taste and Smell. In *Handbook of the Psychology of Aging*, eds. J. E. Birren and K. W. Schiae. New York: Van Nostrand Reinhold, 1977, pp. 554–562.

Feinberg, I., and V. R. Carlson. "Sleep Variations as a Function of Age in Man." *Archives of General Psychiatry* 18 (1968): 239–250.

Fish, F. "Senile Schizophrenia." *Journal of Mental Science* 106 (1960): 938–946.

Frolkis, V. V. Aging of the Autonomic Nervous system. In *Handbook of the Psychology of Aging*, eds. J. E. Birren and K. W. Schaie. New York: Van Nostrand Reinhold, 1977, pp. 177–189.

Gerner, R. H. Depression in the Elderly. *Psychopathology of Aging*, eds. O. J. Kaplan. New York: Academic Press, 1979.

Gurland, B.J. "The Comparative Frequency of Depression in Various Adult Age Groups." *Journal of Gerontology* 31, no. 3 (1976): 283–292.

Havighurst, R. J.; B. L. Neugarten; and S. S. Tobin. "Disengagement and Patterns of Aging." In *Middle Age and Aging*, ed. B. L. Neugarten. Chicago: University of Chicago Press, 1968.

Hendricks, J., and C. D. Hendricks. *Aging in Mass Society.* Cambridge, Mass.: Winthrop, 1981.

Heron, W. "The Pathology of Boredom." *Scientific American.* 196 (1957): 52–56.

Horn, J. L., and G. Donaldson. "On the Myth of Intellectual Decline in Adulthood." *American Psychologist* 31 (1976): 701–719.

Kay, D. W. K. "Epidemiological Aspects of Organic Brain Disease in the Aged." In *Aging and the Brain*, ed. C. M. Gaitz. New York: Plenum, 1972.

Kenshalo, D. R. Age Changes in Touch, Vibration, Temperature, Kinesthesis, and Pain Sensitivity. In *Handbook of the Psychology of Aging*, eds. J. E. Birren and K. W. Schaie. New York: Van Nostrand Reinhold, 1977, pp. 562–579.

Lewinsohn, P. M., and D. MacPhillamy. "The Relationship between Age and Engagement in Pleasant Activities." *Journal of Gerontology* 29 (1974): 290–294.

Niederehe, G. "Interaction of Stressful Events with Locus of Control in Depression of Later Life." Paper presented at the 30th annual scientific meeting of the Gerontological Society, San Francisco, November 20, 1977.

Pfeiffer, E., and E. W. Busse. *Mental Illness in Later Life.* Washington, D.C.: American Psychiatric Association, 1973.

Prinz, P. N.; G. R. Marsh; and L. W. Thompson. "Normal Human Aging: Relationship of Sleep Variables to Longitudinal Changes in Intellectual Function." *Gerontologist* 14 (1974): 41.

Rathbone-McCuan, E., and J. Hashimi. *Isolated Elders.* Rockville, Md.: Aspen systems Corporation, 1982.

Samorajski, T., and J. Hartford. Brain Physiology of Aging. In *Handbook of Geriatric Psychiatry*, eds. E. W. Busse and D. G. Blazer. New York: Van Nostrand Reinhold, 1980, pp. 46–82.

Schaie, K. W. "Biopsychological Aging." In *Psychology and the Older Adult: Challenges for Training in 1980's*, eds. J. F. Santos and G. R. Yandenbos. Washington D.C.: American Psychological Association, 1982.

Schaie, K. W., and J. Geiwitz. *Readings in Adult Development and Aging.* Boston: Little, Brown, 1982.

Schiffman, S. Changes in Taste and Smell with Age: Psychophysical Aspects. In *Sensory systems and Communication in the Elderly*, eds. J. M. Ordy and K. R. Brizzee. New York: Raven Press, 1979.

Schiffman, S.; M. Orlandi; and R. P. Erickson. Changes in Taste and Smell with Age: Biological Aspects. In *Sensory systems and Communication in the Elderly*, eds. J. M. Ordy and K. R. Brizzee. New York: Raven, 1979.

Seligman, M. E. P. *Helplessness.* San Francisco: Freeman, 1975.

Strehler, B. L. *Time, Cells, and Aging.* 2d ed. New York: Academic Press, 1977.

Tomlinson, B. E., and G. Henderson. "Some Qualitative Cerebral Findings in Normal and Demented Old People." In *Neurobiology of Aging*, eds. R. D. Terry and S. Gershon. New York: Raven, 1976.

Watson, W. E. "Inadvertent Processing of Irrelevant Information: Age Equivalence and Differences." Paper presented at the meeting of the Gerontological Society, Dallas, November 1978.

Willis, S. L.; R. Blieszner; and P. B. Baltes. "Intellectual Training in Aging: Modification of Performance on the Fluid Ability of Figural Relations." *Journal of Educational Psychology.* 73 (1981): 41–50.

Woodruff, D. S., and J. E. Birren. "Age Changes and Cohort Differences in Personality." *Developmental Psychology* 6 (1972): 252–259.

Zarit, S. *Aging and Mental Disorders.* New York: Free Press, 1980.

Zemore, R., and N. Eames. "Psychic and Somatic symptoms of Depression among Young Adults, Institutionalized Aged and Non-institutionalized Aged." *Journal of Gerontology* 34 (1979): 716–722.

Chapter 6

Socioeconomic Aspects of Aging

Jeanne E. Bader

The most significant factors that affect older people's attention to their health—in addition to the actual presence of disease or trauma—are economic, environmental, and sociopolitical in nature. The socioeconomic climate is one of increasing fiscal restraint and, possibly, increasing sociopolitical constraint. To better understand and predict older people's attention to their health, the impact of changes in the socioeconomic climate must be examined in conjunction with the examination of cohort differences. In the sense to be used throughout this chapter, a *cohort* refers to a generation of people born within a specified period of time and together experiencing certain life events. The significance of the concept of cohort will emerge in the following discussions.

Importance of the Socioeconomic Aspects of Aging

Professionals, like the lay public, are children of aging parents and grandparents. About 40 percent of U.S. families consist of four or five living generations. An adult child frequently has good reason to care about policies and issues affecting older relatives.

As citizens of a nation that requires most taxpayers to contribute to the support of diverse, economically dependent groups (including the elderly), we have a financial stake in the well-being of members of those groups. The graying of society (one in nine people was 65 or older in 1980) and the graying of the federal budget (about one dollar in every four is spent for some aging-related purpose) increase our interest in

the well-being of the elderly.

A professional needs to practice from a strong knowledge base that includes skills that enhance communication, promotes enlightened policies and procedures, and intelligently guides decision making. For example, because so many more people in the United States are living long and are likely to experience changes in vision, the eye and vision care needs of older people should be expected and understood by eye and vision care specialists.

Finally, most eye and vision care practitioners themselves will live to be "old," no matter what definition of the word is used. As members of a generation who can expect to live longer than our parents, we have a vested interest in understanding and planning for the future for ourselves and others.

The socioeconomic aspects of aging are among the most interesting and important. However, attention to aging itself—let alone its implications for younger people—emerged only recently.

Historical Context

The study of history reveals that aging became recognized as a "national" (Achenbaum 1978) "social" (Fischer 1977) "problem" in the United States beginning early in the 20th century. Such recognition

> simultaneously appeared in the appointment of the first public commission on aging (Massachusetts, 1909), and the first major survey of the economic condition of the aged (Massachusetts again, 1910); in the first federal old age pension bill (1909), and the first state old age

Appreciation is expressed to Celeste Ulrich and Roderic Gillian for their comments on earlier drafts of this chapter. Dedication: H. J. B. and C. L. E.

pension system (Arizona, 1915); in the invention of a new science named geriatrics (1909), and the first published textbook in that field (1914). (Fischer 1977, 157)

The next major event was the passage in 1935 of the Social Security Act (to be discussed later). The Gerontological Society was organized in 1945 with 80 members (now 5,500); the first international congress on aging was held in 1950; the first White House Conference on Aging, in 1961. The first department of geriatric medicine was established in New York in 1983. The call for increased attention on the part of eye and vision care specialists to older patients' needs and eye care habits has just been sounded (Verma 1982).

It should not be assumed that old age was less problematic before the 20th century. The myth of the "good old days" is exactly that—a myth (Hendricks and Hendricks 1978). Few people lived to be old, and their lives were not very comfortable in the 19th and early 20th centuries. For instance, the use of corrective lenses now worn by the great majority of older people (92.1 percent, according to the National Center for Health Statistics 1973, 31) was exceptional at the time of the Civil War (Achenbaum and Kusnerz 1978).

Federal Programs and Policies

Although older individuals tend to focus their attention on immediate family problems, and even as aging-related state-level policies are gradually emerging (National Council of Senior Citizens 1971), it is readily apparent that the federal government has become the chief broker of retirement policies and programs. Since 1935 (that is, since the passage of the Social Security Act), older people have been regarded as legitimate objects of federal concern and legislation. At least 135 federal programs directly or indirectly affect older U.S. citizens (U.S. Congress 1980). Recently, all have undergone severe cuts and rearrangements (Leadership Council of Aging Organizations 1982a).

Federal Legislation and Expenditures

Most federal legislation assumes that older people are dependent and in a state of socioeconomic decline.

Social Security. The largest of the programs designed to respond to this dependency is a direct cash transfer program: Old Age and Survivors Insurance (OASI). Popularly called *Social Security*, OASI benefits or its companion fund Railroad Retirement benefits were paid in 1980 to nearly nine of every ten U.S. families with a head of household who was 65 or older. Social Security is unquestionably the major source of income for the great majority of older people and is in many cases their sole source of income. Initially "weak," "regressive," and "ineffectual" (Fischer 1977), OASI has expanded to include more categories of beneficiaries than were originally intended to benefit from it. A pay-as-you-go program (versus an insurance program), Social Security is payed out to current beneficiaries rather than set aside for taxpayers' own future retirements. "Only" three-fourths of adult U.S. citizens understand the pay-as-you-go nature of Social Security. Half (51 percent) think "Social Security taxes should be raised if necessary to provide adequate income for older people" (National Council on the Aging 1981, 121). Most (59 percent) oppose the notion of raising "the retirement age for full Social Security benefits from 65 to 68 years of age" (National Council on the Aging 1981, 122). Most (76 percent) favor requiring workers who do not now pay Social Security taxes (for example, federal employees) to pay these taxes (National Council on the Aging 1981).

Medicare. Like Social Security, Medicare (Title XVIII of the Social Security Act, enacted in 1965) is an age-entitlement federally administered program. Like Social Security, it has expanded to include additional beneficiaries (the disabled and those suffering from chronic kidney disease). Medicare provides partial reimbursement for hospital and posthospital care, as well as for certain other acute medical care expenditures. Because of the Part A deductible, Part B copayment, and time-limited features of Medicare, recipients must frequently bear extensive out-of-pocket expenses. Explanation of these features of Title XVIII are available from the Social Security Administration. An excellent overview of 1980 health care expenditures appears as Chapter 13 in *Developments in Aging: 1981* (U.S. Congress 1982).

In 1977, Medicare covered 41 percent of the personal health expenses of individuals 65 or over. All federal programs combined financed "only" 67 percent of older people's personal health care expenses (for example, hospital and institutional costs; dental, pharmaceutical, and appliance costs; and physician charges). In the same year, older people's health care costs were nearly three times those of younger people in the United States. Older people's incomes are generally less adequate than their younger relatives'.

Supplemental Security Income. In 1972 Congress passed an amendment to the Social Security Act introducing the Supplemental Security Income (SSI) program. Aged, blind, and disabled citizens become eligible for SSI if their incomes are low. In 1977 about 23,000 "blind" people in the United States who were 65 or over received SSI payments. About 8 percent of households with a head also 65 or older (officially termed *elderly households*) received SSI in 1980.

Medicaid. Like SSI, only the medically indigent are eligible for Medicaid, which is a state-administered program (Title XIX of the Social Security Act, enacted in 1965). Forty percent of Medicaid recipients (the medically indigent of all ages) are 65 or over. States share the costs of Medicaid with the federal government. Arizona is the only state lacking a Medicaid program. California calls its program Medical, and variations exist in other states.

Whereas about 16 percent of older households are covered by Medicaid, by far the greatest percentage of Medicaid expenditures goes to institutional care of older people. Some states (for example, Arkansas, Georgia, New York, and Oregon) are experimenting with noninstitutional uses of Medicaid in the hopes of reducing the number of institutionalized people and lowering overall costs to taxpayers. (U.S. Congress, 1982).

The administration of OASI, Medicare, SSI, and Medicaid is the responsibility of the Social Security Administration. Skyrocketing medical costs and charges of fraud and abuse in these federal and state aid programs (particularly Medicaid) persist. (Hickey 1980).

Designed Housing and Rent Supplements. Like medical assistance and insurance programs, designed housing has been a boon for many lower middle income elderly people. Exemplified by the Section 202 direct loan program and by the Section 236 Federal Housing Administration (FHA) interest subsidy program, federal housing policy for elderly and disabled U.S. citizens has been an on-again, off-again

proposition. Including low-rent public housing, the number of housing units available to older people is far from sufficient to keep up with the demand. Among the best features of federal and state housing programs is that such housing often is designed and managed according to guidelines developed on the basis of extensive research that has studied older tenants and homeowners (Green et al. 1975; Lawton 1975). About 900,000 elderly households (5 percent) lived in subsidized housing in 1979.

Rent supplements also have proved to be very popular among elderly individuals. Rent subsidies are paid directly to landlords in the amount necessary to make up the difference between 30 percent of tenants' incomes and fair market rents. Low-income families of all ages are eligible for Section 8 rent subsidies. The U.S. Department of Housing and Urban Development has chief responsibility for all the housing initiatives discussed.

Food Stamps. The food stamp program is also needs-based. People are eligible for food stamps if their incomes are low (depending on family size) and if they live in communities that participate in the program. Research suggests that many fewer elderly persons receive food stamps than are eligible to receive them. About one million elderly households (6 percent) received food stamps in 1979. The elderly receive 6 percent of total food stamp dollars. The U.S. Department of Agriculture oversees the food stamp program.

Other Federal Programs Benefiting Older People. Certain federal tax provisions benefit the elderly (Allo 1979). The U.S. Senate Special Committee on Aging publishes an annual review of these provisions. Also of benefit to older people are many of the policies, programs, and practices that emerge in the form of recommendations from federally sponsored research. Research on environmental design (Green et al. 1975), on dementia (for example, Mortimer and Schuman 1981), and on healthy aging (Granick and Patterson 1971) has been of immediate benefit to older people. Similarly, the improvements in and extensions of services for older people must be attributed in large part to the efforts of people trained in institutions of higher education. Such efforts frequently gain support from federal agencies (Administration on Aging; National Institute of Child Health and Human Development; National Institute of Mental Health; and, most recently, National Institute on Aging; Schechter 1980), private philanthropic organizations, and individuals (Cohen and Oppedisano-Reich 1977).

Other Relevant Federal Legislation

The Older Americans Act was passed in 1965 and significantly amended in 1973 and 1978. Its intent was to establish a structure and process to enable older people's needs to be serviced. Initially, this meant creating an Administration on Aging (AoA) within the U.S. Department of Health, Education, and Welfare (now the Department of Health and Human Services). In the years that followed the 1973 amendments, a substantial Aging Network of about 55 State Units on Aging (SUAs) and 680 Area Agencies on Aging (AAAs) evolved to coordinate services and advocate when new ones were needed or when existing ones needed improvement. Services in virtually every part of the nation are coordinated by AAAs. Nutrition programs, access programs (for example, information and referral, or I & R, and transportation), legal assistance, and in-home programs have received special support from the act since 1978. Such support has been due, in large part, to lobbying by organizations that expanded in number and power during the 1970s.

The Age Discrimination in Employment Act (ADEA) was enacted in 1967 and amended in 1978 to raise the minimum age at which most people can be retired without further justification from 65 to 70. The ADEA protects most workers 40 to 69 years of age from being forced to retire on the basis of chronological age alone, and it removes the age cap of 70 for federal employees. Other exempted employment categories include highly paid executives and people whose work insures the safety of others. Initially exempted, tenured faculty are no longer exempted under the law (Hansen and Holden 1981). Originally, enforcement was the responsibility of the Department of Labor, but in 1979 a shift of regulatory responsibility was made to the Equal Employment Opportunity Commission (EEOC).

Only 42 percent of U.S. citizens who are 18 or over have heard of the ADEA, including only 47 percent of those protected by the act—the 40- to 69-year-old population. Even more interesting is the fact that only 54 percent of those with responsibility for hiring and firing are familiar with the existence of the ADEA, let alone its

ramifications. Similarly, even among those who have heard of the law, 32 percent have limited or no understanding of its implications (National Council on the Aging 1981).

Representative Claude Pepper of Florida has introduced H.B. 3827 to pay for out-of-hospital prescription drugs, dental care and dentures, eye examinations and eyeglasses, hearing examinations and aids, and biannual physician examinations. If passed, these benefits will be administered by the Social Security Administration as Medicare, Part C.

Expansion of Federal Aging-related Policies

Several explanations for the growth of aging-specific federal legislation and expenditures have been offered (Estes 1979; Gold, Kutza, and Marmor 1976). These include the view that the elderly are economically disadvantaged and require assistance from more advantaged (that is, younger employed) people. Another view holds that the elderly are seen as a political force with which to be reckoned because of the group's increasing membership and regular voting pattern. A third explanation recognizes the effects of societal guilt regarding the treatment of the aged. A fourth explanation suggests societal acceptance of responsibility for the care of the underaged and the retired. A fifth explanation suggests that the elderly deserve to be rewarded with a dignified old age by virtue of their life-long contributions to society. Still another explanation is that it is in the self-interest of those employed in the service of older people in the United States to favor age-specific legislation and expenditures.

Demographic Data

Clearly, the nature and magnitude of the economic, sociopolitical, and environmental resources that older individuals have at their disposal will limit their real and perceived options regarding health-related decisions. Therefore, it is necessary to examine the resources available to older people before attempting to predict their health-related behavior. Most of the information for this section appeared first in the U.S. Congress (1982), Allan and Brotman (1981), and U.S. Congress (1980).

Income

The median income of households with heads who are 65 or older in 1980 was $7,878. About 92 percent of the income received by that population came from Social Security (43 percent), retirement pensions (18 percent), earnings from working (16 percent), and interest on savings (15 percent) (U.S. Congress 1982). One in three individuals 65 or older who are black or Hispanic and one in eleven older whites have no savings reserves.

About 16 percent of the over-65 population had 1980 incomes below the officially defined poverty level, including 38.1 percent of older blacks and 30.8 percent of older Hispanics. An additional 10 percent of the population 65 and older had incomes below the "near-poor" level (defined as 125 percent of poverty). Almost three times as many older women (2,773,000) as older men (1,080,000) were poor in 1981. In 1981, older women had a median income (half above, half below) within $400 of the poverty level, whereas older men had a median income $3,800 above the official poverty line.

Not only their lower work force participation, but also the following contribute to women's lower incomes in later life:

1. Lower earnings ($0.59 for every $1.00 men earn, on the average).
2. Late entry and interrupted participation in the labor force.
3. "Nest egg" depleted by prolonged family illnesses, especially of spouse, parents, and in-laws.
4. Personal resources exhausted by expenses incurred after widowhood (average age of widowhood is 56) and before becoming eligible for Social Security, pension benefits, or both.
5. Differential benefits for women versus men under Social Security and pension programs (this gender-based difference is receiving congressional attention at this time).

For at least two reasons, the economics of aging are likely to worsen, not improve. One reason for the anticipated decline in older people's incomes is that the older female population is already considerably larger—and growing faster—than the older male population. Women make up 57 percent of the population 65 to 74 years old. The population 75 to 84 years old is 63 percent female; the population 85 years old and older is 70 percent female. Because women live longer, are poorer, and live alone much more frequently than older men (80 percent of older people who live alone are women), the economics of aging probably will worsen, not improve. Another reason for the anticipated decline of older

people's incomes has to do with changes in the national birth rate. The declining birth rate forebodes a smaller work force and, hence, fewer taxpayers to share in supporting essential services for a rapidly expanding, increasingly older population.

After Social Security, the next most frequent source of income (without reference to amount) for those 65 years of age or over is income from assets, then earnings, private pensions, government pensions, public assistance, and veterans' benefits (Allan and Brotman 1981). Of the 16.9 million households headed by a person 65 or older, 98 percent receive one or more of the following noncash benefits in 1980 (U.S. Congress): Medicare, food stamps, public housing, and Medicaid. After Medicare, Medicaid was the largest benefit program, serving 2.5 million elderly households.

Various experiments with health insurance are currently under consideration. For example, the Metropolitan Jewish Geriatric Center of Brooklyn has received a foundation grant to design Elderplan, a prepaid health plan that will offer comprehensive health and social services to the well and impaired elderly—ranging from routine eye examinations and dentures to housekeeping services and nursing home care.

Fifty-four percent of U.S. citizens look toward government and 46 percent look toward the children of the aged to assume greater responsibility for the elderly than they now do. Of the national population, 23 percent favors greater self-help on the part of the aged themselves; 19 percent, help on the part of employers; and 14 percent, help on the part of religious and charitable organizations (National Council on the Aging 1981). Most people in the United States favor tax incentives for families who assume responsibility for the aged. It should be noted that family units are already providing 80 percent of the home care of older family members (U.S. Congress 1980).

Employment and Retirement

About one in five males who are 65 or older and one in 12 older females continue to work in the paid labor force (U.S. Congress 1982). Most older people are concentrated in jobs with low pay: part-time, agricultural, and self-employment situations (U.S. Congress 1980). Many older people want to work but cannot find acceptable jobs. This is particularly true for women. Twice as many women as men 55 to 64 years old are unemployed (that is, they are out of work and cannot find work).

A majority of fully retired U.S. citizens say they left the work force by choice (62 percent). However, 37 percent feel they were forced to retire (National Council on the Aging 1981).

Education

In 1980, 38 percent of individuals who were 65 or older had graduated from high school. This was more than double the percentage who graduated in 1950. Whereas the proportion of older people with fewer than five years' formal schooling (that is, the "functionally illiterate") is dropping (about 10 percent in 1980), the rate of college completion is climbing only gradually (about 8 percent in 1980). Older blacks and Hispanics are less than half as likely to have completed high school than whites and more than four times as likely to have completed five years of schooling or less.

In 1980, about 5 percent of older U.S. citizens enrolled in educational programs. Registrants tend to be more highly educated and to have engaged in continuing education throughout their lifetimes (National Council on the Aging 1981; Weinstock 1978).

Relatedness

As was noted at the beginning of the chapter, about 40 percent of U.S. families can boast of four or five living generations. Such generations are not necessarily physically proximate. Eight of every ten older men and six of every ten older women live in family settings. Of these, three in every four men live with a spouse, but only one-third of older women live with a husband. On the average, a woman can expect to live 11 years as a widow. More than one-third of older women live alone, which is three times the rate for men living alone or with nonrelatives.

One in 20 older people lives in an institution. Of these, 84 percent live in nursing homes. The balance live in psychiatric facilities and prisons. Institutionalized elderly tend to be disproportionately childless, female, very old, ill, and alone.

Health Status

Although people 65 or older make up only 11 percent of the total U.S. population, they account for 29 percent of total health costs, 30 percent of acute care beds (in hospitals), 95 percent of nursing home beds, and 20 percent of physicians'

office time. However, only 13 to 14 percent of the older population consider themselves in poor health; 30 percent say their health is "only fair." The majority report their health to be good or excellent (National Council on the Aging 1981). In this regard, Maddox and Douglass (1973) found that older people tend to overestimate their health status in comparison to physician estimates. In reviewing hundreds of studies of aging-related attitudes, Bader (1980) concluded that "unwaivering optimism" (Shanas 1968) and the belief that they are personally better off than their peers and than the "average older person" characterize most older people.

The primary complaint in later life is of chronic disability. Estimates vary: 38 to 44 percent report arthritis; 29 percent, hearing impairments; 20 to 22 percent, vision impairments; 20 to 35 percent, hypertension; and 20 percent, heart conditions. Of the 80 percent of the elderly population who report some chronic condition, fewer than 18 percent report a limitation of mobility due to such conditions: 5 percent stay home (1 percent in bed); 2 percent need the help of another person to get around; and 5 percent use a cane, walker, or wheelchair. About 25 percent of the elderly spend "a lot of time" walking, jogging, or engaged in other forms of exercise (National Council on the Aging 1981).

In general, older people in the United States cite the following as the greatest barriers to health care: the cost of physician visits (18 percent), generally high medical bills (19 percent), and transportation inadequacies (18 percent). It is worth noting that although one-third of the elderly live in the rural United States, fewer than one in five physicians chooses to locate a practice in rural regions.

Older people's extensive use of prescription drugs is striking. Of the total number of prescriptions issued in a single year, about 25 percent is intended for use by older people. Compounding the "problem" is the fact that many medications prescribed for older people are psychoactive (National Institute on Drug Abuse 1979). The amount of drugs alone – averaging about seven medications per elderly individual – suggests possibilities of interactions and side effects. Every health care practitioner should make special note of this fact. In addition, underutilization and overutilization of prescribed medications frequently are reported.

Vision Care

Seventy percent of older people report that they have a personal or family eye care specialist:

[yet two] out of 5 (40% of the senior citizens surveyed) did not visit an eye care specialist at all during the past year (12 months) and over 15% have not done so in the past three years.

Although over half of the elderly are concerned about the cost of eye care, less than one in five say they neglect these services for lack of money. However, among those senior citizens who did not go to an eye specialist the last time they felt the need for eye care, 48% did not go because of lack of money. Forty-five percent of the senior citizens surveyed with limited finances would visit their eye specialist more often if money were no problem. (Eger 1976, 166)

It appears that lack of finances alone does not account for older people's presumed underutilization of the services of eye and vision care practitioners—but personal finances are nonetheless most important in predicting eye care habits.

Among other socioeconomic barriers to proper eye and vision care are the following:

1. Insufficient patient education regarding the benefits of proper eye and vision care.
2. Negative attitudes toward practitioners, toward themselves, and toward the chances of their being helped.
3. Transportation inadequacies (the scheduling and design of vehicles).
4. Competing needs.
5. Inaccessible facilities (for example, too far away, too many steps, or poorly lit parking lots and elevators).
6. Professionals' own behavior (for example, negative attitudes or insufficient training in communicating with older people).

With regard to the barrier to effective eye and vision care that professionals themselves may "cause," practitioner/patient relations undoubtedly would be improved were cohort differences to be adequately appreciated by both practitioner and patient. As has been noted, these differences refer to the inevitable consequences on behavior and attitudes of people's being born in different years. Such differences reflect the unique characteristics, array, and salience of events that characterize a cohort's shared life experience. They are reflected in cohort-specific habits of dress, address, nonverbal communication, values, and goals. Intraspection alone is not a sufficient guide to behavior when dealing with someone decades older or younger.

It is surely obvious that the demographic data cited reflect recent and dramatic population shifts. Whereas a few years ago there were relatively few older citizens, U.S. rates of fertility and infant mortality have changed inversely to produce a graying society. With so many more long-lived people and proportionately fewer taxpayers in the United States, it would be wise to recognize that attitudes and stereotypes related to old age that were prevalent a few years ago are no longer valid (if indeed they ever were). For instance, whereas the following section would have been inaccurate a few years ago, it is accurate now:

Few Old People Are "Old"

The 65+ years of age cutoff used by the U.S. Census Bureau to define the older population may be useful descriptively and politically—but only up to a point. However, "sixty-five or older" is no longer sufficient either to describe the retired population or for policy-planning purposes. Instead, there is increasing agreement that chronological age is not sufficient for most gerontological (that is, scholarly, political, and practice) purposes. And there is agreement that only the old-old resemble those formerly labeled as old.

At least three subpopulations within the 65+ population merit distinctive planning and programming: the young-old, the middle-old, and the old-old. Some federal agencies and organizations are already planning in these terms, for example, the U.S. House of Representatives Select Committee on Aging (U.S. Congress 1980). Eye and vision care practitioners would do well to start thinking in such terms, too.

The young-old (60 percent of the population 65 years old and older) are generally 65 to 74 years of age; new to retirement; and new, in many cases, to leisure. They are aware of their income limitations. Many are newly widowed or divorced women surprised by their sudden change in marital status and not prepared for it. Healthwise, the young-old are in good shape. Fitness, exercise, nutrition, and health maintenance programs may serve to prevent later illness. Many young-old have living parents.

The middle-old (31 percent of the 65 years old and older population) identify and use services available to them in the communities where they live—given the availability of transportation. For those retired from the work force, incomes typically have been halved since retirement. For the majority of people 75 to 84 years of age—women—incomes and benefits are extremely limited and unlikely to increase. Many middle-old people become the elders in their families during these years. Some begin to require extensive aid from families, friends, agencies, and organizations. A few shift their self-identifications from "middle-aged" to "elderly."

The *old-old* (9 percent of the population 65 years old and older) are variously called the *frail, chronically disabled,* and *old-old.* They are generally 85 years of age or older and make up the fastest-growing segment of the total U.S. population. They are disproportionately often institutionalized and are often physically and mentally impaired. Many are women who have outlived their children.

Implications of the Socioeconomic Status of Older People for Communication

Although it is true that many services, policies, and programs are designed to benefit older people, many are unknown to eligible users. Because the burden for identifying resources to meet people's own needs is generally on the people in need, program personnel must make their services known to potential clients and their representatives.

How might we best communicate with the young-old, middle-old, and old-old? Many young-old, might be reached in work, organizational, social, residential, and family settings. Middle-old people might be reached through community-based service agencies (Laurie et al., 1978 100–110), senior centers, their adult children, and congregate living settings. Some old-old live in nursing homes, homes for the aging, and foster homes. Such individuals are probably best contacted through their caretakers and services providers. However, most old-old continue to live in family settings. In general, the old-old are reachable through media that come to them where they live—the print and electronic media.

A majority of older people continue to read newspapers and watch news programs on television (Comstock 1978; Kubey 1977). Some agencies and organizations use these media to their advantage to communicate their messages to older people. For perishable (that is, quickly outdated) information, toll-free 800 numbers; services directories (Bader 1979); public service announcements on radio and television; and brochures, posters, and pamphlets also are used. Of these media for communicating with older

people all but two require literacy and relatively good vision.

When messages are conveyed in writing, not only information but also a permanent record are provided. In fact, the Social Security Administration (1972, 94) found that even those who could not read preferred to be notified by letter regarding changes in Social Security:

> Many respondents stated that benefit changes were a very personal thing and should always be conveyed by letter directly to them. As one respondent said, "I can sit down and read it, figure it out for myself." Because of hearing and sight problems, the recipients feel that they cannot "always believe" what they hear on television or radio, but a letter is a permanent record that can be referred to again and again. Also the problem of individuality comes into play. A broadcast announcement is a mass communications device, but a letter, addressed to the recipient *by name* makes him feel that he hasn't been forgotten as a person.

While it is true that printed materials may serve as relatively low cost memory aids, records, and symbols of privacy and personhood (Bader 1979; Ralph 1982) a sizable group of older people may be better served through other means. Among these may be individuals least able to obtain or use services, no matter how well advertised in the print medium. For these individuals, the electronic media and their family, friends, and advocates may be better informants and motivators.

Political biases aside, we must recognize that the resources that people can call on in their own behalf do decline with advanced age. Among older people's most treasured resources is the independence that adequate vision and socioeconomic stability provide. As has been shown, the one complements the other—and may, in large part, be necessary to the other.

Future Cohorts of Older People

A few years ago, people were "old" at younger chronological ages than they are now. Given the demographics of aging in the United States, the number of jobs necessary to staff services for the elderly in this country, and the cost of such services that taxpayers share, each of us has an investment in the future as well as the present situation of older people.

People born in 1980 will be 70 years old in 2050. Research clearly indicates the salience of cohort-specific events in predicting generation-specific behavior in later life (Cain 1970, 1982). Kastenbaum (1975) predicted the following about successive generations of older people:

• They will be better educated; native born; accustomed to a higher standard of living; less guilty about retirement and leisure time; more interested in continuing education, as well as creative, recreative, and civic activities; and aware of themselves as a social force.

• They will have enjoyed better health longer.

• They will have more adequate incomes.

• They will be more willing than their predecessors to accept programmed assistance.

• They will have thought more about aging and retirement.

• They will have been planned for as never before by professionals, scientists, and elected officials.

We might tentatively add the following to Kastenbaum's list of predictions about future generations of older people:

• They will have more experience living alone.

• They will be more assertive and will have had more experience with self-help movements.

• They may be more geographically mobile than their predecessors.

• They may continue longer in the labor force.

We can note with confidence that future older people will be even more likely to be female than is the case now, cared for at home with a mixture of family and professional services, and increasingly in the position of having to compete with others in need.

At least one of Kastenbaum's predictions may be debated. He suggests that older people increasingly will be regarded as a powerful social force. On the contrary, it appears that they may lose political power in the near future. Although it is true that legislators are increasingly aware of the graying of the population worldwide (Beattie 1977–1978) and of the commitment of the federal budget to programs for the elderly, elected officials are beginning to recognize that older people rarely vote as an age bloc, even though they vote disproportionately often (Maddox 1978). If the graying of the nation further polarizes citizens into age-based competitions (Gustaitis 1980), elected officials may choose to ignore "senior power" in favor of "age-irrelevant" politics (Hall 1980). The beginnings of such a trend were evident at the 1981 White House Conference on Aging (Leadership Council of Aging Organizations 1982b; White House Conference on Aging 1982b).

Personal Significance

Most of the readers of this chapter will live to be old. Many will find the experience of old age to be more positive than they anticipated. A few will be surprised by an unexpected diminution in physical, social, and economic resources. All are urged to become attentive to the socioeconomic and political realities that affect the lives of older people today and of future cohorts of older people. Such realities can be created and recreated by persistent and informed citizens.

Implications for Taxpayers, Professionals, Adult Children of Aging Parents, and Elected Officials

A series of questions flows from this chapter's discussion for consideration by eye and vision care practitioners in the course of their specialized work with older patients. The same questions might well be asked by government officials, personnel managers, taxpayers, and others. Among these questions are the following:

• Who is my "real" patient: the older individual, the taxpayer, older people as a group, my professional colleagues, or older people's family members?

• Who has the right to design policies and programs affecting older people: elected officials, older individuals, taxpayers, older people as a group, or older people's families (Fuchs 1974)?

• Can I support age-segregated programs and policies, in addition to age-integrated ones?

• Can I support senior power movements (for example, the National Council .of Senior Citizens) versus age-irrelevant coalitions (for example, Gray Panthers)?

• Can taxpayers afford to feel responsible for the well-being of older people? Can we afford not to (Jonsen 1976)?

• Should the public sector assume more or less responsibility for the well-being of older people (Cook 1979, 1982)?

• Should the private sector assume more responsibility for the well-being of older people (U.S. Department of State 1982; White House Conference on Aging 1982a)?

• Am I willing to invest more or less in care/cure/maintenance versus prevention/proaction/planning (U.S. Congress 1980)?

• Do I favor age-based or needs-based eligibility criteria for programs benefiting older people (Neugarten 1983)?

• How do I measure sufficiency of service, let alone quality (Winston 1976)?

• What if taxpayers were no longer willing to provide the diversity and coverage of programs for the elderly (Hudson 1978)? What is a tolerable fallback position?

• What should I assume when older people are pictured as competing for scarce resources with others in need and with younger people in general (Gustaitis 1980)? What questions should I ask when the retired population is portrayed as penniless, dejected and impotent? What questions should I ask when it is portrayed as taking advantage of the tax-paying public, as financially solvent, or as politically powerful?

• How will future generations of older people differ from today's older people (Neugarten and Havighurst 1976; Rosow 1975)?

• How much diversity exists within the current group of U.S. citizens 65 and older, and what are the implications of the current trend toward recognition of at least three subpopulations of older people in the United States (the young-old, the middle-old, and the old-old)?

Admittedly, these questions are phrased so broadly that they are thought provoking but not answerable. Respondents' value orientations (Diggs 1976; Jonsen 1976), attitudes (Bader 1980), and information will affect their responses. Respondents will want to identify who is asking each question before venturing a response. Individuals and groups representing competing viewpoints are likely to be soliciting support for their particular views. The nature of the issue, and its visibility, and the probable costs and benefits of responding (versus ignoring or soft-pedaling the issue) will affect respondent behavior.

We can consider these questions in a broad context or solely with respect to the programs, policies, and services regarding the health of older people. We can focus even more specifically on considerations appropriate to our specialties. In each instance, the exercise may prove worthwhile.

References

Achenbaum, W. Andrew. *Old Age in the New World.* Baltimore: Johns Hopkins, 1978.

Achenbaum, W. Andrew, and P. A. Kusnerz. *Images of Old Age in America: 1790 to the Present.* Ann Arbor, Mich.: University of Michigan–Wayne State University, 1978.

Allan, Carole, and Herman Brotman, eds. *Chartbook on Aging in America.* Washington, D.C.: The 1981 White House Conference on Aging, 1981.

Allo, C. D. "Tax Benefits: Income Tax and Property Tax." In *The Rights of Older Persons: An American Civil Liberties Union Handbook,* eds. R.N. Brown, C.D. Allo, A.D. Freeman, and G.W. Netzorg. New York: Avon, 1979.

Bader, Jeanne E. *"The Legibility of Print and the Indexing of Printed Reference Materials Intended for Use by Older Persons."* PhD diss., University of California, San Francisco, 1979.

Bader, Jeanne E. "Attitudes toward Aging, Old Age, and Old People." *Aged Care and Services Review* 2, no. 2 (1980): 1, 3–14.

Beattie, Walter. "Examination of the Impact of the Changing Age Structure on the Institutional and Organizational Arrangement of the Regions and Countries of the World." Paper presented at the Expert Group Meeting on Aging, United Nations Headquarters, New York, 1977–1978.

Cain, Leonard. *The 1916–1925 Cohort of Americans: Its Contribution to the Generation Gap.* Portland: Portland State University, 1970.

Cain, Leonard. "Intemperate Remarks from an Intrepid Observer of the Heretofore Inviolable Gerontology Movement." Paper presented at the annual meeting of the Association for Gerontology in Higher Education, Washington, D.C., 1982.

Cohen, Lilly, and Marie Oppedisano-Reich. *A National Guide to Government and Foundation Funding Sources in the Field of Aging.* Bethesda, Md.: Care Reports, 1977.

Comstock, G. "Television's Four Highly Attracted Audiences." *New York University Education Quarterly* 9, no. 2 (1978): 23–28.

Cook, Fay Lomax. *Who Should Be Helped? Public Support of Social Services.* Beverly Hills, Calif.: Sage, 1979.

Cook, Fay Lomax. "Public Support for Services." *National Forum* 62, no. 4 (1982): 23–25.

Diggs, B. J. "The Ethics of Providing for the Economic Well-being of the Aging." In *Social Policy, Social Ethics and the Aging Society,* eds. B. L. Neugarten and R. J. Havighurst. Washington, D.C.: U.S. Government Printing Office, 1976.

Eger, M. J. "Editorial: Vision Care and Our Senior Citizens." *Journal of the American Optometric Association* 47 (1976): 711–712.

Estes, Carroll L. *The Aging Enterprise.* San Francisco: Jossey-Bass, 1979.

Fischer, David Hackett. *Growing Old in America.* New York: Oxford University Press, 1977.

Fuchs, Victor R. *Who Shall Live? Health, Economics, and Social Choice.* New York: Basic, 1974.

Gold, B.; E. Kutza and T. R. Marmor, "United States Social Policy on Old Age: Present Patterns and Predictions." In *Social Policy, Social Ethics and the Aging Society,* eds. B.L. Neugarten and R.J. Havighurst. Washington, D.C.: U.S. Government Printing Office, 1976.

Granick, S. and R. Patterson, eds. *Human Aging, 2: An Eleven-Year Followup Biomedical and Behaviorial Study.* Washington, D.C.: National Institute of Mental Health, U.S. Department of Health, Education, and Welfare, 1971.

Green, I.; B. E. Fedewa; C A. Johnston; W. M. Jackson and H. L. Deardorff. *Housing for the Elderly: The Development and Design Process.* New York: Van Nostrand Reinhold, 1975.

Gustaitis, Rasa. "Old vs. Young in Florida." *Saturday Review* 7, no. 4 (1980): 11–14.

Hall, Elizabeth. "Acting One's Age: New Rules for Old." *Psychology*, April 1980, 68–80.

Hansen, W. L., and K. C. Holden. *Mandatory Retirement in Higher Education*. Madison: University of Wisconsin, 1981.

Hendricks, C. Davis, and Jon Hendricks. "The Age-Old Question of Old Age." *International Journal of Aging and Human Development* 8, no. 2 (1978): 139–154.

Hickey, Tom. *Health and Aging*. Monterey, Calif.: Brooks-Cole, 1980.

Hudson, Robert B. "The 'Graying' of the Federal Budget and Its Consequences for Old-Age Policy." *Gerontologist* 18 (1978): 428–440.

Jonsen, Albert R. "Principles for an Ethics of Health Services." In *Social Policy, Social Ethics and the Aging Society*, eds. B. L. Neugarten and R. J. Havighurst. Washington, D.C.: U. S. Government Printing Office, 1976.

Kastenbaum, Robert. "Personality Changes in the Older Person Living in the Community or the Institution." Paper presented at Institution on Library Service to the Aging, Wayne State University, 1975.

Kubey, R. W. "Television and the Elderly: A Critical Review." Paper presented at the meeting of the Gerontological Society, San Francisco, 1977.

Laurie, W. F.; T. Walsh; G. L. Maddox and D. Dillinger. "Population Assessment for Program Evaluation." In *Assessment and Evaluation Strategies in Aging: People, Populations and Programs*, ed. George L. Maddox. Durham, N.C.: Duke University Center for the Study of Aging and Human Development, 1978.

Lawton, M. Powell. *Planning and Managing Housing for the Elderly*. New York: Wiley-Interscience, 1975.

Leadership Council of Aging Organizations. *The Administration's 1983 Budget: A Critical View from an Aging Perspective*. Washington, D.C.: Leadership Council of Aging Organizations, 1982. (a)

Leadership Council of Aging Organizations. *Shaping America's Aging Agenda for the 80's*. Washington, D.C.: Leadership Council of Aging Organizations, 1982. (b)

Maddox, George L. "Will Senior Power Become a Reality?" In *Aging into the 21st Century*, ed. Lissy F. Jarvik. New York: Gardner Press, 1978.

Maddox, G. L. and E. B. Douglass. "Self-assessment of Health: A Longitudinal Study of Elderly Subjects." *Journal of Health and Social Behavior* 14 (1973): 87–93.

Mortimer, James A., and Leonard M. Schuman. *The Epidemiology of Dementia*. New York: Oxford University Press, 1981.

National Center for Health Statistics. U.S. Department of Health, Education, and Welfare. *Current Estimates: U.S. 1971*, ser. 10-79. U.S. Department of Health, Education and Welfare Publication no. (HSM) 73-1505, 1973.

National Council on the Aging. *Aging in the Eighties: America in Transition*. Washington, D.C.: National Council on the Aging, 1981.

National Council of Senior Citizens. *Legislative Approaches to the Problems of the Elderly: A Handbook of Model State Statutes*. Washington, D.C.: National Council of Senior Citizens, 1971.

National Institute on Drug Abuse. U.S. Department of Health, Education, Welfare. *Services Research Monograph Series: The Aging Process and Psychoactive Drug Use*. Washington, D.C., 1979.

Neugarten, Bernice, ed. *Public Policies for Older People: Age or Need Based?* Beverly Hills, Calif.: Sage, 1983.

Neugarten, B. L. and R. J. Havighurst. "Aging and the Future." In *Social Policy, Social Ethics and the Aging Society*, eds. B. L. Neugarten and R. J. Havighurst. Washington, D.C.: U. S. Government Printing Office, 1976.

Ralph, J. B. "A Geriatric Visual Concern: The Need for Publishing Guidelines." *Journal of the American Optometric Association* 53, no. 1 (1982): 43–50.

Rosow, Irving. "The Aged in Post-Affluent Society." *Gerontology* 1, no. 4 (1975): 9–22.

Schechter, Irma. *1980 Chartbook of Federal Programs in Aging*. Washington, D.C.: Library of Congress, 1980.

Shanas, E. "Note on Restriction of Life Space: Attitudes of Age Cohorts." *Journal of Health and Social Behavior* 9, no. 1 (1968): 86–90.

Social Security Administration. *The Title XX Recipient: A Communications Study for Title XX Planning*. Baltimore, Md.: Social Security Administration, 1972.

U.S. Congress. House Select Commitee on Aging. Subcommittee on Human Services. *Future Directions for Aging Policy: A Human Service Model*. 96th Cong., 2d sess., 1980.

U.S. Congress. Senate. Special Committee on Aging. *Developments in Aging: 1981*. 97th Cong., 2d sess., 1982.

U.S. Department of State. *U.S. National Report on Aging for the United Nations World Assembly on Aging*. Washington, D.C.: World Assembly on Aging. 1982.

Verma, Satya B. "Geriatric Optometry—Today and Tomorrow." *Journal of Opometric Education* 7, no.4 (1982): 9–11.

Weinstock, Ruth. *The Graying of the Campus*. New York: Educational Facilities Laboratories, 1978.

White House Conference on Aging. *Final Report: The 1981 White House Conference on Aging*. Vol. 3. Washington, D.C.: White House Conference on Aging, 1982. (a)

White House Conference on Aging. *Implementation: Legislative and Administrative Steps to Implement the National Policy on Aging: From the 1981 White House Conference on Aging*. Washington, D.C., 1982. (b)

Winston, E. "Implications for Service Providers." *Aging in America*. Washington, D.C.: National Council on the Aging, 1976.

Suggested Readings
Estes, Carroll L., and Robert J. Newcomer. *Fiscal Austerity and Aging: Shifting Government Responsibility for the Elderly*. Beverly Hills, Calif.: Sage, 1983.

Eustis, Nancy; Jay Greenberg; and Sharon Patten. *Long-Term Care for Older Persons: A Policy Perspective*. Monterey, Calif.: Brooks-Cole, 1984.

Storey, James R. *Older Americans in the Reagan Era: Impacts of Federal Policy Changes*. Washington, D.C.: Urban Institute, 1983.

Chapter 7

Nutrition in Aging: Dietary Recommendations

Marion Nestle

The role of nutrition in health promotion, disease prevention, and longevity for the elderly is of great medical, socioeconomic, and personal interest. Nutrition is essential for normal growth and development and for the maintenance of health throughout life, yet much information about its relationship to these processes remains unknown. Most knowledge of human nutrition has been derived from studies of young, healthy adults. The dietary needs of children, or of the ill or injured, are not so well established.

Our understanding of the nutritional aspects of aging is especially incomplete. We know that aging is accompanied by a gradual deterioration of physical functions and by an increasing incidence of chronic disease, yet we cannot state with certainty how nutrition might prevent or alleviate these problems.

Our lack of information about nutrition in general—and about nutrition and aging in particular—derives primarily from the great difficulties inherent in designing, conducting, and interpreting the results of nutrition research. Nutrition research is expensive; it is often conducted on samples of people that are too small to be statistically significant, and it is especially subject to biases among investigators and to placebo effects among subjects (Twomey 1981). Because the results of nutrition research reveal considerable genetic variation among individuals, correct interpretation demands well-designed control populations.

These problems become even more complicated when studying the elderly (Exton-Smith 1982). Older people in the United States are an extraordinarily diverse group. They vary in social and economic status, educational background, life experience, rate of aging, living arrangements,

and state of health, as well as in dietary behavior. Furthermore, these characteristics are present in individuals whose ages span several decades. It is not yet feasible to conduct research studies that control for all of these variables.

For these reasons, it is difficult to make nutritional generalizations about the elderly that necessarily apply to specific individuals. This situation, however, is by no means unique to this age group. Even with limited information about nutrition, reasonable dietary approaches to health care have been developed for the general public. Present knowledge of the nutritional aspects of aging permits us to develop dietary recommendations that are consistent with general guidelines, yet appropriate for older people in the United States.

Basic Principles of Nutrition

The diet that is best for health and longevity must be one that meets all nutritional needs, maintains adequate (and optimal) body weight, and prevents illness or disability due to deficient or excessive nutrient intake. Because considerable uncertainty still exists about the precise details of these relationships, dietary recommendations are based on current understanding of human nutritional requirements, the nutrient content of food, recent trends in U.S. eating habits, and the effects of these factors on health.

Human Nutritional Requirements

The human diet requires a relatively constant supply of 40 to 50 separate substances that are necessary or useful for health. These substances are listed in Tables 7–1 and 7–2, along with the daily intake levels that are believed to prevent deficiency symptoms in most U.S. adults. These substances include sources of energy and of

Table 7-1
Recommended Daily Dietary Allowances for U.S. Adults Aged 51 and Older, 1980.

Category and Unit Measure	Males	Females
Energy (kilocalories)		
Age 51 to 75	2,000 to 2,800	1,400 to 2,000
Age 76+	1,650 to 2,450	1,200 to 2,000
Protein (g)	56	44
Fat-soluble vitamins		
Vitamin A (μg) retinol equivalents	1,000	800
Vitamin D (μg)	5	5
Vitamin E (mg) α-tocopherol equivalents	10	8
Water-soluble vitamins		
Vitamin C (mg)	60	60
Thiamin (mg)	1.2	1.0
Riboflavin (mg)	1.4	1.2
Niacin (mg niacin equivalents)	16	13
Vitamin B_6 (mg)	2.2	2.0
Folacin (μg)	400	400
Vitamin B_{12} (μg)	3.0	3.0
Minerals		
Calcium (mg)	800	800
Phosphorus (mg)	800	800
Magnesium (mg)	350	300
Trace elements		
Iron (mg)	10	10
Zinc (mg)	15	15
Iodine (μg)	150	150

Source: Data from National Research Council. Food and Nutrition Board. *Recommended Dietary Allowances.* 9th rev. ed. Washington, D.C.: National Academy of Sciences, 1980.

Table 7-2
Estimated Safe and Adequate Daily Dietary Intakes for Selected Vitamins and Minerals for Adults in the United States

Nutrient Category and Unit of Measure	Range
Fat-soluble vitamins	
Vitamin K (μg)	70 to 140
Water-soluble vitamins	
Biotin (μg)	100 to 200
Pantothenic acid (mg)	4 to 7
Minerals	
Sodium (mg)	1,100 to 3,300
Potassium (mg)	1,875 to 5,625
Chloride (mg)	1,700 to 5,100
Trace elements	
Copper (mg)	2.0 to 3.0
Manganese (mg)	2.5 to 5.0
Fluoride (mg)	1.5 to 4.0
Chromium (mg)	0.05 to 0.2
Selenium (mg)	0.05 to 0.2
Molybdenum (mg)	0.15 to 0.5

Source: Data from National Research Council. Food and Nutrition Board. *Recommended Dietary Allowances.* 9th rev. ed. Washington, D.C.: National Academy of Sciences, 1980, p. 178.

carbon, nitrogen, and other inorganic minerals, as well as more than 20 organic molecules— amino acids, fatty acids, and vitamins— whose biosynthetic pathways have been lost during evolution. Such nutrients are considered to be essential if a dietary (or metabolically induced) deficiency results in recognizable disease symptoms that are cured by adding them back to the diet.

Some of the nutrients, however, do not strictly meet this criterion. Instead, they are assumed to be essential because deficiency symptoms have been observed in animals (for example, vitamin E) or because certain drugs produce symptoms of deficiency in human subjects (for example, biotin). Fiber is another such exception. Although it is not truly essential in the diet, fiber improves gastrointestinal function, and its intake is associated with the prevention of cancer and other diseases of the intestine (Spiller and Freeman 1981). Constipation, a frequent complaint of the elderly, is relieved by adding fiber-containing foods to the diet (Hull, Greco, and Brooks 1980).

Excessive intake of nutrients, however, also is associated with disease symptoms. The fat-soluble vitamins (vitamins A, D, E, and K) and many—if not all—of the minerals can become toxic if consumed in amounts much higher than recommended levels (National Research Council 1973). Too much carbohydrate, fat, or protein also may be harmful, leading to obesity and, perhaps, to other disorders. For each nutrient there appears to be an optimal range of intake that is both safe and adequate; healthy diets contain all nutrients within desirable ranges.

Recommended Dietary Allowances

At the present time, the desirable ranges of nutrients for healthy diets cannot be defined precisely for individuals. Instead, recommended intake levels for the population are published every few years by the Food and Nutrition Board of the National Academy of Sciences as Recommended Dietary Allowances, or RDAs (National Research Council 1980a). Table 7–1 presents the 1980 RDAs for the oldest age group. Table 7–2 presents ranges of daily intake levels that are considered both safe and adequate for U.S. adults.

Because the RDAs are used as standards of adequate dietary intake in nutritional status surveys and in food assistance programs for the elderly (and others), it is important to understand their limitations. The RDAs are not pre-cise sets of minimum dietary requirements for individuals. Instead, they are generous overestimations of nutrient intake levels that will prevent deficiency symptoms in the vast majority of healthy people in the United States. In practice, they are established at a statistical level two standard deviations above the mean nutrient requirement as determined by clinical studies.

This method reveals immediately that people with average nutrient requirements may consume perfectly adequate amounts of a nutrient at a level considerably below its RDA. Conversely, a person with unusually high requirements may meet the RDAs but still fail to consume enough nutrients.

Moreover, the RDAs have been developed almost entirely from research studies of young, healthy adults. Although Table 7–1 presents the RDAs for adults aged 51 and over, these figures are, in most cases, the same as those for adults aged 23 to 50. This presentation assumes that the requirements of the elderly are generally similar to those of younger adults; it also assumes that the nutritional needs of 51-year-olds are the same as those of their 95-year-old grandparents. Recommended energy intakes, however, decline markedly with age. This reduction is based on the hypothesis that physical activity declines steadily throughout adult life.

For the nutrients listed in Table 7–2, even less information is available; the Food and Nutrition Board has only defined ranges of daily intake levels that appear to be adequate, yet safe. For these nutrients, one recommended range of intake is presented for adults of all ages.

The limitations of the RDAs, however, do not totally destroy their utility. Although few studies of nutritional needs across the life span have been published, the ones that do exist reveal only minor difficulties in the nutrient requirements of adults of widely varying ages (Todhunter 1980).

Nutritional Quality of Food

The nutritional quality of a food can be assessed by a value referred to as *nutrient concentration* or *nutrient density*. These terms describe the proportion of essential nutrients relative to the calories contained in a food. When we compare two foods with the same number of calories, we assign the higher nutrient concentration to the food with the higher proportion of essential nutrients. In practice, these terms are used nonspecifically; they classify foods into two broad groups—those of relatively high and those of relatively low nutrient density. Foods of high nutrient density contain significant quantities of essential nutrients or fiber along with their calories. Foods of low nutrient density, however, always contain proportionately large amounts of fat (which is high in calories), sugar, refined starches, or alcohol (which contain few nutrients).

Trends in U.S. Food Consumption Practices

Since about 1910, the U.S. Department of Agriculture has collected information on the use of selected food commodities by measuring their disappearance from the U.S. food supply. This method may well overestimate the amounts of food that actually are consumed. Nevertheless, the data reveal five major trends in U.S. eating habits during the 20th century (Brewster and Jacobson 1978):

1. *Increased fat consumption.* People in the United States are eating more vegetable oils, shortenings, and margarines than in 1910. Fats are high in calories; at 9 kilocalories per gram, they contain more than twice the energy value of equivalent portions of protein or carbohydrate and thus lower the nutrient concentration of food. The evidence that links diets high in fat content to development of heart disease and certain cancers makes this trend of special concern (Ahrens and Connor 1979).

2. *Increased consumption of sugars.* In the United States, people consume about 130 pounds per capita per year of sucrose and other sugars and caloric sweeteners, much of it in processed foods and soft drinks. Sugars contain no nutrients. They contribute to the development of tooth decay, a major problem throughout life (Newbrun 1982).

3. *Decreased consumption of complex carbohydrates (starches).* The use of foods such as bread, rice, potatoes, and pasta has diminished steadily throughout this century. These foods are generally rich in vitamins, minerals, and fiber, and they are low in calories. Their consumption is associated with good health (Ahrens and Connor 1979).

4. *Increased consumption of food outside the home.* An increasing proportion of the U.S. food dollar is spent on meals prepared and consumed in restaurants and snack bars. This trend reflects recent societal changes in both family structure and in the food industry; there are more single-parent homes and

working couples, as well as more—and better advertised—fast food products than there were 70 years ago.

5. *Increased consumption of processed foods.* Agriculture Department figures indicate that convenience foods—foods that have been frozen, prepackaged, or altered significantly before sales—are gradually replacing fresh foods in the U.S. diet. Food processing generally lowers nutrient concentration. Cooking, freezing, thawing, and storage of foods all contribute to losses of nutrients; light, oxygen, and heat destroy sensitive vitamins (Harris and Karmas 1975). One vivid example of food processing is the conversion of whole wheat to white flour. In this process, the bran layers and germ are selectively removed from the wheat grain; white flour contains only a small proportion of the original vitamins, trace minerals, and fiber (Harris and Karma 1975). To partially compensate for these losses, white flour is enriched in the United States with three vitamins (niacin, thiamine, riboflavin) and iron. How important are such losses? Preservation and processing methods insure plentiful supplies of fruits and vegetables at all times of the year and a food supply that remains reliable despite fluctuations in harvest yields and world food markets. Processed foods, however, contain fewer nutrients than the fresh foods from which they were derived.

Thus, taken together, these trends suggest that the overall nutritional quality of the U.S. diet has been declining steadily throughout the 20th century.

Nutrition and Disease

Food intake patterns affect overall health, as well as chronic disease incidence. In the United States, nutrient deficiency diseases occur seldom among people whose income is adequate. They are observed chiefly among people in poverty groups or among those with unusually high nutrient requirements, serious illnesses, or diets unusually restricted in the quantity or variety of food. Because these categories apply to many elderly persons, it is not surprising that malnutrition has been identified in older people in the United States; low income and poor health are characteristics of aging in this country.

Some of the ill health, however, is associated with excessive—rather than deficient—food intake. Diseases of overconsumption are quite prevalent in the United States. Many of the common chronic disease conditions of the elderly—among them coronary heart disease, cancer (notably of the bowel and breast), strokes, high blood pressure, cirrhosis of the liver, and tooth decay—have been associated with an imbalanced intake of nutrients (Ahrens and Connor 1979).

Much of the evidence that links diet to chronic disease incidence comes from epidemiologic studies (Hulley et al. 1981). Such studies show, for example, that populations with a high dietary intake of cholesterol or saturated fat exhibit a higher incidence of cornary heart disease than societies whose fat intake is low; when groups with low heart disease rates move to an area where more fats are consumed, the rates increase. Similar studies relate excessive salt intake to hypertension (Ahrens and Connor 1979) and related reduced intake of dietary fiber to cancer and other diseases of the large intestine (Spiller and Freeman 1981).

Such studies demonstrate an association between diet and disease, but they do not necessarily prove causation. This distinction is not trivial; one reason why nutrition information is controversial is the uncertainty that it is diet—and not some other factor—that is responsible for the disease. Despite these concerns, the circumstantial and experimental evidence that relates diet to disease seems consistent enough to permit the development of dietary approaches to health promotion.

Dietary Recommendations for the General Public

To meet the public need for accurate dietary advice and information, numerous governmental and health agencies have incorporated these basic nutritional principles into published dietary recommendations. On occasion, these reports have differed in recommendations and have provided contradictory advice. Despite this controversy, most reports are in surprising agreement on the major principles of healthy diets. Most propose that people in the United States consume a wide variety of foods; increase consumption of foods containing complex carbohydrates (starch and fiber); restrict the intake of sugar, fat (especially saturated fat), cholesterol, salt, and alcohol; and maintain ideal body weight (McNutt 1980).

These recommendations derive directly from our current understanding of nutrition and health. The recommendation to emphasize variety in food intake, for example, evolves from knowledge of food composition. Most foods contain many different nutrients, but in widely varying proportions. Oranges contain more vitamin C than eggs, for example, but eggs have more protein. Consumption of adequate amounts of a variety of foods of complementary nutrient composition is most likely to produce a diet that contains the full range of essential nutrients. The remaining recommendations are directed toward reversing trends in food consumption pat-

Table 7-3
Dietary Goals for the United States

	Current U.S. Diet	Dietary Goals
	Percentage of Total Caloric Intake	
Carbohydrate, total	*46*	*58*
Complex carbohydrate and naturally occuring sugars	28	48
Sugars, refined and processed	18	10
Protein	*12*	*12*
Fat, total	*42*	*30*
Saturated	16	10
Monounsaturated	19	10
Polyunsaturated	7	10
Cholesterol (mg per day)	600	300
Salt (g per day)	6 to 18	5

Source: Data from U.S. Senate Select Committee on Nutrition and Human Needs. *Dietary Goals for the U.S.* 2d ed. Washington, D.C.: U.S. Government Printing Office, 1977, pp. 4–5.

terns that reduce the quality of the food supply and that contribute to high rates of chronic disease.

Dietary Goals for the United States

These principles have been expressed in their most specific form in the report *Dietary Goals for the U.S.* produced by the U.S. Senate Select Committee on Nutrition and Human Needs (1977). These important recommendations form the first public statement by a federal agency on the relationship between diet and disease risk factors.

The specific recommendations of the *Dietary Goals* are listed in Table 7–3. The report identifies the proportion of total calories derived from protein, fat, and carbohydrate in the current U.S. diet, and it presents specific goals for altering these proportions to achieve a healthier food intake. As Table 7–3 shows, the present U.S. diet (according to Agriculture Department disappearance data) contains large amounts of fat and sugar. To improve the nutritional quality of the diet—and the health status of people in the United States—the report proposes significant increases in consumption of food starches (especially those that are unprocessed) and significant decreases in caloric intake from fat and sugars as well as a greatly decreased consumption of cholesterol and salt.

The *Dietary Goals* have generated significant controversy because of their specific recommendations, as well as the major changes in food consumption habits that they require (Harper 1978). To consume a diet consistent with *Dietary Goals* recommendations, people must increase consumption of fruits, vegetables, and whole grain cereals; decrease intake of sugar, fat, and salt; and select lean meats and low-fat dairy products. Such changes, of course, would greatly increase the nutrient density of the diet.

Additional Dietary Recommendations

Despite debate, the *Dietary Goals* have become the standard to which other dietary recommendations are compared. Although they were designed to improve the food intake of healthy people, the *Dietary Goals* turn out to be very nearly indistinguishable from the recommendations of the American Heart Association, whose main nutritional concern has been to reduce the atherogenic potential of the U.S. diet (Grundy et al. 1982). In response to increasing evidence that diets high in starch and fiber control the levels of glucose, insulin, and lipids in blood (Anderson

1981), the American Diabetes Association (1979) now recommends that patients with diabetes mellitus consume a high-carbohydrate, low-fat diet in proportions similar to those of the *Dietary Goals.* Most recently, the National Research Council (1982) report *Diet, Nutrition, and Cancer* stresses the importance of similar dietary principles in cancer prevention.

Nevertheless, several aspects of dietary recommendations remain controversial: the specific levels to which nutrient intake should be restricted; whether it is necessary to restrict cholesterol intake; and—most important—whether dietary restrictions should be applied to everyone, or just to people who carry risk factors for coronary heart disease, obesity, diabetes, or hypertension.

These issues are best illustrated by the recommendations of the Food and Nutrition Board of the National Academy of Sciences (National Research Council 1980b), which argues that dietary modifications are advisable only when necessary to maintain ideal body weight or to prevent or treat specific diseases. Thus, it recommends cholesterol and fat restriction only for people with risk factors for heart disease (for example, high blood pressure or elevated serum cholesterol levels).

Similarly, *Diet, Nutrition, and Cancer* has been criticized for lack of adequate research information to support its specific recommendations and for providing a false sense of security to consumers who might follow its advice ("Whelan Hits NAS Diet-Cancer Advice" 1982).

These kinds of criticisms induced the U.S. Agriculture and Health and Human Services departments to produce *Nutrition and Your Health: Dietary Guidelines for Americans* (U.S. Department of Agriculture 1980), a report that supports the *Dietary Goals* in principle but is much less specific. Despite concern that its provisions are on the one hand too vague and on the other too strong (Greenberg 1980), this report remains available as an educational resource for consumers and patients.

Despite these disagreements, the principles of the *Dietary Goals* have held up rather well, and the report represents a unifying approach to both basic and therapeutic dietary recommendations for the general public. Present information suggests that these recommendations are equally useful for the elderly.

Nutritional Aspects of Aging

Nutritional Status of the Elderly

With this background, we now can examine the nutritional status of the elderly and the ways in which aging affects food consumption and nutrient utilization. A large number of surveys have assessed dietary intake and the extent of malnutrition among elderly people in the United States. These studies consistently report widespread dietary deficiencies of calories, vitamins, and minerals, most frequently citing insufficient consumption of calcium, iron, and certain water-soluble vitamins (O'Hanlon and Kohrs 1978). The reported extent of deficient intake is extraordinarily high; some students have identified dietary deficiencies in as much as 60 to 80 percent of the survey population. These findings are also consistently related to income level; inadequate nutrient intake is reported with far greater frequency among the elderly who are poor and less well educated (Lowenstein 1982).

Although such surveys appear to indicate that the vast majority of the elderly are malnourished, we cannot be certain that this conclusion is correct. Dietary surveys of older people in the United States suffer from well-known methodological and sampling problems that tend to underestimate dietary deficiency (Exton-Smith 1982). Current methods for the assessment of nutritional status are not necessarily appropriate for the elderly. Because normal ranges of values for laboratory tests, anthropomorphic measurements, and heights and weights all have been developed on younger adults, conventional criteria for the diagnosis of malnutrition appear to exaggerate its severity in older adults (Bowman and Rosenberg 1982).

Many surveys determine dietary intake by food recall methods that produce inaccurate data, especially among study subjects with impaired communication skills, hearing, or short-term memory (Campbell and Dodus 1967). Deficient dietary intake almost always is defined as a specific percentage—either 100 or 67 percent—of the RDA. Few elderly people consume 100 percent of the RDAs each day, but even 67 percent may be too high a standard for individuals with average requirements. Thus, such comparisons overestimate the extent of dietary deficiency.

More important, these surveys only rarely reveal correlations between dietary deficiencies and clinical or biochemical signs of malnutrition. The first National Health and Nutrition Examination Survey, for example, reported that 57 percent of elderly black men below poverty level failed to meet the RDA for vitamin A. Fewer than 5 percent of this group was found to have low serum vitamin A levels, however, and only 6 percent showed clinical signs that might have been caused by vitamin A deficiency (Lowenstein 1982). The same study noted deficient energy intake among 84 percent of poverty-level elderly black women, yet it identified 49 percent of this group as obese. Such inconsistencies severely limit the predictive value of dietary intake data as a measure of malnutrition in the elderly (Kerr et al. 1982).

These difficulties also limit present methods for the assessment of nutritional status and the determination of the extent of malnutrition among the elderly. Given this situation, we cannot conclude that malnutrition is a normal concomitant of aging. Instead, it is most likely to be identified in elderly persons who are economically or socially deprived, or who are ill.

Common (Not Necessarily Correct) Assumptions About Aging

Despite the lack of compelling evidence, the elderly are popularly believed to be generally malnourished. This belief derives from direct observation of elderly people who suffer from nutritional deficiencies, as well as from the knowledge that many older people in the United States live on fixed incomes and are of poor health. It also derives, however, from the popular belief that normal aging is inevitably accompanied by a decline in nutritional status. Contributing to this idea are several common assumptions about the physiology of aging that may indeed apply to many elderly persons, but that are not necessarily correct for those who remain healthy and active.

- *"Gastrointestinal function declines with age."* Many physiological functions have been documented to decline gradually throughout the life span (Shock 1961), and it seems reasonable to assume that the ability to digest, absorb, and utilize nutrients should be among them. Remarkably little evidence, however, supports the idea that these functions are lost with age. Instead, gastrointestinal disabilities result most frequently from disease or from chronic drug therapy. Healthy adults well into their 90s have been reported to maintain gastrointestinal function similar to that of much younger individuals (Bhanthumnavin and Schuster 1977).

• *"Taste sensitivity declines with age."* Loss of taste perception would be expected to lead to loss of appetite and enjoyment of food and, therefore, to reduced food intake. It has not been possible, however, to demonstrate a physiologic loss of taste in the elderly in the absence of concurrent disease, drug therapy, smoking, or malnutrition (Kamath 1982).

• *"Basal metabolic rate declines with age."* Classic studies have reported a gradual but consistent decline in basal oxygen consumption with increasing age (McGandy et al. 1966). These studies, however, were performed on adults whose lives had become increasingly sedentary and whose body weights also were increasing; both of these changes would tend to reduce basal energy expenditure. When these factors are taken into consideration, little change in basal metabolism is observed with age (Keyes, Taylor, and Grande 1973).

• *"Lean body mass declines with age."* This widely held assumption is based on numerous studies that have identified a loss of net body protein and a concomitant increase in body fat content with increasing age (Forbes and Reina 1970). These studies also were performed on increasingly sedentary populations, however, and such changes do not take place—or occur at a much slower rate—among elderly people who remain physically active (Sidney, Shephard, and Harrison 1977).

• *"Caloric requirements decline with age."* When basal metabolism and lean body mass decline, fewer calories should be needed to maintain constant body weight. Some studies have reported steadily declining caloric requirements with age (McGandy et al. 1966), but others have not (Calloway and Zanni 1980). Because maintenance of normal body weight demands that caloric intake balance caloric expenditure, caloric requirements will necessarily be greater among people who remain physically active throughout life.

• *"Lack of teeth results in malnutrition."* Loss of teeth is an important problem among the elderly (Lutwak 1976). Teeth are required to chew food, and their absence (or the wearing of ill-fitting dentures) might be expected to result in decreased food intake. Research studies, however, do not support this hypothesis; laboratory and clinical signs of malnutrition do not differ among those who do and those who do not have adequate teeth or dentures (Bates, Elwood, and Foster 1971).

The nutritional implications of these assumptions are extremely important. If, indeed, basal metabolic rates decline with age, fewer calories will be needed to maintain body weight. Requirements for essential nutrients, however, remain the same throughout life. Thus, the elderly would be expected to consume all necessary nutrients within a severely restricted caloric intake. To do so would require an especially careful selection of foods of high nutrient concentration.

The lack of concrete evidence for these assumptions, however, suggests that basic dietary recommendations for younger adults apply equally well to healthy, active, elderly persons. It is only when older people become ill, sedentary, or too poor to purchase adequate food that recommendations must be adjusted to compensate.

Factors That Influence Nutritional Status in the Elderly

Although imbalanced food intake is an obvious cause of malnutrition, it is not sufficient to say that the elderly are malnourished because they do not eat properly. Nonnutritional factors have a major impact on nutritional status. Food must be purchased and prepared, as well as eaten and digested. Nutrients must be absorbed, transported, metabolized, and excreted. Anything that interferes with these processes is likely to cause malnutrition. The most common nonnutritional causes of malnutrition are described in the following sections.

Disease and Disability. Many illnesses affect nutritional status by interfering with mobility, appetite, or absorption and metabolism of nutrients. Malnutrition is observed frequently among patients in hospitals whose ability to recover from their illness may well depend on adequate nutritional support (Tomaiolo, Enman, and Kraus 1981). In severe disease conditions, requirements for protein and calories may greatly increase. Under these circumstances, nutrient intake also must be increased to compensate (Long et al. 1979).

Drug Therapy. The frequency and quantity of drug use increase progressively with age (Greenblatt, Sellers, and Shader 1982). Many drugs used commonly by the elderly interfere with absorption, metabolism, or utilization of nutrients; prolonged drug therapy is likely to induce nutritional deficiencies (Roe 1982). Steroids, diuretics, aluminum-containing antacids, and tetracycline antibiotics, for example, have all been reported to cause increased urinary losses of calcium and are of concern as a factor contributing to the development of osteoporosis (Spencer, Kramer, and Osis 1982). The antituberculosis agent isoniazid induces deficiencies of vitamin B_6 in certain individuals; antacids and phenobarbital induce malabsorption; and thiazides cause excessive excretion of certain minerals (Roe 1982). These effects are often additive; multiple drug regimes are an important cause of malnutrition in the elderly.

Alcoholism. Although moderate drinking has been reported to facilitate social interaction among older people in the United States (Watkin 1979), chronic alcoholism occurs among the elderly, and it is frequently associated with nutritional deficiencies (Barboriak et al. 1978). Because alcohol replaces food calories in the diet, impairs digestion and absorption, and interferes with nutrient metabolism, excessive alcohol intake in an elderly person signals the necessity for special attention to nutritional status.

Poverty. Malnutrition is most frequently identified among the elderly whose income is low. Economic status affects not only the quality and quantity of food purchases, but also living arrangements, cooking facilities, transportation, and general health care—all of which, in turn, affect the ways in which food is purchased and consumed. Low income may well be the single most important predictor of inadequate nutrition in the elderly (Lowenstein 1982).

Social Isolation. Eating is a highly social activity. Social isolation accompanied by depression can produce loss of appetite and an unvarying—and therefore limited—diet (Rao 1973). Nevertheless, one cannot assume that an elderly person who lives alone is necessarily malnourished; studies of single—but healthy and independent—individuals identify adequate nutritional status among them and refute the "tea and toast" stereotype (Krondl et al. 1982).

Institutionalization. Malnutrition is documented to occur at extraordinarily high rates among elderly residents of nursing homes (Shaver, Soper, and Lutes 1980) and hospitals (Tomaiolo, Enman, and Kraus 1981). Such people, of course, are often ill and may not eat properly; their disease conditions may well interfere with nutritional status. It is difficult, however, to make generalizations that apply to all institutionalized elderly. Institutions vary in standards of care, health status of the patient population, and quality of dietary provisions. Comparative studies of institutionalized elderly demonstrate that their diets can be at least as adequate as those of their noninstitutionalized counterparts (Brown et al. 1977).

Physical Inactivity. Many studies have documented the gradual loss of physical performance with age (Shock 1961). Nevertheless, many older individuals are able to work better than their younger counterparts. As in all aspects of aging, there is much individual variation in physical strength and endurance. This observation suggests that at least some loss of function might be prevented by adequate physical activity throughout life. A considerable body of evidence supports this idea. Moderate exercise has been demonstrated to improve work capacity (Barry et al. 1966), to increase lean body mass and reduce body fat content (Sidney, Shephard, and Harrison 1977), and to improve cardiac capacity (Kavanagh 1977) among the elderly. Exercise burns calories; active people must eat more to maintain body weight. Because it is easier to meet nutritional requirements when caloric intake is adequate, a physically active person would be expected to have better nutritional status. Many of the changes commonly attributed to old age may, in fact, result from the increasingly sedentary life-style of the elderly; it seems likely that adequate exercise throughout life might prevent or alleviate many of the common complaints of old age (Bortz 1982).

Thus, present knowledge of the common assumptions about aging and the many factors that affect nutritional status in the elderly does not permit us to make simple generalizations that necessarily apply to all older individuals. Declining nutritional status does not appear to be an invariant aspect of aging, but it is likely to appear when social, economic, and health status are compromised. The more compromising factors present, the more an older person is likely to require nutritional—as well as social, financial, or medical—intervention. In most cases of malnutrition in the elderly, these factors are inextricably linked.

Popular Dietary Advice for the Elderly: A Critical Evaluation

The media, best-selling books, and health food advocates, as well as the federal government and health organizations, all produce abundant dietary information for the elderly. This information is often contradictory or incomplete. With current knowledge of basic dietary recommendations and the factors that affect nutritional status in the elderly, however, it is possible to examine popular dietary advice and evaluate its efficacy and safety.

Caloric Restriction

Studies of laboratory animals have demonstrated conclusively that the single most important nutritional factor in increased longevity is caloric deprivation; rats restricted in infancy or early adulthood to 60 to 80 percent of normal caloric intake live 20 to 30 percent longer than their well-fed littermates (Ross 1976). It is not immediately obvious, however, how these results might apply to human nutrition. Starvation produces well-known adverse physical and behavioral effects in both children and adults (Kerndt et al. 1982) that are especially deleterious in the elderly (Tomaiolo, Enman, and Kraus 1981). Moreover, the animal data are inconsistent with recent reports that suggest that optimum body weights for maximum longevity are actually somewhat higher than those currently considered ideal (Andres 1980). For these reasons, severe caloric restriction is unlikely to produce beneficial health effects and should not be recommended to the elderly.

Low-Fat Diets

The Pritikin (Leonard, Hafer, and Pritikin 1974) and similar diets carry the recommendations of the *Dietary Goals* to their most extreme values. They advocate severe restriction of dietary fat (to about 10 percent of total caloric intake), along with a greatly increased intake of complex carbohydrate (to 70 to 80 percent of the calories). The long-term effects of such diets on health have not yet been established. As long as food intake is sufficiently varied and caloric intake remains adequate, such diets should provide the necessary protein, vitamins, minerals, and essential fatty acids. Iron may be an exception; its status should be monitored by laboratory tests. Because very low-fat diets are not readily available in restaurants and may be difficult to prepare, they require special attention to food purchase and preparation that may be difficult for people who lack mobility or adequate cooking facilities, or those who generally eat meals prepared by others.

Vegetarian Diets

Vegetarian diets vary greatly in food restrictions. They range from diets that simply exclude red meat to those that restrict all meats or all animal foods (including dairy products). Although the meat and dairy content of vegetarian diets differs, all are perfectly capable of meeting nutritional needs (ADA Reports 1980). Vegetable foods provide ample quantities of protein; the quality (that is, the content of essential amino acids) of the protein, however, is not as appropriate for human nutrition as that of animal foods. Fortunately, vegetable foods vary sufficiently in their composition of essential amino acids so that when they are consumed in proper combination—grains and beans, for example—they complement each other's amino acid content. This principle of protein complementarity illustrates the importance of variety in food intake. Even with adequate variety and quantity of food intake, however, strict vegetarians—who eat no animal foods—can become deficient in vitamin B_{12} and should supplement their diet with this vitamin. Because vegetarian diets are sometimes deficient in iron, it is also useful to monitor iron status.

Vitamin and Mineral Supplements

Nutrient supplements are desirable in those rare elderly persons who show signs of nutrient deficiencies or in those who take drugs that interfere with nutritional status. Many studies, however, have documented a widespread use of nutritional supplements among the elderly (Todhunter 1980). Although it seems reasonable that supplements should produce recognizable health benefits, improved health seems only to be observed among people who exhibit clinical signs of malnutrition. In general, health benefits have not been demonstrated among asymptomatic elderly subjects (Mickelsen 1976). Most vitamin and mineral supplements actually are consumed by individuals whose diets are adequate; when people with inadequate diets take supplements, however, they often take those that are inappropriate (Garry et al. 1982; Yearick, Wang, and Pisias 1980). Megadose supplements have not yet been demonstrated by controlled trials to prevent or cure illness and should not, therefore, be recommended. More important, fat-soluble vitamins (vitamins A, D, E, and K) are toxic when taken at levels greater than 10 to 20 times the RDA; excessive intake of minerals also should be avoided (National Research Council 1973). Thus, the most reasonable supplement to recommend for "insurance" purposes is a standard multivitamin/mineral preparation that contains no more than the RDA level for each included nutrient.

Calcium Supplements

In contrast, the use of calcium supplements as a preventive measure for osteoporosis may be highly beneficial. Although the precise relationship of nutrition to osteoporosis has not been established (Avioli 1981), several lines of evidence support a role for calcium. Calcium intake is frequently low among adult women, and it becomes lower after menopause, especially among those who do not consume milk products (Heaney et al. 1982). Many drugs taken frequently by the elderly—diuretics, antacids, and alcohol—increase calcium excretion (Spencer, Kramer, and Osis 1982). Reduced physical activity also is associated with calcium losses (Bortz 1982). More important, clinical studies have demonstrated improved bone mineralization among postmenopausal women taking calcium supplements; one recent study has reported a 50 percent reduction in bone fractures among osteoporotic women taking 1500 mg of calcium per day (Riggs et al. 1982). This therapy is well worth further investigation. Calcium supplements are inexpensive and harmless at this level of intake; they certainly would appear to be an excellent investment for women at risk for osteoporosis.

Choline Supplements

On autopsy, patients with senile memory disorders of the Alzheimer's type have been found to have greatly decreased brain concentrations of choline acetyltransferase, an enzyme that catalyzes the synthesis of acetylcholine. Furthermore, feeding choline or lecithin—precursors of acetylcholine—to experimental animals has been demonstrated to increase neurotransmitter levels in the brain (Bartus et al. 1982). These observations immediately suggest that feeding choline or lecithin to patients with senile dementias would increase acetylcholine biosynthesis and, therefore, improve the symptoms.

The results of many such studies, however, have been disappointing. In only a few cases have memory or cognitive or communication skills improved (Bartus et al. 1982). At the present time, the use of these supplements in elderly patients remains experimental.

Antioxidant Supplements

Harmon (1981) and others have proposed that free-radical chemical reactions constitute the major aging process. They suggest that the healthy life span could be extended by preventing free-radical reactions with antioxidants (such as the nutrients vitamin C, vitamin E, selenium, and cysteine) or with antioxidant food additives (such as butylated hydroxytoluene, or BHT). Nutrient antioxidants are certainly essential for health. Studies in laboratory animals, however, have failed to demonstrate significant beneficial effects of supplemental antioxidants on mortality (Tappel, Fletcher, and Deamer 1973). Because the health effects of BHT are controversial (Jacobson 1976) and excessive intake of vitamin E (a fat-soluble vitamin) produces documented toxic effects (Roberts 1981), excessive antioxidant intake should be avoided. A diet that contains adequate amounts of essential nutrients—including those that are antioxidants—seems the one most reasonable to recommend for good nutrition in the elderly.

Aluminum-free Diets

Symptoms of mental disturbances similar to those of senile dementias of the Alzheimer's type have been observed in renal failure patients treated by chronic hemodialysis; thus dialysis encephalopathy can be reversed by removing aluminum from the dialysis solutions (Rozaz, Port, Rutt 1978). Further association of aluminum with symptoms of Alzheimer's disease derives from X-ray evidence of aluminum deposits in focal regions of the brains of patients who died with this condition (Perl and Brody 1980). The amount of aluminum has been reported to be higher in the brains of Alzheimer's patients than in the brains of controls (Trapp, Miner, et al. 1978).

Aluminum enters the food supply from tap water that has been treated with aluminum sulfate to precipitate out sulfate particles, as well as from aluminum cooking pots (Trapp, Cannon, and Koning 1981). By far the most important sources of ingested aluminum, however, are drugs that contain aluminum salts (for example, antacids). The average daily intake of aluminum in the United States is about 20 mg; a single antacid tablet, however, may contain more than 200 mg *(Physicians' Desk Reference* 1981). Aluminum is at least partially absorbed from the gastrointestinal tract (Kachny, Hegg, and Alfrey 1977). The association of aluminum intake with Alzheimer's symptoms does not, of course, prove causation. Much more research is needed to determine whether this relationship is significant. In the meantime, avoidance of aluminum can be recommended to those concerned. Because the amounts of aluminum obtained from water and cooking pots are so small, attention should focus on the elimination of as many aluminum-containing drugs as possible from the regimens of elderly patients.

Conclusion: Dietary Recommendations for the Elderly

Our discussion thus far has emphasized the great variation in the effects of aging on individuals and the inadequacy of current generalizations about the role of nutrition in maintaining health, preventing disease, and prolonging life in the elderly. Much information on these processes has yet to be discovered. More–and better–research on nutrition and aging is needed urgently to provide the data on which to base appropriate dietary recommendations for the elderly. The formation of the Department of Agriculture's new research center on nutrition and aging ("New Center" 1982) should be a major step toward that goal.

In the meantime, dietary recommendations for the general public seem entirely applicable to the elderly, especially if they are modified slightly to emphasize the special nutritional concerns of older people in the United States. Thus, the principal recommendations should include the following precepts:

1. Consume sufficient calories to maintain normal body weight.
2. Emphasize the consumption of foods of high nutrient concentration.
3. Consume a wide variety of fruits and vegetables, whole grain cereals, and legumes.
4. Choose lean meats and low-fat dairy products.
5. Select foods that have been processed as little as possible.
6. Increase food consumption to compensate for disease or for drug therapy.
7. If dietary supplements are taken, choose those that are appropriate for nutritional needs.
8. Remain physically active.
9. Whenever possible, correct social, medical, and economic impediments to good nutrition.

Diets consistent with these guidelines automatically will contain adequate amounts of the necessary nutrients and of fiber. They will contain minimal amounts of saturated fat, cholesterol, sugar, and salt (unless it is added deliberately) and, therefore, will be consistent with current guidelines on nutrition and health. It is useful to note that these recommendations are readily adaptable to individual nutrient requirements, food preferences, and cultural traditions.

Aging, of course, is a lifelong process. The sooner in life these recommendations are followed, the better will be health in old age.

References

ADA Reports. "Position Paper on the Vegetarian Approach to Eating." *Journal of the American Dietetic Association* 77 (1980): 61–69.

Ahrens, E.H. and W.E. Connor. "Symposium Report on the Task Force on the Evidence Relating Six Dietary Factors to the Nation's Health." *American Journal of Clinical Nutrition* 32 (1979): 2621–2748.

American Diabetes Association. "Principles of Nutrition and Dietary Recommendations for Individuals with Diabetes Mellitus." *Diabetes* 28 (1979): 1027–1029.

Anderson, J.W. "The Role of Dietary Carbohydrate and Fiber in the Control of Diabetes." *Advances in Internal Medicine* 26 (1981): 67–96.

Andres, R. "Effect of Obesity on Total Mortality." *International Journal of Obesity* 4 (1980): 381–386.

Avioli, L.V. "Postmenopausal Osteoporosis: Prevention vs. Cure." *Federation Proceedings* 40 (1981): 2418–2422.

Barboriak, J.J.; C.B. Rooney, T.H. Leitschuh; and A.J. Anderson. "Alcohol and Nutrient Intake of Elderly Men." *Journal of the American Dietetic Association* 72 (1978): 493–495.

Barry, A.L.; J.W. Daly; E.D.R. Pruett; J.R. Steinmetz; H.F. Page; N.C. Birkhead; K. Rodahl. "The Effects of Physical Conditioning on Older Individuals: 1. Work Capacity, Circulatory-Respiratory Function, and Work Electrocardiogram." *Journal of Gerontology* 21 (1966): 182–191.

Bartus, R.T.; R.L. Dean; B. Beer; and A.S. Lippa. "The Cholinergic Hypothesis of Geriatric Memory Dysfunction." *Science* 217 (1982): 408–417.

Bates, J.F.; P.C. Elwood; and W. Foster. "Studies Relating Mastication and Nutrition in the Elderly." *Gerontologia Clinica* 13 (1971): 227–232.

Bhanthumnavin, K. and M.H. Schuster. "Aging and Gastrointestinal Function." In *Handbook of the Biology of Aging*, eds. C.E. Finch and L. Hayflick. New York: Van Nostrand Reinhold, 1977.

Bortz, W.M. "Disuse and Aging." *Journal of the American Medical Association* 248 (1982); 1203–1208.

Bowman, B.B. and I.H. Rosenberg. "Assessment of the Nutritional Status of the Elderly." *American Journal of Clinical Nutrition* 35 (1982): 1142–1151.

Brewster, L. and M.F. Jacobson. *The Changing American Diet.* Washington, D.C.: Center for Science in the Public Interest, 1978.

Brown, P.T.; J.G. Bergan; E.P. Parsons; and I. Kroll. "Dietary Status of Elderly People." *Journal of the American Dietetic Association* 71 (1977): 41–45.

Calloway, D.H. and E. Zanni. "Energy Requirements and Energy Expenditure of Elderly Men." *American Journal of Clinical Nutrition* 33 (1980): 2088–2092.

Campbell, V.A. and M.L. Dodus. "Collecting Dietary Information from Groups of Older People." *Journal of the American Dietetic Association* 51 (1967): 29–33.

Exton-Smith, A.N. "Epidemiological Studies in the Elderly: Methodological Considerations." *American Journal of Clinical Nutrition* 35 (1982): 1273–1279.

Forbes, G.B. and J.C. Reina. "Adult Lean Body Mass Declines with Age: Some Longitudinal Observations." *Metabolism* 19 (1970): 653–663.

Garry, P.J.; J.S. Goodwin; W.C. Hunt; E.M. Hooper; and A.G. Leonard. "Nutritional Status in a Healthy Elderly Population: Dietary and Supplemental Intakes." *American Journal of Clinical Nutrition* 36 (1982): 319–331.

Greenberg, D.S. "Nutrition: A Long Wait for a Little Advice." *New England Journal of Medicine* 302 (1980): 535–536.

Greenblatt, D.J.; E.M. Sellers; and R.I. Shader. "Drug Disposition in Old Age." *New England Journal of Medicine* 306 (1982): 1081–1088.

Grundy, S.M.; D. Bilheimer; H. Blackburn; W.V. Brown; P.O. Kwiterovich; F. Mattson; G. Schonfeld; and W.H. Weidman. "Rationale of the Diet-Heart Statement of the American Heart Association: Report of the Nutrition Committee." *Circulation* 65 (1982): 839A–854A.

Harmon, D. "The Aging Process." *Proceedings of the National Academy of Sciences of the USA* 78 (1981): 7124–7128.

Harper, A.E. "Dietary Goals: A Skeptical View." *American Journal of Clinical Nutrition* 31 (1978): 310–321.

Harris, R.S. and E. Karmas, eds. *Nutritional Evaluation of Food Processing,* 2d ed. Westport: AVI, 1975.

Heaney, R.P.: J.C. Gallagher; C.C. Johnston; R. Neer; A.M. Parfitt; G.D. Whedon. "Calcium Nutrition and Bone Health in the Elderly." *American Journal of Clinical Nutrition* 36 (1982): 986–1013.

Hull, C.; P.S. Greco; and D.L. Brooks. "Alleviation of Constipation in the Elderly by Dietary Fiber Supplementation." *Journal of the American Geriatrics Society* 28 (1980): 410–414.

Hulley, S.B.; R. Sherwin; M. Nestle; and P.R. Lee. "Epidemiology as a Guide to Clinical Decisions: 2. Diet and Coronary Heart Disease." *Western Journal of Medicine* 135 (1981): 25–33.

Jacobson, M.F. *Eater's Digest: The Consumer's Factbook of Food Additives.* New York: Anchor Books, 1976.

Kachny, W.D.; A.P. Hegg; and A.C. Alfrey. "Gastrointestinal Absorption of Aluminum from Aluminum-Containing Antacids." *New England Journal of Medicine* 296 (1977): 1389–1390.

Kamath, S.K. "Taste Acuity and Aging." *American Journal of Clinical Nutrition* 36 (1982): 766–775.

Kavanagh, T. and R.J. Shepard. "The Effects of Continued Training on the Aging Process." In *The Marathon: Physiological, Medical, Epidemiological, and Psychological Studies,* ed. P. Milvy. *Annals of the New York Academy of Sciences* 301 (1977): 656–670.

Kerndt, P.R.; J.L. Naughton; C.E. Driscoll; and D.A. Loxterkamp. "Fasting: The History, Pathophysiology, and Complications." *Western Journal of Medicine* 37 (1982): 379–399.

Kerr, G.R.; E.S. Lee; M.–K. M. Lam; R.J. Lorimer; E. Randall; R.N. Forthofer; M.A. Davis; and S.M. Magnetti. "Relationships between Dietary and Biochemical Measures of Nutritional Status in HANES I data." *American Journal of Clinical Nutrition* 35 (1982): 294–308.

Keyes, A.; H.L. Taylor; and F. Grande. "Basal Metabolism and Age of Adult Man." *Metabolism* 22 (1973): 579–587.

Krondl, M.; D. Lau; M.A. Yurkiw; and P.H. Coleman. "Food Use and Perceived Food Meanings of the Elderly." *Journal of the American Dietetic Association* 80 (1982): 523–529.

Leonard, J.N.; J.L. Hafer; and N. Pritikin. *Live Longer Now.* New York: Charter Books, 1974.

Long, C.L.; N. Schaffel; J.W. Geiger; W.R. Schiller; and W.S. Blakemore. "Metabolic Response to Injury and Illness: Estimation of Energy and Protein Needs from Indirect Calorimetry and Nitrogen Balance." *Journal of Parenteral and Enteral Nutrition* 3 (1979): 452–456.

Lowenstein, F.W. "Nutritional Status of the Elderly in the United States of America." *Journal of the American College of Nutrition* 1 (1982): 165–177.

Lutwak, L. "Periodontal Disease." *Nutrition and Aging,* ed. M. Winick. New York: Wiley, 1976.

McGandy, R.B.; C.H. Barrows; A. Spanias; A. Meredith; J.L. Stone; and A.H. Norris. "Nutrient Intakes and Energy Expenditure in Men of Different Ages." *Journal of Gerontology* 21 (1966): 581–587.

McNutt, K. "Dietary Advice to the Public: 1957 to 1980." *Nutrition Reviews* 38 (1980): 353–360.

Mickelsen, O. "The Possible Role of Vitamins in the Aging Process." In *Nutrition, Longevity, and Aging,* eds. M. Rockstein and M.L. Sussman. New York: Academic Press, 1976.

National Research Council. Committee on Diet, Nutrition, and Cancer. *Diet, Nutrition, and Cancer.* Washington, D.C.: National Academy Press, 1982.

National Research Council. Committee on Food Protection. Food and Nutrition Board. *Toxicants Occuring Naturally in Food.* 2d ed. Washington, D.C.: National Academy of Sciences, 1973.

National Research Council. Food and Nutrition Board. *Recommended Dietary Allowances.* 9th rev. ed. Washington, D.C.: National Academy of Sciences, 1980.

National Research Council. Food and Nutrition Board. *Toward Healthful Diets.* Washington, D.C.: National Academy of Sciences, 1980.

"New Center Explores Links Between Nutrition, Aging." *Journal of the American Medical Association* 248 (1982): 2801.

Newbrun, E. "Sugar and Dental Caries: A Review of Human Studies." *Science* 217 (1982): 418–423.

O'Hanlon, P. and M.B. Kohrs. "Dietary Studies of Older Americans." *American Journal of Clinical Nutrition* 31 (1978): 1257–1269.

Perl, D.P. and A.R. Brody. "Alzheimer's Disease: X-ray Spectrophotometric Evidence of Aluminum Accumulation in Neurofibrillary Tangle-Bearing Neurons." *Science* 208 (1980): 297–299.

Physicians Desk Reference. 35th ed. Oradell, N.J.: Medical Economics Company, 1981.

Rao, D.B. "Problems of Nutrition in the Aged." *Journal of the American Geriatrics Society* 21 (1973): 362–367.

Riggs, B.L.; E. Seeman; S.F. Hodgson; D.R. Taves; and W.M. O'Fallon. "Effect of the Fluoride/Calcium Regimen on Vertebral Fracture Occurrence in Postmenopausal Osteoporosis." *New England Journal of Medicine* 306 (1982): 446–450.

Roberts, H.J. "Perspective on Vitamin E as Therapy." *Journal of the American Medical Association* 246 (1981): 129.

Roe, D.A. "Dietary Control of Human Studies Related to Aging and Drug Disposition or Response." *Journal of American College of Nutrition* 1 (1982): 199–205.

Ross, M.H. "Nutrition and Longevity in Experimental Animals." In *Nutrition and Aging,* ed. M. Winick. New York: Wiley, 1976.

Rozaz, V.V.; F.K. Port; and W.M. Rutt. "Progressive Dialysis Encephalopathy from Dialysate Aluminum." *Archives of Internal Medicine* 138 (1978): 1375–1377.

Shaver, H.J.; J.A. Loper; and R.A. Lutes. "Nutritional Status of Nursing Home Patients." *Journal of Parenteral and Enteral Nutrition* 4 (1980): 367–370.

Shock, N.W. "Physiologic Aspects of Aging in Man." *Annual Review of Physiology* 23 (1961): 97–119.

Sidney, K.H.; R.J. Shephard; and J.E. Harrison. "Endurance Training and Body Composition of the Elderly." *American Journal of Clinical Nutrition* 30 (1977): 326–333.

Spencer, H.; L. Kramer and D. Osis. "Factors Contributing to Calcium Loss in Aging." *American Journal of Clinical Nutrition* 36 (1982): 776–787.

Spiller, G. A. and H. J. Freeman. "Recent Advances in Dietary Fiber and Colorectal Disease." *American Journal of Clinical Nutrition* 34 (1981): 1145–1152.

Tappel, A.; B. Fletcher; and D. Deamer. "Effect of Antioxidants and Nutrients on Lipid Peroxidation Fluorescent Products and Aging Parameters in the Mouse." *Journal of Gerontology* 28 (1973): 415–424.

Todhunter, E. N. "Nutrition of the Elderly." In *Human Nutrition: A Comprehensive Treatise.* 3A, *Nutrition and the Adult,* eds. R. B. Alfin-Slater and D. Kritchevsky. New York: Plenum Press, 1980, pp. 397–416.

Tomaiolo, P. P.; S. Enman; and V. Kraus. "Preventing and Treating Malnutrition in the Elderly." *Journal of Parenteral and Enteral Nutrition* 5 (1981): 46–48.

Trapp, G. A.; J. B. Cannon; and J. H. Konin. "Correspondence: Aluminum Pots as a Source of Dietary Aluminum." *New England Journal of Medicine* 304 (1981): 172–173.

Trapp, G. A.; G. D. Miner; R. L. Zimmerman; A. R. Mastri; and L. L. Heston. "Aluminum Levels in Brain in Alzheimer's Disease." *Biological Psychiatry* 13 (1978): 709–718.

Twomey, P. "Getting Started in Clinical Nurtrition Research." Baltimore: American Society of Parenteral and Enteral Nutrition (ASPEN), 1981.

U.S. Department of Agriculture, U.S. Department of Health and Human Services. *Nutrition and Your Health: Dietary Guidelines for Americans.* Washington, D.C.: U.S. Government Printing Office, 1980.

U.S. Senate Select Committee on Nutrition and Human Needs. *Dietary Goals for the U.S.* 2d ed. Washington, D.C.: U.S. Government Printing Office, 1977.

Watkin, D. M. "Role of Alcoholic Beverages in Gerontology." In *Fermented Food Beverages in Nutrition,* eds. C. F. Gastiniau, W. J. Darby, and T. B. Turner. New York: Academic Press, 1979.

"Whelan Hits NAS Diet-Cancer Advice." *CNI Weekly Reports* 12, no. 46 (1982): 6.

Yearick, E. S.; M. –S. L. Wang; and S. J. Pisias. "Nutritional Status of the Elderly: Dietary and Biochemical Findings." *Journal of Gerontology* 35, no. 5 (1980): 663–671.

Chapter 8

Vision Problems of the Aging Patient: An Overview

Jay M. Enoch

The role of the vision care practitioner is to improve the patient's visual quality of life. As people age, vision becomes increasingly important and its maintenance, more critical. Advancing age brings increased visual problems from physiological and pathological causes. Corrective bifocals or trifocals are commonly prescribed to counteract the loss of amplitude of accommodation with age (presbyopia). Such corrections assist people in performing the myriad near tasks so essential to everyday living.

The incidence of diseases of the eye increases with age. Included in this group of diseases are open angle glaucoma, diabetic retinopathy, cataract, and age-related macular degeneration. There is also an increasing incidence of retinal detachment and peripheral retinal changes. Another common, although poorly understood, problem is the increasing number of individuals with dry-eye syndromes, in which both tear volume and content are altered. These highly uncomfortable anomalies are particularly common in people with arthritic conditions and present a major problem to the contact lens fitter.

Thus, good vision care is crucial to aging individuals. Their senses become less sharp, so what remains must be able to operate at or near capacity. It is obvious that there is a certain amount of redundancy, or excess capacity, in the system. This can be deduced from the great overlap of receptive fields in the visual system. Sommer et al. (1984) pointed out that before visual field changes are detected in glaucoma, approximately half the optic nerve fibers in a given eye are no longer functional. Although diagnostic techniques clearly require improvement, this finding points out the fact that even with substantial ganglion cell loss, visual function shows only modest degradation.

The Uniqueness of Each Aging Patient

One of the cornerstones of success in handling elderly patients is to remember that each is unique. Give each person adequate time to respond, and if possible, use vision test targets of higher luminance. These simple steps can greatly improve patient performance. Furthermore, take the time to listen carefully to the complaints of these patients. Elderly patients are often acute observers but either cannot properly express their concerns or hesitate to do so.

When studying elderly patients, we should not just study individuals who show ocular anomalies and diseases; we also should study those who maintain their visual and other capabilities to determine what is unique about them. In that uniqueness may well lie the means of improving performance among those showing visual loss. The same principle can be applied to the study of those who have lost sight, have low vision, or have experienced blindness. Some adapt to their conditions remarkably well and lead rich and meaningful lives, whereas others cannot be reconciled to their situations. Again, we must ask what is unique about those who succeed as a guide for those who are less successful.

There is no typical older individual, and there are vast differences between individual responses. Too much of our clinical knowledge is based on simple experience and too little, on orderly experimental investigation. Furthermore, in dealing with the aging population, we must not lose sight of the total individual. In the busy clinic or practice, we need to be sure that there is full commitment to the needs of these patients. Practitioners who serve the aging patient need to work with each other to optimize the success of individual patient care. We need to achieve not only visual goals, but also life goals. A case study of one of the author's patients illustrates this point in both a lesson and a warning (the names are fictitious):

> Mr. Brown had long-standing Fuchs' corneal dystrophy, dry-eye problems, some retinal problems, and a dense cataract in one eye. The second eye was essentially nonfunctional. An ophthalmologist had performed combined corneal transplantation and cataract surgery on the first eye. The first corneal transplant had failed, and the second had succeeded in the sense that part of the transplant remained clear; however, the corneal surface was highly irregular and astigmatic.
>
> Mr. Brown's problem had existed for some years, and prior to the surgical intervention in the one eye, he had been essentially blind. In that period Mr. Brown, a widower, had lived in a small flat above some stores in a rural Florida town. Each morning Mrs. Green brought him breakfast and chatted with him. Later in the morning the letter carrier brought up his mail, read it to him, and visited with him for a bit. At lunch Mrs. Black brought him a hot meal and stayed to chat. Most afternoons some other retired people came to visit, and in the evening Mr. Brown managed to find diversion with his radio.
>
> After surgery Mr. Brown was referred to me for visual correction. I managed to combine a piggyback hard contact lens system on top of a special soft contact lens with an inset well. The hard contact lens was contained in the well, centered on the eye, overlying the relatively clear area of the graft. Remarkably, I was able to take this man from hand motion detection (a very low visual response level) to something approximating 20/25 or 20/30 visual acuity in the one eye. With an occasional drop of saline to help the dry-eye condition and a pair of spectacle reading additions, he was able to read ordinary newsprint. In short, I had been successful in changing an essentially blind person to one capable of living a reasonably adequate and normal visual life. I was very pleased with myself for achieving this result, and Mr. Brown was pleased as well.
>
> Mr. Brown returned periodically for brief checkups to be sure the contact lenses and other visual corrections were performing properly, the corneal transplant did not show signs of rejection and remained clear, and the correction did not cause irritation. We would chat briefly about his situation and his visual condition, and he always assured me that he was doing just fine.
>
> However, now that he was seeing so well, Mrs. Green no longer brought him breakfast. The letter carrier put the mail in the mailbox, and Mrs. Black no longer brought lunch. His friends did not feel the social obligation of visiting him nearly as regularly. His entire social life changed, and Mr. Brown committed suicide.

This story illustrates a crucial concept: the vision care practitioner treats the individual, not just the eyes. I often think of this case when I have a moment of pride of achievement to make sure I have not forgotten some critical element in the care of a patient. Obviously, the goal is not just visual acuity, not just the extended field, not just the fit of the contact lens, and not just the advantage made possible by an aid to vision; the goal is the successful use of these corrections in the life process.

The key to quality of life is the optimization of function, the optimization of life-style, and the integrated whole being. Somehow, practitioners must insure that in achieving their goals, they do not overlook larger questions.

Special Problems with Pharmaceuticals

Pharmacology is an area that needs serious consideration by practitioners. Unfortunately, many elderly patients become nearly overwhelmed by the number of pharmaceutical agents they take and are often made ill by the side reactions. Furthermore, prescribers often pay too little attention to possible interactions between medications, the optimal schedule, and the form of drug delivery. This can result in frank personality changes, effects on the patient's alertness, disruption of daily schedules, and the like. The problem is often exacerbated by the fragmentation of care among providers and the patient's sometimes inadequate reporting of all medications taken.

Special Considerations in Correcting Vision Problems

Effects of Cataract Formation

A point often overlooked in the assessment of patients with monocular or binocular cataracts is the fact that in the process of cataract formation, the lens may absorb considerable water, swell, and then change yet again as fluid content varies in time. Changes of several diopters in the monocular refraction can occur. For each diopter of change in one eye, there can be up to 1.5 percent of binocular refractive aniseikonia. Thus, although often not considered, aniseikonia may well be part of the symptomatology of these patients. This is, of course, in addition to the veiling glare and other effects encountered with cataract.

It is often pointed out that patients with sub-capsular cataract have greater vision problems than those with nuclear cataract. This is true, but the reason has been poorly understood. If a bright point of light is shown to such patients, they often see multiple images. The lens must swell in segments (much like an orange is divided), and presumably the spokes of the cataract define these segments. In turn, these segments must act as prisms. A small pinhole pressed close to the eye will generally limit the image to one.

On the same subject, the visual acuity loss (and, no doubt, contrast sensitivity function alteration) can be surprisingly large for what seems to be modest corneal endothelial change. Such visual losses need to be studied. They may involve local lenslike, prismatic, or scattering effects. The greater the distance such changes occur from the retina, the more disruptive they can be for vision. The flip side of this argument is the sometimes surprisingly limited effects on vision of floaters or debris near the retina. Incidentally, the clinician should allow the patient with a modest retinal bleed to sit quietly in the office for a half-hour prior to the examination to allow gravity to act upon the debris and blood residue. Vision often appears to increase dramatically over such a time span.

Evaluation of Surgical Outcomes

One of the greatest challenges to the ophthalmic surgeon is to anticipate resultant vision after surgery. This is a major concern among corneal and cataract surgeons, as well as those performing vitrectomy. There are a dozen techniques for evaluating visual potential prior to surgery, each of varying value. In general, a negative finding on any test is noninformative, but a good result is promising. Available techniques include simple tests of projection of lights; two-point resolution threshold measures; blue-field entoptoscopy; flash ERG; visually evoked potential (VEP); analysis of speckle patterns; two-point interference tests; Maxwellian view projection of acuity charts (Potential Acuity Meter, or PAM); and, most recently, tests of hyperacuity (vernier visual acuity).

Why is this determination important? Simply put, the expectation of good vision by both the patient and surgeon after uncomplicated surgery is very high. There are few things more disruptive in the ophthalmologist's office than an unhappy patient—with a clear corneal graft and crystal sharp media (after cataract removal) with virtually no vision— passing through the busy waiting room. The waiting patients ("There but for the grace of God go I"), the patient ("the surgeon failed me"), and the physician ("I failed") are all agitated. These patients return again and again seeking a magic that is just not there. Thus, there is great pressure to anticipate the surgical result before the fact.

Given this, what do we mean by *good vision?* The whole literature is predicated on anticipating postsurgical Snellen visual acuity. However, this is really not enough. The clinician actually wants to know whether patients will be able to perform functionally those tasks of special importance to them. Will they be able to drive, read, sew, watch television, and so on? Thus, at issue is not only the few minutes of arc defining central foveal function and single-letter Snellen acuity; rather, the issue is whether there is reasonable visual acuity, central vision, and a workable visual field on the one hand or whether there is scotoma, eccentric viewing, possible poor prognosis, and any hint of metamorphopsia (possible retinal detachment, tumor, and so forth) on the other hand.

In our own laboratory we have been successfully studying hyperacuity or vernier acuity techniques as applied to this set of issues. Vernier acuity differs from Snellen acuity in that the clinician asks *where* one object is relative to a second one (and assumes the presence of two objects at the outset). In Snellen acuity tasks the clinician asks *how many* details are seen (resolution). Even in the presence of enormous image degradation, a person retains the capability to make vernier judgments. Unlike all other methods, no window through an opacity is needed for response (Enoch et al. 1985).

Corrections for Aphakia

Aphakia is a special area of interest to practitioners dealing with elderly patients. This field has changed rapidly with the advent of intraocular implant lenses to replace the eye's natural lens. In the future the vision care practitioner may deal less with the aphakic visual correction per se and more with induced aniseikonia after placement of the intraocular implant. Size differences can be the result of mixed anterior and posterior chamber implants, differences between an implanted lens and the natural eye lens, and so forth. Such effects as tilting and displacement of the implant also must not be overlooked. In fact, if one portion of an implant is not located in the lens capsule (posterior chamber implant), it is not unusual for the haptic to locate in the area of the ciliary sulcus and migrate into the ciliary body near or into contact with the great arterial circle of the iris. This results in displacement and tilt of the pseudophakic lens, which often can be detected by resultant spherical and cylindrical refractive changes that are unaccounted for. The small induced astigmatic component will have its plus corrective axis 90 degrees from the axis of lens alignment and insertion (Lakshminarayanan et al. forthcoming).

One set of issues not generally appreciated is the satisfaction of patients following surgery for cataract, vitrectomy, or corneal transplants (noncomplicated surgery, such as that for patients without resultant Irvine-Gass syndrome, graft clouding or rejection, metamorphopsia, and so on). The results of these surgeries are often dramatic; the change in vision, enormous; and, not without reason, the appreciation of the patient for the surgeon's capabilities, very substantial. However, often substantial monocular and binocular visual problems remain. Image sizes are altered; wavelength transmission may be quite different; and problems may be caused by binocular vision from cataract or other defects in the other eye or from resultant anisometropia, aniseikonia, induced astigmatism, and so forth. To make sure that such impediments to visual comfort and functional satisfaction do not limit a fine surgical result, the vision care practitioner should pursue such matters and seek to provide relief as needed. If there is anisometropia, it is important not to exacerbate possible aniseikonia. This can be achieved by matching base curves and lens thicknesses in both eyes, keeping vertex distances to a minimum, fitting bifocals a bit high, and having cylinders ground on the rear surface (minus format). If refractive aniseikonia is present, it should be addressed using the methods outlined by Brown and Enoch (1970). Slab-offs and Fresnel stick-on prisms should be considered as needed.

The maintenance of binocularity also may be a problem. Often these patients have experienced monocular vision for years because of their ocular condition and would benefit from the adjustment of one eye for seeing at the far distance and one eye, for near distance. Adequate ultraviolet filtering should be provided. The practitioner needs to help the patient adjust to changes in object size, mobility problems, and so on.

A common complaint of patients with spectacle refractive corrections for aphakia is that the spectacles are uncomfortable, slide down the nose, or both. Spectacle design is important to the success of optical corrections. Contemporary design considerations of frames and lenses are covered at length in Chapter 18.

A very common problem experienced by aphakic elderly people fitted with contact lenses is relatively dry eyes and a frank lessening of tolerance to discomfort. However, when a corneal section is made during the course of cataract surgery, the contact lens fitter encounters an interesting set of reactions. A corneal section or corneal transplant severely affects the sensory nerves serving the cornea. Contact lens fitting should not begin until the eye is quiet following surgery, but the initial fitting of the contact lens turns out to be simplified because of lack of corneal sensitivity. However, this makes it important to follow the patient closely to be sure there are no adverse reactions. At a certain time (many months to a year after surgery), corneal sensitivity returns, and the patient experiences a characteristic period of modest discomfort even though an excellent contact lens fit has been achieved. The optometrist must be sensitive to these changes.

Another special problem of the aging patient is manual dexterity and stability and their effect on the patient's ability to insert the contact lens. The visibility of the contact lens once it is off the eye is also a concern. Of course, extended wear contact lenses offer a ready solution to these problems. Unfortunately, all too often dry-eye syndromes or a contact lens correction that is too thick makes such an option of limited use. Great suction may build up between a soft contact lens and the cornea of the dry-eye patient and cause considerable difficulty for the patient seeking to remove the lens from the eye. A drop or two of saline often does wonders, saves the corneal epithelium, and promotes considerable patient comfort. The problems of fitting aging patients with contact lenses are considered in Chapter 19.

The practitioner should never overlook cosmetic factors. The elderly have great pride and are concerned about their appearance and apparent vitality. In every instance they will opt for a visual aid that is less visible or that sets them off less from others, if at all possible. In this sense they are no different from younger patients. Practitioners should not overlook these patients' desires to seem attractive to individuals of the opposite sex and should never make light of them. In all phases of the care of the aged, the individual needs to be handled with dignity and understanding.

Finally, eye and vision care practitioners need to consider hearing as well as vision in optimizing patient performance. Adjusting the response in both ears to provide correct spatial localization is important if hearing is to play a major part in mobility. Questions of compliance with instructions, assistance with medications and visual aids (insertion and removal of contact lenses, lens cleaning, and so forth), and teaching the use of aids are all crucial factors in successful patient management.

Institutions and Other Patient Care Settings
When treating aging patients, among the complications encountered is the necessity of sometimes dealing with an institution within which they reside. The optometrist must be prepared to interact with the administration and the service personnel of the institution, as well as with the patient, if good vision care is the goal (see Chapter 16).

The practitioner must also be willing to travel to the patient's home or to some external setting to provide services for the special needs of at least some of these patients. Practitioners become so fixed in their ways that they often overlook this simple approach to problems. Not only can this flexibility help the individual patient; it also can help the practitioner gain added insights into patient handling. For example, the author once examined a quadruple amputee and found little visually wrong when testing the patient in the office. A visit to the home setting, however, revealed that the problem was not one of clear vision but of not being able to see through the spectacle correction. While the patient lay prone or semiprone, the glasses were pointed the wrong way, and the patient could not adjust them. This issue was not considered in the office setting, where the patient was seated upright and comfortably in a wheelchair. Problems and their solutions associated with examination methods out of the office are described in Chapter 20.

Need for Interdisciplinary Cooperation
The fragmentation of the delivery of health care to the elderly is extremely serious. If there is a single area most lacking in research, it is the general question of how to handle the rehabilitation of elderly visually impaired patients. The optometrist, ophthalmologist, rehabilitation counselor, social worker, and other professionals must coordinate their efforts and communicate. Health care practitioners have no clear idea of when it is best to start certain therapeutic measures. For example, when vision is lost in age-related maculopathy, should visual rehabilitative therapy be initiated immediately or only after a period of time? When is eccentric viewing best taught, and what are the preferred strategies? Too much of the approach to these patients is based on anecdotal reports. Another area of concern, the functional rehabilitation of the patient with binocular coordination problems, is discussed in Chapter 21.

Another important area demanding coordination of effort is the development and provision of visual aids for the visually impaired. This complex area has been in the backwaters of research for years but is served by dedicated people. It requires major infusions of effort and money. Often the patients' resources do not match our capability to help them. Practitioners are frequently frustrated by their inability to invest in devices of substantial cost that may be of assistance but for which there are no funds available.

Often the development of new procedures and devices is chaotic, with no orderly thought given to the special needs of the patient. Engineers or well-meaning scientists develop devices they think will benefit patients. Such devices may or may not meet specific needs, may be limited in use to a few individuals, and may or may not be cost effective. Here is an opportunity for an orderly scientific approach that involves interdisciplinary contact, a specific review of the needs of the patients, and development designed to meet those needs. This area has been neglected far too long. Well-defined research and development needs are described in Chapter 22.

At a time in history exploding with technological advances—where all manner of electronic interfaces are available for modulating, altering, and interacting with images and where the use of voice synthesis is common—we should be farther along in the development of appropriate aids for the elderly visually impaired. We need to find adequate resources to provide the necessary equipment, visual aids, and additions to people's lives to maintain their life quality and productiveness to the greatest extent possible. More effective institutions, centers of research, and centers of learning are necessary to seek meaningful ways for ameliorating the conditions of the elderly and helping them meet life's challenges.

References

Brown, R., and J. M. Enoch. "Combined Rules of Thumb in Aniseikonic Prescriptions." *American Journal of Ophthalmology* 69 (1970): 118.

Enoch, J. M.; R. A. Williams; E. A. Essock; and M. Fendick. "Hyperacuity: A Promising Means of Evaluating Vision through Cataract." In *Progress in Retinal Research,* Vol. 4, eds. N. N. Osborne and G. J. Chader. Elmsford, N.Y.: Pergamon Press, 1985, pp. 67–88.

Lakshminarayanan, V.; J. M. Enoch; T. Raasch; B. Crawford; and R. W. Nygaard. "Refractive Changes Induced by Intraocular Lens Tilt Longitudinal Displacement." *Archives of Ophthalmology.* Forthcoming.

Sommer, A.; H. Quigley; N. Miller; A. Robin; and S. Arkell. "Prospective Assessment of the Nerve Fiber Layer in Glaucoma." *Investigative Ophthalmology and Visual Science 25 (1984): 193.*

Chapter 9

Ocular Implications of Systemic Disease in the Elderly

David M. Cockburn

Man's alloted span of three score years and ten remains little altered since biblical times, the most significant change being that many more people live out this span to reach four score years and confirm the further prophesy that these years shall be lived in sorrow and pain. The age-related changes in bodily function appear to occur in a linear manner, interrupted at times by disease, which then superimposes a steplike deterioration. Disease in the aged is frequently a complex of multiple disease states, perhaps commencing with one organ system but affecting other systems in a cascading sequence. The ocular system, of course, is included in this process. The burden of these diseases, added to the social and mobility problems of the aged, bring in turn depression, mental degeneration, and rapidly increasing senility. Indeed, the first manifestations of systemic disease in the elderly are likely to mimic senility, but they have the potential to be reversed by appropriate care.

Problems that occur in the diagnosis of disease in the aged include a tendency for patients to ignore the symptoms because they believe these are inevitable consequences of aging. Decreased cognizance, which is often an early sign of systemic disease, also may cause patients to ignore their symptoms and fail to seek attention. The mode of presentation of both systemic and ocular diseases is likely to be different in the aged patient from that which is typical in younger subjects. This is particularly true of diabetes, drug intoxication, and thyroid disease. Another group of diseases is common only in elderly patients and occurs only rarely in the mature or younger-age groups; examples of these diseases are basal cell carcinoma, Paget's disease, Parkinson's disease, and temporal arteritis. A well-designed program of screening for disease in the

elderly must reflect these factors.

Samples of patients seeking optometric care are not necessarily similar to those seeking general medical, hospital, or even ophthalmologic care; in consequence, epidemiologic data derived from these sources may not apply to optometric patients. Patients of optometrists tend to be older than the general population; a consecutive series of patients of one optometrist in private practice had a mean age of 55.2 years (Cockburn 1982), whereas the community from which it was drawn had a mean age of 32 years (Cameron 1982, 91). It is also reasonable to expect that patients of optometrists are more healthy than those seeking other health care, since they are a self-selecting group who are not yet subject to being monopolized by the medical system. These unique characteristics of optometric patients point to the need to be aware of the very early signs and symptoms of the diseases that are likely to occur in the aged. Of course, special attention should be given to the detection of those ocular signs that suggest systemic disease.

The selection of diseases to be discussed in this chapter was influenced by a number of factors, which include the following:

- The disease should be significantly associated with the processes of aging and be found most commonly in the aged.
- The samples of patients attending optometrists should contain a reasonable yield of the disease state.
- The disease should be capable of being recognized during an optometric examination by techniques that are appropriate to the optometric role in the health care services of developed countries.
- The disease should have a potential to cause

significant morbidity or mortality.

- Some form of effective therapy to cure or relieve the effects of the disease should exist.

Optometrists have an obligation to insure that their patients do not suffer any avoidable visual loss or systemic effects of diseases that can be recognized during the ocular examination and that can be treated successfully. To discharge this obligation requires a detailed knowledge of the diseases of the elderly and constant vigilance.

Cardiovascular Disease

Stroke

Stroke is the condition in which failure of cerebral vascular supply results in permanent neurological damage. Stroke has an incidence of approximately 1 case in every 500 people each year (Howells 1982, 170; McDowell 1975, 647; Warlow 1981), and it is more likely to occur in older age groups. Some 92 percent of all strokes occur in patients aged 50 years or over (McDowell 1975, 647). One-third of stroke cases recover to the extent that they can resume a normal life, one-third are seriously and permanently incapacitated, and one-third die (McDowell, 1975, 647; Warlow 1981). Cerebrovascular disease is the cause of approximately 13 percent of all deaths, based on the 1979 international classification of diseases. It was second only to ischemic heart disease as a cause of death in Australia during 1980 to 1981, and 85 percent of these deaths occurred in subjects aged 65 years or older (Howells 1982, 170).

Many subjects who subsequently develop stroke experience early symptoms over a period of time; these symptoms result from brief episodes of cerebral ischemia of a duration or extent that falls short of causing permanent neurological damage. The attacks last from a few minutes to several hours; they are characterized by their sudden onset, patterns of neurological involvement, and complete recovery. Often the attacks are repeated several or many times in an individual. These episodes are referred to as *transient ischemic attacks (TIAs)*.

There is ample and convincing evidence that TIAs are forewarnings of more serious cerebrovascular compromise leading to stroke (Acheson and Hutchinson 1964; Duncan et al. 1976; Fein 1978; Field and Lemak 1976; Herman et al. 1980; Wishnant, Matsumoto, and Elueback 1973). There is a special risk of stroke

in the first few weeks following the initial TIA (Warlow 1981).

The effectiveness of treatment to prevent stroke in patients having TIAs is still subject to controversy (Muuronen and Kaste 1982). However, there is evidence that anticoagulation therapy—usually aspirin in small quantities—is effective (Harrison et al. 1971; Muuronen and Kaste 1982; Olsson, Muller, and Berneli 1976), especially in males (Canadian Cooperation Study Group 1978). Surgical repair of atheromatous lesions in the internal carotid artery (endarterectomy) is effective in the elimination of TIAs and the delay or prevention of stroke (McDowell 1975, 647).

The vascular supply to the brain derives from the right and left internal carotid arteries anteriorly, whereas the posterior portion is supplied by the vertebral arteries, which join to form the basilar artery. Insufficiency of supply in one of these vessel systems results in neurological deficits, the nature of which is determined by the watershed of the involved artery. However, the signs and symptoms are modified by the availability of an alternative blood supply through anastamosing vessels distal to the site of obstruction. The most important anastamosis, which is at the base of the brain, takes the form of the arterial circle of Willis; by way of the two posterior communicating arteries and the anterior communicating artery, effectively links the vertebrobasilar and carotid artery distributions. Likened to building practices, it could be said that this arrangement is architecturally brilliant, but the plumber misread the plans, since the communicating arteries are frequently absent or so poorly represented that they are ineffective should one of the major channels be blocked (Sedzimer 1959). There is also considerable anatomic variation in the vascular arrangement of many of the major cerebral vessels (Riggs and Rupp 1963).

The signs and symptoms of TIA are determined by the cerebral distribution of the affected vessel and the extent to which alternative blood supply is available. It follows that attacks experienced by an individual follow a similar pattern, but that attacks vary between individuals, even when the site of obstruction is similar.

Visual symptoms frequently are experienced during TIAs, a fact that might be expected in view of the extreme sensitivity of the visual system to oxygen deficits and its dependence for supply on both the vertebrobasilar system and the carotid arteries. The classic TIA of carotid origin is ipsilateral amaurosis fugax and contralateral paresthesia, or paresis of the face and/or upper or lower limbs. When the dominant hemisphere is involved, speech disorders are also common (dysarthria). These symptoms do not necessarily occur at the same time. In vertebrobasilar-induced TIA, the visual disturbance tends to take the form of homonymous hemianopias or photopsias as a result of cortical ischemia; the nonvisual symptoms are chiefly the result of brain stem ischemia and involve the disruption of muscle coordination. Drop attacks commonly occur in basilar territory TIAs; the patient falls without losing consciousness because of loss of postural tone. Figure 9–1 illustrates the signs and symptoms that might be suspected in TIAs associated with insufficiency of the individual arteries. Table 9–1 shows the prevalence of the various signs and symptoms

of TIAs and of cervical bruits experienced by 82 subjects selected from 1,000 consecutive patients aged 50 years of more who visited an optometrist (Cockburn 1983).

Symptoms of TIA are unlikely to be mentioned voluntarily by patients during history taking, particularly when they are other than visual in nature. Even previous attacks of amaurosis fugax are readily forgotten by the patient; only in 1 of 17 cases was this symptom volunteered prior to the clinician's asking a specific question relating to the symptom (Cockburn 1983). If patients having TIAs are to be identified, it is important that history taking include questions designed to elicit the symptoms of TIA, including those having a transient visual nature.

Showers of emboli derived from ulcerated atherosclerotic lesions of the heart or great vessels proximal to the cranium may cause stroke or TIAs when they lodge in cerebral vessels. Those that traverse the carotid system

Figure 9–1

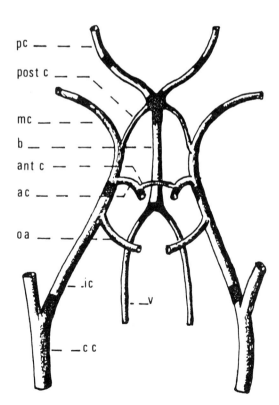

**Vertebrobasilar System
TIA Involving
Homonymous Field Loss**

Posterior Cerebral Artery
Homonymous hemianopia
  with sparing of fixation
Disturbance of visual
  recognition and memory

Basilar artery
Dizziness
Diplopia
Vertigo
Drop attacks
Oscillopsia
Nystagmus

**Carotid Artery System
TIA Involving Unilateral
Hemiplegia Ischemic Pain**

Middle cerebral artery
Homonymous hemianopia
  with splitting of fixation
Hemiplegia or hemiparesis;
  hemiparesthesia of
  contralateral face, hand or
  arm

Anterior cerebral artery
Hemiplegia or hemiparesis;
  hemiparesthesia of
  contralateral leg

Ophthalmic artery
Amaurosis fugax or unilateral
  blindness
Central retinal artery
  occlusion
Venous stasis retinopathy
Ischemic optic neuropathy
Unilateral cataract
Rubeosis iridis

Schematic Drawing of the Cerebrovascular Arterial Supply Showing Common Sites for Occlusions to Develop (Solid Black) and the Signs and Symptoms Resulting from Occlusions of Major Arterial Branches. pc = posterior cerebral artery; post c = posterior communicating artery; mc = middle cerebral artery; b = basilar artery; ant c = anterior communicating artery; ac = anterior cerebral artery; oa = ophthamic artery; ic = internal carotid artery; v = vertebral artery; and cc = common carotic artery.

Table 9-1
Prevalence of the Symptoms of TIAs and of Cervical Bruits Detected
in 82 Patients Selected from 1,000 Consecutive Patients Aged 50 or Older

Symptom	Prevalence	Percentage of Sample
Cervical bruit (carotid, 27; transmitted, 3)	30	3.0
Paresthesia of hands or feet	28	2.8
Drop attacks	23	2.3
Transient visual field disturbance	22	2.2
Dysarthria	20	2.0
Paresis	18	1.8
Amaurosis fugax	17	1.7
Dizziness	6	0.6
Syncope	6	0.6
Numbness of lips or tongue	4	0.4
Ischemic pain	3	0.3
Diplopia	1	0.1
Hearing loss	1	0.1
Memory loss	1	0.1

Source: Adapted with permission from D. M. Cockburn. "Signs and Symptoms of Stroke and Impending Stroke in a Series of Optometric Patients." *American Journal of Optometry and Physiological Optics* 60, no. 9 (1983): 749–753.

may enter the ophthalmic artery to cause temporary, permanent, or incomplete blockage of the short posterior ciliary arteries or the central retinal artery. Emboli lodging in the ciliary and choroidal vessels cause anterior ischemic optic neuropathy (Hayreth 1975, 115), since the region of the optic disc depends on the choroidal circulation for its nutrition. The emboli that reach the central retinal artery may be seen as white fibrinous deposits in the vessel (Fisher plugs) or as bright crystals of cholesterol (Hollenhorst's plaques) located at arterial bifurcations (see Figure 9-2).

Larger emboli lodging in the central retinal artery cause sudden visual loss and the ophthalmoscopic picture of a white infarcted inner retinal layer with retention of the normal red color at the macula as a cherry red spot. The emboli may be seen at major bifurcations, but they usually lyse rapidly and disappear after several days (see Figure 9-3).

Atherosclerotic lesions may affect that intraocular portion of the central retinal artery close to the disc, since this portion of the vessel retains a lamina. These lesions occasionally appear as dense yellow sheathing that replaces the normal vessel wall; the lumen of the vessel may remain patent, although no blood column is visible (see Figure 9-4). The finding of atherosclerotic changes in retinal vessels suggests widespread intracranial atherosclerosis.

The gradual reduction of the vascular supply to the retina may lead to retinal ischemia and venous stasis retinopathy. The most common cause of the restriction of flow is atheromatous disease of the carotid artery, which results in ipsilateral ocular ischemia that resembles central retinal vein thrombosis. The retinal veins are dilated, tortuous, and often have hemorrhages lying parallel to their courses. Other retinal hemorrhages (predominantly dot and blot hemorrhages in the deeper retinal layers), together with microaneurysms and cotton wool patches, complete the retinal picture. The optic disc is usually hyperemic (see Figure 9-5).

The absence of hard exudate and the unilateral presentation should differentiate venous stasis retinopathy and diabetic retinopathy, which would be bilateral in presentation at this florid stage of development (Kearns and Hollenhorst 1963). The clinician should consider a diagnosis of carotid artery insufficiency when these signs are present. Retinal signs of vascular insufficiency were found in 24 of 1,000 consecutive patients aged 50 or over; the prevalence of individual signs is shown in Table 9-2.

The most consistent clinical finding in atheromatous disease of the carotid artery is the presence of a carotid bruit (Wilson and Ross-Russell 1977). This is a sound that is heard on auscultation of the region overlying the caro-

Figure 9–2

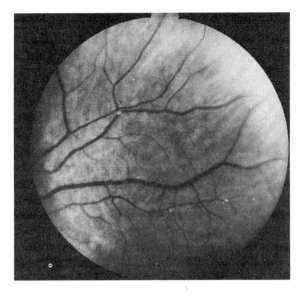

Multiple Bright Refractile Cholesterol Emboli Located at Arteriolar Bifurcations (Hollenhorst's Plaques)

Figure 9–4

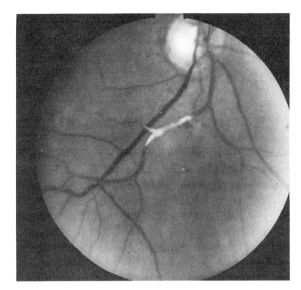

Bright, Scintillating, Yellow Opacification of a Retinal Arteriolar Wall.

Figure 9–3

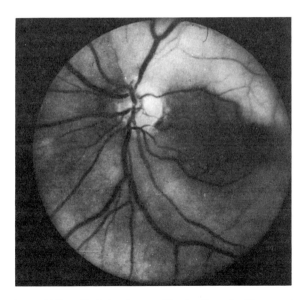

Large Yellow Embolus Located in the Superior Temporal Arteriole Where It Crosses under the Vein. Note the pale infarcted retina in the region served by this occluded vessel.

Figure 9–5

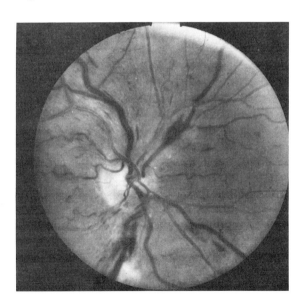

Venous Stasis Retinopathy Resulting from Restriction of the Internal Carotid Artery. Note the dilated retinal veins, nerve fiber layer hemorrhages, and a cotton wool patch inferior to the disc.

tid artery bifurcation. This sign was detected in 61 (6.1 percent) of the 1,000 patients 50 years or over (Cockburn 1983). These sounds may be due to a lesion in the carotid artery or be transmitted from the heart, aorta, or innominate or subclavian arteries. The distinction is usually possible on the grounds that a bruit of carotid origin is louder over the site of bifurcation in the neck, whereas transmitted bruits are heard with greater intensity lower in the artery and at a maximum in the region of the subclavian fossa at the base of the neck. Of the carotid bruits just mentioned, 44 (4.4 percent) were carotid; the remaining 17 (1.7 percent) were judged to be transmitted. In 27 cases of carotid bruit, the patient also experienced TIAs. The high yield of this important sign in an aging population of patients of an optometrist justifies the inclusion of carotid auscultation in the examination of patients, especially those in older age groups and those having the additional risk factors of stroke.

Table 9-2
Prevalence of Retinal Signs of Vascular Insufficiency Detected in 24 of 1,000 Consecutive Patients Aged 50 or Older

Sign	Prevalence
Hollenhorst's plaques	6
Venous stasis retinopathy	5
Central retinal artery plaques or emboli at or proximal to second bifurcation	5
Central retinal vein thrombosis	4
Occlusion of central retinal artery	3
Occlusion of branch retinal artery	3
Tributary retinal vein thrombosis	2
Hemorrhage on the disc	1

There are a number of risk factors for or causes of stroke, the more common being athero-sclerosis, diabetes, hypertension, heart disease and dysrhythmias, and the various forms of peripheral arteritis (Kannel 1971; McDowell 1975, 647; Veshima et al. 1980; Warlow 1981). Atherosclerosis, probably a universal and inevitable aging change in the major arteries, is undoubtedly the principal cause of nonhemorrhagic stroke. Atheromatous disease is very commonly present in advanced form in association with both diabetes and hypertension. In fact, diabetes or hypertension is present in over two-thirds of all stroke patients (McDowell 1975, 647). It follows that all patients having these diseases, especially patients of advanced years, should be carefully examined for evidence of impending stroke. This implies a careful evaluation of the history in searching for TIAs, routine cervical auscultation, and evaluation of fundus signs of vascular changes.

The clinician who is aware of the risk factors of stroke and who carefully assesses elderly patients will be rewarded by a relatively high yield of positive findings; as a result of

appropriate referral and treatment, the optometrist retains a grateful patient whose declining years are accompanied by retained physical and mental faculties.

Hypertension
Because hypertension is a disease defined in terms of a continuous variable, its prevalence in a community will depend largely on the definition adopted. The World Health Organization (1962) recommends the adoption of a broad standard in which hypertension is defined as systolic pressure of 160 mm Hg or more and/or diastolic pressure of 95 mm Hg or more. Surveys of the prevalence of hypertension also will be influenced by the selection of subjects; the methods used to measure blood pressure; and environmental, psychological, and geographic considerations. It is also necessary to take into account subjects who are being treated for the condition and whose pressures would be classed as within normal limits as a result of successful therapy. A survey of adults in the small community of Queenscliff, Australia, encompasssed 74 percent of the population of 1,456 adults. Using the WHO criteria and including hypertensives already under treatment, it was found that 437 (30 percent) were hypertensive; of these, 161 (11 percent) of the sample were previously unaware of their condition (Christie, McPherson, and Vivian 1976). In the United States the situation is similar: Stamler (1970, 8) summarizes the evidence of several surveys as follows: "Of the almost 20 million persons with hypertension in the United States, about half are undetected; of the half known, no more than half are receiving long term care from physicians; and of those on therapy, only about half are receiving satisfactory care in terms of the simplest minimum criterion, reduction of blood pressure below hypertensive levels."

The prevalence of hypertension is related to age; in the Queenscliff study, the prevalence was lowest in the group aged 25 to 34 (4.8 percent); it rose to 24.4 percent in the group aged 55 to 64, but declined again to 19.6 percent in subjects aged 65 or over. Especially in its early years, hypertension is symptomless; the patient is comfortable and appears to be well. This benign presentation, together with the high prevalence of hypertension, insures a continuing diagnostic challenge. The significance of this challenge will depend on the morbid effects that untreated hypertension has on its victims and the ability of treatment to delay or prevent these effects. In the special case of the aged, practitioners should examine critically the diagnostic criteria, signs, prognosis, and treatment of hypertension, since these may not be the same as in young and middle-aged subjects.

The levels of both diastolic and systolic blood pressures have long been recognized by life insurance companies as an excellent predictor of life expectancy. Actuarial figures indicate that there is no point at which increased risk of death commences; the risk of cardiovascular-related mortality simply increases as blood pressure rises. The lowest mortality was found in subjects having systolic pressures 5 to 15 mm Hg below average for their age and among those having below-average diastolic pressures (Society of Actuaries 1959). There is no dividing line between normotension and hypertension (Pickering 1972).

The problems of establishing treatment strategies for hypertension are compounded by the rise of diastolic and, more particularly, systolic pressures with age (Page and Sidd 1972), as well as the fact that females have a higher threshold for resultant cardiovascular damage than males. The actuarial figures relate to predictions mainly for young to middle-aged males. However, these figures show that for moderate to severe hypertension, the risk for aged subjects, as a percentage of increased mortality is actually less than for the younger subjects (Society of Actuaries 1959). It is as though high blood pressure in youth and middle-age imposes a serious threat to middle and long-term survival because of the length of time it has to cause complications, whereas its acquisition in old age is less serious, since other cases of death intervene before hypertensive complications occur. It appears that there is a well-established association between high blood pressure and increased morbidity, but does this association imply a true cause-and-effect relationship? Does the reduction of blood pressure improve the patient's prognosis, and does any improvement extend to the aged hypertensive?

Treatment of moderate to severe hypertension in males has been shown to markedly reduce cardiovascular-related morbidity (Veterans Administration 1970). However, it should be noted that in this trial, the treated subjects had a mean age of 50.5 years, and treatment appeared to benefit those subjects under 50 years of age more than those aged 50 or over. Similar trials conducted in samples drawn from an aged population are not available, and we must rely on clinical experience rather than firm evidence to evaluate the benefit of reducing blood pressure in the aged patient. Chalmers (1977, 7) advises treating diastolic pressures in excess of 110 mm Hg "except perhaps the very old"; Beevers (1982), while pointing out that there is no evidence to suggest that treatment is beneficial in the age group over 70, also recommends treating diastolic pressure in excess of 110 mm Hg.

Treatment of hypertension in the age group over 70 frequently is administered because of symptoms that are not related to the hypertension; in fact, these symptoms can be made worse by potent hypertensive drugs (Peart 1975, 989). Some physicians believe that in the absence of proof, treatment is effective in providing a more comfortable and longer life for the elderly. Raised blood pressure in aged patients should not be treated unless it is the result of malignant hypertension. This advice is underscored by the finding that 10 percent of all admissions to geriatric departments in the United Kingdom were caused by drug side effects and that it is not uncommon for geriatricians to find that their greatest therapeutic successes are achieved by stopping drugs prescribed by other physicians (Denham 1981). The opposing view is that hypertension in the elderly should be reduced to around 160/90 mm Hg (Niarchos 1980), and that this therapy will reduce the incidence of stroke and congestive heart failure (Welzel 1982).

The controversy surrounding treatment of an elderly patient must be resolved by the attending physician after the patient's overall condition has been considered rather than a set of numbers representing blood pressure. To make correct decisions, the physician needs as much evidence as is available on the state of the organs that are the targets for damage caused by hypertension. The retinal tissues and their supporting vascular system are such a target organ and provide a unique opportunity for direct and noninvasive assessment of complications. The ability to make useful assessments of this kind is built upon continuing experience in examining the fundus, reinforced by knowledge of intercurrent disease, level of blood pressure, and the patient's age. Upon weighing these factors, the optometrist is in a position to assist the physician in the management of the elderly hypertensive patient.

Ocular Involvements. The retina is limited in its response to the various insults to which it can be subjected by disease; as a consequence, no ophthalmoscopic signs can be said to be pathognomonic of systemic hypertension. Moreover, many of the signs that in the more youthful eye have high specificity for hypertension are commonly found in the eyes of elderly subjects having blood pressure at or below mean levels for their age. Similarly, an acute rise in blood pressure may affect younger, more adaptable retinal arterioles in a quite different fashion from that of the sclerosed vasculature of the aged fundus. The indications of damage sustained by the retinal vasculature in the aged are therefore somewhat different from those found in the young and middle-aged hypertensive subject. Table 9–3 lists the retinal signs of systemic hypertension, together with indications of the efficiency of each sign in ophthalmoscopic detection of hypertension and its allied conditions. The table shows these estimates for young to middle-aged and elderly patients separately.

In the aged patient, the most significant signs are those that demonstrate advanced damage to the retinal vasculature; these may be the direct result of hypertension or be due to arteriosclerosis and arteriolarsclerosis, metabolic disease, or disorders of blood constituents. Whatever the primary cause of the vascular lesions, hypertension is a frequent accompaniment. In the presence of such lesions, blood pressure status should be reviewed carefully. Where blood pressure levels are above 110 diastolic, 170 systolic, or both, a gradual and moderate reduction of these levels is likely to benefit the patient. Whereas cotton wool patches and papilledemas are the hallmarks of severe and malignant hypertension, these developments are exceedingly rare in the elderly (Hodkinson 1981). The valuable signs of vascular breakdown are those that herald impending thrombosis of the veins or occlusion of arteries. Therefore, the practitioner should search carefully for banking of the retinal veins distal to arteriovenous crossings, arterial/arteriolar plaques, the development of shunt vessels, or microaneurysms. When the blood-retinal barrier already has been compromised, the important and common signs in the aged are hemorrhages of both dot and blot and nerve fiber layer types, although the latter are the more typical of hypertensive damage. Macular edema also may be caused by leakage of retinal vessels; however, it is more likely that the source of this

problem is the choriod as a result of senile changes in Bruch's membrane. Venous thrombosis typically results in sheathing of the vessel, which remains long after compensation has taken place (see Figure 9–6). Should these signs be discovered in an elderly patient, the attending physician should be informed of the findings in order to review the patient's overall condition in the light of evidence of vascular involvement.

Figure 9–6

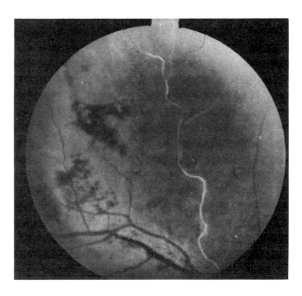

Venular Sheathing Following Thrombosis of the Vessel Approximately 12 Months Previously. Hemorrhages indicate current venular obstruction in adjacent vessels.

Whether or not to treat the elderly hypertensive and to what therapeutic goals remains a matter of controversy. However, in view of the general clinical impression that lowering of the blood pressure reduces vascular and renal complications, it appears reasonable to lower pressures gradually in the elderly patient (Tucker 1980). A general guide might be to treat patients having diastolic pressures of 105 mm HG or greater and those having diastolic pressures between 90 and 104 mm Hg if there is target organ damage, a family history of hypertensive complications, diabetes, raised cholestrol levels, elevated systolic pressures, or the patient smokes (Lucas and Omar 1980). The therapeutic aims of the internist should be a symptom-free patient having blood pressure around 160/90 (Niarchos 1980).

Table 9–3

Ocular Fundus Signs of Hypertension and Related Systemic Disease Showing the Pathophysiological Correlates of the Signs and an Estimate of Diagnostic Efficiency for Subjects Young to Middle-Aged and the Elderly

Ophthalmic Sign of Hypertension or Associated Condition	Pathophysiolocial Correlates	Efficiency as a Sign in Young to Middle-Aged	Efficiency as a Sign in the Aged
Diffuse arteriolar narrowing	Narrowing due to spasm of the vessel wall. Potentially reversible in young subjects.	A difficult sign to evaluate.	Attenuation of vessels occurs commonly with age. Not a reliable indicator.
Focal constriction of arterioles	Localized regions of passive arteriolar dilation alternating with local spasm.	A very specific and sensitive sign of hypertension in this age group.	Aged but otherwise healthy vessels often have this sign. Not a reliable indicator.
Straightening of arterioles	Occurrence in conjunction with diffuse narrowing from constriction of vessel; also secondary vascular occlusion and following compensation. May also occur in toxic states.	Only reliable if comparison is possible with previous appearance.	Not a reliable indicator.
Venular tortuosity	Stasis of flow through arterial insufficiency or venous occlusion. May signify macular edema when at posterior pole.	Difficult to evaluate, but very significant when present. Occurs in diabetes and many blood dyscrasias.	A reliable sign, especially in association with other signs (banking and hemorrhages).
Silver wire reflexes	Reflection of light from arteriolar wall accentuated in sclerosis of the vessel, which often is associated with hypertension.	Very poor specificity and difficult to assess. Of use only when noted in younger subjects.	Occurs in age as a senile change.
Arterial/arteriolar plaques	Atheromatous change in the artery on the disc or adjacent to the disc. Thrombi from heart carotid or great vessels. Arteriolar sclerosis due to hyalinization of vessel wall.	Very important indication of vascular damage, often associated with hypertension.	An important and reliable sign. Treatment of associated hypertension is justified.

Table 9-3 continued

Sheathing of veins	Fatty degeneration of vein following an occlusion or inflammation. The channel may recanalize and be associated with the development of shunt vessels.	Venous occlusions occur commonly in association with hypertension. An important sign of local and/or systemic disease.
Microaneurysms	Localized ballooning of the capillaries, venules, or arterioles. Occurs in diabetic retinopathy and following venous occlusions.	Uncommon in hypertension alone, but very common in diabetes. A useful sign of possible accompanying hypertension in diabetes and other vascular disorders. A highly significant sign.
Arteriovenous nicking (Gunn's sign)	Vein compressed at the point of arteriovenous crossing by a sclerosed arteriole or venule. The vein may be depressed into the retinal layers, which obscure it at the point of opacification of the arteriolar wall. Due to hyaline changes that obscure the vein.	Occurs in almost all senile fundi. Of little use as an indicator of disease unless associated with banking.
Banking	Restriction of the venous return distal to the site of arteriovenous crossing. Causes distension of the vessel. Commonly precedes thrombotic occlusion.	Confirms Gunn's sign (see the previous category) and is a very reliable sign of impending retinal vascular damage, which is often due to hypertension or related disease.
Shunt vessels	Dilation of capillary channels to form shunts to compensate for partial or total venous occlusions. Often seen in association with banking or sheathing.	Indicates serious previous or current vascular insufficiency. Often associated with hypertension.
Dot and blot hemorrhages	Leakage of blood into the outer plexiform layer or nuclear layers of the retina. Indicates breakdown of blood retinal barrier in the deep capillary plexus.	Common in diabetes and in venous thrombosis. These diseases commonly are associated with hypertension. An important sign that requires evaluation.
Flame hemorrhages	Bleeding from superficial capillary layer.	Hypertension is the most common cause, but it also occurs in diabetes, venous thrombosis, anemia, papillidema, papillitis, sickle cell disease, and the blood dyscrasias.

Subretinal hemorrhages	Leakage of blood through Bruch's membrane from a choroidal source or from new vessels that have penetrated under the retinal pigment epithelium.	A serious sign often indicating the onset of disciform degeneration. May be associated with hypertension.	An indication of serious underlying vascular disturbance. May be associated with hypertension.
Preretinal hemorrhages	Hemorrhages that are usually due to rupture of newly formed vessels arising from the retina or the disc, and occasionally due to breakthrough by a large choroidal hemorrhage.	Part of the spectrum of diabetic retinopathy. Diabetes and hypertension often coexist, making this an important sign. May occur subsequent to venous thrombosis.	Proliferative diabetic retinopathy is rare in the elderly. Usually denotes old venous thrombosis or fragility of retinal vessels from arteriosclerosis; both may be associated with hypertension.
Papilledema	Noninflammatory swelling of the nerve head because of stasis of circulation, interruption of axoplasmic transport, or both. Commonly associated with increased intracranial pressure.	Rarely seen in clinical practice as a sign of hypertension, but is a serious sign in advanced cases. Other causes should be assumed in mild to moderate hypertensives.	In the elderly, it probably never occurs as a result of hypertension. Seek other causes.
Cotton wool patches (soft exudates)	Edema of the nerve fiber layer resulting from microinfarcts of this region. Potentially reversible.	Most common cause is accelerated hypertension and diabetes. Not likely to be found in mild to moderate hypertension. Also occurs in venous stasis retinopathy, papilledema, and systemic lupus erythematosus.	Not found in the moderately elevated blood pressures usual in the aged. However, it is a sign that requires investigation.
Hard exudates	Serum lipid deposits in the outer plexiform layer or partly phagocytosed remains of this layer. May remain permanently or resolve over a long period.	Most common in diabetes, but they appear also in hypertension, when they appear more white than the yellow deposits found in diabetes. A significant sign, since the damage is irreversible. In the absence of diabetes, they may be due to vascular occlusions associated commonly with hypertension.	Relatively common in the elderly patient having multiple-system disease, which may include hypertension.
Retinal edema	Leakage of serum from retinal vessels or from the choroid through Bruch's membrane.	An occasional complication of untreated hypertension, more common in diabetes.	An occasional complication of untreated hypertension, more common in diabetes.

Infective Endocarditis
(Bacterial Endocarditis)

Infective endocarditis is a disease in which there is inflammatory involvement of the heart endocardium, the heart valves, or the aorta. There is usually a focus of infection at the site of previous damage to these structures. The most common infective organisms are streptococci or staphylococci, although other bacteria and fungi are becoming increasingly implicated (Gribbin 1983, 13.221).

Until fairly recent times, infective endocarditis was chiefly a disease seen in adolescents or young adults as a sequel to previous attacks of rheumatic fever or congenital heart defects. Better control of these predisposing causes has dramatically reduced the number of young people at risk of infective endocarditis, especially in developed countries. However, the increasing number of older people having open heart surgery, including the insertion of prosthetic heart valves, has created a new high-risk population in which the disease occurs much later in life (Geddes 1982). The clinical features of infective endocarditis in the elderly differ from the classical descriptions of the disease in the younger age groups. In young subjects the organisms that affect the heart and great vessels are most commonly introduced during dental surgery and lodge at sites of previous damage to the heart. For this reason, patients having a history of rheumatic fever or congenital heart defects should have prophylactic antibiotic cover prior to undergoing even simple dental procedures. In aged patients, especially males, the introduction of the infection commonly follows urinary tract instrumentation (Gribbin 1983, 13.221).

The probable overall incidence of infective endocarditis in the United Kingdom is 6 per 10,000 per annum. However, these figures vary in different socioeconomic settings, with those countries having less well developed medical services tending toward a greater incidence and a lower age of onset for the disease.

The course of infective endocarditis usually is categorized as acute or subacute, although no clear-cut difference exists over a spectrum of clinical presentation. The chief nonophthalmic signs and symptoms are fever, headache, malaise, muscle and joint pains, nausea, and heart murmurs. Osler's nodes (small raised and tender nodes approximately 5 mm in diameter) may develop on the pads of the fingers or toes in approximately 5 percent of cases, and small hemorrhagic lesions (Janeway's lesions) appear on the palms of the hands and the soles of the feet in a similar proportion of subjects (Gribbin 1983, 13.221). There may be splinter hemorrhages in the fingernails, and in chronic disease the fingers are clubbed. Neurological involvement may occur in as many as one-third of patients; this is particularly likely in elderly patients (Geddes 1982) and may be due to embolic occlusions of ocular or cerebral vessels.

In the eye and its adnexa, petechial hemorrhages are common in the conjuctiva, and similar lesions may appear in the mouth. Hemorrhages are found in the retinal nerve fiber layer and are commonly associated with a white exudative center (Roth's spot; see Figure 9–7). In addition to these ocular signs, Duke-Elder (1976, 53) lists spastic mydriasis, optic neuritis, venous thrombosis, and choroiditis as occasional complications of infective endocarditis.

Infective endocarditis is not rare in the elderly, although its presentation is frequently atypical and difficult to recognize. The elderly patient may be lethargic, confused, and disoriented, with loss of short-term memory. Any fever may be slight or intermittent. A heart murmur is very common and usually will be heard during routine cervical auscultation as a transmitted bruit, particularly on the left side. The erythrocyte sedimentation rate may be raised, appetite is diminished, and weight loss occurs in chronic disease. These findings in elderly patients should suggest the possibility of infective endocarditis, especially when there is history of previous heart damage or open heart surgery; a careful search for conjunctival and retinal hemorrhages could provide valuable corroborative evidence. Prompt referral to a physician will enable effective treatment to be given and avoid the very high mortality associated with untreated endocarditis. Treatment consists of antibiotic administration, preferably using drugs specifically chosen for their effectiveness against the invading pathogen. Surgical repair of underlying physical heart abnormalities may be appropriate in some cases.

Carotid Artery/Cavernous Sinus Fistula

A fistula of the internal carotid artery may develop within the cavernous sinus as a result of the rupture of a small previously asymptomatic aneurysm. Middle-aged and elderly females are particularly susceptible, although the more common cause is trauma in younger

Figure 9-7

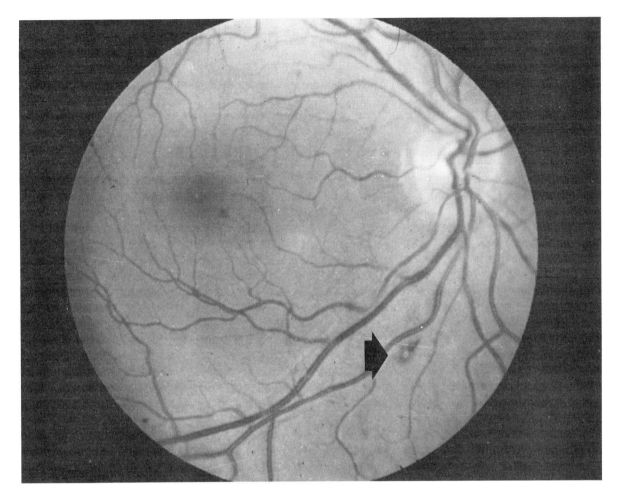

Small Splinter Hemorrhage in the Nerve Fiber Layer with Roth's Spot.

subjects. Because the cavernous sinus serves the ophthalmic venous drainage system and also contains both the ocular motor nerves and the ophthalmic and maxillary divisions of the trigeminal nerve, there is potential for diverse ocular signs and symptoms as a result of rupture of the internal carotid artery within the sinus.

A fistula between the artery and the sinus allows arterial blood to enter the sinus and raise the venous pressure to near-arterial values. The increased venous pressure is transmitted to the ophthalmic venous system, causing conjuctival congestion, chemosis, dilation of the conjuctival veins, and raised episcleral venous pressure, which in turn causes raised intraocular pressure. A dramatic feature of the disease is a pulsating exophthalmos, which is usually unilateral at first but becomes bilateral, since the sinuses are joined by the connecting circular sinus, and the effect of raised venous pressure is transmitted to both sinuses. In the retina, the veins become dilated and tortuous as a result of back pressure; microaneurysms develop, leading to hemorrhages and the typical picture of venous stasis retinopathy.

The marked changes in hemodynamics that result from a carotid cavernous sinus fistula give rise to a bruit with a swishing or blowing character that can be heard by auscultation over the orbit or brow. A pediatric stethoscope attachment is ideal for auscultation of the orbit. The patient may also be aware of this sound, which is synchronous with the heart and disappears when the carotid artery in the neck is compressed.

When the intra sinous course of the oculomotor nerves is affected, diplopia may result from paresis of the muscles, most commonly the lateral rectus. Facial and ocular pain occur because of the effect on the sensory nerves.

The differential diagnosis should include cavernous sinus thrombosis; however, this disease occurs most commonly as a complication of well-established and serious sepsis, which spreads via the cerebral and intracerebral veins or from adjacent structures.

A carotid cavernous sinus fistula may heal spontaneously; however, the progress is usually poor, and treatment is not without hazard. Treatment consists of carefully graded partial ligation of the cervical portion of the internal carotid artery on the side of the fistula. This reduces the arterial pressure transmitted to the sinus and — provided there is sufficient colateral supply available to the ocular and cerebral regions — the signs and symptoms are relieved and sufficient circulation is maintained to preserve normal function.

Vascular Occulsive Disease: Temporal Arteritis

Temporal arteritis (cranial arteritis, giant cell arteritis, or Rumbold's disease) is a self-limiting form of generalized granulomatous arteritis that has a special predilection for the carotid arteries and their cranial branches. It is rare in patients under 50 years of age, and most affected people are between 60 and 80 years of age (Cogan 1974, 132). Both sexes are equally affected. When the symptoms of temporal arteritis occur in their classic form, it is more likely that the patient will seek medical rather than optometric treatment, and the relatively low incidence of the disease insures that optometrists do not see many cases. However, on occasion the ocular symptoms may be the first to appear and cause the patient to seek optometic advice. These early symptoms may occur singly or in various combinations, and the very high risk of blindness from temporal arteritis demands vigilance on the part of the optometrist.

The pathology of temporal arteritis consists initially of degeneration of the smooth muscle cells of major arteries, followed by damage to the elastic lamina and generalized inflammation of the wall of the vessel (Reinecke and Kuwabara 1969). Macrophages respond to these changes by conversion to giant cells within the artery wall; fibroblasts proliferate, and consequently there is restriction or total occlusion of the lumen of the affected artery (Greer 1972, 10). These changes may be present in patches or over the entire course of the major arteries, including the aorta and hepatic and renal vessels (Beeson 1975, 175).

In the classic presentation of the disease, the watershed of the facial artery and, particularly, the superficial temporal artery becomes extremely tender to the touch. The superficial temporal artery becomes prominent as a tortuous, beaded, and swollen vessel under locally reddened skin. The early signs and symptoms of temporal arteritis are a general malaise, low-grade fever, weight and appetite loss, and a headache that may be very severe and unresponsive to analgesic treatment (Beeson 1975, 175).

Insufficiency of arterial supply may give rise to ischemic ocular pain or pain in the face, jaw, tongue, temple, or neck. Many patients report pain on chewing as an early sign; this condition is brought about by the failure of an adequate vascular supply to the muscles used in mastication. The tongue may become necrotic, and gangrene of fingers and toes has been reported (Andrews 1966).

The extrocular muscles are affected by the disease in approximately 15 percent of patients (Gombos 1977, 264), causing paresis or paralysis of any or all these muscles. A diagnosis of temporal arteritis should be considered in all elderly patients having diplopia of recent onset.

Retinal complications of temporal arteritis are common and occasionally may be the presenting signs. These most commonly occur in the first 1 to 4 weeks of the disease and are due to vascular insufficiency brought about by occlusion or significant restriction of the ophthalmic, central retinal, or short posterior ciliary arteries. The classic fundus picture of central retinal artery occlusion — a pale, infarcted inner retinal layer, grossly attenuated arterioles, and a red macula — is a common tragic feature of this disease. Central retinal artery occlusion sometimes occurs in spite of treatment (Beeson 1975, 175), and, on occasion, as an initial sign. When the short posterior ciliary arteries are occluded, there may be pale overall or sectoral swelling of the disc, with a few retinal hemorrhages and choroidal infarction at the posterior pole. The disc becomes pale and atrophic following regression of the inflammatory process. On the rare occasions in which the iris is affected by the ischemic process, rubeosis iridis and secondary glaucoma may follow (Gartner and Henkind 1978).

Occult temporal arteritis may occur in elderly subjects when the presenting symptom is a sudden loss of vision and there is either an absence of other signs and symptoms or only vague indications of the underlying arteritis. Cullen (1967) considers the occult form to be a common cause of blindness in the elderly and believes it occurs more frequently than the classic form of the disease.

The diagnosis of temporal arteritis is confirmed by a raised erythrocyte sedimentation rate (ESR) and biopsy of the temporal artery that demonstrates the presence of giant cells, histocytes, lymphocytes, and other inflammatory evidence. A raised ESR may occur in many conditions other than arteritis, and a biopsy may be negative during the disease because of the patchy nature of the inflammation in some cases (Eshaghian 1979). Treatment relies on the use of 60 to 80 mg of prednisone daily, and a tapering of this quantity after several weeks (Field and Lemak 1976). Treatment should be continued for several months. Unfortunately, blindness from arterial occlusion may occur in spite of this treatment and may be in the contralateral eye rather than in the eye that apparently is involved clinically (Merck Manual 1982, 557). Bilateral blindness is not uncommon.

Endocrine Disease

Diabetes Mellitus

Rather than a specific disease, diabetes mellitus is a complex syndrome of biochemical anomalies caused by a deficiency of production of biologically active insulin or a hindrance of its action at the receptors on cell membranes. Whereas the signs and symptoms of this disease are protean and encompass almost every aspect of medicine, the predominant clinical feature is hyperglycemia. In addition to its role in the metabolism of glucose, insulin is also essential for amino acid and lipid uptake, storage, and later release for use. The spectrum of the diabetes syndrome as determined by the assessment of these metabolic functions ranges from clearly normal to levels incompatible with life; between these two extremes lies an area in which a precise diagnosis is not possible. Blood glucose levels—either during fasting, after meals, or following challenge by large oral doses of sugar—are used by the clinician in diagnosing diabetes. The presence of other abnormal signs or symptoms makes this judgment more reliable in the event that blood assays are within the equivocal range. Table 9-4 show the generally accepted values of blood glucose for the clinical diagnosis of diabetes (Keen 1981).

Diabetes is now classified as insulin-dependent diabetes mellitus (IDDM) or noninsulin-dependent diabetes mellitus (NIDDM); this replaces the previous classification of juvenile or mature age onset diabetes (National Diabetes Data Group 1979). Table 9-5 shows the further subclassification of diabetes. There are shortcomings to this classification, since the underlying etiology has not yet been elucidated, and individual cases may change in status between and within the two major classifications during the natural course of the disease.

Diabetes is clearly an inheritable disease (Urrets-Zavalia 1977, 1); concordance for diabetes in identical twins approaches 100 percent for NIDDM acquired in later life; however, for IDDM acquired in early life, the concordance is less. Subjects at special risk are those having two parents with diabetes, those with a diabetic family history, or those who are the identical

Table 9-4
Diagnostic Levels of Capillary Blood Sugar (Millimoles per Liter)

Diagnosis	Fasting Level	Random Blood Sugar Test Level (Postabsoptive)	2-hour Blood Sugar Level Following 75 gm Oral Glucose
Normal	—	<6	<6
Equivocal	—	6–10[a]	—
Impaired glucose tolerance	—	—	6–12[b]
Diabetic	≥8	>11	>12

[a]Requires 2-hour blood sugar screening test.
[b]Requires standard glucose tolerance test.

twin of a diabetic. Whereas the propensity for diabetes appears to be inherited, it frequently is precipitated through overnutrition; 90 percent of noninsulin-dependent diabetics are overweight at the time of diagnosis (*Merk Manual* 1982, 1038).

Table 9–5
Classification of Diabetes Mellitus

1. Insulin-Dependent Diabetes Mellitus (IDDM)

2. Noninsulin-dependent Diabetes Mellitus (NIDDM)
   Nonobese
   Obese
   Secondary NIDDM
       Pancreatic disease
       Hormonal disorders
       Drug induced
       Insulin receptor abnormalities
       Genetic syndromes
       Miscellaneous

3. Impaired glucose tolerance
   Nonobese
   Obese
   Drug or disease induced

Source: Adapted with permission from H. Keen, "The Nature of the Diabetic Syndrome." *International Medicine* 8 (1981): 328.

The prevalence of diabetes is approximately 2.5 percent in Western population groups (Duke-Elder 1967, 412). It is estimated that a further 1 to 2 percent are as yet undiagnosed diabetics. There is a peak age of onset between 40 and 60 years (National Diabetes Data Group 1979), and between 40 and 60 percent of subjects in the ninth decade have abnormal glucose tolerance (Cahill 1975, 1599). Since diabetes has a peak age of onset that coincides with the onset of presbyopia, optometrists see and have the opportunity to recognize patients having the early manifestations of the disease. In a sample of 483 consecutive patients of an optometrist, 16 (2.7 percent) were established diabetics, and 44 (9.2 percent) had a parent or sibling with the disease. This patient sample ranged in age from 4 to 93 years and had a median age of 53 years (Cockburn 1974).

The eye, brain, kidney and lower limbs appear to be the major targets for the pathological

changes of diabetes. Diabetes is the most important systemic disease giving rise to blindness, and the majority of the diabetic blind are middle-aged or elderly (Caird, Pirie, and Ramsell 1969, 7). Ocular involvement may occur in the early stages of diabetes; indeed, between 20 and 40 percent of diabetic subjects had ocular involvement at the time of diagnosis of their disease (Caird, Pirie, and Ramsell 1969, 8). The high prevalence of diabetes in an aging population, together with frequent and early ocular involvement, justifies the inclusion in the eye examination of a specific search for the signs and symptoms of diabetes.

History Taking. History taking provides a useful guide to the presence of diabetes. All patients should be questioned for a family history of diabetes; when their answer is positive, they should be further questioned to find evidence of other relevant symptoms. The early diabetic may have an increase fluid intake (polydipsia) and consequent increased micturition (polyuria). Younger subjects especially have an increased appetite (polyphagia). In spite of the increased food intake, the untreated diabetic may lose weight although generally remaining obese. Fluctuating vision and changes in refractive errors are fairly common in uncontrolled diabetics.

The history taking should include an investigation of the patient's current medication, since glucose tolerance may be significantly reduced by the action of a large number of therapeutic substances. These drugs include many of the commonly prescribed diuretics; mood-altering drugs; hormones (particularly the glucocorticoids); indomethacin (which is used for the treatment of osteoarthritis); and neurologically active drugs, including levodopa (which is used to regulate blood pressure) (Treleaven 1982, 237). Even the humble niacin, a vitamin complex frequently prescribed for psychopathological conditions, is implicated in the impairment of glucose tolerance (Duke-Elder 1971, 765). Elderly patients are particularly at risk, because of their lowered tolerance to toxicity and the common use of these classes of drugs in the aged population.

Although it is not a common early manifestation of diabetes, a form of neuropathy may involve those nerves serving the extraocular muscles and the iris. Complaints by elderly patients of difficulties related to binocular vision, especially diplopia, should initiate a search for diabetes. The neuropathy involving the extraocular muscles usually resolves spontaneously after about 12 weeks.

Cataracts. Cataracts occur in a high proportion of elderly nondiabetic patients. Diabetes appears to accelerate the progression of cataracts so that they appear at an earlier age than usual or are more advanced for the patient's age than would be expected. The acute onset of snowflake opacities, which characterize diabetic cataracts, occurs only in diabetics under 30 or 40 years of age. An increase in the density of the lens nucleus may cause a shift toward myopia or lessened hypermetropia. Although this occurs in many nondiabetic subjects, a special search for diabetics is warranted under these conditions.

Duke-Elder (1969b, 323) cites a number of studies that demonstrate that asteroid bodies frequently are associated with abnormal glucose tolerance or frank diabetes. In spite of the controversy regarding this association (Topilow et al. 1982), asteroid bodies are sufficiently unusual to make reasonable special efforts to seek other signs of diabetes in patients having this sign.

The retinal vasculature is commonly, if not invariably, involved in diabetic angiopathy. These changes occur predominantly in the small vessels of the retina and involve loss of the nuclei of the intramural pericites (Cogan and Kuwabara 1963). At the same time the basement membrane becomes thickened, the lumen narrows and occlusions of small vessels become common (Scheie and Albert 1977, 434). These processes lead to relative ischemia of the retina and a breakdown of the blood-retinal barrier, culminating in the characteristic fundus lesions of diabetic retinopathy. Similar changes have been noted in the choroid (Saracco et al. 1982).

Diabetic Retinopathy. Diabetic retinopathy is generally classified as preretinopathy, simple or background retinopathy, and proliferative retinopathy. However, it might prove useful for clinical purposes to include a transitional stage between simple and proliferative retinopathy, which would include retinas that possess the hallmark of the transition from the simple to the proliferative stage. The treatment of proliferative retinopathy is most successful if applied at an early stage of this complication (Hercules et al. 1977), and it could be argued that the transitional phase represents the most important clinical diagnosis and warrants separate emphasis. Table 9–6 summarizes the clinical signs associated with these forms of diabetic retinopathy and includes notes regarding their treatment.

The onset of diabetic retinopathy is closely related to the duration of the diabetes (West, Erdreich, and Stober 1980). It is common after 10 years' duration and almost universally present after 20 years' duration. Its incidence does not appear to be related to the severity of

Table 9–6
Classification of Diabetic Retinopathy Based on Clinical Data and Showing Appropriate Treatment

Diabetic Complication	Description (in Most Common Sequential Order)	Treatment
Preretinopathy	Dilated tortuous veins, venous loop formations	None proved, possibly anticoagulants (aspirin)
Simple retinopathy as above, plus	Retinal microaneurysms, dot and blot hemorrhages, waxy hard yellow exudates, retinal edema	Photocoagulation of leaking vessels near macula to possibly reduce macular edema in selected cases
Transition stage as above, plus	Multiple large blot hemorrhages, venous beading, duplication of blood vessels, cotton wool patches	Panretinal or focal photocoagulation to reduce oxygen demand and resolve new vessels
Proliferative retinopathy as above, plus	New vessels at the disc in the retina and in the vitreous, especially above the disc; preretinal hemorrhages; formation of fibrinous strands; retinal detachment; rubeosis iridis; secondary glaucoma	Panretinal coagulation Vitrectomy, detachment surgery, pituitary ablation

the diabetes (Newell 1982, 439) or the method of blood glucose control. In many cases, retinopathy occurs in spite of good blood sugar control. However, there is a strong clinical impression that good early control of blood sugar levels delays or reduces the extent of retinal damage (Kohner et al. 1969). The Steno Study Group (1982) reported that continuous infusion of insulin had considerable value in the control and prevention of diabetic retinopathy. However, this question cannot be considered to be settled, since Lawson et al. (1982), in a similar study, found that in spite of good blood sugar control, the treatment did not provide protection against or reduce the effect of diabetic retinopathy. Unfortunately for the vast majority of diabetics, ocular involvement becomes inevitable, the aged diabetic being affected after a shorter duration of the disease than younger subjects.

Preretinopathy. Preretinopathy is difficult to identify, since dilated veins and tortuosity are common in normal subjects and in eyes of patients having other vascular diseases. It is probably safe to make this diagnosis only for a confirmed diabetic or a patient for whom there is a fundus photographic record that establishes a change in status.

Simple Retinopathy. Simple retinopathy is heralded by the appearance of microaneurysms (Chuna-Vaz 1978), preferentially in the area outside the capillary-free macular zone and extending for about 10 degrees from the posterior pole. They may appear in clusters or as isolated dense dark red spots, which are easily overlooked unless specifically sought (Figure 9–8). Later, dot and blot hemorrhages and the hard yellow diabetic exudates appear (Figure 9–9). Retinal hemorrhages are confined by the orientation of the tissues into which the blood seeps; in the outer plexiform layer, this pools the blood into vertical columns, which then appear as dark red, discrete dots (dot hemorrhages). The loosely packed and predominantly horizontally coursing fibers in the nuclear layers allow the blood to spread irregularly and form thin sheets (blot hemorrhages). Leakage of serum may occur in some eyes, causing retinal edema and severe visual loss when it occurs near the macula.

Although diabetes appears to affect the deep capillary layers preferentially, signs of retinal nerve fiber layer involvement in the form of flame hemorrhages and cotton wool patches are

not unusual. These, along with exacerbation of the size and number of deep retinal hemorrhages, may herald the onset of the proliferative stage of retinopathy.

Figure 9–8

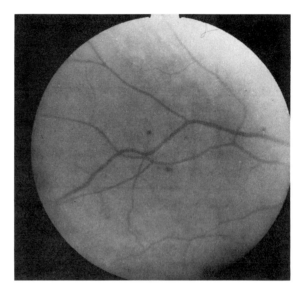

Large Microaneurysms without Other Visible Retinal Signs of Diabetes. Microaneurysms are usually much smaller than these and are easily overlooked.

Figure 9–9

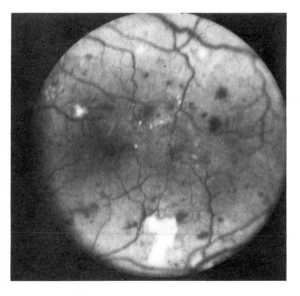

Advanced Simple Diabetic Retinopathy Featuring Microaneurysms, Dot and Blot Hemorrhages, and Exudates. This patient subsequently developed proliferative diabetic retinopathy.

Proliferative Retinopathy. Ballantyne and Michaelson (1973, 235) cite studies that indicate that between 2 and 16 percent of diabetics progress through the simple form of retinopathy to the proliferative stage. The emergence of new vessels marks this transformation and may commence at the disc or in any portion of the retina, including the periphery (Figure 9–10). It is believed that a vasogenic factor (at present not identified) is produced in response to retinal ischemia, which in turn is brought about by closure of large areas of the retinal capillary bed. These areas may be visualized in fluorescein angiograms as dark patches of capillary nonperfusion.

Figure 9–10

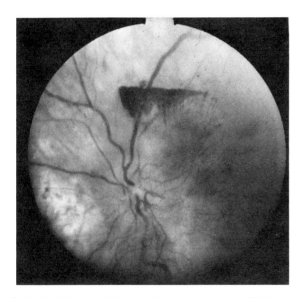

Early Proliferative Diabetic Retinopathy in a 32-Year-old Female. Numerous new vessels arise from the disc, and a small preretinal hemorrhage lies superior to the disc.

The newly formed vessels are immature and readily break down to cause preretinal hemorrhages (Figure 9–11) and vitreal hemorrhages (if the vessels have penetrated the vitreous). The growth of vitreal channels is accompanied by a fibrous matrix, which after resolution of the vessels may remain a dense strand (Figure 9–12). Contraction of these strands causes retinal detachment in the late stage of proliferative retinopathy.

In association with retinal and vitreal neovascularization, new vessels may form on the iris, beginning with the pupillary margin and

Figure 9–11

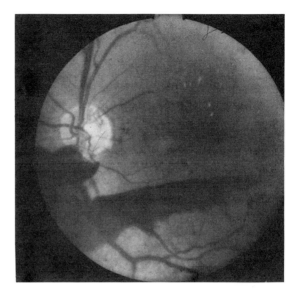

Large Preretinal Hemorrhages in a Diabetic Patient (Same Patient as Illustrated in Figure 9–8). Note that the hemorrhages overlie all retinal features, and new vessels are present on the disc.

Figure 9–12

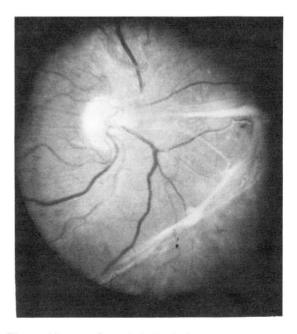

Fibrous Vitreous Strands in Partly Resolved Proliferative Diabetic Retinopathy.

spreading to invade the anterior chamber angle. The vessels in the angle are accompanied by a fibrovascular membrane similar to that which develops in association with vitreal neovascularization. This membrane may occlude the trabecular spaces, denying access of aqueous humour to the canal of Schlemm and causing a steep rise in intraocular pressure. This form of secondary glaucoma is particularly difficult to treat, but it may respond to panretinal photocoagulation, direct goniophotocoagulation, or pancryotherapy (Ward 1982, 162).

It is fortunate that the proliferative form of diabetic retinopathy occurs only in a relatively small proportion of the overall diabetic population. It is chiefly confined to IDDM patients in whom the disease becomes manifest before age 40 and after many years of its duration. The majority of older patients develop the NIDDM form of the disease, and it is uncommon for elderly subjects to have this added complication.

Treatment. Elderly NIDDM patients are treated with oral hypoglycemic drugs, which include sulfonylurea, biguanides, and sulfapyrimidine derivatives. Apart from occasional gastrointestinal side effects, these drugs are well tolerated and do not appear to cause ocular side effects.

Optometric Management of the Diabetic Suspect. Although there is at present no effective treatment for simple retinopathy, the physician in charge of overall mangement of the patient should be informed of the ocular status and be assured of cooperation should retinopathy progress to the proliferative stage. At the first indication of the transition stage, or the appearance of frank proliferation, the patient should be referred to an ophthalmologist for possible panretinal photocoagulation designed to reduce oxygen demand. Ophthalmologic attention is also necessary on the appearance of macular edema or sensory retinal detachment.

Arguably, the most important role for the optometrist is the early detection of previously undiagnosed diabetes at a stage before it causes brain, kidney, or eye damage or an acceleration of atherosclerosis with its consequences for stroke and coronary disease. Vigilance in the history taking and ophthalmoscopy may be complemented by the use of blood glucose estimates. Instruments for this purpose are readily available, simple to use, and provide valid and reli-able estimates. However, whenever any doubt remains, the patient should be referred for a standard glucose tolerance test. Figure 9–13 is an algorithm intended as a guide to the extended investigation of the person suspected of having diabetes using blood sugar analysis as a diagnostic criterion.

Hyperthyroidism (Thyrotoxicosis, Toxic Goiter, Basedow's Disease)

Thyroid hormones control the metabolism of oxygen and the synthesis of proteins; as a consequence, they regulate the metabolic activity in most of the body's tissues. This system is influenced and controlled by the pituitary through the production of thyroid-stimulating hormone, which in turn is subject to modulation according to the level of circulating hormones. Other organ systems, notably the liver, are involved in this regulatory system, the nature of which is not yet fully understood. Considering the complexity of the system, it is hardly surprising that the etiology of many of the thyroid abnormalities is not yet clear. In clinical terms, *thyroid disease* is classified as hyperthyroidism or hypothyroidism (myxedema) and a number of less–common varieties such as Hashimoto's thyroiditis; virus-induced granulomatous thyroiditis; tumors of the thyroid; and euthyroid goiter, in which there is painless and symptomless enlargement of the thyroid gland in association with normal concentrations of thyroid hormones. The ocular signs of interest to the optometric clinician may occur in either hyperthyroidism or, less commonly, in hypothyroidism and in the euthyroid state. The term *Graves' disease* is appropriate when ophthalmic symptoms occur in any form of the thyroid disease (Duke-Elder 1976, 63). Table 9–7 lists both the ocular and general signs and symptoms of Graves' disease.

The peak age of onset of thyroid disease is 30 to 50 years. The disease has an incidence of 3 per 10,000 adults per year and a female-to-male ratio of 5 to 1 (De Groot 1975, 1703). However, some 15 percent of patients having hyperthyroidism are aged 65 or older (*Merck Manual* 1982, 997); in this age group the classic signs may be confined to a single organ system to produce a confusing clinical picture referred to as *occult* or *masked thyrotoxicosis.* The diagnosis is easily missed, especially when there are no signs of thyroid enlargement; therefore, the presence of any ocular signs in Table 9–7 should raise the issue of thyroid disease in the differential

Figure 9–13

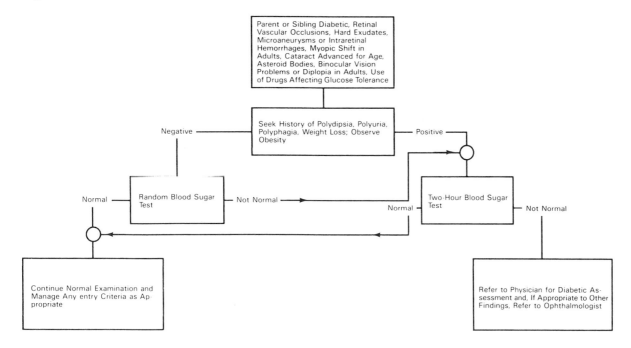

Algorithm Showing Suggested Management of Ophthalmic Patients Having Risk Factors for Diabetes

Table 9–7
Ocular and General Signs and Symptoms of Hyperthyroidism (Graves' Disease),
with the Special Diagnostic Indicators of the Occult Form Found in Aged Patients

Ocular Signs	General Signs	Occult Form Signs
Lid retraction and staring gaze	Weakness, fatigue, weight loss, breathlessness on exertion	Muscle weakness
Lid lag on downward gaze		Depression
Proptosis		Inactivity
Reduced blink rate	Insomnia	Apathy
Lid edema	Hyperactivity	Mental confusion, senile-dementialike state
Bulbar and conjunctival swelling or hyperemia	Tremor	
	Excessive perspiration, moist fine skin	Low-grade fever
Tearing or burning sensation		Wizened, wrinkled appearance
Exposure keratitis, corneal ulceration	Thinning hair, brittle nails	Weight loss
Weakness of convergence	Heat intolerance, cold tolerance	Congestive heart failure
Diplopia, phoria, or ophthalmoplegia	Swelling of thyroid gland	Arrhythmias, atrial fibrillation
Retrobulbar pain	Heart palpitations, systolic murmur	Constipation
Reduced visual acuity		Liver enlargement
Retrobulbar neuritis (central and arcuate)	Tachycardia, arterial fibrillation	Bone pain
Visual field defects	Abdominal pain, loose bowel motions, pruritus	
Papilledema	Absence or irregularity of menstrual periods	
Secondary glaucoma	Anxiety, restlessness	
	Absence of forehead wrinkling on upward gaze	

diagnosis. Other signs that may support the diagnosis of occult thyrotoxicosis in an aged patient are tachycardia (which should be detected during carotid auscultation) and a patient who is wrinkled, apathetic, lethargic, and apparently prematurely senile. These and other signs and symptoms more common in the aged thyrotoxic patient are shown separately in Table 9–7. Note that in the aged subject, inactivity rather than hyperactivity is common.

In the more common form of presentation of hyperthyroidism, the variety and combinations of symptoms and signs bear no relationship to the metabolic state (Sachdev, Chatterji, and Sharma 1979) and may precede, occur in conjunction with, or only become manifest after remission of the hormonal disturbance. Furthermore, the ocular signs may recede or progress in spite of treatment that normalizes the thyroid hormonal balance (Bouzas 1980). The rare, but important, complication of optic neuropathy should be considered when visual field losses are discovered. These defects may be central scotomas or nerve fiber bundle defects (Henderson 1958). The increased bulk of retrobulbar tissue that gives rise to the proptosis of thyrotoxicosis also may restrict the episcleral vessels, which in turn compromises aqueous outflow. The resulting increase in intraocular pressure may be sufficient to lead to secondary glaucoma (Stone 1982, 222). Temporary and less serious rises in intraocular pressure tend to occur when the patient attempts eye movements against the restrictions imposed by extraocular muscle hypertrophy and orbital adhesions. The optometric review of these patients should include a search for signs of optic nerve compression. When the disease presents in a classic form, diagnosis may be simple. However it should be confirmed by the physician after laboratory testing; this is particularly important in the aged patient having atypical signs or the occult form of hyperthyroidism.

Propranolol is effective in controlling tachycardia, tremor, and psychiatric symptoms, but it must be used with caution in patients having a tendency to congestive heart failure. Otherwise, treatment involves the use of radioactive iodine and other thyroid suppressants (*Merck Manual* 1982, 997). Support treatment by the optometrist may be directed toward correcting any ocular muscle defects, using prisms where appropriate and providing methylcellulose drops for any dry eye problem that is due

to exposure in proptosis. Drying of the cornea may occur during sleep from a failure of lid closure. The patient may benefit from the use of a shield similar to a Buller's shield, which fits closely over the eye to maintain high humidity and prevent corneal dehydration.

Neurological Disease

Parkinson's Disease (Paralysis Agitans)
Parkinson's disease is a term that embraces a group of neurological disorders involving degeneration of the region of the brain stem, particularly the substantia nigra (Escourolle and Poirer 1978, 137). It is said to have a prevalence of 1,000,000 cases in the United States, with the addition of a further 50,000 new cases each year. The disease has an insidious onset in later years, usually becoming manifest between the ages of 50 and 65 (Yahr 1975, 636). Although variably progressive, most cases run a slowly worsening course during which the patient remains mobile for some 10 to 20 years before death or major incapacity occurs.

Disease that occurs at the extrapyramidal level involves the complex of nerve fibers and nuclear masses that runs from the motor cortex to the brain stem. Descending motor fibers then descend the spinal cord to control muscle activity. Lesions at the extrapyramidal level cause a delay in the initiation of and poverty of movement, together with a large-amplitude tremor and repetitive involuntary movements (MacLeod 1979, 272). It is generally held that lesions of the extrapyramidal pathways interfere with involuntary and stereotyped movements without being directly involved with voluntary movements (Barr 1979, 276).

The clinical picture of parkinsonism is unmistakable. An early and obvious sign involves a coarse, repetitive movement of the thumb across the tips of the fingers in a "pill-rolling" movement that stops when the patient attempts a voluntary movement involving the hands. The patient's face tends to be expressionless, with the facial muscles smoothed out and almost immobile. Speech is slow and monotonous, yet occasionally interspersed with a very rapid series of words, the whole delivered at such a low level that it may be impossible to hear. The blink rate is much reduced, yet the glabellar tapping blink reflex is exaggerated. In the normal subject, repetitive tapping over the bridge of the nose results in the subject's blinking synchronously for the first 5 or 6 taps and then reverting to the normal blink pattern. The parkinsonian patient will continue to blink synchronously for as long as the tapping is continued.

The gait of patients have Parkinson's disease is characteristic: they tend to lean forward and almost fall from one short, shuffling step to the next while the hands are held flexed and at the sides. There is a pronounced slowness of all voluntary movements and, frequently, a muscular rigidity in passive movements that results in a series of jerks as a limb is moved (cogwheel rigidity). The patients also tend to be unable to continue or initiate a movement; this may be quite striking when they attempt to walk but find that they are unable to move their feet.

The tremor characteristic of Parkinson's disease has a rate of between 4 and 8 cycles per second; it is most severe at rest and when fatigued but will diminish with voluntary movement and disappear in sleep (*Merck Manual* 1982, 1130). It may affect the mouth or tongue, with resulting rhythmic sucking, whistling, or lip movements. The patient's handwriting may deteriorate, causing previously flowing writing to become spidery, diminished in size, and wandering from straight lines.

In addition to alteration of the blink reflex previously noted, other ocular signs are common in Parkinson's disease. A form of facial spasm affects some patients. The lids are tightly clamped together, and the other facial muscles develop irregular jerks without order or rhythm; this performance is repeated at regular intervals interspersed with periods of repose. The optometric examination of these patients can be most frustrating; however, a show of impatience by the clinician will only worsen the problem. Frequently, a paresis of the upper lids causes them to remain fixed when the patient looks downward. When the lower lids are also affected, the eyes adopt the staring appearance of the typical parkinsonian victim. In contrast, ptosis may result from rigidity of the levator muscle (Treleaven 1982, 237).

Ocular movements may become involved in the disease so that eye movements become slow and irregular, with a slowing of saccades and deficiency of convergence. Patients having Parkinson's disease frequently have difficulty turning the eyes upward; this may be noted when the optometrist attempts to instill eyedrops. Eventually, myostatic paralysis may cause

the eyes to assume a locked position in which any attempt at voluntary movement gives rise to ineffective cogwheel movements (Duke-Elder 1973, 851).

Optometric management is largely supportive but requires initiative in meeting the special needs of these patients. Bifocal segments may be placed much higher than is usual to allow effective use of the reading segment, since a forward head tilt usually is adopted. A stand on which reading material can be rested will relieve the problem of shaking from tremor of the upper limbs. Fixed-focus stand magnifiers also should be considered for people with low vision. Binocular vision problems may be alleviated initially by the use of prisms, but monocular occlusion is probably a better solution in advanced cases. Ocular lubricants will provide relief from the discomfort of the dry eye resulting from paucity of blinking.

Medical Treatment and Prognosis. Levodopa, the metabolic precursor of dopamine, relieves the symptoms of Parkinson's disease, presumably through replenishment of dopamine, which is deficient in the corpus striatum of patients having this disease. Carbidopa inhibits the breakdown of levodopa in extracerebral tissues, thus making more levodopa available to the brain. Treatment consists of using levodopa alone or in combination with carbidopa titrated to achieve satisfactory control of symptoms. The dosage may be reduced in geriatric patients with liver or kidney disease, since these organs are responsible for the breakdown and excretion of dopamine. Because dopamine in turn is the precursor of epinephrine and norepinephrine, this drug tends to dilate the pupils and may precipitate angle closure glaucoma in susceptible patients, especially when used in combination with monoamine oxidase inhibitors (Mandelkorn and Zimmerman 1982, 248). Management of patients with Parkinson's disease is very complex and should be under the direction of a competent physician.

Psychiatric Illness

Psychopathology is the study of the abnormal function of personality (abnormal in that the expression is an exaggeration of characteristics present in the normal personality). It follows that the clinical appearance of psychiatric illness is a continuum from what would be regarded as a clearly normal personality to frank psychotic behavior in which all contact with reality has been lost. Optometrists occasionally are consulted by patients having psychiatric illnesses in early or moderately advanced form; however, the visual problems of these people generally differ little from those of other patients. Patients having psychiatric disorders, however, may have functional visual defects in the form of lowered visual acuity or visual field defects. These symptoms are unresponsive to spectacle or placebo treatment and persist for lengthy periods (Kathol et al. 1983). Since the possibility of an unrecognized underlying organic disorder always exists, it is important that these patients receive a complete ophthalmologic assessment.

The patients of optometrists tend to include a high proportion of elderly people, since some degree of failing sight is almost universal in the aged. Advanced age brings not only failing sight, but also increasing forgetfulness, lethargy, and an inability to adjust to change. These characteristics are accepted as a natural and inevitable part of aging; however, at some point that is almost impossible to define, these and other behavioral characteristics decline to the point where the patient is said to suffer dementia. Although there are no ocular changes specific to the condition, the optometrist needs to recognize dementia to successfully manage the patient's visual problems.

Senile Dementia

Dementia is a state in which there is a reduction of intellectual ability from a previous stable level. In the early stages it manifests itself as defective self-criticism or capacity to make fine discriminations involving moral and social issues and as a lessening of the ability to use abstract concepts and to learn new procedures. Short-term memory loss is an early and obvious feature of dementia. In the aged these initial changes may be quite subtle and the progress of the condition so gradual that the individual and the family adapt to the changes without difficulty. The majority of patients finally die from an unrelated cause without serious behavioral problems having arisen.

The course of dementia may be interrupted by a sudden exacerbation following an increase in emotional or physical stress. Commonly, this additional life stress is caused by bereavement, the onset of physical disease, trauma, ingestion of medication having central nervous system effects, or drastic changes in living patterns.

With worsening of the dementia, there may be serious lack of initiative, apathy, depression, a deterioration of personal hygiene, and a worsening memory problem. Abstract concepts become more difficult to grasp; verbal communication tends to be introspective, repetitive, and often failing to reach the intended conclusion because the subject loses the thread of thought. Emotional instability may appear as fits of anger or euphoria, although apathy and depression are more common. The patient may fail to answer questions or answer only after several repetitions, after which the reply may be inappropriate as the result of the patient's diminished capacity for judgment and expression.

With the progress of dementia, the patient's previous character traits tend to become exaggerated. For example, an exacerbation of previous obsessive states of hyperchondriasis could lead the patient into a miserable existence, which in turn could accelerate the dementia through added emotional stress. These changes impose nearly intolerable burdens upon family, friends, and health care practitioners. However, the reactions of people close to the patient are crucial to the containment of dementia; kindness, understanding, and gentle persuasion reduce the rate of deterioration, whereas the opposite occurs when the subject is abandoned by family and friends.

Obviously, the patient with dementia will cause special problems for the optometrist. During the ocular examination the patient is in an unfamiliar place surrounded by complex equipment and is subjected to a history taking that taxes his or her defective memory for details that cannot be recalled. The patient is required to maintain a fixed posture and attention while unfamiliar procedures are carried out. During the subjective refraction, the patient is expected to follow complex instructions in order to make many fine discriminatory judgments in rapid succession. It is hardly suprising that patients having even a minor degree of dementia retreat into an apathetic state and either fail to provide answers or provide quite unreliable responses to the questions directed to them.

When examining an elderly patient having dementia, the optometrist should adapt the investigation to the intellectual capacity of the subject. History taking can be made to appear a relatively casual series of questions asked intermittently during the course of the examination rather than a rapid-fire preliminary to the physical examination. The information being sought should be relevant to the patient's special circumstances; it need not necessarily explore for conditions usually found in younger subjects nor search for hereditary ocular disease that would have become manifest many years earlier.

During the physical examination the patient may have difficulty maintaining concentration or keeping the eyes in a fixed position. Elderly patients tend to slump during the refractive examination, and if they are placed behind a phoropter, they eventually begin to look through the extreme lower edge of the lens or even slip into a position where they cannot see through the lens aperture at all. The use of a trial frame during both retinoscopy and the subjective refraction prevents this problem and also allows large changes of lens power to be introduced in a single step and with greater speed.

The patient having dementia may be dissatisfied in spite of appearing to have reasonable vision with glasses. Reading requires a high level of intellectual capacity and concentration, which the patient may lack. To the patient and the immediate family, it seems most likely that a reading difficulty is due to poor vision; they can be disappointed when new spectacles do not allow easy reading. The optometrist should be sure there is an appreciable benefit from changes made to spectacles and that the use of any special aids is within the capacity of the patient.

Although there is no treatment for idiopathic dementia, the optometrist should insure that these patients are under medical care, since almost identical changes can be caused by subdural hemorrhage, alcohol abuse, lead and carbon monoxide poisoning, and inappropriate drug therapy. A similar clinical picture occurs in Alzheimer's dementia, Pick's disease, and occasionally as a result of viral encephalitis. A steplike deterioration of intellect may accompany multiple infarcts of the brain caused by intermittent showers of small emboli. Early recognition and treatment of the underlying cause may prevent serious brain damage and death. Because dementia may be secondary to a treatable disease, patients not already under medical care should be referred for examination by a physician. Even in cases where no causative disease can be found, antidepressant drugs may be valuable and intercurrent medical problems managed to the overall benefit of the

patient's life style; hence, an improved prognosis may be possible for the dementia itself.

Connective Tissue Disease

The connective tissue diseases are a complex and heterogeneous group of diseases in which the common factor is pathological changes in the main supporting tissues of the body (in particular, skin, tendons, cartilage, bone, and the vascular system). Although classified as inflammatory or degenerative, the distinction is seldom clear, since prior inflammation renders the supporting tissue vulnerable to the stresses it must bear in its functional role. However, inflammation is a common, if not universal, response to the degenerations resulting from these stresses.

Arthritis

The collagen diseases that have ocular manifestations are chiefly those of the rheumatoid arthritis group and those affecting blood vessels (scleroderma, systemic lupus erythematosus, and polyarteritis). Osteoarthritis is the most common connective tissue disease; it is universally present to some degree in the aged population. It has no recognized ocular complications. Many of the rheumatoid arthritis group are diseases having an onset in the early or middle years of life; however, the victims of these diseases may carry their disease with its complications into old age, and it is important that the clinician have a knowledge of these conditions. Table 9–8 lists the ocular complications of a number of the connective tissue diseases.

Rheumatoid Arthritis

Rheumatoid arthritis is an inflammatory disease of unknown etiology that affects principally the joints but may result in multisystem complications in which the eyes may be involved. Although any of the synovial joints may be affected, those of the hands, wrists, and feet are most consistently involved. The changes are primarily due to synovial swelling and the accumulation of granulomatous tissue within the joints. Bone changes consist of periarticular osteoporosis and areas of bone erosion leading to distortion through weakening of their structure and subluxation of smaller joints.

The onset of rheumatoid arthritis is most commonly between the ages of 20 and 50 years; however, the disease may appear at any age (*The Merck Manual* 1982, 1177). Although there are no internationally accepted criteria for the

Table 9-8
Ocular Complications of Selected Connective Tissue Diseases

Ocular Complication	Marfan Syndrome	Pseudo-xanthoma Elasticum	Sjögren Syndrome	Systemic Lupus Erythematosus	Dermato-myositis	Myotonic Dystrophy	Myasthenia Gravis	Erythema Multiform	Ankylosing Spondylitis	Rheumatoid Syndrome Juvenile	Rheumatoid Syndrome Adult	Reiter Syndrome	Sarcoidosis	Progressive Systemic Scleroderma
Ectopia lentis	+													
Lens dislocation	+													
Glaucoma	+									+			+	
Retinal detachment	+													
Angioid streaks		+												
Retinal hemorrhages		+		+	+								+	+
Keratoconjunctivitis			+	+	+									+
Scleritis or episcleritis			+	+	+			+	+		+	+	+	+
Cotton wool patches				+	+									+
Optic atrophy				+										
Retinal vascular occlusions				+										+
Ophthalmoplegia or ocular paresis					+		+						+	+
Cataracts	+					+		+		+	+			
Color vision defects						+								
Peripheral retinal pigmentation						+								
Impaired dark adaptation						+								
Ptosis						+	+							
Uveitis					+			+	+	+	+		+	+
Symblepharon								+						
Band-shaped keratopathy										+	+		+	
Dry eye			+	+				+			+		+	+
Keratoconus	+													
Papilledema													+	+
Keratitis or corneal furrowing				+				+						+
Conjunctival telangiectasis														+

diagnosis of rheumatoid arthritis, the four-tier classification of the American Arthritis Association (Rodman 1973) provides a practical basis for clinical diagnosis. These classifications are classical, definite, probably, and possible rheumatoid arthritis. The nonlaboratory criteria for the system follow:
1. Stiffness in the joints.
2. Pain in the joints on movement.
3. Joint swelling that is symmetrical on the two sides of the body.
4. Subcutaneous nodules over bony prominences, on the extensor surfaces, or in regions close to joints.

Because of the looseness of the criteria and the lack of an international standard definition of the disease, the reported prevalence of rheumatoid arthritis varies considerably but appears to be approximately 1 to 2 percent of males and 2 to 4 percent of females.

The mode of onset of rheumatoid arthritis varies widely; it may be slow and insidious, or it may occur painfully and precipitously in the course of a single day (Christian 1975, 142). Up to 75 percent of sufferers will improve with conservative treatment within a year, 10 to 20 percent will have virtually complete remissions, and 5 to 10 percent are eventually disabled by the disease (*The Merck Manual* 1982, 1177).

Clinical Presentation. The small bones of the hands and feet are most commonly first affected in the classical form of rheumatoid arthritis. The finger joints particularly become swollen and distorted (Figure 9–14), the skin becomes fragile, and the hands bruise easily. Firm nodules approximately 1 cm in diameter develop beneath the skin; these may break down, ulcerate, and heal only with difficulty. Systemic complications affect the heart, the lungs, and the dura mater (Hayson and Grennan 1983, 165). Entrapment of nerves within the distorted bony tissue may produce neurological signs, including paresis of muscles; the combination of these changes and loss of mobility of the joints evenually leads to muscle wasting.

Patients suffering from rheumatoid arthritis have more severe pain and stiffness in the

Figure 9–14

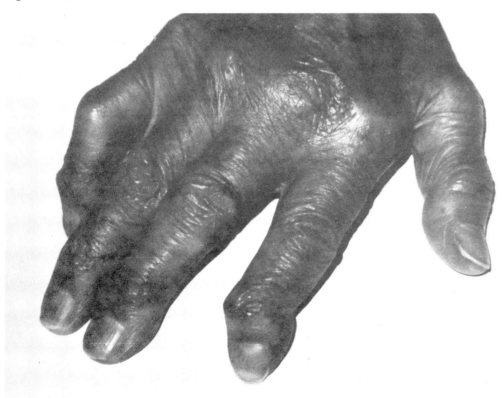

Typical Changes in the Hand of a Patient Having Rheumatoid Arthritis. Note distortion of the joint in the index finger.

morning on rising and after periods of inactivity; these symptoms are worse in cold weather. The patient is easily fatigued; suffers loss of appetite; is more sensitive to cold; and may experience numbness, particularly in the hands and feet.

Ocular Signs. The most common eye complication is keratoconjunctivitis sicca, either alone or in combination with paucity of saliva (Sjögren syndrome). The lacrimal secretion reserve may be estimated from the height of the tear meniscus at the lower lid. In the normal eye, this meniscus has a height of approximately 0.1 to 0.3 mm (Lamberts, Foster, and Perry 1979). Schirmer test is usually considered to be positive if less than 10 mm of the strip wets within 5 minutes in an eye that is not anesthetized. In dry eyes, Bengal Rose frequently stains the conjunctiva and filamentous threads of mucous secretion, whereas there may be punctate staining of the inferior portion of the corneal epithelium. Some 10 to 15 percent of rheumatoid arthritis sufferers develop keratoconjunctivitis sicca; this disease is the most common cause of dry eyes (Pavan-Langston 1980, 99).

The less common, albeit more serious, ocular complications tend to occur when the disease has been present in severe form for a long time. Table 9–9 summarizes these signs, together with their special features and sequelae. Elderly subjects having rheumatoid arthritis are especially prone to develop scleral nodules. In the early stages it

is difficult to differentiate between relatively benign, although possibly quite painful, rheumatic nodules and early necrotizing nodular scleritis. Both forms are raised yellowish nodules in the sclera surrounded by hyperemic conjunctiva. Rheumatic nodules go through remissions and exacerbations more or less in synchrony with the underlying systemic disease, whereas necrotizing nodules develop into extremely painful areas that become thinned to the degree that the uvea becomes ectatic. Uveitis is common in eyes having necrotizing scleral nodules. The aged subject having rheumatoid arthritis is at risk of developing scleromalacia perforans. This is an insidious, usually painless condition that develops from a scleral nodule; the sclera melts away, leading to perforation and the complications of cataract, uveitis, panophthalmitis, and glaucoma (Duke-Elder 1965, 1042).

Sorsby and Gomaz in 1946 drew attention to the prevalence of a mild anterior uveitis in patients having rheumatoid arthritis. In their series of 332 subjects, 15 (4.5 percent) had uveitis.

Treatment. Because of its largely unpredictable course, the treatment of rheumatoid arthritis is difficult to evaluate. Spontaneous remissions are frequently ascribed to whatever fad diet or conventional treatment was in use at the time improvement commenced. The mainstay of treatment is aspirin (Leak 1983) because of its combined anti-inflammatory and analgesic

Table 9–9
Ocular Complications of Rheumatoid Arthritis, Their Features, and Possible Sequelae

Complication	Features and Possible Sequelae
Keratoconjunctivitis	Occurrence in 10 to 15 percent of rheumatoid arthritis. lacrimal insufficiency; foamy tears; corneal and conjunctival erosion (part of Sjögren syndrome)
Scleritis and episcleritis	Painful red eye
Rheumatic nodules of sclera	Raised nodules surrounded by hyperemic sclera; pigmented areas on resolution
Necrotizing nodules	Uveitis; gross hyperemia; pain; scleral ectasia
Scleromalacia perforans	Perforation of the globe; panophthalmitis; cataract; glaucoma; often symptomless in early stage
Corneal marginal degeneration	Corneal ulceration; new vessel growth
Band keratopathy	Occurrence in long-standing corneal involvement
Anterior uveitis	Very mild, often symptomless; occurrence in 4 to 5 percent of subjects; usually resolution without serious damage; may be recurrent
Cataract	Complicated cataract; rarely polychromatic
Paresis of extraocular muscles	Usually transient, causing diplopia

effect. Other drugs commonly used include indomethacin, phenylbutazone, chloroquine, hydroxychloroquine sulfate, gold compounds, adrenocorticosteriods, and penicillamine. These drugs may be useful when salicylates prove ineffective; however, the complications associated with both nonsteroidal anti-inflammatory drugs and the corticosteriods can cause greater morbidity than the disease itself (Christian 1975). The eyes are frequently involved in these side effects. Corticosteroids may cause sharply increased intraocular pressure (Armaly 1963; Becker and Mills 1963) and posterior capsular cataract (Oglesby, Black, Allmann, and Bunim 1961), as well as precipitate diabetes mellitus in susceptible subjects (Irvine, Cullen, Eward, Baird, and Harcourt-Webster 1974). Indomethacin and chloroquine have been implicated in damage to the cornea and retina, particularly the macular and paramacular regions (Burns 1968). Patients undergoing treatment with these drugs merit careful ocular examination at regular intervals, particularly as they age and cumulative effects become more likely.

Paget's Disease (Osteitis Deformans)
Paget's disease is a noninflammatory, slowly progressive bone disease of insidious onset. It is characterized by an absorption of bone alternating with its replacement by a chemically, structurally, and architecturally abnormal material that produces skeletal deformities. The condition, except for a rare juvenile form, is unknown in subjects of less than 30 years of age; it has an increasing prevalence in older age groups, and about 10 percent are affected by age 90. Both sexes are affected, and it appears to have a peculiar geographic distribution, being unusually common in Australia and New Zealand (Saville 1975, 1841). Patients of optometrists are largely drawn from older population groups and, consequently, provide a sample in which Paget's disease is not uncommon. This trend is exaggerated by the fact that in most patients the disease does not cause mobility problems or intellectual impairment, leaving the subject capable of seeking private eye care rather than that provided in institutions.

Paget's disease has an unknown etiology. In spite of a rapid turnover and reabsorption of calcium, serum levels of calcium remain normal, although the serum alkaline phosphatase level becomes elevated (Holvey 1972, 1236). Decalcifi-

cation of bone results in softening, which in turn causes deformities, especially of the long bones and other weight-bearing structures. This becomes most obvious in a marked bowing of the legs. In advanced cases there may be spontaneous fractures of these bones. X-ray studies show enlarged and irregular contours, abnormal strands in the bone structure, and dense zones chiefly extending from the ends of the affected bones. Severe impairment of hearing is common.

From the optometrist's viewpoint, the importance of Paget's disease is its frequent involvement of the bones of the skull. These changes may produce headaches, which vary greatly for different patients. They are usually severe and accompanied by back pain and tenderness of other bony structures. The compression of nerves entering the orbit may lead to extraocular muscle palsies and diplopia. The lateral recti are the muscles most commonly affected. In extreme and long-standing cases, the development of bony material along the facial midline causes lateral displacement of the orbits, with a consequential increase in pupillary distances (Duke-Elder 1974b, 999).

Angioid streaks are a more dramatic ocular manifestation of Paget's disease and occur in about 10 percent of cases (Cogan 1974, 97). As the name implies, these streaks have a superficial resemblance to blood vessels in the retina. However, on inspection with the slit lamp and fundus contact lens, they are readily identified as being situated deep in the retina in Bruch's membrane. They consist of breaks along lines of stress in the fibroelastic layer of this membrane and have a characteristic radiating pattern that tends to originate from an incomplete ring surrounding and close to the optic disc (Figure 9–15). There may be hemorrhages into the streaks or the exudation of serum, which causes sensory retinal detachment or a disciform macular lesion (Greer 1972, 174). Angioid streaks are commonly associated with retinal pigment epithelial abnormalities and the formation of drusen.

The diagnosis of asymptomatic Paget's disease is not urgent, since a treatment has yet to emerge; the most effective help to the patient is supportive measures if and when the symptoms develop, as well as treatment of intercurrent disease. Frequently, widespread cardiovascular disease is associated with Paget's disease of long standing, consisting of systemic hypertension, intermittent claudication, and gastrointestinal

Figure 9-15

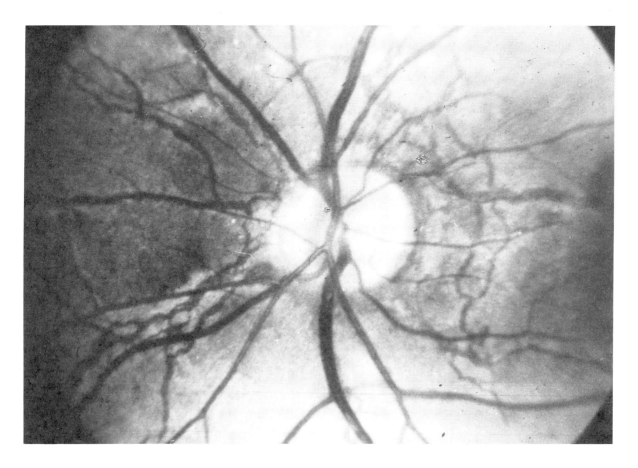

Angioid Streaks. These breaks in Bruch's membrane have a superficial resemblance to blood vessels and occur occasionally in Paget's disease.

bleeding (Cogan 1974, 97). The disease is associated with extensive development of new vascular channels in the bone structure, which leads to high-output cardiac stress and ultimately death from heart failure (Holvey 1972, 1236).

Treatment consists of the adminstration of calcitonin, mithramycin, and drugs of the diphosphonate group (Greenburg 1976). Calcitonin is the least toxic of these drugs, having few, usually transient side effects; nevertheless, treatment should be reserved for those cases having pain that proves refractory to analgesics and those with neurological involvement (Peabody 1980, 331). Patients having angioid streaks require ophthalmologic attention, since neovascular tufts within the choroidal breaks can be destroyed by photocoagulation, thus preventing bleeding and retinal edema.

Tumors of the Eyelids, Conjunctiva, and Skin

Subjects living in and exposed to sunny environments are particularly at risk of epibulbar and adnexal tumors (Irvine 1972), especially aged subjects who have been exposed to actinic radiation for many years (MacRae 1980). Elderly, fair-complexioned people, especially males who have worked outdoors in sunny climates for most of their lives, are rarely spared some form of skin lesion. The following discussion will emphasize the commonly seen benign lesions, premalignant tumors, and malignant tumors that most commonly occur in the elderly patient.

Tumors of the eyelids, conjunctiva, and the skin surrounding the eyes present a formidable diagnostic challenge, since a clinical differentiation between benign and malignant forms is frequently impossible, and only a biopsy and cytological study of the tissues will allow identification. In the early stages of tumor growth, the difficulty of diagnosis is even more marked, yet it is at this stage that treatment of malignancies is most effective. Naturally, an advanced fulminating and disfiguring tumor will cause the patient to consult a medical rather than optometric clinician. The optometrist will be more likely to observe early tumors of which the patient is either unaware or that are not sufficiently advanced to cause concern. For these reasons, optometrists should be alert to the possibility of tumors on and about the eye and accept a relatively high overreferral rate of these lesions in return for the confidence that early, treatable cancers are not neglected until they have caused serious damage.

It is customary to classify tumors into the broad categories of *malignant* and *benign*. Malignant tumors tend to invade adjacent tissues, they may metastasize, and the cells may become undifferentiated or may revert to more primitive forms than those cells from which they derived. In contrast, benign tumors do not invade other tissues or metastasize; they more closely retain the characteristics of the cells of origin, and they usually are enclosed in a connective tissue capsule. This classification is not absolute, and some tumors exhibit mixed characteristics.

Tumor types are named according to the cells from which they develop, to which the suffix *-oma* is added. The term *carcinoma* denotes that the tumor is epithelial in nature; this term may be interchanged with *epithelioma*. Thus, *basal cell carcinoma* is a tumor that arises from the basal cell layer of the dermis. A *sarcoma* derives from connective tissue. Where the tumor cells can be identified as being of a primitive form, *blast* is inserted into the description (for example, *retinoblastoma*), whereas a more mature cell form has the addition of *cyto* (for example, *astrocytoma*). If two or more cell types are involved, the less prominent cell type is named first and the more prominent, second (for example, *neurofibrosarcoma*).

Common Benign Tumors

Papillomas are the most common benign eyelid tumors. They tend to occur on the lid margin as raspberrylike growths or pedunculated (being attached by a stalk) lesions (MacRae 1980) that have a smooth, flat surface continuous with the palprebral conjunctiva. They usually cause no symptoms and grow very slowly. Less commonly, fleshy papillomas develop on the conjunctiva, where they appear in villiform (protruding), sessile (being attached by a base), or pedunculated configurations. They may have a viral origin (Irvine 1972). The possibility of misdiagnosis of conjunctival papillomas is greater than for those on the eyelids, and these cases should be referred for further examination. Treatment is by simple excision.

Skin tags are common in the aged. They are harmless, soft, pedunculated protrusions usually constricted at their base. They commonly are found on the upper lid and on the skin of the neck. Treatment is not necessary except for cosmetic reasons.

Seborrheic keratoses are symptomless and harmless, slowly growing, flat-fissured and slightly raised plaques having a characteristic greasy texture. They are most commonly brownish, appear to be merely stuck to the surrounding skin, and typically reach a size of 1 or 2 cm. These are very common in elderly patients and usually occur on the face and arms. They may be removed for cosmetic reasons but commonly re-form after removal.

Keratoacanthomas usually occur as single lesions on the hands, arms, face, or lids of elderly patients. These are rapidly growing, benign tumors growing in an elevated fashion but having a characteristic crusted central crater with a keratinized plug. They resolve spontaneously in approximately 6 to 8 weeks but may be removed by simple excision. Kerarocanthoma and squamous cell carcinoma may have a similar appearance (Greer 1972, 95).

Pingueculae are yellowish, raised limbal lesions that are very common in the aged and probably represent a degeneration of subepithelial collagen that results from long exposure to the sun and other irritating factors. Very occasionally the epithelium covering a pinguecula will undergo carcinomatous change (Greer 1972, 95). A prominent pinguecula may cause the eyelid to rise above a portion of the cornea during blinks. This results in dehydration and thinning of the corneal stroma to form dellen. Dellen are readily treated by drops containing polyvinyl alcohol or methylcellulose. Uncomplicated pingueculae do not require treatment.

Pterygiums are wedge-shaped degenerative lesions arising from the proliferation of fibrovascular tissue at the limbus, usually from the site of pingueculae (Figure 9–16). A wing of tissue invades the cornea, causing degeneration of Bowman's level and edema of the underlying stromal tissue. To a large extent the virulence of a pterygium can be judged by the degree of vascularization; rapidly developing lesions have an abundant network of vessels. Infiltration of the stroma is visible as a dark shadow seen with the retinoscope against the retinal reflex. When this shadow extends more than about 1 mm beyond the superficial growth, the pterygium is probably developing rapidly.

Figure 9-16

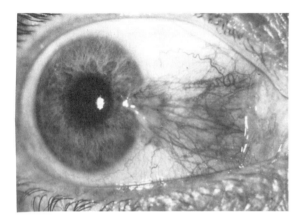

Active Pterygium Accompanied by a Prominent Bank of Conjunctival Vessels.

Treatment of pterygiums can be delayed in the very old, provided the growth is not rapid and the pterygium is not encroaching on the optic zone of the cornea. Removal should be considered when the lesion is on the only good eye and the growth is rapid. A large change in the cylindrical component of the refractive error is also a good indication that the growth should be removed.

Common Premalignant Tumors

Solar Keratoses. Solar keratoses take the form of slowly developing, multiple dry scaly plaques on exposed skin. They are very common in elderly whites who have been exposed to years of sunlight. The clinician often will feel rather than see the scaly lesions on the forehead while steadying the ophthalmoscope during the ocular examination. Their importance lies in reports that between 12 percent (MacRae 1980) and 25 percent (Greer 1972, 95) develop into squamous cell carcinomas. Less frequently, basal cell carcinomas may arise from these lesions (Boink

1964, 239). Patients having solar keratoses should be strongly encouraged to have these lesions removed, to use ultraviolet filtering creams on exposed surfaces, and to wear protective clothing and headwear to prevent continued skin damage from actinic radiation.

Carcinoma in situ (Intraepithelial Carcinoma, Bowen's Disease). A carcinoma in situ is a squamous cell carcinoma that is confined to the epithelial layer of the conjunctiva and the cornea. It has a gelatinous elevated and vascularized appearance with fingerlike processes (Figure 9-17). When on the bulbar conjunctiva it may resemble a conjunctival papilloma. However, carcinoma in situ is found predominantly in elderly males and rarely, if ever, in children, whereas papillomas are relatively common in children (Duke-Elder 1969a, 1154). Although these tumors only occasionally become malignant, they should be removed when they invade the cornea or become particularly exuberant. The differential diagnosis includes papilloma, pterygium, and corneal pannus.

Figure 9-17

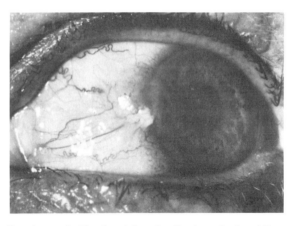

Carcinoma in Situ Involving the Conjunctival and Corneal Epithelium. Note the gelatinous-looking mass on the conjunctiva and keratinized plaque. The tumor has involved the cornea and has a superficial resemblance to a pterygium.

Common Malignant Tumors

Basal Cell Carcinoma. A basal cell carcinoma is the most common malignancy affecting the eyelids and is reported to occur in 0.8 percent of ophthalmic patients (Morax, cited in Duke-Elder 1974a, 421). It has a peak incidence in subjects between 60 and 69 years old, and the lower lid or medial canthus was the site in 75 percent of cases (Collin 1976). Males are said to be more likely to have a basal cell carcinoma than females (Scheie and Albert 1977, 450), although one large series involved almost equal sex distribution (Payne et al. 1969). The early appearance of a basal cell carcinoma is a raised, pearly nodule or a flat, hard, scarlike plaque; the lesion is symptomless and grows slowly. Eventually, the tumor develops a roughly circular, raised border leaving a central crater that may develop a small scab from the breakdown of a blood vessel within the tumor (Figure 9–18). The edges of the raised tumor are shiny, and small telangiectasias can be seen on slit lamp examination. If the lesion is pinched between the thumb and idex finger, the deep portion will be found to be harder than the normal surrounding tissue.

appears that the size of the tumor is the critical factor in bringing the patient for attention, and careful history taking to assess the age of the lesion will help the clinician make the correct diagnosis. Discovery of a basal cell carcinoma should alert the optometrist to the likelihood of multifocal basal cell tumors; in one series of 30 consecutive ocular basal cell carcinoma patients, 18 (60 percent) had one or more additional lesions (Wesley and Collins 1982).

Although basal cell carcinomas rarely, if ever, metastasize, they can become locally invasive and cause extensive tissue destruction (Figure 9–19). Lesions that develop in the medial canthus carry the worst prognosis, and the absence of metastasis should not be a cause for complacency, since basal cell carcinoma still can be a fatal disease (Collin 1976).

Figure 9–18

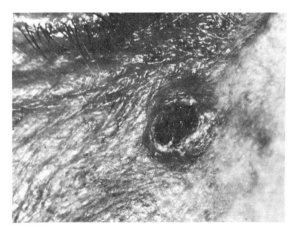

A Typical Basal Cell Carcinoma below the Lid Margin Showing Raised Crenated and Pearly Edges with a Central Depression in Which There Is an Accumulation of Dried Blood.

Figure 9–19

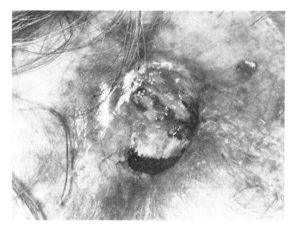

Neglected Basal Cell Carcinoma That Has Extended to Involve Deeper Tissues, Including the Frontal Bone.

Errors of diagnosis are common. In a series of 273 cases of histologically proved basal cell carcinomas, the clinical diagnosis was correct in 60 percent of the cases. The most common misdiagnosis was papilloma (Payne et al. 1969). Basal cell carcinoma may contain pigment cells and be confused with malignant melanoma as a result of their dark color. Patients typically seek professional examination when the lesion has been present for approximately 5 years and has reached a diameter of 4 or 5 mm. Squamous cell carcinomas, in contrast, grow more rapidly and reach this size in approximately 1 year. It

Treatment of basal cell carcinomas is by excision, preferably under frozen section control by means of which the margins of the excised tissue are examined for abnormal cells and the incision is enlarged until all margins contain normal cells (Doxanas, Green, and Iliff 1981). However, good results also are claimed for cryotherapy (Allen et al. 1979) and radiation treatment (Lederman 1976).

Squamous Cell Carcinoma. A squamous cell carcinoma is another tumor that is more common in aged subjects (MacRae 1980), although it is much less prevalent than basal cell carcinomas. It has a predilection for developing on the bulbar conjunctiva, particularly at the transition zone between the conjunctival and corneal epithelium; when it occurs on the lids, the upper lid is more likely to be the site of the lesion. As has been noted, this form of tumor grows more rapidly than a basal cell carcinoma, and patients tend to seek consultation when the tumor reaches approximately 5 mm and has been present for 12 months.

In its early stages a squamous cell tumor on the lid is similar in appearance to a basal cell carcinoma; it has papular or plaquelike form with an indurated base. However, it is generally whitish and is more likely to be keratinized before the ulcerative stage has been reached. These tumors frequently evoke an inflammatory response, which can lead to the misdiagnosis of hordeola. Squamous cell carcinomas that develop on the conjunctiva form gelatinous-looking masses, usually at the caruncle or the limbal margin, and they are easily confused with papillomas. Squamous cell carcinomas eventually metastasize by extension through the lymphatic system, where they become rapidly invasive, often causing an inflammatory response and considerable pain (Peabody 1980, 331). Early treatment of squamous cell carcinoma is desirable and may be by excision, radiation, or chemotherapy (MacRae 1980).

Management Decisions

When elderly patients have clinical evidence of conjunctival, lid, or skin tumors, the optometrist should temper management decisions with a knowledge of and experience with these lesions. *When in doubt, assume the diagnosis having the worst prognosis, and refer the patient for a second opinion.* A very frail, elderly patient having a terminal illness and short life expectancy may elect to remain untreated. Forgoing treatment is reasonable for precancerous lesions and perhaps for early basal cell carcinomas; however, squamous cell carcinoma may cause painful and destructive lesions within 12 months and should not be neglected.

Conclusion

No single professional group has the capacity to provide a comprehensive support service for the aged. Trained, dedicated, and caring professionals from many disciplines who are prepared to work as a team offer the greatest prospect of meeting the needs of these people. Although high-level technology has a place in some areas

of medical care, the instruments of good geriatric medicine are simple and universally available; they are the ears, the heart, and the time of the clinician. In many cases, the ability to listen, empathize, and show concern for the elderly patient is all that is required to produce therapeutic dividends. If the clinician can dispel false apprehensions, add a little genuine reassurance, and accentuate the more positive aspects of the prognosis, the vast majority of aged patients will live out their last years in tranquility.

Optometrists have the potential to become an important part of the caring team for the aged; they are uniquely equipped to optimize the vision of elderly patients, yet not so remotely professional and exalted that they cannot relate to their patients. Both the value of their contribution and the acceptance of their role depend on the extent of their clinical skills, their humanitarian approach, and particularly their depth of knowledge of the common systemic diseases encountered in age.

The optometrist also must understand and respect the scope of service available through other professionals and be prepared to refer patients when appropriate. Frequently, a decision must be made about whether to advise further medical investigation or treatment of systemic disease noted during the ocular examination or to simply provide support and comfort without further intervention. The burden of this decision should be shared with patients to the limits of their ability to understand the alternatives, but clinicians must never abrogate their responsibility to fully and accurately inform the patients so that the decisions can be soundly based. However, it does no service to the elderly patient to draw attention to or initiate uncomfortable procedures merely to confirm the presence of a disease for which treatment is ineffective. The vast majority of the ambulatory elderly who make up patient samples are capable of and have the inalienable right to make informed choices involving their own life styles and medical care.

It should be remembered that in age, illness becomes more easily tolerated through the blunting of the senses. Physical incapacity is accepted as the desire for activity diminishes, and even death becomes less frightening when the challenges of life are behind and there is assurance of understanding and caring support.

References

Acheson, J., and E. C. Hutchinson. "Observations on the Natural History of Transient Ischemic Attacks." *Lancet* 11 (1964): 871–874.

Allen, E. D., et al. "Cryotherapy of Basal Cell Lesions." *Transactions of the Ophthalmological Society of the United Kingdom* 99 (1979): 264–268.

Andrews, J. M. "Giant Cell (Temporal) Arteritis." *Neurology* 16 (1966): 963–971.

Armaly, M. F. "Effect of Corticosteriods on Intraocular Pressure and Fluid Deficiencies." *Archives of Ophthalmology* 70 (1963): 482–499.

Ballantyne, A. J., and I. C. Michaelson. *Textbook of the Fundus of the Eye.* Edinburgh: Churchill Livingstone, 1973.

Barr, M. L. *The Human Nervous System.* 3d ed. Hagerstown, Md.: Harper & Row, 1979.

Becker B., and D. W. Mills. "Corticosteroids and Intraocular Pressure." *Archives of Ophthalmology* 70 (1963): 500–507.

Beeson, P. B., "Polymyalgia Rheumatica and Cranial Arteritis." In *Textbook of Medicine,* 14th ed., eds. P. B. Beeson and W. McDermott. Philadelphia: Saunders, 1975.

Beevers, D. G. "Hypertension." *Internal Medicine* (Australian ed.) 19, part 3 (1982): 892–902.

Boink, M. *Ocular and Adnexal Tumors.* St. Louis: Mosby, 1964.

Bouzas, A. G. "Endocrine Ophthalmology." *Transactions of the Ophthalmological Society of the United Kingdom* 100 (1980): 511–520.

Burns, A. "Indomethacin Reduced Retinal Sensitivity and Corneal Deposits." *American Journal of Ophthalmology* 66, no. 5 (1968): 825–835.

Cahill, G. F. "Disorders of Carbohydrate Metabolism: Diabetes Mellitus." In *Textbook of Medicine,* 14th ed., eds. P. B. Beeson, and W. McDermott. Philadelphia: Saunders, 1975.

Caird, R. I.; M. A. Pirie; and T. G. Ramsell. *Diabetes and the Eye.* Oxford, England: Blackwell, 1969.

Cameron, R. J. *Year Book Australia.* No. 66. Canberra: Australian Government Publication, 1982.

Canadian Co-operation Study Group. "A Randomized Trial of Aspirin and Sulfinpyrazone in Threatened Stroke." *New England Journal of Medicine* 299 (1978): 53–59.

Chalmers, F. P. "Treatment of Uncomplicated Essential Hypertension." *Australian Prescriber,* 2, no. 1 (1977): 6–8.

Christie, D.; L. McPherson; and V. Vivian. "The Queenscliff Study: A Community Screening Programme for Hypertension." *Australian Medical Journal* 2 (1976): 678–680.

Christian, C. L. In *Textbook of Medicine,* 14th ed., eds. P. B. Beeson and W. McDermott. Philadelphia: Saunders, 1975.

Chuna-Vaz, J. G. "Pathophysiology of Diabetic Retinopathy." *British Journal of Ophthalmology* 62 (1978): 351–355.

Cockburn, D. M. "Detection of Diabetic Signs in Optometric Practice." *Australian Journal of Optometry* 57 (1974): 243–250.

Cockburn, D. M. "The Prevalence of Ocular Hypertension in Patients of an Optometrist and the Incidence of Glaucoma Occurring during Long-Term Follow-Up of Ocular Hypertensives." *American Journal of Optometry and Physiological Optics* 59, no. 4 (1982): 330–337.

Cockburn, D. M. "Signs and Symptoms of Stroke and Impending Stroke in a Series of Optometric Patients." *American Journal of Optometry and Physiological Optics* 60, no. 9 (1983): 749–753.

Cogan, D. G. *Ophthalmic Manifestations of Systemic Disease.* Philadelphia: Saunders, 1974.

Cogan, D. G., and T. Kuwabara. "Capillary Shunts in the Pathogenesis of Diabetic Retinopathy." *Diabetes* 12 (1963): 293–300.

Collin, J. R. O. "Basal Cell Carcinoma in the Eyelid Region." *British Journal of Ophthalmology* 60 (1976): 806–809.

Cullen, J. F. "Occult Temporal Arteritis." *British Journal of Ophthalmology* 51 (1967): 513–525.

De Groot, L. J. "The Thyroid." In *Textbook of Medicine,* 14th ed., eds P. B. Beeson and W. McDermott. Philadelphia: Saunders, 1975.

Denham, M. "Diagnostic Differences in Old Age." *Medicine Australia,* series 1, no. 35/36 (1981): 2578–2580.

Doxanas, M. T.; W. R. Green; and C. E. Iliff "Factors in the Surgical Management of Basal Cell Carcinoma of the Eyelids." *American Journal of Ophthalmology* 91 (1981):726–736.

Duke-Elder, S. *System of Ophthalmology.* Vol. 8, part 2. London: Henry Kimpton, 1965.

Duke-Elder, S. *System of Ophthalmology.* Vol. 10. London: Henry Kimpton, 1967.

Duke-Elder, S. *System of Ophthalmology.* Vol. 8. London: Henry Kimpton, 1969. (a)

Duke-Elder, S. *System of Ophthalmology.* Vol. 11. London: Henry Kimpton, 1969. (b)

Duke-Elder, S. *System of Ophthalmology.* Vol. 12. London: Henry Kimpton, 1971.

Duke-Elder, S. *System of Ophthalmology.* Vol. 6. London: Henry Kimpton, 1973.

Duke-Elder, S. *System of Ophthalmology.* Vol. 13, part 1. London: Henry Kimpton, 1974. (a)

Duke-Elder, S. *System of Ophthalmology.* Vol. 13, part 2. London: Henry Kimpton, 1974. (b).

Duke-Elder, S. *System of Ophthalmology.* Vol. 15. London: Henry Kimpton, 1976.

Duncan, G. W.; M. S. Pessin; J. P. Mohr; and R. D. Adams. "Transient Cerebral Ischemic Attacks." *Advances in Internal Medicine.* 21 (1976): 1–20.

Escourolle, R., and J. Poirer. *Basic Neuropathology.* Philadelphia: Saunders, 1978.

Eshaghian, J. "Controversies Regarding Giant Cell (Temporal, Cranial) Arteritis." *Documenta Ophthalmologica* 47 (1979): 43–67.

Fein, J. M. "Microvascular Surgery for Stroke." *Scientific American* 238, no. 4 (1978): 59–67.

Field, W. S. and L. A. Lemak. "Joint Study of Intracranial Arterial Occlusion: Part 9. Transient Ischemic Attacks in the Carotid Territory." *Journal of the American Medical Association* 235, no. 24 (1976): 2608–2610.

Gartner, S. and P. Henkind. "Neovascularization of the Iris (Rubeosis Iridis)." *Survey of Ophthalmology* 22 (1978): 291.

Geddes, M. "Infective Endocarditis." *Internal Medicine* 19, no. 3 (1982); 878–884.

Gombos, G. M. *Handbook of Ophthalmological Emergencies.* 2d ed. Flushing, N.Y.: Medical Examination Publishing, 1977.

Greenberg, P. P. "Calcitonin in Paget's Disease." *Australian Prescriber,* 2, no. 1 (1976): 26–27.

Greer, C. H. *Ocular Pathology.* 2d ed. Oxford England: Blackwell, 1972.

Gribben, B. "Infective Endocarditis." In *Oxford Textbook of Medicine*, Vol. 2. eds. D. J. Weatherall, J. G. G. Ledingham, and D. A. Warrell. Oxford: Oxford University Press, 1983.

Harrison, M. J. G.; J. Marshall; J. C. Meadows; and K. W. Russ-Russell. "Effect of Aspirin in Amaurosis Fugax." *Lancet* 2 (1971): 743–744.

Hayreh, S. S. *Anterior Ischemic Optic Neuropathy.* Berlin: Springer-Varlag, 1975.

Hayson, M. I. V. and D. M. Grennan. "Clinical Features of Rheumatoid Arthritis." In *Oxford Textbook of Medicine*, eds. D. J. Weatherall, J. G. G. Ledingham, and D. A. Warrell. Oxford: Oxford University Press, 1983.

Henderson J. W. "Optic Neuropathy in Exophthalmic Goiter (Graves' Disease)." *Archives of Ophthalmology* 59 (1958): 471–480.

Hercules, B. L.; I. I. Gayed; S. B. Lucas; and J. Jeacock. "Peripheral Retinal Ablation in the Treatment of Proliferative Diabetic Retinopathy: A Three Year Interim Report of a Randomized Study Using Argon Laser." *British Journal of Ophthalmology* 61 (1977): 555–563.

Herman, B.; B. P. M. Schulte; J. H. van Luijk; A. C. M. Leyton; and C. W. G. M. Frenken. "Epidemiology of Stroke in Tilburg, The Netherlands." *Stroke* 2, no. 2 (1980): 162–165.

Hodkinson, M. "Diagnostic Differences in Old Age." *Medicine Australia*, series 1, no. 35/36 (1981): 2578–2580.

Holvey, D. N., ed. *The Merck Manual of Diagnosis and Therapy.* 12th ed. Rathway, N.J.: Merck, Sharp and Dohme, 1972.

Howells, G. *Annual Report of the Director-General of Health, 1981–82.* Canberra: Australian Government Printer, 1982.

Irvine, R. A. "Epibulbar Squamous Cell Carcinoma and Related Lesions." International Ophthalmology Clinics 71 (1972): 83.

Irvine, W. J.; D. R. Cullen; R B. L. Eward; J. D. Baird; and J. N. Harcourt-Webster. "Diseases of the Endocrine Glands." In *A Companion to Medical Studies*, Vol. 3, eds. R. Passmore, and J. S. Rotron. Oxforu, England: Blackwell, 1974, pp. 23–76.

Kannel, W. B. "Current Status of the Epidemiology of Brain Infarction Associated with Occlusive Arterial Disease." *Stroke* 2, no. 4 (1971): 295–318.

Kathol, R. G.; T. A. Cox; J. J. Corbett; and H. S. Thompson. "Functional Visual Loss: Follow-up of 42 Cases." *Archives of Ophthalmology* 101 (1983): 735–739.

Kearns, T. P., and R. W. Hollenhorst. "Venous-Stasis Retinopathy of Occlusive Disease of the Carotid Artery." *Proceedings of the Mayo Clinic* 38 (1963): 304–312.

Keen, H. "The Nature of the Diabetes Syndrome." *International Medicine* 8 (1981): 327–333.

Kohner, E. M.; T. R. Fraser; G. F. Joplin; and N. W. Oakley. "The Effect of Diabetic Control on Diabetic Retinopathy." In *The Treatment of Diabetic Retinopathy*, eds. M. F. Goldberg and S. L. Fine. U. S. Public Health Service Publication no. 1890. Washington, D.C.: U. S. Government Printing Office, 1969, pp. 119–128.

Lamberto, D. W.; C. S. Foster; and H. D. Perry. "Schirmer Test after Topical Anaesthesia and the Minimum Height in Normal Eyes." *Archives of Ophthalmology* 97 (1979): 1082–1085.

Lawson, P. M.; M. C. Champion; C. Canny; R. Kingsley; M. C. White; J. Dupre; and E. M. Kohner. "Continuous Subcutaneous Insulin Infusion Does Not Prevent Progression

of Proliferative and Preproliferative Retinopathy." *British Journal of Ophthalmology* 66 (1982): 762–766

Leak, A. M. "Advances in the Treatment of Rheumatic Disease." *Practitioner* 227 (1983): 1139–1145.

Lederman, M. "Radiation Treatment of Cancer of the Eyelids." *British Journal of Ophthalmology* 60 (1976): 794–805.

Lucas, C. P., and M. Omar. "Pretreatment Assessment." *Geriatrics* 35 (1980): 51–55, 59.

McDowell, F. H. "Cerebrovascular Diseases." In *Textbook of Medicine*, 14th ed., eds. P. B. Beeson and W. McDermott. Philadelphia: Saunders, 1975.

McLeod J., ed. *Clinical Examination.* 5th ed. Edinburgh: Churchill Livingstone, 1979.

MacRae, D. W. "Tumors and Related Lesions of the Eyelids and Conjunctiva." In *Principles and Practice of Ophthalmology*, Vol. 3, eds. A. P. Gholam, D. R. Sanders, and M. F. Goldberg. Philadelphia: Saunders, 1980.

Mandelkorn, R. M., and T. J. Zimmerman. "Effects of Nonsteroidal Drugs on Glaucoma." In *The Secondary Glaucomas*, eds. R. Ritch and M. B. Shields. St. Louis: Mosby, 1982.

The Merck Manual. Rathway, N.J.: Merck & Co., 1982.

Muuronen, A., and M. Kaste. "Outcome of 314 Patients with Transient Ischemic Attacks." *Stroke* 13, no. 1 (1982): 24–31.

National Diabetes Data Group. "Classification and Diagnosis of Diabetes Mellitus and Other Categories of Glucose Intolerance." *Diabetes* 28 (1979): 1039–1057.

Newell, F. W. *Ophthalmological Principles and Concepts.* 5th ed. St. Louis: Mosby, 1982.

Niarchos, A. O. "Hypertension in the Elderly." *Modern Concepts of Cardiovascular Disease* 49 (1980): 49–54.

Oglesby, R. B.; R. L. Black; L. Allmann; and J. J. Bunim. "Cataracts in Patients with Rheumatic Diseases Treated with Corticosteroids." *Archives of Ophthalmology* 66 (1961): 625–630.

Olsson, J. E.; R. Muller; and S. Berneli. "Long-term Anticoagulant Therapy for TIAs and Minor Strokes with Minimum Residual." *Stroke* 7, no. 5 (1976): 444–451.

Page, L. B. V., and J. J. Sidd. "Medical Progress: Medical Management of Primary Hypertension." *New England Journal of Medicine* 287, no. 19 (1972): 960–966.

Pavin-Langston, D., ed. *Manual of Ocular Diagnosis and Therapy.* Boston: Little, Brown, 1980.

Payne, J. W.; J. R. Duke; R. Butner; and D. E. Eifrig. "Basal Cell Carcinoma of the Eyelids: A Long-term Follow-up Study." *Archives of Ophthalmology* 81 (1969): 553–558.

Peabody, R. R. "Angioid Streaks." In *Current Ocular Therapy*, eds. F. Fraunfelder and F. T. Roy. Philadelphia: Saunders, 1980.

Peart, W. S. "Arterial Hypertension." In *Textbook of Medicine*, 14th ed., eds. P. B. Beeson and W. McDermott. Philadelphia: Saunders, 1975.

Pickering, G. "Hypertension, Definitions, Natural Histories and Consequences." *American Journal of Medicine* 52 (1972): 570–583.

Reinecke, R. D., and T. Kuwabara. "Temporal Arteritis." *Archives of Ophthalmology* 82 (1969): 446–453.

Riggs, H. E., and C. Rupp. "Variation in the Form of Circle of Willis." *Archives of Neurology* 8, no. 1 (1963): 8–31.

Rodman, G. P., ed. "Primer on the Rheumatic Diseases: Criteria for the Diagnosis and Classification of Rheumatic Diseases." *Journal of the American Medical Association* 224, no. 5 (1973): 799–800.

Sachdev, Y.; J. C. Chatterji; and R. C. Sharma. "Hetrogenicity of Failure of Visual Acuity in Graves' Disease." *Postgraduate Medical Journal* 55 (1979): 241–247.

Saracco, J. B.; P. Castaud; B. Ridings; and C. A. Ubaud. "Diabetic Choroidopathy." *Journal Français d'Ophthalmologie* 5 (1982): 231–236.

Saville, P. S. "Paget's Disease of Bone: Osteitis Deformans." In *Textbook of Medicine*, 14th ed., eds. P. B. Beeson and W. McDermott. Philadelphia: Saunders, 1975.

Scheie, H. G., and D. M. Albert. *Textbook of Ophthalmology*, 9th ed. Philadelphia: Saunders, 1977.

Sedzimer, C. B. "An Angiographic Test of Collateral Circulation through the Anterior Segment of the Circle of Willis." *Journal of Neurology, Neurosurgery and Psychiatry* 22, no. 1 (1959): 64–68.

Society of Actuaries. *Build and Blood Pressure Study*. Vols. 1 and 2. Chicago: Society of Actuaries, 1959.

Sorsby, A. and A. Goma. "Iritis in Rheumatoid Disease." *British Journal of Medicine* (1946): 597–600.

Stamler J. *Comprehensive Treatment of Essential Hypertensive Disease: Why, When, and How*. Monographs on Hypertension. Rathway, N.J.: Merck, 1970.

Steno Study Group. "Effect of 6 Months of Strict Metabolic Control of Eye and Kidney Function in Insulin Dependent Diabetics with Background Retinopathy." *Lancet* 1 (1982): 121–124.

Stone, R. A. "Glaucoma Associated with Systemic Disease." In *The Secondary Glaucomas*, eds. R. Ritch, and M. B. Shields. St. Louis: Mosby, 1982.

Topilow, H. W.; K. R. Kenyon; M. Takahashi; H. M. Freeman; F. I. Tolentino; and L. A. Hanninen. "Asteroid Hyalaosis: Biomicroscopy Ultrastructure and Composition." *Archives of Ophthalmology* 100 (1982): 964–968.

Treleaven, G. K. ed. *Prescription Proprietaries Guide*. Melbourne: Australian Pharmaceutical, 1982.

Tucker, R. M. "Is Hypertension Different in the Elderly?" *Geriatrics*, May 1980, 28–32.

Urrets-Zavalia, A. *Diabetic Retinopathy*. New York: Masson, 1977.

Veshima, H.; M. Lida; T. Shimamoto; M. Konishi; K. Tsujioka; M. Tanigaki; N. Kakanishi; W. Ozawa; S. Kojima; and Y. Komachi. "Multivariate Analysis of Risk Factors in Stroke." *Preventative Medicine* 9 (1980): 722–740.

Veterans Administration Co-operative Study Group on Antihypertensive Agents. "Effects of Treatment on Morbidity in Hypertension: 2. Results in Patients with Diastolic Blood Pressure Averaging 90 through 114 mm Hg." *Journal of the American Medical Association* 213, no. 7 (1970): 1143–1152.

Wand, M. "Neovascular Glaucoma." In *The Secondary Glaucomas*, eds. R. Ritch and M. B. Shields. St. Louis: Mosby, 1982.

Warlow, C. "Management of Cerebrovascular Disease." *Medicine Australia* 32, no. 3 (1981): 2300–2308.

Welzel, G. "Antihypertensive Treatment in the Elderly." *Gerontology* 28, supp. 1 (1982): 83–92.

Wesley, R. E., and J. W. Collins. "Basal Cell Carcinoma of the Eyelid as an Indicator of Multifocal Malignancy." *American Journal of Ophthalmology* 94 (1982) 591–593.

West, K. M.; L. J. Erdreich; and J. A. Stober. "A Detailed Study of the Risk Factors for Retinopathy and Nephropathy in Diabetes." *Diabetes* 29 (1980): 501–508.

Wilson, L. A., and R. W. Ross-Russell. "Amaurosis Fugax and Carotid Artery Disease: Indications for Angiography." *British Medical Journal* 2 (1977): 435–437.

Wishnant, J. P.; N. Matsumoto; and L. R. Elueback. "Transient Cerebral Ischemic Attacks in a Community; Rochester, Minnesota, 1955 through 1969." *Proceedings of the Mayo Clinic* 48 (1973): 194–198.

World Health Organization. *Arterial Hypertension and Ischemic Heart Disease*. World Health Organization Technical Report no. 231. Geneva, WHO, 1962.

Yahr, M. D. "The Parkinsonian Syndrome." In *Textbook of Medicine*, 14th ed., eds. P. B. Beeson and W. McDermott. Philadelphia: Saunders, 1975.

Chapter 10

Changes in Visual Function in the Aging Eye

Meredith W. Morgan

This chapter will be limited to changes in visual function in the normal, healthy aging eye free from obvious structural or pathological anomalies. This restriction may raise some practical as well as philosophical problems, since few eyes that have survived 60 or more years of life are free from at least some slight sign of deterioration, degeneration, or past or present disease that can escape a scientific, sophisticated search. This chapter will use the concept of "normal" in much the same way as the average clinician states that an amblyopic eye is "normal" in that it has no apparent structural or pathological defect that could account for the reduced acuity. Such an eye is obviously not normal, since it has less than normal acuity. In an amblyopic eye there is just no readily apparent cause for the reduced acuity. Conditions that apply to most aged eyes, such as miosis and the absence of accommodation, will be considered normal rather than abnormal or pathological.

This approach is used for two main reasons: (1) pathological and degenerative conditions affecting the aging eye are discussed in other chapters, and (2) departure from normal function is often a clue that a more detailed and critical examination and search need to be made. This requires that the examiner know what normal function is. Unfortunately, most clinical optometric norms have been established by data from prepresbyopic subjects.

The major thrust of the discussion will be about the aspects of vision that are of chief concern to clinicians and ordinarily measured by them. Some attention, however, will be given to phenomena that today are primarily of interest to visual scientists, but that will someday also be of concern to clinicians. As a matter of fact, most of the significant changes in visual func-

tion of the aging eye, except for the loss of focusing ability and the increase in variability of measured functions, are not quantified by clinicians in the usual vision examination. As yet, nearly all ophthalmologists, as well as a majority of optometrists, assume that aging patients without significant motor imbalance and with good corrected visual acuity at distance and near must have satisfactory or normal visually controlled behavior. Some visual scientists, as well as some optometrists, are suggesting that there is a more sophisticated and comprehensive view of vision (Leibowitz 1980).

The increase in variability or dispersion of measured function with increasing age applies to nearly all visual functions. This makes it extremely difficult to identify performance that is clearly subnormal. There are almost always some older persons who function as well as younger ones, but the number at "best performance" usually declines with age. For example, Weymouth (1960), using data supplied by Hirsch, reported that in the age bracket from 40 to 44, 93.5 percent of patients had a corrected visual acuity of 20/20 or better; in the age bracket from 70 to 74 however, only 41.9 percent had a corrected visual acuity of 20/20 or better, whereas 56.1 percent had a corrected visual acuity of 20/40 or better. Most of this decrease in the percentage of individuals with maximum acuity and the greater variability in best-corrected acuity is due to the effects of degeneration or disease conditions. Some of the decrease, however, cannot be accounted for on this basis. In the 70-to-74 age group just referred to, 14.5 percent of the patients with corrected visual acuity of less than 20/25 had no clinically reportable degenerative or disease conditions—the eyes were clinically normal.

A good many of the apparent physiological or psychological changes in visual function have a physical cause. Consequently, this chapter first will discuss changes in the structure of the eye that could result in a change in visual function and that are detected by clinicians in routine vision examinations.

Changes in the Cornea with Age

Corneal sensitivity to touch decreases with age. According to Millodot (1977), the threshold for touch almost doubles between the ages of 10 and 80, increasing rapidly after the age of 40. The cause for this decrease is not known. It is both an advantage and a disadvantage in fitting contact lenses—an advantage in that older patients adapt more readily to contact lenses, but a disadvantage in that corneal lesions may occur without creating significant subjective symptoms of pain. The practitioner, particularly with older patients, should not depend on the presence of symptoms to suggest that the integrity of the cornea need be examined carefully.

There have been reports of the increase in against-the-rule astigmatism in older people since before Helmholtz. Most cross-section studies of refractive error and age confirm this trend. Does this change in the meridian of greatest refractive power of the eye from the 90-degree meridian in youth to the 180-degree meridian in old age signify that the curvature of the cornea changes with age? Helmholtz (1924) believed that the natural form of the cornea was such that the meridian of greatest curvature was horizontal, but that the cornea was deformed in youth by the pressure of the lids so that the greatest curvature was vertical in youth. As the lid tension decreases and the ocular tissues harden with age, the cornea escapes back to its natural form.

Helmholtz's armchair physiology is not exactly borne out by experimental evidence. According to Wilson et al. (1982), lid retraction from corneas having more than 1.00D of with-the-rule astigmatism resulted in less with-the-rule astigmatism as measured with a keratometer. The major change in curvature obtained was an increase in curvature of the horizontal meridian rather than a decrease in curvature of the vertical, as predicted by Helmholtz.

The concept that the corneal curvature changes with age seems to be confirmed by the studies of Kratz and Walton (1949) and Phillips (1952). Kratz and Walton reported from a study of clin-

ical records that the best estimate for the correction of astigmatism based on keratometric findings was achieved when the allowance for physiological astigmatism in Javal's formula remained at a 0.50D for all ages. They argue that since the total astigmatism increases against-the-rule throughout life, the cause of the increase must be a change in corneal astigmatism. Their actual data, originally presented in graphic form, are summarized in Table 10–1. The data seem to support the concept that the number of patients having with-the-rule astigmatism decreases with age. Phillips' data from a clinical practice in Great Britain are shown in Table 10–2.

These data of Kratz and Walton and Phillips are unfortunately in relative terms showing the difference in power of the two principal meridians. It cannot be stated categorically that the vertical power, and hence the curvature, decreased or that that horizontal power, and hence the curvature, increased.

In a longitudinal study of 46 patients over a period of 0.5 to 20 years, Exford (1965) reports that corneal power in both the horizontal and vertical meridians increased at a rate slightly less than 0.25D per decade and that there was no observable trend that either meridian changed more rapidly than the other.

Mason (1940, 400–401) reported on 475 eyes of people between the ages of 12 and 39 and 475 eyes of people between the ages of 45 and 79. All eyes had at least a 0.25D with-the-rule corneal astigmatism as measured using a keratometer. Of the younger group, 22 percent required against-the-rule corrections, whereas 41 percent of the older group required such corrections. Mason's data in graphic form are restated in Table 10–3.

The data of Mason indicate that the increase in against-the-rule astigmatism with age must be accounted for on some other basis than changes in corneal curvature, since even with matched corneal astigmatisms, more of the older group have against-the-rule astigmatism than do the younger group.

The meager evidence indicates that the corneal curvature probably changes slightly with age and that in spite of the appearance of a larger percentage of individuals with against-the-rule astigmatism in the older age bracket, it cannot be stated categorically that the curvature of the horizontal meridian increases or that the curvature of the vertical meridian decreases with increasing age.

Table 10–1
Corneal Astigmatism in Kratz and Walton Study

Decade	Against-the-Rule Corneal Astigmatism	With-the-Rule Corneal Astigmatism	No Corneal Astigmatism
2	18%	80%	2%
5	11	78	11
8	30	20	50
9	75	25	0

Note: The number of patients at each decade is unknown.

Source: Based on J. D. Kratz and W. G. Walton. "A Modification of Javal's Rule for the Correction of Astigmatism." *American Journal of Optometry and Archives of American Academy of Optometry* 26 (1949): 302. *American Journal of Optometry and Physiological Optics.* Copyright 1949. American Academy of Optometry.

Table 10–2
Corneal Astigmatism According to Phillips

Age	Against-the-Rule Astigmatism	With-the-Rule Astigmatism	No Astigmatism	Number of Patients
10 to 20	6.8%	75.5%	12.7%	164
20 to 30	8.2	72.3	19.5	268
30 to 40	17.7	64.1	18.2	204
40 to 50	25.6	46.9	27.5	320
50 to 60	31.7	40.5	27.8	356
60 to 70	33.9	37.7	28.4	239
70 to 80	35.0	37.2	27.8	140

Source: Based on R. A. Phillips. "Changes in Corneal Astigmatism." *American Journal of Optometry and Archives of American Academy of Optometry* 29 (1952): 379. *American Journal of Optometry and Physiological Optics.* Copyright 1952. American Academy of Optometry.

Table 10–3
Comparison of Corneal and Ametropic Astigmatism

With-the-Rule Corneal Astigmatism	Ametropic Astigmatism				
	Ages 12–39 years		Ages 45–75 years		
	Against	With	Against	With	
0.25D	40%	22%	50%	10%	
0.50	21	41	41	30	
0.75	15	52	20	45	
1.00	9	67	10	55	
1.25	5	70	9	65	
1.50	2	87	1	66	
1.75	1	90	1	67	
2.00	1	99	1	88	

Note: The percentage of those with 0.00D cylindrical correction for astigmatism has been omitted.

Source: Based on F. L. Mason. *Principles of Optometry.* San Francisco: Carlisle, 1940, pp. 400–401.

Changes in the
Anterior Chamber with Age

Weale (1962), quoting Johansen and Raeder, states that the depth of the anterior chamber decreases from an average of 3.6 mm in the age range of 15 to 20 years to an average of 3.0 mm by the age of 70 because of growth of the lens. A decrease in the depth of the anterior chamber must tend to make the angle of the anterior chamber at the root of the iris more acute, thus increasing the possibility of interference with aqueous outflow. Likewise, if all other factors remain constant, a decrease in the anterior chamber depth slightly increases the refractive power of the eye, making the eye relatively more myopic. The chemical composition and refractive index of the aqueous appears to be independent of age.

Changes in the Iris with Age

One of the most significant changes in the older eye is senile miosis (Girren, Casperson, and Botwineck 1960; Weale 1963). In addition, the difference in diameter of the pupil in the light- and dark-adapted states becomes less and less. The cause of the miosis is not known, but it is thought to be due to atrophy of the dilator muscle fibers, an increased rigidity of the iris blood vessels, or both. In any event, the pupil becomes smaller at all levels of illumination, with only a slight increase in the latency of pupillary responses (Feinberg and Podolak 1965).

This miosis reduces retinal illuminance and the diameter of retinal blur circles when the eye is out of focus. Consequently, at high levels of illumination, uncorrected visual acuity may appear to improve with age rather than decrease. Likewise, the range of clear vision at near through any addition appears to increase with age, giving the appearance of accommodative change.

This miosis makes it difficult to examine the fundus or other structures of the eye through the undilated pupil. Subjective refraction becomes more difficult, since changes in lens power do not change the diameter of retinal blur circles as much as a similar change in eyes with larger pupils. This means that the optometrist must be prepared to use a 0.50 or 0.62D instead of the usual 0.37D crossed cylinder in the determination of the magnitude and the axis of any astigmatism. In other words, the older patient may be less sensitive to lens changes than the younger because of optical reasons rather than because of a decrease in observational abilities due to supposed senility.

Changes in the Lens with Age

The lens of the eye continues to grow throughout life. Weale (1962), quoting Johansen and Raeder, states that the axial thickness of the lens increases by about 28 percent by age 70 over that which existed at age 15 to 20 years. This means that if the lens is assumed to be 3.6 mm thick at age 15 to 20 (the Gullstrand standard), then by age 70 it will be approximately 4.6 mm thick. The nuclear thickness remains constant while the cortical thicknesses increase. On the average, the anterior cortex increases by 0.6 mm and the posterior, by 0.4 mm.

As the lens increases in size, the curvature would be expected to decrease. According to Mellerio (1971) quoting Fisher, however, the growth of the lens is not uniform, and the equatorial diameter to polar thickness decreases with age, resulting in a conical bulging of the posterior lens surface. If this observation is correct, it can be assumed that the anterior lens surface becomes flatter with age; it is less certain, however, that the posterior lens surface likewise becomes flatter.

The lens substance is not crystal clear, but is yellow; thus, as the lens thickens, it absorbs light selectively (Coren and Gergus 1972; Mellerio 1971; Said and Weale 1959; Weale 1973). This increase in absorption is mainly due to the increased thickness rather than to any increase in pigment density per unit thickness. As the lens grows, it accumulates two fluorogens, one of which is activated by light of wavelength 345 nm and emits light of wavelength 420 nm (Lerman and Borkman 1976; Satchi 1973). In addition, the mass of some protein molecules of high molecular weight increases toward the nucleus of the lens. In some cases, the index of refraction of these high-mass molecules is greater than the index of their environment, and they can, under some conditions, act as scatter points for light (Spector 1983).

The miosis and the growth of the lens does alter visual performance. According to Weale (1961, 1962, 1963), the amount of light reaching the retina in a normal 60-year-old is only about one-third that reaching the retina of a 20-year-old. This means that an older person must use significantly more light to achieve the same level of retinal illuminance as that achieved by a younger person. Mesopia and scotopia occur at higher levels of ambient luminance. In addition, the useful light reaching the retina may be attenuated by fluorescence and scatter. Both fluorescence and scatter tend to reduce contrast. The visual performance of an older person usually will be impaired at twilight.

The yellow pigment of the lens absorbs the short wavelengths more than the long. Thus, older people have a decreased sensitivity at the blue end of the spectrum. White objects may appear yellow, and the distinction between blues and greens is decreased. For example, the distinction between a light green wall and a blue green carpet will become less marked with age. Since there is great variation between older individuals of the same age, it is not possible to state that any given 70-year-old will have significant difficulty with color perception. This means that color vision of those over 55 or so should be checked at regular intervals.

Contrary to the assumption of many clinicians, there does not seem to be much evidence that the index of refraction of the lens substance changes with age in the normal eye as defined in the introduction of this chapter (Parsons 1906, 929).

The common clinical concept that the lens substance becomes significantly harder and less pliable with age is supported by the fact that the amplitude of accommodation decreases with age and ultimately becomes essentially 0 by the sixth decade of life. There is, however, little direct research data to support this concept. Likewise, there is little or no evidence of atrophy or sclerosis of the ciliary muscle (Weale 1962, 1963). In fact, the evidence seems to indicate hypertrophy of the ciliary muscle. Depending somewhat on the supporting pressure exerted by the vitreous, the mechanical aspects of the suspension of the crystalline lens in relationship to the ciliary muscle must change as the lens increases in size with age. However, a change great enough to reduce the amplitude of accommodation to practically 0 should increase the static power of the eye as well as reaction time.

The static power of the eye does change with age (Exford 1965; Hirsch 1959; Walton 1950), but in the normal eye free from cataract and diabetes, the change is toward hypermetropia at a rate of little more than 0.25D per decade after the age of 40. As has been discussed, against-the-rule astigmatism increases with age. The increase in hypermetropia found clinically is consistent with the increase in axial thickness of the crystalline lens and the flattening of the lens surfaces, but contrary to an apparent increase in corneal curvature and the decrease in depth of the anterior chamber.

There does seem to be a slight increase in the reaction time for positive accommodation, but not for negative for those over 45 (Allen 1956).

Assuming the changes previously described (anterior chamber depth, 3.0 mm and lens thickness, 4.6 mm) and that the corneal curvature remains constant, and further assuming the radius of curvature of the anterior lens surface to be 10.6 mm and that of the posterior surface to be 6.4 mm, the author has calculated, using Gullstrand's simplified eye as a model, that the refractive power of the eye should decrease by somewhat less than 1.00D by age 70. This is very near the actual average change, but it does not take into account any change in corneal power or any change in the index of refraction of the vitreous.

Changes in the Vitreous with Age

Millodot (1976) has found that the magnitude of the chromatic aberration of the eye decreases with age in both the phakic and aphakic eye. Millodot and Leary (1978) have found that the discrepancy between the magnitude of the ametropia determined by skiametry and subjective methods changes from plus to minus with increasing age of patients. Both of these observations can be explained if it is assumed that the index of refraction of the vitreous increases with age. This would also help explain the loss of reflectance of the fundus observed with an ophthalmoscope. Goodside (1956) has presented evidence that supports this hypothesis.

If the index of the vitreous increased enough to introduce a concave surface into the refractive system of the eye, in order to account for the decrease in chromatic aberration, the refractive power of the eye would become markedly reduced, and the increase in hypermetropia would be much greater than that reported for the aging eye. This decrease in power could be compensated for if there were a corresponding increase in the refractive index of the nucleus of the crystalline lens or a slight increase in power of the cornea. These changes must be investigated more fully before it can be stated that Millodot's hypothesis is correct or not.

In addition to a possible change in the refractive index, the vitreous appears to be subject to liquefaction and syneresis with age, which results in an increase in the speed and amplitude of the movements of vitreous floaters and a decreased support for the posterior lens surface. Ordinarily, muscae volitantes have no effect on vision except to give older people something to watch in an otherwise empty field or when bored. Sometimes, however, they can be very distracting during reading.

Retinal and Neural Connection Changes with Age

The changes in the retina and the neural connections that can accompany the normal aging process are largely inferential rather than directly observable in the normal eye. Consequently, this section will discuss the changes in visual function rather than the changes in the retina or neural connections.

Clinicians usually assess the integrity of the retina and the visual system by direct observation (ophthalmoscopy and biomicroscopy) and by the determination of corrected visual acuity and the size and shape of the visual fields using various methods, including the Amsler grid. On occasion, stereo-acuity may be determined, and even less frequently, performance on one of the color vision screening devices may be determined.

In the absence of pathology, there is little decline in static visual acuity with age that cannot be accounted for by miosis and the increased density of the lens (Pitts 1982). In general, however, the number of individuals achieving 20/10 to 20/25 visual acuity declines with age. According to the Framingham study (Kahn et al. 1977), 95.4 percent of individuals in the age group from 52 to 64 years have corrected acuity between 20/10 and 20/25. In the age group from 65 to 74 years, this percentage declines to 91.9, and in the age group from 75 to 85, it becomes 69.1. The major causes of this decline for the 75 to 85 age group are cataract (46 percent), macular degeneration (28 percent), glaucoma (7.2 percent), and general retinal pathology (7 percent). A number of studies have shown that an increase in illuminance is required to maintain vision in older subjects viewing high-contrast targets such as visual acuity optotypes (Pitts 1982). (See also the introduction to this chapter).

The size of the visual field as measured under standard conditions decreases with age. That is, the $1/1,000$ isopter for the average normal 60-year-old will be inside that of an average normal 20-year-old (Burg 1968; Dannheim and Drance 1971), even when the pupil is controlled (Carter 1982; Drance Berry, and Hughes 1967). This does not necessarily mean that neural function is diminished, since the density of the lens will reduce retinal illuminance even when pupil size is controlled. The retinal illuminance will be reduced even more by light scatter within the eye. Consequently, a slightly reduced field cannot be taken as positive evidence that there is reduced neural function. The presence of scotomas or areas of reduced sensitivity, as well as sudden changes in the visual field, are more important than a slightly reduced field. The clinician must make comparisons between recent fields. This means that the visual field should be determined and recorded at regular intervals in the aging patient.

Although individuals with excellent stereopsis do not necessarily have a good ability to judge distance, they do have good binocular motor and sensory integration. Thus, the determination of stereo-acuity can aid the optometrist in judging whether or not a patient's visual neural system is functioning properly. Likewise, the integrity of the monocular visual neural system can be judged from a determination of vernier acuity. Vernier acuity can be more easily determined in eyes with a poor optical system (with corneal or lenticular opacities) than can visual acuity, and hence it should prove useful in cataractous eyes.

Hofstetter and Bertsch (1976) have reported that stereo-acuity does not decline with age (up to age 42 at least) in individuals with good visual acuity. Pitts (1982) suspects that stereopsis would decrease with age after 50 years in a randomly selected sample of the population. Unfortunately, the author is not aware of a published study of the effect of aging on vernier acuity.

The changes in the ability to discriminate colors already have been discussed. Briefly, there is a shortening of the spectrum on the blue end, a loss of ability to discriminate blues from blue-greens, and a yellowing of white objects so that the older individuals may have difficulty discriminating between white and yellow and between pastel violets and yellow-greens. These changes occur in the absence of disease and degeneration. Since subtle changes in color vision may be the first sign of disease, it is important that the color vision of aging patients be determined at regular intervals and that comparisons be made between the eyes of the same individual as well as with some normal standard.

The fact that mesopia and scotopia occur at lower levels of ambient illuminance in older individuals than in younger means that the difficulty with color discrimination that occurs after sunset occurs earlier in the evening for older persons.

It may well be that all the usual tests of sensory neural integrity show small but definite decrements in the absence of disease or degeneration.

Motor Systems Changes with Age

Accurate, steady fixation by either eye and by both eyes together is essential for normal binocular vision. Dannheim and Drance (1971) reported that under scotopic conditions, aging subjects had difficulty with fixation. In contrast, the evidence derived from the maintenance of relatively good static visual acuity and good stereo-acuity, as well as the clinical evidence that aging patients usually have normal binocular vision, indicates that under photopic conditions, aging individuals maintain good, steady fixation. Mesopia occurs at higher levels of ambient illuminance in older people (Carter 1982).

Version Eye Movements

Sharpe and Sylvester (1978) compared the monocular pursuit eye movements of 15 subjects between the ages of 19 and 32 with those of 10 subjects between the ages of 65 and 77. Even at relatively slow target movements, the older subjects showed a decreased gain (increased lag) and consequently an increased number of saccades in order to maintain fixation.

Leigh (1983) claims that with advancing age, the range of voluntary eye movements becomes limited. If the individual follows a moving target, the restrictions are less marked. Vertical version movements seem to be restricted more than movements in other directions (Chamberlain 1971).

In the author's clinical experience, however, most normal, vigorous, aging patients do not exhibit marked restrictions of version movements, whether voluntary or following. In those instances in which the movements have appeared somewhat restricted, clinically acceptable version movements were restored by simple home vision training. In those instances in which the voluntary and following movements were markedly restricted, the patient either had or was discovered to have neurological disturbances.

Vergences

Tonic Vergence: Distance Heterophoria. Tonic vergence appears to increase somewhat with increasing years, as evidenced by increasing esophoria for distance fixation. The increase is about 0.03Δ per year after age 30. Hirsch, Alpern and Schultz (1948) found the mean heterophoria to be just over a 0.5Δ exophoria at age 30 and nearly 0.4Δ esophoria by age 50. This variation has no clinical significance and is less than the error of measurement used in clinical testing.

Fusional (Disparity) Vergence. According to Sheedy and Saladin (1975), positive fusional vergence decreases with age, but negative fusional vergence does not. The decrease in positive fusional vergence is far greater than the increase in the near exophoria and thus appears to be a real loss in amplitude. In the author's clinical experience, however, positive fusional vergence in the elderly responds well to training; thus, the decrease in positive fusional vergence with age does not necessarily represent a permanent or serious loss.

Total Vergence. The total vergence as determined from the far point to the near point of convergence does not appear to change significantly with age (Duane 1926; Mellick 1949), but some reduction is to be expected.

Accommodative Convergence and Proximal Convergence

It is generally accepted that the loss of accommodation with age is due to changes in the lens substance, ciliary body, or both. As already mentioned, Weale (1962, 1963) states that there is hypertrophy rather than atrophy of the ciliary muscle with age. Shirachi et al. (1978) believe that the loss of accommodation is due to the continued growth and hence the decreasing curvature of the lens itself and with a corresponding decrease in mechanical advantage of the ciliary muscle. This does not seem probable as an explanation of the total loss, since it would result in a greater change in the static power of the eye than that actually found.

The loss of accommodation appears to be due to changes in the lens or ciliary body rather than to changes in the underlying neural mechanisms. There does not appear to be any evidence that the appreciation of blur or the appreciation of nearness decreases with age. The fact that convergence is less effective in producing accommodation as age increases (Fincham 1955; Kent 1958; Morgan 1954) may be explained by a reduction in the response of the lens to the forces that deform it in accommodation rather than by a reduction in the neural input to the effector mechanism. Thus, it appears that aging affects neither the sensory output of the reflex nor the motor neural input to the ciliary muscle.

There is some direct evidence supplied by impedance cyclography (Saladin and Stark 1975; Swegmark 1969) that neural impulses reach the ciliary muscle of presbyopic subjects who have little or no accommodative response. In other words, presbyopic subjects attempt to accommodate even when there is no direct feedback in the form of clearer retinal images. It is not known whether the origin of these impulses is reflex in nature due to blurring, nearness, or convergence, or whether it is voluntary.

There is also indirect evidence that the accommodative mechanism is probably activated in presbyopic individuals even though there is little or no gain in clearness of the retinal image. Sheedy and Saladin (1975) found that the mean near phoria of a group of young subjects was 2.8Δ exophoria whereas that for a group of presbyopes using a +2.50D addition was 8.7Δ exophoria, or only approximately 6Δ greater than that for younger subjects. If this increase in near exophoria were due entirely to the loss of accommodation, the difference should be nearly 10 to 12.8Δ exophoria, since the average AC/A ratio is about 4Δ/1.00D. Sheedy and Saladin also reported that the near fixation disparity for the younger subjects increased from 0.17 minutes of arc of exo disparity to 6.62 minutes of arc through a +2.50D addition. The older subjects exhibited only 1.48' of exo fixation disparity through the same addition. In other words, presbyopic subjects exhibit greater proximal convergence both in the disassociated and associated conditions than do nonpresbyopic subjects under similar conditions. This increased proximal convergence could be gradually conditioned as accommodative convergence is lost with age, or it could be due, at least in part, to convergence stimuli derived from attempted accommodation.

Although it is really not germane to a discussion of accommodative convergence in individuals whose accommodative amplitude is no greater than the depth of focus, it is interesting to speculate about the changes that do occur in accommodative convergence as the amplitude of accommodation decreases with age. The AC/A ratio in younger individuals appears to be essentially linear in the middle ranges of accommodation, omitting the first 0.75D and the last 1.00D or so of accommodation (Alpern, Kincaid, and Lubeck 1959; Flom 1960).

The first 0.75D or so should be omitted partly because of the difficulty of determining 0 on the scale. The condition of emmetropia representing the 0 point between myopia and hypermetropia and the 0 level of accommodation usually is established by a clinical process that is usually the maximum convex or minimum concave lens power that does not cause a decrement in best corrected accuity; consequently, the actual correction may be 0.50D or more too much plus. The difficulty with the last 1.00D or so of the response is apparent from Figures 10–1 and 10–2. As the absolute maximum amplitude is reached, the AC/A ratio appears to become almost infinitely

Figure 10–1

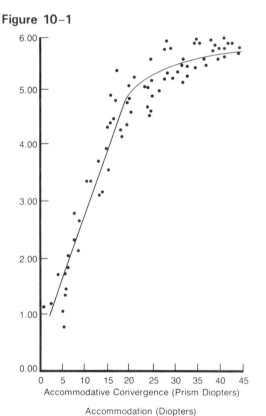

Accommodative Convergence (Prism Diopters)

Accommodation (Diopters)

AC/A Ratio. Amplitude of accommodation is approximately 5.75D. Convergence is expressed in prism diopters and accommodation, in diopters. Source: M. W. Morgan. "The Ciliary Body in Accommodation and Accommodative Convergence." *American Journal of Optometry and Archives of American Academy of Optometry* 31 (1954): 222. *American Journal of Optometry and Physiological Optics.* Copyright 1954. American Academy of Optometry.

Figure 10-2

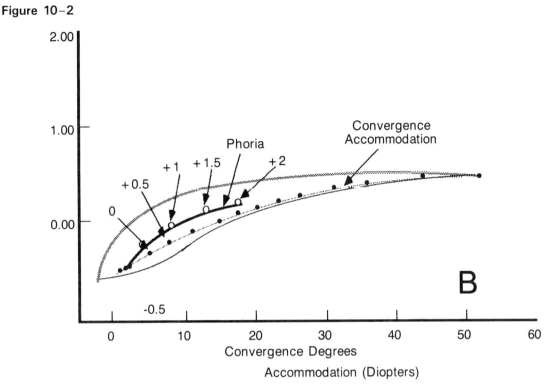

AC/A Ratio (Phoria Line). Change in accommodation, and hence the amplitude, is approximately 0.75D. Convergence is expressed in degrees and accommodation, in diopters. Source: M. H. Balsam and G. A. Fry. "Convergence Accommodation." *American Journal of Optometry and Archives of the American Academy of Optometry* 36 (1959): 573. *American Journal of Optometry and Physiological Optics.* Copyright 1959. American Academy of Optometry.

large.

This relatively horizontal portion of the curve, especially the portion that extends beyond the limits of positive relative convergence (base-out to blur) to the limit of convergence, is sometimes referred to as the *spike* (Alpern) of the zone of single binocular vision. One explanation for this phenomenon is that accommodative response stops because it has reached its capacity (amplitude), but convergence continues because it has not yet reached its capacity. It is not known whether the innervation to this "extra" convergence is due to continued accommodative convergence impulses or whether the maximum accommodative convergence is supplemented by a latent form of convergence. As Fry (1983, 419) has noted, subjects who can demonstrate the spike "are very much aware that a great deal of voluntary effort is being expended." Unfortunately, it is not possible to be certain of the nature of this effort. Is it the effort to continue to accommodate more and more, even though there is no feedback information arising from a decrease in target blur? (The target remains blurred after the depth of focus has been exceeded.) Is it the effort of

voluntary convergence, even though the fixation point is not visible to the nonfixating eye? When the data for Figure 10-1 were taken (Morgan 1954), it was the author's impression that the spike was generated by voluntary convergence and that there was a shift from accommodative convergence to convergence accommodation. In any event, the effort was accompanied by micropsia of the fixated object.

As accommodation diminishes with age, the spike occurs at lower and lower levels of accommodation, and the whole plot of the AC/A ratio (the phoria line) becomes less and less linear (compare Figures 10-1 and 10-2) and more and more indeterminate as a simple ratio. The phoria line of Figure 10-2, taken from Balsam and Fry (1959), represents Fry's AC/A ratio at age 50. The author estimated that the total change in accommodation was slightly more than 0.70D, whereas the change in the phoria was about 32Δ, an overall AC/A ratio of 45Δ/1.00D. The actual ratio varies from 5.5Δ/1.00D to 210.0Δ/1.00D, depending on which segment of the curve is taken. Fry has calculated his AC/A ratio as 32.5Δ/1.00D for these data.

Cross-sectional clinical studies of the AC/A ratio indicate that it remains fairly constant with increasing age. In addition to the report of Fry (1959) on the change in the response AC/A ratio (the actual level of accommodation measured rather than assumed from the optics), there are two other studies, a cross-sectional one by Breinin and Chinn (1973) and a longitudinal one by Eskridge (1973, 1983). All three of these response investigations indicate that the AC/A ratio increases slightly up to about the age of 40, but thereafter it increases markedly and no longer can be expressed with any degree of certainty as a simple ratio after about the age of 50.

The difference between the clinical stimulus AC/A ratio and the laboratory response AC/A ratio is accounted for by the fact that subjects under clinical conditions underaccommodate for near fixation distances: hence, the amount of accommodation is always underestimated, and the closer the fixation distance, the greater the error. As Breinin and Chinn (1973) remarked, subjects seem to exert no more than some comfortable effort of accommodation, regardless of their amplitude of accommodation or the nearness of the target.

In the case of convergence accommodation, the situation is clearer (Fincham 1955; Kent 1958; Morgan 1954). Here, the amount of accommodation induced per unit of convergence decreases year by year until it becomes essentially 0. It also appears that the response is almost linear for most of the range of accommodation. This has been interpreted to mean that the effort to induce accommodative change increases with age, but that at any given amplitude, the last diopter requires no more effort than does the first.

Fisher (1977), using an ingenious in vitro method, presents evidence that the accommodative response in diopters is proportional to the square root of the radial force exerted through the zonule by the ciliary muscle. Such an effort-response relationship results in curves that look similar to the top portion of the curve in Figure 10-1 and all of the curve in Figure 10-2. Fisher also has determined that the coefficient of proportionality was 0.41 for a 15-year-old and 0.07 for a 45-year-old. Thus, his evidence implies that not only is more effort required for the last diopter than for the first, but that as age increases, the effort for the first diopter also increases.

If the effort to induce the last diopter or so of change in accommodation is proportional to the change in convergence per unit of accommodation, as shown in Figures 10-1 and 10-2, the effort to accommodate the last portion of the range must be greater than that required for the first and middle portions. Consequently, there is a third alternative in the effort-response relationship in accommodation; namely, the first portion of accommodative response takes less effort than the last, and since the total range of accommodation declines with age, the cut-off level of accommodation between less and more effort also decreases with age.

As a clinician and as one who has gone through the process of the loss of accommodation, the author is impressed by the fact that presbyopia is virtually free from asthenopia. The major problems that occur indicating that more addition is needed follow: Print is blurred, the contrast of the print with the background is not great enough, the print is too small, or the reading distance is too long. The reading distance is adjusted rather than the accommodation. The rule of thumb that half the amplitude should be kept in reserve does not help differentiate between the possibilities (1) that every bit of accommodation requires excessive effort or (2) that only the last portion requires excessive and increasing effort. In either case, keeping half the amplitude in reserve would be "playing it safe."

As already stated, this discussion concerning accommodative convergence, convergence accommodation, and the effort required for accommodation is purely academic for individuals over 55 years of age. This is probably just as well, since the author finds himself, after nearly a lifetime spent in the study of accommodation, at a loss to explain a great many aspects of this function.

In summary, the usual clinical tests and measurements of the visual system of older individuals in the absence of degenerative and pathological changes reveal little difference in function that cannot be accounted for by three changes common to all aging individuals: miosis, growth of the lens, and loss of accommodation. There are, however, some real losses that are not disclosed by the usual clinical evaluation, but even here at least one is probably due to miosis and lens growth.

Changes in Dark Adaptation with Age
Most investigators report that the absolute level of adaptation reached by the elderly is less than that reached by younger individuals. Whether

there is a difference in the rate of adaptation, however, is unclear (Birren and Shock 1950; Domey, McFarland, and Chadwick 1960). This change in the level of adaptation is probably due to the miosis and lens growth (Weale 1962). Mesopia and scotopia occur at higher levels of ambient luminance in the elderly than in the young (Carter 1982).

Changes in Recovery from Glare with Age

Paulson and Sjostrand (1980) and Reading (1968), among others, have reported that elderly subjects are more sensitive to glare than are younger subjects. This is indicated by an increase in reaction and redetection time in the presence of a glare source.

Severn, Tour, and Kershaw (1967a, 1967b) among others, have advocated a "photostress" test measuring the time required for functional recovery to a specified visual acuity after exposure to a measured flash of light. Unfortunately, none of these glare recovery tests that have been proposed from time to time have become standardized and acceptable as a part of routine clinical procedures.

Contrast Sensitivity Changes with Age

Even in the absence of a glare source, Sekuler (1980) and Sekuler and Hutmann (1980) have reported that older individuals are only one-third as sensitive to low spatial frequencies (below 4 cycles/degree) as younger subjects. This loss of contrast sensitivity at low frequencies has not been borne out by a more carefully controlled investigation by Sekuler, Owsley, and Hutmann (1983). If care is used to be certain that the subjects have the proper optical correction and are free from disease and degenerative conditions, it becomes apparent that older people exhibit sensitivity losses predominantly at intermediate and high frequencies. This also reduces peak sensitivity and shifts it to lower frequencies. Most, but not all, of this loss is due to the decreased retinal illuminance found in older subjects.

In addition, these same investigators report that older subjects experience difficulty in detecting and differentiating between relatively large complex targets, such as faces, at low contrast.

The investigation of the variations of the relationship between spatial frequency and contrast sensitivity and its meaning in visual perception is important. It brings to mind the pioneering work of Luckiesh and Moss (1983) and Guth

(1957, 1981). They developed a number of methods of determining the relationship between luminance, contrast, and target size (Luckiesh and Moss 1983). Clinicians need a simple test that has meaning to them in order to assess these relationships. Perhaps as more experience is gained with Arden's plates (Arden and Jacobson 1978), a test will be developed.

Attention Factors

Older individuals appear to have a decreased resistance to distraction and a decreased ability to selectively attend to one source of information in the presence of competing messages. They exhibit a decreased flexibility in observing all aspects of reversible figures (Hartman and Sekuler 1980; Kline and Birren 1975).

Temporal Resolution Changes with Age

Kline and Orme-Rogers (1978) have presented evidence that indicates that the ability to separate visual events that happen serially declines with age. Events that appear as separate to younger individuals may be reported as smeared together by older observers.

Dynamic Visual Acuity Changes with Age

It is well known that visual acuity for moving targets is less than for stationary targets and that the more rapidly a target moves, the greater is the decrease in dynamic visual acuity. Both Burg (1966) and Reading (1972) have reported that this decline in acuity with target velocity increases with increasing age. The cause for this decline is not known, but Goodson and Morrison (1979) have shown that dynamic acuity can be improved by training. The decline may be related to the decrease in the rate of smooth following movements, and the improvement with training may be due to the improvement in these movements following visual training.

Variability

The variability in visual performance between individuals appears to increase with age for virtually all tasks (Ratwinick 1978). This alone tends to make it more difficult for a clinician to assess whether a below-normal performance on some visual task should be attributed to some optical or neural defect of an aging visual system or to just a normal decrease. As has been mentioned several times, such things as a decrease in dark adaptation, a shift in color perception at the blue end of the spectrum, and a report of increased sensitivity to glare may be attributed to miosis and growth of the lens rather than to a neural defect. However, these changes, although not indicative of degenerative conditions or disease, are nevertheless real and do represent actual decreases in function that may not be apparent from a routine visual examination. Consequently, elderly patients, in the absence of pathology, will have some decreased visual function that is reported by them but undetected by the clinician in routine examination.

The usual clinical procedures do not reveal such conditions as decreased contrast sensitivity and reduction of temporal resolution, yet these losses may result in subjective symptoms that, although real, are vague and poorly described by the elderly patient and not properly interpreted by the optometrist, ophthalmologist, or internist. The elderly patient may know that something is wrong, and it is not helpful to be informed by an optometrist or physician that everything is normal. For this reason alone, a good simple clinical test of contrast sensitivity is needed that can be used to assess the visual performance of elderly patients.

All of these changes in visual function become much more critical under reduced visual conditions such as driving at night or in fog, where a further decrease in intermediate- and high-frequency information would be especially troublesome; when the rapid interpretation of successive visual stimuli are important, such as in reading road signs or detecting the shape of the sign in a unfamiliar location; or when reading poor-contrast printing or crowded printing under less-than-optimum levels of illumination.

Many of these conditions that result in decreased or more difficult visual performance cannot be avoided or corrected, but they can be explained to the elderly patient. Most elderly astute patients already know before they seek optometric care that they perceive more "slowly" and with less certainty than they did when younger. They seek vision care to eliminate or improve their visual performance or to seek assurance that nothing critical is wrong. The optometrist should be certain that patients understand the cause for their symptoms, and they should be advised about ways and means of improving their visual performance by using more light, substituting incandescent for fluorescent light, reducing driving speeds, avoiding looking directly into the headlights of oncoming cars at night, and closing one eye in the presence of momentary glare. With age, the best optical correction becomes increasingly important, as does the utilization of home visual training where appropriate to keep ocular movements free and full. Perhaps most important is understanding and sympathetic optometrists, who will themselves someday be aging viewers of the world and its wonders.

References

Allen, M. J. "The Influence of Age on the Speed of Accommodation." *American Journal of Optometry and Archives of American Academy of Optometry* 33 (1956): 201–208.

Alpern, M. "Zone of Clear Single Binocular Vision at the Upper Limits of Accommodation and Convergence." *American Journal of Optometry and Archives of American Academy of Optometry* 27 (1950): 491–513.

Alpern, M.; W. M. Kincaid; and M. J. Lubeck. "Vergence and Accommodation: 3. Proposed Definitions of the AC/A Ratios." *American Journal of Ophthalmology* 48 (1959): 141–148.

Arden, G. B., and J. Jacobson. "A Simple Grating Test for Contrast Sensitivity: Preliminary Results Indicate Value for Screening Glaucoma." *Investigative Ophthalmology and Visual Science* 17 (1978): 23–32.

Balsam, M. H., and G. A. Fry. "Convergence Accommodation." *American Journal of Optometry and Archives of American Academy of Optometry* 36 (1959): 567–575.

Birren, J. E., and N. W. Shock. "Age Changes in the Rate and Level of Dark Adaptation." *Journal of Applied Psychology* 26 (1950): 407–411.

Breinin, G. M., and N. B. Chinn. "Accommodation, Convergence, and Aging." *Documenta Ophthalmologica* 34 (1973): 109.

Burg, A. "Visual Acuity as Measured by Dynamic and Static Tests: A Comprehensive Evaluation." *Journal of Applied Psychology* 50 (1966): 460–466.

Burg, A. "Lateral Visual Fields as Related to Age and Sex." *Journal of Applied Psychology* 52 (1968): 10–15.

Carter, J. H. "Predictable Visual Responses to Increasing Age." *Journal of the American Optometric Association* 53 (1982): 31–36.

Chamberlain, W. "Restriction in Upward Gaze with Advancing Age." *American Journal of Ophthalmology* 71 (1971): 341–346.

Coren, S., and J. S. Gergus. "Density of Human Lens Pigmentation: In Vivo Measures over an Extended Age Range." *Vision Research* 12 (1972): 343–346.

Dannheim, F., and S. M. Drance. "Studies of Spatial Summation of Central Retinal Areas in Normal People of All Ages." *Canadian Journal of Optometry* 6 (1971): 311–319.

Domey, R. G.; R. A. McFarland; and E. Chadwick. "Threshold and Rate of Dark Adaptation as Functions of Age and Time." *Human Factors* 2 (1960): 109–119.

Drance, S. M.; V. Berry; and A. Hughes. "Studies on the Effects of Age on the Central and Peripheral Isopter of the Visual Field in Normal Subjects." *American Journal of Ophthalmology* 63 (1967): 1667–1672.

Duane, A. "The Norms of Convergence." In *Contributions to Ophthalmic Science,* eds. W. Crisp and W. C. Finnoff. George Banta, 1926, pp. 24–46.

Eskridge, J. B. "Age and the AC/A ratio." *American Journal of Optometry and Archives of American Academy of Optometry* 50 (1973): 105–107.

Eskridge, J. B. "The AC/A Ratio and Age: A Longitudinal Study." *American Journal of Optometry and Physiological Optics.* 60 (1983): 911–913.

Exford, J. "A Longitudinal Study of Refractive Trends after Age Forty." *American Journal of Optometry and Archives of American Academy of Optometry* 42 (1965): 685–692.

Feinberg, R., and E. Podolak. "Latency of Pupillary Reflex to Light Stimulation and Its Relationship to Aging." In *Behavior, Aging and the Nervous Systems,* eds. A. T. Welford and J. E. Birmen. Springfield, Ill.: Charles Thomas, 1965.

Fincham, E. F. "The Proportion of Ciliary Muscular Force Required for Accommodation." *Journal of Physiology* (London) 128 (1955): 99–122.

Fisher, R. F. "The Force of Contraction of the Human Ciliary Muscle during Accommodation." *Journal of Physiology* (London) 270 (1977): 51–74.

Flom, M. C. "On the Relationship between Accommodation and Accommodative Convergence: 1. Linearity." *American Journal of Optometry and Archives of American Academy of Optometry* 37 (1960): 474–482.

Fry, G. "The Effect of Age of the AC/A Ratio." *American Journal of Optometry and Archives of American Academy of Optometry* 36 (1959): 299–303.

Fry, G. A. "Basic Concepts Underlying Graphical Analysis." In *Vergence Eye Movements,* eds. C. M. Schor and K. J. Cuiffreda. Boston: Butterworths, 1983, pp. 403–434.

Girren, J. E.; R. C. Casperson; and J. Botwineck. "Age Changes in Pupil Size." *Journal of Gerontology* 5 (1960): 267–271.

Goodside, V. "The Anterior Limiting Membrane and the Retinal Light Reflexes." *American Journal of Optometry* 41 (1956): 288–292.

Goodson, J. E., and T. R. Morrison. "Effects of Surround Stimuli upon Dynamic Visual Acuity." Paper presented at Tri-Service Aeromedical Research Coordinating Panel, Pensacola, Fla., December, 1979.

Guth, S. K. "Effects of Age on Visibility." *American Journal of Optometry and Archives of American Academy of Optometry* 34 (1957): 463–477.

Guth, S. K. "Prentice Memorial Lecture: The Science of Seeing–A Search for Criteria." *American Journal of Optometry and Physiological Optics* 58 (1981): 870–885.

Hartman, L. P., and R. Sekuler. "Spatial Vision and Aging: 2. Criterion Effects." *Journal of Gerontology* 35 (1980): 700–706.

von Helmholtz, H. In *Physiological Optics,* Vol. 1, ed. James P. C. Southall. Optical Society of America, 1924.

Hirsch, M. J. "Changes in Astigmatism after the Age of Forty." *American Journal of Optometry and Archives of American Academy of Optometry* 36 (1959): 395–405.

Hirsch, M. J.; M. Alpern; and H. L. Schultz. "The Variation of Phoria with Age." *American Journal of Optometry and Archives of American Academy of Optometry* 24 (1948): 535–541.

Hofstetter, H. W., and J. D. Bertsch. "Does Stereopsis Change with Age?" *American Journal of Optometry and Physiological Optics* 53 (1976): 644–667.

Kahn, H. A., et al. "The Framigham Eye Study: 1. Outline on Major Prevalence Findings." *American Journal of Epidemiology* 106 (1977): 17–41.

Kent, P. "Convergent Accommodation." *American Journal of Optometry and Archives of American Academy of Optometry* 35 (1958): 393–406.

Kline, D., and J. E. Birren. "Age Differences in Backward Dichoptic Masking." *Experimental Aging Research* 1 (1975): 17–25.

Kline, D., and C. Ormee-Rogers. "Examination of Stimulus Persistence as a Basis for Superior Visual Performance among Older Adults." *Journal of Gerontology* 33 (1978): 76–81.

Kratz, J. D., and W. G. Walton. "A Modification of Javal's Rule for the Correction of Astigmatism." *American Journal of Optometry and Archives of American Academy of Optometry* 26 (1949): 295–306.

Leibowitz, H., et al. "The Role of Fine Detail in Visually Controlled Behavior." *Investigative Ophthalmology and Visual Science* 19 (1980): 846–848.

Leigh, R. J. "The Impoverishment of Ocular Motility in the Elderly." In *Aging and Human Visual Function,* eds. R. Sekuler, D. Kline, and K. Dismukes. New York: Liss, 1983, pp. 173–180.

Lerman, S., and R. Borkman. "Spectroscopic Evaluation and Classification of Normal, Aging and Cataractous Lens." *Ophthalmic Review* 8 (1976): 335–353.

Luckiesh, M. and F. K. Moss. *Seeing.* Baltimore: Williams and Wilkins, 1983.

Mason, F. L. *Principles of Optometry.* San Francisco: Carlisle, 1940.

Mellerio, J. "Light Absorption and Scatter in the Human Lens." *Vision Research* 11 (1971): 129–141.

Mellick, A. "Convergence: An Investigation into the Normal Standards of Age Group." *British Journal of Ophthalmology* 33 (1949): 755–763.

Millodot, M. "The Influence of Age on the Chromatic Aberration of the Eye: 5." *Grafes Archiv fur Klinische und Experimentelle Ophthalmologie* 198 (1976): 235–243.

Millodot, M. "The Influence of Age on the Sensitivity of the Cornea." *Investigative Ophthalmology and Visual Science* 16 (1977): 240–272.

Millodot, M., and D. Leary. "The Discrepancy between Retinoscopic and Subjective Measurements: Effects of Age." *American Journal of Optometry and Physiological Optics* 55 (1978): 309–316.

Morgan, M. W. "The Ciliary Body in Accommodation and Accommodative Convergence." *American Journal of Optometry and Archives of American Academy of Optometry* 31 (1954): 219–229.

Parsons, J. H. *The Pathology of the Eye.* Vol. 3. London: Hodder and Staughton, 1906, p. 929.

Paulson, L. E., and J. Sjostrand. "Contrast Sensitivity in the Presence of a Glare Light." *Investigative Ophthalmology and Visual Science* 19 (1980): 401–406.

Phillips, R. A. "Changes in Corneal Astigmatism." *American Journal of Optometry and Archives of American Academy of Optometry* 29 (1952): 379–380.

Pitts, D. G. "The Effects of Aging on Selected Visual Functions: Dark Adaptation, Visual Acuity, and Stereopsis, and Brightness Contrast." In *Aging and Human Visual Function,* eds. R. Sekuler, D. Kline, and K. Dismukes. New York: Liss, 1982, pp. 131–159.

Pitts, D. G. "Visual Acuity as a Function of Age." *Journal of the American Optometric Association* 53 (1982): 117–124.

Ratwinick, J. *Aging and Behavior: A Comprehensive Investigation of Research Findings.* New York: Sprenger, 1978.

Reading, V. M. "Disability Glare and Age. *Vision Research* 8 (1968): 207–214.

Reading, V. M. "Visual Resolution as Measured by Dynamic and Static Tests." *Pflugers Archiv fur die Gesamte Physiologie* 338 (1972): 17–26.

Said, F. S., and R. A. Weale. "Variation with Age of the Spectral Transmissivity of the Living Human Crystalline Lens." *Gerontologica* 3 (1959): 1213–1231.

Saladin, J. J., and L. Stark. "Presbyopia: New Evidence from Impedance Cyclography Supporting the Hess-Gullstrand Theory." *Vision Research* 15 (1975): 537–541.

Satchi, K. "Fluorescence in Human Lens." *Experimental Eye Research* 16 (1973): 167–172.

Sekuler, R. "Human Aging and Spatial Vision." *Science* 209 (1980): 1255.

Sekuler, R., and L. Hutman. "Spatial Vision and Aging: 1. Contrast Sensitivity." *Journal of Gerontology* 35 (1980): 692–699.

Sekuler, R.; C. Owsley; and L. Hutman. "Assessing Spatial Vision of Older People." *American Journal of Optometry and Physiological Optics* 59 (1983): 961–968.

Severn, S. L.; R. L. Tour; and R. H. Kershaw. "Macular Function and the Photostress Test: 1. *Archives of Ophthalmology* 77 (1967): 2–7. (a)

Severn, S. L.; R. L. Tour; and R. H. Kershaw. "Macular Function and the Photostress Test: 2." *Archives of Ophthalmology* 77 (1967): 163–167. (b)

Sharpe, J. A., and T. O. Sylvester. "Effect of Aging on Horizontal Smooth Pursuit." *Investigative Ophthalmology and Visual Science* 17 (1978): 465–468.

Sheedy, J. E., and J. J. Saladin. "Exophoria at Near in Presbyopia." *American Journal of Optometry and Physiological Optics* 52 (1975): 474–481.

Shirachi, D.; J. Liu; M. Lee; J. Jang; J. Wong; and L. Stark. "Accommodation Dynamics: 1. Range of Nonlinearity." *American Journal of Optometry and Physiological Optics* 55 (1978): 631–641.

Spector, A. "Aging of the Lens and Cataract Formation." In *Aging and Human Visual Function,* eds. R. Sekuler, D. Kline, and K. Dismukes. New York: Liss, 1983, pp. 27–43.

Swegmark, G. "Studies with Impedance Cyclography on Human Ocular Accommodation at Different Ages." *Acta Ophthalmologica* 47 (1969): 1186–1206.

Walton, W. G., Jr., "Refractive Changes in the Eye over a Period of Years." *American Journal of Optometry and Archives of American Academy of Optometry* 27 (1950): 267–286.

Weale, R. A. "Retinal Illumination and Age." *Transactions of the Illuminating Engineering Society* 26 (1961): 95–100.

Weale, R. A. "Presbyopia." *British Journal of Ophthalmology* 46 (1962): 660–668.

Weale, R. A. *The Aging Eye.* London: Lewis, 1963.

Weale, R. A. "The Effects of the Aging Lens on Vision." *Ciba Foundation Symposium* 19 (1973): 5–20.

Weymouth, F. "Effect of Age on Visual Acuity." In *Vision of the Aging Patient,* eds. M. J. Hirsch and R. E. Wick. Philadelphia: Chilton, 1960, pp. 37–62.

Wilson, G.; C. Bell; and S. Chotai. "The Effect of Lifting the Lids on Corneal Astigmatism." *American Journal of Optometry and Physiological Optics* 59 (1982): 670–674.

Chapter 11

Ocular Disease in the Aged

David D. Michaels

Each age has its virtues and its defects, its chores and its delights. The defects, unhappily, multiply disproportionately as we grow older. A dismal list of cumulative incapacities and imbecilities fills the geriatric literature. We progress, according to the latest statistics, in ever-increasing numbers toward second childhood. We are embalmed from birth, it seems, by the genetic limits of our protoplasm. Therefore, little can be said for old age, even less can be asserted for the alternative. We cling to our universe for fear of finding something worse; however poor may be the start, few are anxious to depart.

Aging: A Perspective

What is aging? Decay of the flesh, loss of vital substance, entropy, the victory of catabolism over anabolism. It is the stage when other people look old who have reached our age. It is wisdom without tranquility, compassion without passion. All definitions incorporate the element of time; every night we are poorer by a day. Aging is universal, progressive, inescapable, mainly intrinsic, and generally deleterious. It is evolution's way of getting rid of the superfluous. Its features, after centuries of inquiry, continue to attract because of our awe of life and fear of death. The chronicle of the care of the elderly is the history of civilization.

What causes aging? Theories of aging are rather vague. Most concentrate on the genetic apparatus, the intercellular substance, and the noxious effects of the environment. Cellular hypofunction is illustrated by a decline in DNA and RNA synthesis. A hereditary influence on life expectancy is demonstrable by twin and familial studies. Sustained sublethal injury leads to intracellular inclusions of glycogen, complex lipids, and pigments. Intercellular accumulations of amyloid are seen in aging tissues. Some tissues grow old as a direct result of wear and tear, which is evident in teeth, bone, cartilage, and joints.

Is aging inevitable? Current evidence suggests that it is. The life span of normal human cells (in contrast to malignant ones) is only about 50 doublings before they are no longer capable of replication. Nor does transplanting the cell into a fresh environment alter these limits. Not only do genetic factors regulate life cycle, they also affect how and to what degree a cell responds to injury. For example, patients with xeroderma pigmentosa have a genetically determined enzyme deficiency that prevents repair of DNA in squamous epithelium after ultraviolet exposure.

Is aging a disease? Normal aging affects all body functions, and it is difficult to separate the physiologic from the pathologic. Ischemia, for example, increases the rate of anaerobic glycolysis, causing a sodium-potasssium imbalance that leads to intracellular edema and eventual death. The same effect can be produced by trauma, infection, toxins, and metabolic disorders. The similarity of the biochemical and structural end result—whatever the cause of cellular injury—has been termed the final common path. Aging and disease are but collateral channels to this terminal goal.

Can aging be prevented? From a therapeutic point of view, differences between normal aging and disease are largely irrelevant. If the loss of immunologic and hormonal mechanisms reduces the body's ability to repair itself, such deficiencies can be medically replaced, toxic agents can be removed, infections can be combated, and harmful radiations can be filtered. In fact, the increased longevity we enjoy today is largely the result of intervention at the environmental level. No one knows what controlled genetic manipulations hold for the future. In the meanwhile, many complications of aging can be postponed to achieve that contentment which is the nectar, if not the spice, of life.

The Aging Eye

Senescence is inevitable, but not identical, for everyone; the strands of life unravel at different rates for the eye as well as other organ systems. Ocular morphologic changes are usually bilateral; often symmetrical; and, although not constant, fairly typical. Functional visual deficits exhibit a spectrum ranging from those that restrict daily activities to some that can be demonstrated only in the laboratory. These changes deserve close scrutiny, for they place the ophthalmic diseases of later life in proper perspective.

The enophthalmos of aging is more apparent than real. Although orbital fat may shrink and fascial connections loosen, the primary factor is flaccidity of the lids. Older people exhibit a decrease in appositional tension between the eyeball and the ease with which the lid may be lifted off the globe. With advancing age, the lateral canthus drifts inward, shortening the palpebral aperture. The increased flaccidity of the lower lid may result in an inward flip (senile entropion) or an outward sag (senile ectropion). Vertical dimensions of the palpebral aperture also diminish due to reduced function of the levator and sagging skin. Flaccid lids may not adequately support a hard contact lens and make its removal from the eye more difficult.

In older eyes, the distance between preseptal and pretarsal portions of the obicularis is reduced; hence, the force exerted on the lacrimal fascia is diminished. Failure of the lacrimal pump coupled with displacement of the lacrimal punctum results in epiphora. Since tear production decreases with age, the older eye cries less but waters more.

The skin of the lids, like skin elsewhere, dries out from loss of oily secretions. The hair grays, and eyebrows and lashes thin out. The dermis becomes dehydrated and loses its elasticity and vascularity. Atrophy of subcutaneous fat leads to wrinkling and deepens the lid folds. Sagging skin may rest on the lashes to produce pseudoptosis. Orbital fat prolapses to form the typical bulge at the inner half of the upper lid. Freckles and lentigo are common, and the skin itself

acquires a yellow tinge. Melanophore migration sometimes involves both lids and resembles ecchymosis. Baggy lower lids may represent not only relaxed tissue, but accumulation of fluid from cardiac or renal failure. Benign tumors such as papillomas, xanthelasma, and keratoses are common in the elderly. Cosmetic surgery may be indicated in the eternal struggle to remain young or, at least look young.

The aging conjunctiva becomes thinner, more friable and acquires a yellow color. Loss of transparancy results from hyaline and fatty changes. Hyaline degeneration refers to the deposition of a homogeneous eosinophilic material—either within cells or in the interstitial spaces—probably from excess glycoproteins. Fatty deposits probably are derived from damaged tissues. Two common conjunctival lesions in the aged are pingueculae and pterygiums. A pinguecula is a small, yellowish, elevated mass in the interpalpebral fissure and represents degenerated collagen fibers. Pterygiums are probably further progressions to form the characteristic triangular fold of tissue that invades the cornea. The prevalence of these lesions in the exposed areas of the bulbar conjunctivea supports the concept of an external irritant. Areas of keratinization produce the pearly appearance of Bitot's spots and may result not only from malnutrition, but also from chronic exposure, as in lagophthalmos and exophthalmos. Inspissated concretions in the upper tarsus can feel like a foreign body.

Tear production diminishes with age and can be recognized by a smaller-than-normal tear film meniscus and a positive Schirmer test (less than 15 mm wetting). The normal tear film is composed of an outer lipid layer, a middle aqueous layer, and an inner mucin layer. The lipid layer prevents evaporation, and the mucin layer aids in maintaining adhesion to the corneal epithelium. Each of the three layers may be selectively involved by disease. Aqueous deficiency is most common and is termed *keratitis sicca* (as contrasted to Sjögren syndrome, characterized by dry eyes, xerostomia, and rheumatoid arthritis). The effect of the aqueous deficiency on the cornea include desiccation, dry spots (dellen), erosions, neovascularization, and scarring. Tear deficiency may preclude satisfactory adjustment to contact lenses. Recent evidence suggests that excess tear evaporation plays a significant role in dry eye syndromes.

Aging changes in the cornea include stippling

of Bowman's membrane (crocodile shagreen), destruction of Bowman's membrane near the limbus (white limbus girdle), excrescences on Descemet's membrane (Hassall-Henle bodies), and arcus senilis. Hassall-Henle bodies appear as dark holes in the endothelium when observed by specular reflection with the biomicroscope. Annular accumulations of lipids in the peripheral cornea produce the arcus senilis, which may be complete or incomplete. The cause is probably local, induced by sclerosis of the perilimbal vascular plexus. The fatty deposits are separated from the limbus by a characteristic clear interval. Optical changes in the aging cornea consist of increased light scatter and an overall flattening, most marked in the vertical meridian.

The sclera becomes more transparent and yellowish with age, due to dehydration and lipid deposits. The yellow color should not be confused with jaundice. Local areas of excessive translucency (hyaline plaques) may be mistaken for tumors or inflammation. Intrascleral nerve loops are sometimes misdiagnosed as melanomas. Increased scleral rigidity with age has clinical application in interpreting Schiötz tonometry and tonography.

The anterior chamber becomes progressively shallower with age due to growth of the crystalline lens. The potential risks of angle closure following mydriatics therefore increase, and a flashlight estimate of chamber depth should be made before drugs are instilled. Increased hyalinization of the trabeculae, changes in the trabecular ground substance, and loss of endothelial lining cells make the older eye more susceptible to glaucoma. There is no definite evidence, however, that aqueous outflow decreases with age in normal eyes.

Atrophic changes in the iris are evident as depigmentation, pigment migration, and opacification of the supporting tissue. Surface markings and crypts may be obliterated, resulting in partial color change. The collagen fibers aggregate and hyalinize, so tissue elasticity decreases. The pupil therefore becomes more rigid and does not dilate as readily in the dark. Liberated pigment is carried by aqueous convection currents and deposited on the posterior corneal surface (Krukenberg's spindle), on the lens, and in the lower portion of the chamber angle.

Failure of the pupil to dilate well is one factor in the complaint of poor night vision by older people. Contributing to the pathophysiology are reduced retinal illumination, crystalline lens discoloration and opacification, increased light scatter, uncorrected senile myopia, and a slower rate of dark adaptation. Changes in adaptation are probably the result of slower photoreceptor processing and nerve conduction, but the exact cause is not known. Increased reaction time and perceptual delays perhaps also play a role.

The ciliary muscle atrophies with age, but this does not appear to contribute to presbyopia, and the AC/A ratio does not increase. Thus, phorias tend to shift to an exo rather than an eso direction. An eso shift would represent increased ciliary effort to drive the accommodative mechanism. Interestingly, the circular part of the ciliary muscle undergoes marked degeneration, whereas the longitudinal fiber bundles that attach to the scleral spur remain practically unchanged.

Morphologically, the ciliary processes become hyalinized, and these areas may contain granular calcium deposits. The thickness of the external limiting membrane increases with age, and the blood vessels undergo sclerosis and eventual obliteration. Aqueous secretion diminishes somewhat in older eyes.

The crystalline lens continues its growth throughout life, although the rate slows with age. Sclerosis of the lens substance and decreased elasticity of its capsule are the main factors causing loss of accommodation. Progressive lens surface flattening is compensated by compaction of the nucleus, so no significant change in refraction occurs. Perhaps most remarkable is that these changes occur in all lens meridians symmetrically and in both eyes simultaneously.

Cataract is superimposed on the normal aging of the lens, and, indeed, differences may be imperceptible in early stages. Among well-established age changes are an increased proportion of insoluble proteins, yellow discoloration, and increased lens weight. Biochemical alterations reflect a progressive decrease in metabolic activity. Yellowing represents an oxidation by-product—perhaps of tryptophan and tyrosine—in which ultraviolet exposure may play a role. Lens fluorescense is also greater. Lens weight increases three times or more from birth to old age.

Age changes of the vitreous consist of liquefaction, cavitation, shrinkage, and detachments. Fibrillar aggregates may cast a shadow on the retina if the pupil is small and become visible as muscae volitantes. Contraction of the vitreous gel with a separation of solid and liquid components is termed *syneresis*. This may occur 10 to 20 years earlier in myopic eyes.

The choroid is the vascular and pigmented tunic of the eye. Blood vessels reach it from both anterior and posterior vessels and nourish the outer half of the retina and all of the fovea. The thickness of the choroid gradually diminishes with age due to arteriolar sclerosis, even in the absence of systemic vascular disease. Atrophic changes are particularly prominent around the optic disc (senile peripapillary atrophy). Diffuse attenuation of pigment occurs regularly with age and gives the senescent fundus its tessellated appearance.

The retina is the central nervous system outpost of the brain. Since it cannot regenerate, retinal disorders are always sight threatening. The aging retina becomes thinner due to loss of neural cells. In the periphery actual spaces appear, which may coalesce to form vacuoles (peripheral cystic degeneration). Lipofuscin, the degradation product of photoreceptor discs, accumulates in pigment epithelial cells and displaces melanin. The glistening ophthalmoscopic reflexes of the youthful fundus disappear, and the foveal reflex is lost. Degenerative changes in the optic nerve include corpora amylacea and arenacea. These basophilic staining bodies are visible only on histologic specimens and have no clinical significance.

Our list of changes peculiar to each ocular tissue would tend to suggest that the older eye does not see because nothing is as it used to be. In fact, visual function remains remarkably efficient in the absence of disease. Acuity declines very little, visual fields remain full, ocular motility stays brisk, and night vision is only slightly impaired. Of course, there are annoyances, fortunately mostly minor. We must learn to put up with presbyopia and bifocals, with color deficiencies under reduced illumination and fluorescent lights, with spots and dots in our visual field, and with assorted cosmetic blemishes. Overall, however, if work is less fun and fun is more work, we must blame ourselves rather than our eyes.

Clinical Evaluation of the Aged Eye

Examination of the aged eye does not differ in essentials from any other eye, except it takes more time, more tact, and more patience. It takes more time, because older people frequently have many nonspecific complaints, poorly expressed and sequentially muddled. Some symptoms may go unreported because of memory loss, fear, or indifference. It takes more tact, because, in the nature of things, some senescent diseases are not only chronic, but irreparable. Clinicians must suppress their own feelings of impotence and stress the positive aspects. It takes more patience, because the aged eye often suffers multiple defects that must be sorted out. For example, a person with reduced acuity may have some corneal endothelial changes, some lens vacuoles, some macular pigment dispersion, some amblyopia, and some misplaced spectacles. These causes must be partitioned, since each can contribute to the decreased vision, which may not even be the chief complaint.

Older patients should never be treated condescendingly, called by their first name, or addressed by fatuous words of endearment. It gives me great pleasure to converse with the aged, wrote Plato. They have been over the road that all of us must travel, and know where it is rough and difficult, and where it is level and easy.

To define an illness, goes the proverb, don't ask the doctor—ask the patient. Expert diagnosticians consistently emphasize listening to patients for they are telling you the diagnosis. But listening must be analytic to develop the sequence of the disease process, and it must be informed to group the findings into recognizable syndromes. Psychogenic complaints are not unusual and often represent attempts to gain attention, affection, or respect. The office visit can be a major event in the life of the elderly, and the clinician should seize this opportunity to bolster their confidence and dignity.

Much information can be obtained by simple observation—indeed, as soon as the patient walks into the room. Skin color and texture, posture and gait, cranial and facial features, ptosis and ectropion, head tilt and strabismus—all have diagnostic meaning to the alert examiner. A shrewd guess of the life course can be made by comparing apparent and stated age. Old photographs are sometimes helpful to separate acute from chronic afflictions.

Of all the criteria of visual performance, acuity is the simplest, the most widely used, and the most clinically rewarding. It is true that the Snellen chart is poorly standardized and poorly calibrated, and the test is sometimes poorly administered. But it is surprisingly accurate, and it has maintained that reputation after a century of practical use. The responses of patients with scotomas, hemianopia, amblyopia, latent nystagmus, ptosis, myopia, and presbyopia—although not diagnostic—are highly suggestive. Some lens opacities interfere with acuity more in dim light; some, more in bright light. Subcapsular opacities tend to compromise near vision more than distance vision. The decreased acuity of macular edema may be accompanied by metamorphopsia; that of corneal edema, by halos and coronas. Of course, all this information will be missed if the acuity examination is delegated to an assistant.

The absence of light perception is a serious diagnosis and carries with it many therapeutic limitations. Patients tend to confabulate invisible targets because hope springs eternal, and surgical procedures to restore function will be disappointing for all concerned if light perception is absent. The diagnosis, therefore, should be made not only on the basis of subjective responses, but on objective evidence of an amaurotic pupil.

Contrast sensitivity is a new method of evaluating acuity. Unlike high-contrast optotypes, gratings can be adjusted spatially and temporally to analyze high- and low-frequency loss. But, the tests take more time and are not easily understood by older patients. Clinical correlations with disease also have not been established. Moreover, no optical aids are available to correct low-frequency loss.

The aging crystalline lens creates the effect of looking through a yellow filter. Although color discrimination is not seriously affected, aging of the lens sometimes leads to peculiar responses in duochrome refractive tests. More important, by checking color vision for each eye separately, one occasionally can pick up supporting evidence for macular or optic nerve disease.

Vision takes time, a factor usually ignored in practice, not because it is irrelevant, but because there are no convenient clinical tests to measure it. Dynamic visual acuity, flicker fusion frequency, perceptual span, reaction time, light adaptation, and masking are examples of theoretically important, but clinically unexplored functions. Exceptions are the time delay in optic nerve conduction manifest as the Marcus Gunn pupil or the analogous Pulfrich phenomenon, the time delay of glare recovery in macular disease, and the inertia patients complain of in early presbyopia.

In contrast to central acuity, perimetry measures the peripheral field of vision. Ideally, every patient should have fields recorded, but this is not always practical. Perimetry is indicated, however, in any elderly patient who gives headache as a primary complaint; who reports flashes, floaters, or curtains in the field of vision; who has episodes of transient visual loss or transient refractive changes; who exhibits personality and cognitive changes, diplopia, or other neuro-ophthalmic signs and symptoms; whose visual deficit cannot be explained by external or ophthalmoscopic findings; and whose intraocular tensions are outside the normal range. Although different parts of the visual field interact to function as a whole, it is useful to separate the central and more peripheral fields. Each can be studied independently by tangent screen and perimeter. Central fields should be done with optical correction; peripheral fields without spectacles. One must use larger-than-average targets for older patients; the stimulus size should also be commensurate with available vision. Central fields find the greatest utility in detecting early glaucomatous damage; peripheral fields, in detecting neuro-ophthalmic disorders. Central fields are usually unrewarding in the very old, those with poor vision, and aphakics. In unreliable or bedridden patients, a good confrontation field will identify any significant hemianopia or quadrantic defect. The double-finger counting technique provides rapid information with minimal effort. Senescent changes in isopter dimensions are common and mostly artifacts due to poor or unsteady fixation, slow reaction time, limited attention span, large nose, overhanging brow, sagging lids, or thick spectacle frames. Another common error in glaucoma follow-ups is to attribute progressive field loss to poor pressure control when increasing lens opacities are actually responsible. To guard against this, fields should be periodically repeated with the pupil dilated.

The pupil is of signal importance not only in neuro-ophthalmic diseases, but also in the evaluation of any eye with media opacities. If the fundus cannot be seen, one can still formulate an estimate of retinal integrity by noting whether the consensual reflex is present in the other eye.

Pupillary reflexes (direct and consensual) should be obtained with a good light. The best near reflex target is the patient's own finger. Responses are graded from 1+ to 4+. Anisocoria can be detected only if the eyes are inspected in both dim and bright light. A spurious anisocoria results from a bound-down pupil following an old injury or uveitis. In Horner's syndrome, the abnormal pupil is miotic; in Adie's syndrome, the abnormal pupil is mydriatic. A blind eye still exhibits a near and consensual reflex. Light-near dissociation is not always luetic; more common causes are pituitary lesions, myotonic dystrophy, Adie's syndrome, and aberrant regeneration of the third nerve. The afferent pupillary defect (Marcus Gunn pupil) is best elicited with the swinging flashlight test. Shining the light from one eye to the other, one sees a pupil dilation instead of constriction – an apparent paradoxical reaction. The significance of the Marcus Gunn pupil is that it practically always means a conduction defect in the optic nerve. Macular disease, media opacities, and amblyopia do not cause afferent pupil defects. A fixed dilated pupil is usually caused by drugs or by third nerve palsy or compression. Myopathies never involve the pupil.

Intraocular tensions should be obtained in every older patient at every routine examination. Applanation tonometry is preferred over Schiötz, because it is not influenced by ocular rigidity. At any ocular pressure level, however, the risks of glaucomatous damage increase with age. The debate whether ophthalmoscopy or perimetry detects the earliest glaucoma changes ignores the fact the the two methods are complementary, not exclusive. Selective perimetry may save time by concentrating on paracentral scotomas and nasal steps.

Biomicroscopy is a unique method of ophthalmic examination not duplicated by any other technique. It affords visibility of anatomic details not only magnified, but in depth and stereoscopically. It serves as a guide in diagnosis, prognosis, and treatment. The cornea, anterior chamber, iris, and crystalline lens of the aged eye deserve obvious attention and are best evaluated with the biomicroscope. Vitreous prolapse and adhesions may follow lens dislocation or cataract extraction. Iris atrophy, discoloration, adhesions, ruptures, nodules, new vessels, and tumors are readily seen. The classification of senile cataracts is based on slit lamp appearance. The location and fixation of intraocular implants can only be studied biomicroscopically. For general examination, the low power ($10\times$ to $12\times$) is most useful. Methods of illumination include diffuse, focal, scatter, retroillumination, indirect,

specular, and tangential. Switching from one technique to the other, coupled with oscillations of the beam, becomes automatic after some practice.

Loss of corneal luster is common in older eyes. Sometimes is simply represents a tear deficiency, but in many cases it reflects pathologic surface changes. These might include epithelial edema, erosions, dry spots, scars, infiltrates, tumors, dystrophies, foreign deposits, and neovascularization. Simple flashlight inspection, therefore, can reveal a great deal about the state of corneal health. Corneal curvature can be further documented by keratometry coupled with photographic keratoscopy. Such measurements are useful in following postsurgical healing, fitting contact lenses, analyzing corneal molding by contact lenses or pterygiums or modifying curvature by radial incisions and wedge resections.

Fundus details are best analysed with direct and indirect ophthalmoscopy. Both methods are based on illuminating the patient's fundus and observing this area with an appropriate optical system. The direct method uses the optics of the patient's eye to obtain a real image; in the indirect method, the reflected rays are focused by the condensing lens to produce an inverted aerial image. Magnification is inversely proportional to the power of the condensing lens. The usual magnification obtained by the direct method is about $15\times$; with the indirect about $3\times$. The field of view, is thus about 2 disc diameters with the direct technique and 8 disc diameters with the indirect. The direct method can be compared to the high power and the indirect to the low power of the microscope. The indirect method is indispensable for observation of peripheral degenerative changes common in the elderly. A third method of examination is fundus biomicroscopy with a preset Hruby or contact lens. This technique combines the optical advantage of the slit beam with the magnification of the biomicroscope and might be compared to the oil-immersion power of the microscope. The Hruby lens needs no topical anesthetic; contact lenses require both topical anesthesia and gonioscopic solution. A wide-angle contact lens (Pansunduscope) has recently become available, that gives an excellent overall view of the fundus almost up to the ora serrata without mirrors or scleral depression. Subtle vitreous changes can be observed with the biomicroscope, including cells, cavities and detachments. Fundus areas of elevation and depression are seen in optic sections, and hemorrhages, exudates, and pigments can be localized in depth.

Fundus features of the aged eye that deserve special emphasis are those related to diseases common in later life—namely, the optic disc changes of glaucoma and ischemic neuropathies, the vascular changes of hypertension and arteriosclerosis, diabetic retinopathy in all its variations, macular degeneration, peripheral retinal degenerations, retinal detachment, and the normal aging changes of the choroid and retina previously described.

The integrity of macular function is frequently compromised in the elderly, and the diagnosis may not be obvious from ophthalmoscopic inspection, even under high magnification. A few simple tests are available, however, that can help localize disease to this area. The Amsler grid is a self-administered tangent screen test confined to the central 20 degrees. A reasonably intelligent patient can be instructed to report any distortions in the grid. The test is especially applicable in serous macular detachments and also can be used to follow the progress of the disorder by giving the patient some graph paper for home use. The photostress test is a measure of macular glare recovery. One compares the time it takes, after exposure to a strong light, for each eye to recover the maximum acuity of which it is capable. In macular disease, recovery time is significantly prolonged, presumably because photopigment regeneration is delayed. Neutral density filters can differentiate between organic and functional amblyopia. The filter reduces acuity more severely in macular and optic nerve disease than in functional amblyopia.

In contrast to macular disease, optic neuritis causes a decrease in vision characterized by a central scotoma on the Amsler grid, defective color vision, and a normal photostress test. In comparing brightness, the patient may report that it appears reduced on the side of the neuritis. This is the subjective analogue of the Marcus Gunn pupil. The swinging flashlight test is, of course, positive in neuritis and normal in macular disease. Red-free ophthalmoscopy may also reveal nerve fiber dropout, atrophy of the disc, and fewer disc capillaries.

Gonioscopy is indicated in the initial work-up of every glaucoma patient. It differentiates open- from closed-angle mechanisms, the treatment for each of which is fundamentally different. The most popular technique utilizes the biomicro-

scope and a mirrored contact lens applied to the topically anesthetized eye. The mirror makes an angle of 64 degrees so that the lower chamber angle is seen when the mirror is placed above. Slit lamp magnification of 16 to 20× is most suitable, and both broad and narrow beams help define the configuration of the angle. The goniolens is then rotated to study the angle circumferentially. The angle is classified from Grade IV to Grade 0, the latter representing a closed angle. Peripheral anterior synechiae may also block aqueous outflow and can result from uveitis, trauma, previous angle closure, and intraocular surgery. Thus, a combined mechanism may result from a flat chamber following a procedure for open-angle glaucoma. One can observe the presence of new vessels, blood, pigment, tumor cells, and foreign bodies. Congenital adhesions are present in iridocorneal dysgenesis syndromes.

Refraction of the elderly patient proceeds at a more leisurely pace with more tolerance for indecision. Refractive errors are the most common cause of blurred vision, and their rehabilitation has probably added as much to the quality of life and extended its usefulness as any advance in biology. But ametropia and presbyopia also occur in diseased eyes, and it is not unusual to confuse blurred vision with loss of vision. Many patients with cataract or macular disease can have useful vision restored by proper refraction with or without low-vision aids. The examination of such combined disorders may require stronger light, higher contrasts, and nearer test distances.

Transient refractive changes can only be detected by repeated examination. They may result from drugs used topically or systemically, lens swelling from electrolyte imbalances, and corneal edema from endothelial decompensation or contact lens overwear. Fluctuating ametropia may also occur in retinal edema, with orbital masses and following ophthalmic surgical procedures.

Binocular motility disturbances may result from progressive loss of accommodative vergence in presbyopia. The increased exophoria in cases of fusional deficits may cause intermittent diplopia. Convergence insufficiency is not unusual and may require reducing the add, or utilizing base-in prisms. The latter can sometimes be achieved by spectacle lens decentration or separate reading glasses. Aniseikonia can become symptomatic when unilateral lens swelling induces sudden anisometropia. Such optical incongruities may interfere with stereopsis. Patients wearing aphakic spectacles seldom achieve true binocularity, though they may not complain. Aphakic contact lenses cause about a 6 percent image disparity, and the binocular potential is somewhat better, but unpredictable. Best results are reached with intraocular implants. Vertigo and spatial distortions are not uncommon complaints in uninitiated bifocal wearers. Aphakic spectacles also cause field restrictions, ring and roving scotomas, and magnification and prismatic displacements with consequent eye-head and eye-hand incoordination and lack of confidence. Unilateral blindness results in sensory exotropia.

Monocular diplopia is a fairly common complaint in the elderly. The usual cause is an improperly positioned bifocal seg. Another common mechanism is a lens vacuole or cleft that acts as a beam splitter. This can be confirmed with a card or pinhole. Other causes are tear film debris, corneal irregularities, oily topical medications, and macular edema.

It may perhaps be useful to summarize this section on examination by re-emphasizing some clinical points. Unlike pathology textbooks, patients seldom present with the names of their disease. Diagnosis proceeds from signs and symptoms, not the other way around. Moreover, textbook descriptions tend to emphasize advanced, or at least typical, features of disease, whereas in practice one often deals with minimal signs. Classic patterns of disease are also altered in the elderly because of greater response variability and concurrent illnesses. Older patients may forget or mix up therapeutic admonitions and instructions. Finally, compliance in diagnostic tests is seldom perfect; hence, cross-checks should be incorporated in the examination to confirm validity.

Age-related Ocular Disease: Topical Aspects

One advantage of aging is that it need not be repeated. But this is not true for diseases. For example, clinical manifestations of retinitis pigmentosa, keratoconus, migraine, diabetes, and multiple sclerosis may recur and progress in later life. It follows that not only are the elderly prone to diseases of old age, but also to the aggregate effects of illnesses whose onset is earlier and that may even be congenital. Although we consider only some age-related dis-

eases, this pathologic background must always be remembered in the differential diagnosis. In all instances, moreover, vision-threatening conditions get priority. Obviously, it is also more important to identify disorders for which effective treatment is available. Thus, papilledema is a critical diagnosis; recognition of optic atrophy can be placed on the back burner. Fortunately, medical and surgical therapy is constantly evolving; many diseases for which no treatment was available only a few years ago can now be controlled or even cured.

Orbital Diseases

Cardinal features of orbital disease are proptosis, ptosis, pain, pulsation, and restricted ocular motility. Other manifestations include choroidal wrinkling and transient hyperopia from pressure on the globe. Neuropathies or myopathies cause diplopia. Trigeminal involvement produces corneal and periorbital anesthesia. Lacrimal complications lead to tear deficiency. Pressure on the optic nerve may cause blindness; extension into the cranial cavity may cause death.

In evaluating orbital disorders, one notes rate of onset, progression, and systemic features of endocrine disease. In addition to inspection, palpation, compression, auscultation, visual fields, forced ductions, plain X-ray, and biopsy, a variety of specialized diagnostic techniques are now available. These include tomography, ultrasonography, venography, arteriography, pneumography, and contrast injections into orbital soft tissues. Computerized tomography has revolutionized noninvasive methods of visualizing orbital tissues; natural high-density differences allow clear distinctions between fat, nerves, muscles, and vessels.

The most prominent presenting feature of orbital disease is proptosis (or exophthalmos). It may be unilateral or bilateral, and globe displacement may be axial or eccentric. Quantitative measurement with a Hertel-type exophthalmometer document progression and help rule out enophthalmos on the opposite side or an apparent proptosis due to lid retraction. In recording such measurements, one should specify both the degree of protrusion and the interorbital distance, making due allowance for facial asymmetry and parallax. The differential diagnosis usually centers around endocrine exophthalmos, inflammation, pseudotumor, vascular anomalies, true neoplasms, and trauma (for example, hematomas and foreign bodies). Since neoplasms may be primary, metastatic, or involve the orbit by extension from adjacent areas, neurologic, ENT and general medical evaluation are often necessary. Laboratory tests for thyroid function, blood dyscrasias, sarcoidosis, diabetes, lues, and systemic infections are part of the work-up.

Infection (cellulitis) causes rapidly developing proptosis with swelling, redness, pain, tenderness, lid edema, chemosis, fever, and leukocytosis. The source may be a foreign body, adjacent sinuses, the eye or its adnexa, or a systemic infection. Chronic cellulitis can occur with dacryadenitis (Mikulicz syndrome), sarcoidosis, tuberculosis, or lues. An important cause to recognize (because it is potentially lethal) is mucormycosis. This fungus infection occurs in debilitated or diabetic patients, or following cancer chemotherapy. The infection starts in the nose and spreads rapidly as a black gangrenous mass through the soft tissue. Thrombophlebitis and cavernous sinus thrombosis may develop with alarming speed.

Pseudotumor is a nonspecific, chronic inflammatory process that mimics neoplasms. Unlike true tumors, the inflammation eventually involves both sides, some signs of inflammation may be found, there are usually no bone erosions, and it tends to respond to steroids. Indolent inflammation may involve the superior orbital fissure and produce a painful ophthalmoplegia (Tolosa-Hunt syndrome).

Vascular anomalies such as carotid-cavernous fistula or aneurysms exhibit pulsation, and the patient may complain of a bruit. Pulsations also occur because of defects in the orbital roof or angioma and may vary with head position.

Endocrine exophthalmos is considered in a subsequent section. It is important to point out, however, that although this is a systemic illness, the exophthalmos is often unilateral. Eye signs can occur in the absence of obvious thyroid dysfunction.

Orbital tumors in the elderly may be benign or malignant. These include hemangiomas, lymphomas, neuromas, carcinomas, and meningiomas. The diagnosis depends on clinical features and biopsy. X-ray changes in the optic canal may explain compressive optic neuropathy. A- and B-scan ultrasonography can often identify the size, location, configuration, and density of the lesion.

Trauma to the orbit can occur at any age. Like the proverbial broken egg, a fractured orbit is hard to put together again. Deformity, muscle entrapment, persistent diplopia, neural involvement, and enophthalmos are major complications of blow-out fractures of the orbital floor. Optic nerve function must be carefully monitored. Proper surgical repair, properly performed, can usually, but not always, restore normal function.

Diseases of the Lids
Patients with lid disorders may complain of pain, red eyes, itching, tearing, dryness, a sleepy sensation, swelling, tics, and cosmetic deformity. Common lid disorders in the elderly include inflammation, skin problems, ectropion and entropion, ptosis and pseudoptosis, anomalies of lid closure, trauma, and neoplasms.

Examination of the lids includes inspection of the skin, lashes, caruncles, puncta, and eyebrows; palpation for cysts and tumors; compression to determine Meibomian secretions and lacrimal sac regurgitation; evaluation of lid-globe apposition; and estimates of levator and orbicularis function. Since the posterior layer of the lids is continuous with the globe, inflammation of one affects the other, as in allergic dermatoconjunctivitis. The lids also participate in generalized skin diseases such as atopic dermatitis, in metabolic disorders such as diabetes, in collagen diseases such as disseminated lupus, in myopathies such as myasthenia, and in neurologic afflictions such as parkinsonism.

Infection of the lid margin (blepharitis) is common in the elderly and is usually associated with seborrhea of the eyebrows, skin of the nose, cheeks, and scalp. It is a chronic, annoying, sometimes disabling, often disfiguring disorder. The lid margins are red, thickened, may develop ectropion, and dusted by fine dandrufflike flakes. Scarring may result from the lashes rubbing against the cornea. Secondary staphylococcus infections cause styes, ulceration, chalazia, and abscesses. The patient complains of itching, burning, scratching, tearing, and intolerance to light, smoke, and dust. The wrinkled skin, especially at the canthi, predisposes to retention of moisture and tears, causing cracking and further irritation. All this is often complicated by allergic reactions to a variety of prescribed medications and assorted home remedies. This may include steroids used for long periods, causing iatrogenic glaucoma, cataract, superinfection, or reactivation of herpetic ulcers.

Allergies result from local interaction of antibodies and antigens, causing release of chemical mediators that act on blood vessels to produce vasodilation and attract additional cells capable of responding to the foreign intruder. Clinical signs and symptoms are lid edema, redness, swelling, itching, eruptions, scaling, eczema, crusting, and lichenification. Of particular importance in the elderly is contact dermatitis caused by drugs, chemicals, cosmetics, and other substances applied to the skin surface. Atopic eczema is caused by pollens, dust, animal substances, and bacterial products in patients predisposed to hay fever and asthma. Finally, some reactions are not allergic, but are direct toxic effects of drugs such as atropine, eserine, phospholine iodide, and assorted antibiotics.

Skin disorders frequently involve the lids of the elderly. Xanthelasma is a yellowish lipoidal degenerative condition typically presenting as a discrete, slightly elevated mass, often symmetrical, near the inner angle. It grows slowly and requires excision only for cosmetic reasons. Large defects may need skin grafting. Papillomas are elevated, localized warty lesions that should not be confused with infectious verrucae found in the young. Senile keratoses are flat, irregular, slightly brownish lesions, presumably due to long exposure to the sun, and important because they are potentially malignant. Lentigines are senile freckles commonly known as liver spots, though they have nothing to do with liver function. Seborrheic keratoses are elevated, fleshy papules having a stuck-on appearance with a characteristic greasy scale resembling candle wax drippings. Small cysts or milia have an easily recognizable, pearly white appearance; clear cysts of occluded sweat glands disappear when punctured. The eyelids may be involved in psoriasis, pseudoxanthoma elasticum, acne rosacea, and sebaceous adenomas of the face. Senile pruritus from dry, brittle skin is a common complaint that often persists despite all local treatment.

Laxity of the lid margins may lead to eversion or ectropion. Chronic ectropion causes thickening of the lid margins, epiphora, excoriation of the skin, and exposure keratitis. The degree of laxity can be estimated by the force required to pull the lower lid away from the globe. Senile flaccidity is the most common cause of ectropion. In contrast, loose tissue may cause the border of the tarsus to swing in, giving rise to senile (spastic) entropion. The chief symptoms are due to the constant rubbing of the lashes against the cornea, which produces a painful keratopathy. Both ectropion and entropion can be corrected by relatively simple surgical procedures.

Ptosis (blepharoptosis) may be congenital or acquired. The acquired forms can be neurogenic, myogenic, inflammatory, mechanical, or spurious (pseudoptosis). Neurogenic ptosis is seen in oculomotor nerve palsy and Horner's syndrome; myogenic ptosis, in senile loss of levator tone, progressive external ophthalmoplegia, and myasthenia; inflammatory ptosis, in chronic lid edema; mechanical ptosis in lid tumors and scarring; and pseudoptosis, in phthisis and dermatochalasis. In evaluating ptosis, measurements are obtained of the vertical diameter of the palpebral aperture in the primary position, and in up- and down-gaze. The presence of Bell's phenomenon should be noted. A Tensilon test is indicated in a patient with ptosis and diplopia. Photographs are useful to document progression.

Anomalies of lid closure interfere with the tear film and may fail to protect the eye, particularly during sleep. A common cause in the aged is Bell's palsy due to inflammation of the facial nerve in the stylomastoid foramen. Although spontaneous resolution is the rule, a tarsorrhaphy may be needed to protect the cornea in the meanwhile. Orbicularis weakness associated with trigeminal anesthesia, hearing loss, and sixth nerve palsy should lead to intensive investigation for acoustic neuroma.

Blepharospasm is not unusual with a corneal foreign body, keratitis, uveitis, or any condition associated with intense photophobia. It is also a sequel to facial nerve palsy or stroke. It sometimes appears as an isolated, presumably psychogenic phenomenon for which no cause can be discovered. Some of these patients eventually manifest signs of parkinsonism.

Lid lacerations require prompt treatment if they are not to result in corneal exposure, deformity, and disfigurement. The most important part of examining a traumatized lid is to check the eyeball for wounds or foreign bodies. Contusion injuries often cause massive hematomas, which may make examination of the globe difficult without special retractors. Orbital and skull fractures must always be considered. Thermal, radiation, and chemical injuries will require special attention.

The most common malignant lesion of the lid is the basal cell carcinoma. Other neoplasms such as squamous cell carcinoma, adenoacanthoma, cancerous melanosis, and melanoma are rare. In examining a lid lesion, one evaluates size, shape, color, consistency, degree of elevation, ulceration, surrounding hyperemia, location, draining lymph nodes, and associated lesions elsewhere on the skin. The typical basal cell lesion occurs in the lower lid or inner canthus. It presents as a nodule with a central necrotic ulcer that has rolled, raised, pearly borders. Early lesions are nodular without ulcers; atypical lesions may be diffuse, multicentric, or even pigmented. Basal cell carcinomas are slowly progressive and do not metastasize. The diagnosis is established by biopsy.

Diseases of the Conjunctiva

Many factors that normally protect the eye from infection and injury are absent or diminished in the elderly: the flushing action of sufficient tears, the bactericidal action of lysozyme, the mechanical barrier of normal blinking, and the presence of unimpaired immune mechanisms.

The causes of conjunctival disease are numerous; infectious, allergic, toxic, mechanical, traumatic, metabolic, degenerative, vascular, and neoplastic. Symptoms and signs might include hyperemia, exudates, scratchy or burning sensations, tearing, and chemosis. Symptoms may be out of proportion to apparent severity of disease. Pain, photophobia, and decreased vision occur if the cornea is involved, itching, if there is an allergic component.

Evaluation should include a thorough history with respect to acute or chronic onset, the use of drugs or home remedies, predisposition to atopy and blephorrhea, and exposure to either environmental toxins or allergens. A sequential plan of examination is helpful: periorbital skin, lids, lashes, tear film debris, tear break-up time, draining lymph nodes, bulbar and tarsal conjunctiva proper, sclera, cornea, and the remainder of the anterior segment. Specific features of conjunctivitis might include type of exudate, petechiae, membranes and pseudomembranes, granulomas, pigmentation, corneal staining, infiltrates, or neovascularization. The type of conjunctival reaction—papillary or follicular—is most important. Finally, one evaluates the lacrimal sac as a source of infection. Scrapings, culture, and biopsy may be required for a definitive dagnosis.

Bacteria may involve the eye in several ways; they may grow upon the surface and cause damage by liberating exotoxin, they may invade the epithelium, they may grow beneath the epithelium and proliferate in the subepithelial stroma, or they may produce inflammation from a distance by an allergic mechanism. Viruses cause damage within the cell, cause proliferative changes in other cells, or act as antigens. The conjunctival response to infection may be categorized into two broad types; papillary and follicular. Papillae are tufts of new capillaries that rise perpendicularly in the tarsal conjunctiva. Their diameter is about 0.1 mm, and they are separated by colorless, threadlike spaces. Papillae are therefore the direct result of vascular irritation. Follicles represent a lymphiod hyperplasia of the adenoid layer of the tarsal conjunctiva. They are directly proportional to the degree of inflammation. The follicles consist of a dense collection of mononuclear cells separated by clear areas. They are several times larger than papillae and appear as translucent, hemispheric protuberances. Small vessels may climb over their surface but do not appear in the center, as in papillae. While both papillae and follicles are nonspecific and may occur together, the follicular response predominates in viral and toxic disorders.

A common cause of catarrhal conjunctivitis in the elderly is *Staphylococcus* infection. The conjunctiva is edematous and hyperemic, and the papillary response gives it a velvety appearance. Hyperacute infections, as seen in children, are uncommon in adults. The usual symptoms are tearing, discharge, and irritation. Both eyes are generally involved. Lower corneal ulceration is common and may represent a reaction to exotoxins, though this is in dispute. Seborrhea predisposes the eye to chronic infection. Chronic irritation and maceration of the outer canthi may resemble angular conjunctivitis caused by *Moraxella*. Gram negative infections occur in elderly debilitated individuals, not infrequently from chronic dacryocystitis or contaminated contact lenses.

In contrast to bacterial infections, viruses produce a follicular reaction and regional lymphadenopathy. Corneal involvement is common and often characteristic. The most important viral infection from an epidermiologic viewpoint is adenovirus (epidemic) conjunctivitis. This disease is now endemic, as well as intermittently epidemic. There is marked hyperemia; a follicular reaction; lymphadenopathy; hemorrhages; lid edema; and, in severe cases, pseudomembranes. The clinical picture may resemble an injury. One week after onset, the cornea may show superficial punctate erosions producing a foreign body sensation and photophobia. In about half the cases, this is followed by subepithelial nonstaining corneal infiltrates that reduce vision and may last for months. The smear/scraping shows predominately lymphocytes. There is no satisfactory treatment for this infection. Recognizing it is important because it can be transmitted by fingers or instruments to one's own eye and to the eyes of other patients. Care should therefore be taken to examine these eyes with a cotton applicator, and hands should be frequently and thoroughly washed.

Toxic follicular conjunctivitis is caused mainly by miotics such as eserine and antiviral agents such as idoxuridine. Occasionally, molluscum contagiosum may shed toxic material into the conjuctival sac and produce a follicular reaction. These conditions are chronic as long as the inducing agent persists. The smear shows as lymphocytic rather than the eosinophilic reaction found in allergy. If chronic corneal involvement occurs, it may result in pannus and scarring.

Not every red eye is caused by infection. Conjunctival congestion can also result from air pollution, ultraviolet exposure, alcohol, and lack of sleep. Passive congestion may be caused by venous obstruction that is due to orbital tumors or dysthyroid ophthalmopathy, as well as by hyperviscosity syndromes such as multiple myeloma. Cavernous sinus fistulas and carotid stenosis produce active congestion. In uveal and scleral disease, the deeper vascular networks are involved, and these may be mistaken for conjunctival vessels.

Allergic conjunctivitis is generally characterized by itching, occasionally burning, and eosinophils in the smear. There is a watery discharge, redness, and papillary reaction, and this may be accompanied by an eczematous skin response. Two major types of allergic mechanisms are recognized: the immediate immunoglobulin-mediated response and the delayed cell-mediated response. The immediate reaction might be caused by grasses, pollens, dust, or similar allergens in predisposed (often atopic) individuals with a family history of allergy and other allergic symptoms such as hay fever, hives, or asthma. The delayed response is commonly precipitated by drugs, chemicals, cosmetics, or even eyeglasses in patients who have no atopic history but may report previous contact with the offending agent. A variant of this is the giant papillary conjunctivitis that occurs in response to a foreign body such as contact lenses. Giant papillae are not lymphoid tissue and rather resemble those seen in children with vernal catarrh.

Injuries to the conjunctiva are common and may be mechanical or chemical. Foreign bodies lodged in the fornix can easily be overlooked; even contact lenses have been "lost" in the upper fornix. It is most important to estimate the speed of a particle that struck the eye. Drilling, nailing, and similar acitivities may allow perforation of the globe; this is not likely with something that "blows" into the eye. If, in addition, there is a conjunctival laceration, soft tissue X-rays and exploration may be advisable.

Chemical burns can be industrial, agricultural, or from the use of household agents. Alkali burns are especially dangerous, because they do not delimit themselves. If the cornea is involved, hospitalization and intensive therapy may prevent permanent scarring. Finally, mild and often unrecognized injuries can cause subconjunctival hemorrhages that, though asymptomatic, greatly alarm the patient. The condition is benign and resolves within a few days. Repeat hemorrhages, however, should trigger an evaluation of drug use and hemotologic disorders.

Diseases of the Cornea
The cardinal features of corneal disease are pain, photophobia, lacrimation, and impaired vision. Pain from corneal disease may be described as sandy, scratchy, burning, or gritty. True photophobia is ocular pain induced or exacerbated by light. It differs from dazzling or glare, in which discomfort results from excessive illumination. Lacrimation is a reflex response to trigeminal stimulation. Impaired vision follows excessive light scatter, clouding of the stroma, epithelial edema, and scarring. Corneal disease in the elderly may result from infections, toxins, metabolic changes, tear deficiency, exposure, trigeminal involvement, trauma, degenerations, and neoplasms.

Corneal examination is best done with the biomicroscope. One notes shape; size; curvature; thickness; luster; opacities; infiltrates; vesicles; ulcers; filaments; pannus; neovascularization; pigmentation; edema; keratic precipitates; hypopyon; blood staining; and involvement of adjacent sclera, conjuctiva and lids. Corneal sensitivity is checked with a wisp of cotton. Staining characteristics are helpful. Fluorescein stains the stroma where epithelial cells are absent. Rose bengal stains devitalized epithelial cells themselves. The staining pattern may suggest a possible mechanism: linear in abrasions, dendritic in herpes, 3 and 9 o'clock with hard contact lenses, filamentary for keratitis sicca, punctate for many viral diseases, geographic in drug reactions, craterlike in ulcers, involving aqueous in perforating wounds, vesicular in bullous keratopathy, and stippled with topical anesthetics or contact lens overwear. The staining distribution is also helpful: lower cornea in Staphylococcus infections and exposure keratopathy and upper cornea in trachoma, verruca, or a foreign body under the lid.

Corneal ulcers are uncommon but may become an emergency in older patients who are diabetic, debilitated, or immune suppressed. Failure to find and treat the cause may lead to corneal scarring at best, or perforation and endophthalmitis at worst. Pyogenic ulcers are gray with poorly defined margins, and there may be iritis, hypopyon, and intense cirumcorneal injection. Fungus ulcers have feathery edges and may have satellite lesions. Smears and cultures are mandatory; they are the only ways to identify the specific organism.

Herpes simplex viruses are a leading cause of corneal disease. The epidemiology is worldwide, and people seem to be the only natural reservoir. Two viral types are recognized; Type I is responsible for ocular and skin infections, while Type II causes neonatal and genital disease. In adults the ocular disease usually causes dendritic ulcers confined to the corneal epithelium. Attacks may be recurrent, so a history of prior eye or skin lesions is important. In early stages or as a recurrence variant, the infection may present as a superficial punctate keratitis or a localized stromal edema with or without epithelial involvement. The reason for the dendritic pattern is not known. A number of trigger mechanisms may lead to recurrence: fever, sunburn, mechanical trauma, contact lenses, emotional stress, and topical steroids. Stromal disease may be accompanied by iritis and elevated intraocular pressure. In some cases it results in a permanent discoid opacity.

Herpes zoster is caused by the same virus that causes chickenpox but has serious implications in the elderly. First, it often occurs in patients who may have underlying malignancy; second, it can produce severe uveitis, as well as keratitis;

third, the corneal lesion may resemble herpes simplex; and fourth, long after cutaneous lesions heal, neuralgic pains may persist and last for months and even years.

Toxic disorders of the cornea may follow the use of antimalarial drugs such as chloroquine, which produce a characterisic whorllike pattern; hyphema with elevated intraocular tension, which produces blood staining; the use of silver preparations, which cause argyrosis; and retained iron foreign bodies, which cause siderosis. Corneal changes also occur in disorders of fat, protein, copper and calcium metabolism. Thus, the Kayser-Fleischer ring is pathognomonic of Wilson's disease.

Disorders of the mechanisms that maintain normal corneal deturgescence alter optical homogeneity and therefore transparency. The marked affinity of the cornea for water is counteracted by an active metabolic pump within endothelial cells. Thus, endothelial disease (from dystrophy, trauma, or improper irrigating solutions during intraocular surgery), elevated intraocular pressure, or severe hypotony cause corneal edema. On the epithelial side, water may enter the stroma if the epithelial barrier is broken, the tear film loses its isotonicity, or there is chronic anoxia. Since the cornea swells perpendicular to its surface, edema can be quantified by measuring thickness (pachometry). Biomicroscopically, edema is evident as vertical striae; folds or breaks in Descemet's membrane; increased relucency; and, eventually, by epithelial vacuolization, cysts, and erosions. An important example of endothelial disease is cornea guttata. This is an extension of the process of Hassall-Henle body formation on Descemet's membrane. As the endothelial cells are stretched over these excrescences, they become thinned and eventually disappear with endothelial pump decompensation. Water from the aqueous enters the stroma and percolates into and between epithelial cells. The swollen epithelial cells form vesicles, which burst to cause painful erosions, photophobia, and visual impairment. At this stage, the clinical picture resembles that of any other bullous keratopathy. Causes might include glaucoma, keratoconus, mechanical trauma, inflammation, vitreous touch syndromes, corneal graft failure, and contact lens overwear.

Dry eye syndromes are an important cause of disability in the elderly. Tear volume is reduced, and so is the force and completeness of blinking.

This is frequently complicated by lid-cornea incongruities (ectropion, trichiasis, pterygiums, contact lenses, lid margin hypertrophy), or orbicularis weakness. Finally, corneal sensitivity may be decreased. The problem, therefore, is not only that the patient has a dry eye, but that he or she does not blink normally in response to the dryness. This results in dry spots (dellen), which may progress to erosion and ulceration. Symptoms include irritation, foreign body sensation, intolerance to dust and smoke, and, occasionally, excessive tearing. Biomicroscopy reveals an irregular tear meniscus containing mucous debris, corneal filaments, punctate staining in the lower half of the cornea, a rapid tear breakup time (less than 10 seconds), and a positive Schirmer test. In some cases, the clinical picture resembles papillary conjunctivitis.

Exposure keratopathy is a variant of dry eye syndromes in which, because of proptosis or lagophthalmos, the cornea is inadequately protected from tear evaporation. When exposure is coupled to loss of corneal sensitivity, trophic effects can quickly lead to disaster (neuroparalytic keratopathy).

Corneal injuries are common; some causes are abrasions, foreign bodies, chemicals, ultraviolet exposure, and contact lens overwear. Most heal uneventfully and, if not too deep, without significant scarring. In some cases, however, the patient suffers recurrent erosions that present a clinical challenge. In this condition, the epithelium repeatedly breaks down following some minor injury such as a fingernail scratch. Strangely, the recurrence is sometimes at a site different from that of the initial surgery. The clinical picture is characteristic and the diagnosis can almost be made from the history. The patient, weeks or months after the original injury has healed, notes a sudden, sharp pain in the eye on awakening associated with all the other features of an abrasion. The pathology is not clearly understood but is apparently related to some defect in basement membrane synthesis, which holds epithelial cells to the underlying Bowman's membrane.

Corneal neoplasms are rare. Important in the elderly are papillomas, Bowen's disease, and melanomas. Bowen's disease generally occurs at the limbus as an elevated, highly vascularized, gelatinous tissue. Diagnosis is confirmed by biopsy.

The normal cornea is avascular and this protects it from immune mechanisms. Pathologic neovascularization diminishes this isolation and makes prognosis of keratoplasty less favorable. Indications for corneal grafting might include keratoconus, advanced corneal guttata (Fuchs' dystrophy), dense corneal scars, trauma, degenerative ulcers, and neoplasms. Grafts may be total or partial and designed to achieve optical and/or therapeutic goals. Risks are warranted only when vision is considerably impaired.

Diseases of the Lens

Cataracts are naturally a major topic in any discussion of ocular disease in the aged. The histopatholoy, despite multivaried clinical appearance, is remarkably uniform: degeneration and atrophy of epithelium, water clefts in the cortex, lens fiber fragmentation, and deposits of crystals such as calcium and cholesterol. Whatever the means, the symptomatic end is equally simple: progressive visual impairment. The rate of progression can be months to years. Patients should therefore be reassured that one or two opacities do not require immediate or even eventual surgery.

The causes of cataract can be congenital, toxic, metabolic, traumatic, or senescent. Although our discussion will be limited only to the last, other causes should be kept in mind in the differential diagnosis. For example, diabetes may induce a specific type of cataract, but also predisposes to ordinary senile cataracts at an earlier age.

The lens has a high potassium and low sodium concentration, which is maintained by active epithelial pumps. Glucose diffuses into the lens and is metabolized by anaerobic glycolysis and, to a limited extent, by aerobic Krebs cycle enzymes. A pentose shunt and sorbitol path is implicated in diabetic cataracts. The lens also contains large amounts of ascorbic acid, glutathione, inositol, and taurine. The biochemistry of cataract is complex, and the causes of opacities remain elusive. In some cases, an understanding of biochemical mechanism has proved of great value (for example, in galactosemia, renal failure, and drug-induced cataracts). As for senile cataract, however, neither cause nor prevention is known, and the only effective treatment is surgical. Fortunately, cataract extraction is progressively safer and effective. Even aphakia is no longer inevitable, as intraocular lenses have become practical alternatives to contact lenses and spectacles.

Senile cataract is the most common disorder of the crystalline lens. The opacities may be classified as cortical, subcortical, and nuclear. In advanced stages, these coalesce. Cortical cataracts are characterized by translucent grayish spokes, flakes, and dots arranged radially. Subcapsular opacities usually involve the posterior poles and appear as irregular granules, vacuoles, and crystals of various colors. Nuclear cataracts are an exaggeration of the yellow aging change and may cause a myopic shift in refraction, due to swelling. Although senile cataract is a bilateral disorder, it is usually asymmetric; one eye may be involved months to years before the other.

In evaluating visual disability from a cataract, the usual distance acuity test is insufficient. Some cataracts interfere more with far vision; others, with near vision. Glare may also be more incapacitating outdoors. A cleft or vacuole can cause monocular diplopia. Lens swelling produces transient refractive changes, and the patient may even be able to read without glasses. Sequential spectacle changes may restore useful vision for a time. A record of such refractive changes is most helpful in choosing proper intraocular lens power.

The presence of a cataract does not preclude other disorders. Many concurrent causes of poor vision are common in this age group. The differential diagnosis would certainly include corneal disease; macular degeneration; optic neuropathy; amblyopia; glaucoma; diabetic retinopathy; and, occasionally, psychogenic factors. In most cases these can be ruled out by history, tonometry, perimetry, and careful ophthalmoscopy. The indirect method often allows better visualization of the fundus despite lens opacities. One can also formulate an estimate by comparing the patient's acuity with the clarity that the fundus can be seen ophthalmoscopically. Nevertheless, in some cases the cataract is so dense that fundus visualization is not possible. Several tests are available to bypass the opacities, thus allowing some judgment of retinal function. Such tests also apply to opacities from an opaque cornea, vitreous membranes, or vitreous hemorrhage. No matter how dense the cataract, the patient should be able to see light, some color, and shadow movements. Light projection can be faulty in vitreous hemorrhage where no image is produced because of diffusion. With cataracts, however, projection generally is accurate. Pupillary reflexes are normal with cataracts. Shadow recognition may permit a simple hand confrontation field.

Entoptic visualization of retinal vessels or of leukocytes against a blue field is reassuring, but it may be absent if light is greatly diffused. Bright flash eletroretinography and visual evoked potentials are sometimes useful. Ultrasonography can provide information about the vitreous cavity and retinal detachments. Laser interference fringes are a new method, useful if available.

The decision to operate for cataracts is based on three quesitons: What is the patient's disability? Will the operation reduce this disability? and What are the risks of adding to the disability? The primary indication is when patients can no longer carry out activities important to them. This will depend on age, occupation, driving, avocation, mental status, whether they must care for themselves, and soon. It follows that cataract surgery is sometimes necessary on an eye that is not in perfect health, in patients who are not in the peak of condition. Balancing risks and rewards is, of course, the essence of surgical judgment. The choice between a visual result that may not be ideal versus a procedure that is never totally innocuous is always an individual matter. Results must be calculated not by what is taken, but by what is left.

Surgical planning naturally includes considerations regarding acceptability of spectacle correction, feasibility of contact lens wear, or advisability of an intraocular implant. Each has advantages and disadvantages that vary for different patients. Indication would certainly change for someone who has only one eye, a retinal detachment, poorly controlled glaucoma, repeated episodes of uveitis, or chronic tear deficiency.

Evaluation of the aphakic eye must consider the coherence of the wound, the functions of the anterior segment, the clarity of the optical media, and the integrity of the macula and optic nerve. Thus, corneal curvature fluctuates during the healing period, the aqueous may be filled with protein and red cells, the iris is somewhat inflamed, the vitreous may be prolapsed, the choroid may be detached, the macula may be edematous, and intraocular tension may fluctuate. Distinguishing the normal from the pathologic and deciding what, when, and how to treat are responsibilities the surgeon is committed to when undertaking to perform the procedure.

Several postoperative complications require immediate surgical or medical attention. These include loss of the anterior chamber, particularly if the corneal endothelium contacts an intraocular implant; wound leakage, which sets the stage for ciliochoroidal detachment; hypotony and potential infection; epithelial downgrowth; pupillary block glaucoma; vitreous touch syndromes; endothelial decompensation and corneal edema; implant dislocation; the "ugh" syndrome of pseudophakia (uveitis, glaucoma, and hyphema); ischemic optic neuropathy; endophalmitis; cystoid macular edema; and retinal detachment. The differential diagnosis of these and related conditions requires experienced judgment, since the welfare of the eye hangs in the balance. In addition, a number of elective procedures are sometimes indicated to improve the visual result. For example, careful keratometric monitoring of corneal wound healing may require cutting or adding sutures or wedge resections to reduce or eliminate astigmatism. Retained lens material or posterior capsular opacification can be treated with lasers.

Cystoid macular edema is a condition of unknown etiology that is, unfortunately, a common complication of cataract surgery. Typically, one to three months after surgery, acuity decreases several lines and the eye becomes irritable and photophobic with circumcorneal injection. Ophthalmoscopy may show little, or there may be some yellow deposits and cysts in the macula. The cystoid spaces are best seen with fluorescein angiography, which demonstrates the characteristec honeycomb leakage. Despite the extensive macular pathology, acuity is surprisingly good, and functional recovery is the rule. The pathogenesis remains obscure. Vitreous traction has been implicated but does not seem to be a major cause. Permanent macular degeneration may follow persistent edema.

Cataract extraction nowadays is commonly followed by an intraocular implant. The refraction of such eyes deserves special mention. First, there are considerably more reflections, which makes retinoscopy difficult. These reflections occur because the crystalline lens with its lamellar structure has been replaced by a homogeneous plastic. Second, healing of the corneal incision takes several weeks, with considerable variability in refraction findings (particularly astigmatism). Third, the pupil of eyes supporting an iris-clip pseudophakos must not be dilated, as dislocation may result. Fourth, the refractive power of the eye is deliberately altered either toward emmetropia or iseikonia, depend-ing on estimated future status of the opposite eye. This fifth, makes binocular vision possible in a high percentage of cases, so analysis of fusion and binocular reflexes requires maximum care.

Optical correction of aphakia may involve spectacles or contact lenses. Spectacles may be spheric or aspheric; glass or plastic; full-field or lenticular; with round, flat top, or multifocal segs. Contact lenses may be hard or soft; daily or extended wear; of high or low water content; single vision or bifocal; and with variable oxygen transmission. The clinician should be aware of the indications and contraindications for each that will best suit the visual needs of the patient. Many optical problems remain unresolved, including aphakic lens design, the best bifocal style, the need for ultraviolet protection, and how to reestablish iseikonia with the phakic eye.

Diseases of the Uveal Tract
Although uveitis is common, its prevalence decreases with age. It may be classified as anterior or posterior. The division into granulomatous and nongranulomatous may be confusing, since the two forms are not the result of different causes and may, in fact, appear sequentially during the same disease. Uveitis in the aged might be associated with surgical trauma, hypersensitivity to drugs or crystalline lens material, reactions to degeneration products in chronically sick eyes, intraocular tumors, systemic infections, severe ischemia, herpes zoster ophthalmicus, and intraocular foreign bodies.

The signs and symptoms of anterior uveitis are rather typical. Pain results from irritation of the ciliary nerves and is referred to the eye or periorbital area. It is aggravated by light and pressure. Pain and photophobia are more severe in acute than in chronic iridocylitis. Tearing is a minor feature and is secondary to reflex irritation of the corneal and ciliary nerves. Circumcornial injection differs from conjunctival hyperemia by its violet hue and the fact that the vessels do not blanch with topical vasoconstrictors. Blurred vision may be due to ciliary spasm, exudation into the anterior chamber, or macular edema. Prolonged inflammation may result in pigment deposits and fibrous proliferation from the iris onto the lens capsule. This and an associated glaucoma with corneal edema further blurs vision. Keratitis can result from extension of inflammation into the peripheral cornea from the limbal circulation or through damaged endothelium. This may result in band keratopathy, which is characterized by a progressive superficial deposition of calcium across the central cornea. Persistent corneal edema is usually followed by pannus and neovascularization. Keratic precipitates are deposits of inflammatory cells on the corneal endothelium. They may vary in size, number, and disposition, depending on the aqueous current and composition. Thus, aqueous containing fibrin and large amounts of protein circulates poorly and traps the cells so that they cannot adhere to the cornea. Macophages tend to form larger precipitates (mutton fat keratic precipitates), whereas lymphocytes and plasma cells tend to be white and smaller and are typical of nongranulomatous uveitis. Aqueous flare is a Tyndall phenomenon and represents disease activity. It is due to protein in the aqueous and is readily detected by the narrow slit of the biomicroscope in a dark room. Various cells may appear in the slit lamp beam, including inflammatory cells, macrophages, pigment cells, and granules. They originate from adjacent tissue or from capillaries. The number of cells per field is graded like the aqueous flare. Precipitates may be found in the chamber angle and on the surface of the iris (Koeppe's and Busacca's nodules). Aqueous containing much fibrin may clot, or in some cases, an inflammatory exudate forms in the floor of the chamber (hypopyon).

Bleeding into the anterior chamber is not unusual in traumatic or herpetic uveitis. Iris atrophy results from prolonged inflammation. The loss of pigment is especially evident in heterochromic cyclitis. Synechiae in the chamber angle are detected by gonioscopy. Cataracts may result from the toxic effects of uveal inflammation (complicated cataracts). Hypotony is characteristic of active uveitis; late glaucoma is due to sequelae of inflammation.

The signs and symptoms of posterior uveitis are also characteristic. Vitreous opacities are inflammatory cells, red blood cells, tissue cells, and debris, best seen with fundus biomicroscopy and retroillumination. Vitreous exudate produces a positive Tyndall phenomenon. If the vitreous is detached, a flare still appears in the retrovitreal space. Vitreous detachment is due to liquefaction and shrinkage. With vitreous collapse, a ring floater may be visible to the patient, representing previous attachment to the optic disc. Retinal edema is common in posterior uve-

itis and, if the macula is involved, causes reduced vision. Prolonged macular edema leads to cystic changes and permanent loss of central vision. Disc edema is usually transitory and is the result of irritation, particularly when the inflammatory process is nearby (for example, Jensen's juxtapapillary choroiditis). Active chorioretinal lesions appear gray or white and vary in size, shape, depth, and outline. Poorly defined edges indicate infiltration. Deeper lesions are obscured by overlying tissue, and associated vitreous haze is less marked. Satellite lesions may appear in the vicinity of older, healed areas. Retinal detachment follows serous exudation, but holes are generally absent. Perivasculitis may occur from cellular infiltration or by retrograde inflammation into the perivascular spaces. Exudates, bleeding, and occlusion are secondary complications. Visual disturbances are often associated with photopsia, metamorphopsia, and scotomas.

Serous choroidal detachment is a complication of intraocular and retinal detachment surgery. The combination of trauma and hypotony causes an abnormal aqueous flow into the space between the ciliochoroid and sclera. The result is a dramatic ophthalmoscopic picture of a large, dark bulge protruding into the vitreous, which may be mistaken for a tumor or retinal detachment. Central vision is usually unaffected unless the posteriorfundus is involved, but some pain is common. The effusion tend to subside after one or two weeks. The most serious complication is a flat anterior chamber, which, if there is an intraocular implant, becomes a surgical emergency.

Choroidal melanomas are the most important malignant intraocular tumors of the elderly. Approximately half of all uveal melanomas occur in the fifth and sixth decades of life. The chief symptom is a change in visual acuity, and this depends on tumor size and position and associated retinal detachment. Scotomas may be interpreted as blurred vision. Macular edema may cause metamorphopsia. Pain and redness are uncommon. The chief sign is the discovery of a mass in the fundus. Appearance can vary from a small, flat lesion resembling a nevus to a large, protuberant mass that invades the retina and vitreous. Retinal detachment invariably occurs, which may make visualization of the underlying solid tumor difficult. Pigmentation can vary greatly and may be absent. The differential diagnosis, besides nevi and melanocytomas, includes metastatic neoplasms, hemangiomas, and disciform degeneration. Since so much depends on a proper diagnosis, patients exhibiting a suspected mass in the fundus must be referred to an ophthalmologist who has experience with gradations of appearance and malignancy and who can promptly initiate ancillary diagnostic tests.

Diseases of the Retina

Retinal disease is a dominant cause of visual disability in the elderly. It is also a topic of extraordinary interest for several reasons. First, one can usually relate visual impairment to the ophthalmoscopic picture. Second, the histologic substrate can often be deduced from fundus appearance. Third, recent advances such as fluorescein angiography and electrophysiologic tests have clarified the basis for both pathologic and clinical findings. And fourth, new therapeutic techniques such as photocoagulation, vitrectomy, and retinal microsurgery have brought about exciting changes in prognosis.

Despite its histologic and functional complexity, most diseases produce rather stereotyped retinal changes. These include edema, infarcts, exudates, hemorrhages, pigment dispersion, vascular changes, atrophy, deposits of foreign cells or material, cysts, holes, breaks, schisis, and detachments. In interpreting retinal lesions, one notes size, shape, location, color, border, depth, effect on adjacent tissue, translucency, and elevation.

Retinal edema may be localized or general, chronic or evanescent. The retina appears boggy, pale red or white, and more or less thickened. Color changes are most evident when contrasted to a normal area. The cherry red macular spot of central retinal artery occlusion is a classic example. Macular edema is suggested by a loss of transparency, thichening of Henle's layer, and distortion of the narrow beam of the slit lamp on the fundus biomicroscopy. The patient may report metamorphopsia.

Infarcts, or cotton wool spots, are sometimes called "soft exudates." They are white, fluffy, located mostly in the posterior pole, invariably superficial (that is, they often cover retinal vessels), and do not stain with fluorescein. Histopathologically, infarcts represent focal swelling of nerve fibers (cytoid bodies).

Exudates (also called hard exudates) are yellow to white lesions with sharp margins that are most abundant in the posterior poles. Occasion-

ally, they are arranged in a circinate or star-shaped pattern. They occur in the middle retinal layers and consist of fatty material. Hard exudates should be differentiated from drusen of Bruch's membrane. The latter are not associated with retinopathy and may fluoresce, whereas exudates obscure background choroidal fluorescence. Hemorrhages may be subretinal, intraretinal, or preretinal. Subretinal blood has a gray green color. Intraretinal hemorrhages are punctate or rounded when in the deeper layers and flame shaped when in the nerve fiber layer. Preretinal blood tends to form large masses and may have a fluid level. Extensive retinal hemorrhages are usually the result of venous congestion. Hemorrhages with a white center (Roth spots) occur in leukemia and endocarditis. Vitreous hemorrhage may result from breaks in proliferating new vessels or from a retinal tear and detachment. Every vitreous hemorrhage should be assumed to hide a retinal detachment in older people until proved otherwise.

Pigment dispersion is a reaction to injury and may represent pigment epithelium cell migration or loss, or phagocytosis. Although nonspecific, the pigment distribution sometimes presents as a diagnostic pattern as in retinitis pigmentosa. Vascular changes consist of alterations in the pattern, reflexes, diameters, and crossings of retinal arteries and veins. Narrowing, tortuosity, congestion, sheathing, obstruction, vascular shunts, and new vessels are adaptations to pressure changes, ischemia, and infection. *Atrophy* refers to loss of cells or diminution of cell size. Repair may be complete or incomplete, resulting in holes, cysts, or glial proliferation. If pigment epithelium and choroid are absent, the white sclera is visible. Areas of atrophy frequently are surrounded by pigmented margins, which distinguish them from colobomatas.

Foreign cells are illustrated by metastatic tumors; foreign material is usually endogenous and might include cholesterol, hemosiderin, melanin, and lipoids. Bright, scintillating spots overlying an artery are atheromatous emboli. Breaks in Bruch's membrane are illustrated by angioid streaks, lacquer cracks, and traumatic ruptures. Schisis represents splitting within the retina, usually the result of a merger of cystic areas. Detachments represent a splitting between the neural and pigment epithelial layers. Fluid or vessels may cause pigment epithelium to detach from Bruch's membrane.

In evaluating retinal lesion one may make use of shadowing, parallax, focusing the ophthalmoscope, red-free light, and observing what structures overlie or are in turn obscured by it. The depth of the lesion may also be evident from limitations imposed by surrounding tissue, as in flame-shaped hemorrhages and macular star exudates. The slit beam of fundus biomicroscopy confirms elevations or depressions.

Fluorescein angiography has greatly aided the interpretation of fundus pathology and made purely descriptive discussions in older textbooks obsolete. Intravenous injection of fluorescein allows observation of ocular circulation and adequacy of blood-aqueous barriers. A permanent record is obtained by sequential photography. Normally, fluorescein does not stain the retina, because retinal vessels and pigment epithelium have tight junctions that act as barriers. Fluorescein does escape from normal choriocapillaries (background fluorescence). Detachment of pigment epithelium allows dye to puddle in the involved area. Areas where pigment is lost act as windows to the underlying choroidal fluorescence (window defects). Blood and exudates in the retina obscure background fluorescence. Damaged retinal vessels leak dye into the retina proper. Fluorescein angiography might be indicated in diabetes, macular edema, nonrhegmatogenous detachments, disciform degeneration, vascular occlusion syndromes, sickle cell disease, presumed histoplasmosis, and whenever neovascularization is suspected.

Macular degeneration is by far the most important retinal disease in the aged. The average age of onset is 65, and the second eye is generally involved within four years. Loss of central vision results from exudative detachment of pigment epithelium, choroidal neovascularization and hemorrhage, and geographic atrophy of the pigment epithelium. Although the disease is primarily an aging phenomenon, a hereditary dystrophy may also be implicated. We have already seen that there is progressive loss of choroidal capillaries with age. Secondary changes develop in Bruch's membrane, characterized by drusen and irregular pigment changes. Drusen usually increase in size and number and may cause minor visual loss. This may be followed by direct progression to geographic atrophy, or there may be intermediate stages of serous detachment. Thinning of the retina may result in a macular hole. In another

form of this disease, there is an ingrowth of fibrovascular tissue from the choroid through breaks in Bruch's membrane. The presence of new vessels is suggested by clinical observation of a yellow to gray circular patch, subretinal pigment, and a ring of hemorrhage or exudates. Rupture and bleeding of these new vessels causes sudden, total loss of central vision. Repair may be followed by a disciform atrophic scar that varies in color from white to brown or even black. Further hemorrhages may occur at the margins of the disciform lesion. Current interest centers around photocoagulating leaking vessels, providing the branches are sufficiently distant from the fovea.

A number of other conditions may be associated with neovascularization in the elderly. In degenerative myopia, hemorrhage with pigmentary and atrophic scarring results in Fuchs' spot. Drusen of the optic nerve may be associated with macular edema. Angioid streaks represent breaks in Bruch's membrane through which choroidal vessels can gain access to the retina.

Occlusive disease of the retinal circulation may involve either arteries or veins. Central artery occlusion is the most dramatic, the most sudden, and the most catastrophic of all ocular diseases. There may be a history of previous transient ischemic attacks. The cause can be thrombotic or embolic. Most, but not all, patients have accompanying systemic vascular disorders (carotid atheromas, giant cell arteritis, valvular heart disease, hypertension, or diabetes). Branch retinal artery occlusion usually involves the temporal vessels, and visual loss depends on macular involvement. Central retinal vein obstruction is also a disease of older people with a peak incidence in the sixth decade. The pathogenesis remains unknown, but concomitant arterial disease and local thrombotic factors are implicated. Inflammatory causes are unusual. The clinical picture in central retinal vein obstruction is a sudden, painless decrease of vision, but not as profound as with arterial occlusion. The ophthalmoscopic picture of massive hemorrhages with dilated vessels is characteristic. Pathologic changes are due to hemorrhagic infarction with destruction of neural elements. The most dreaded complication is neovascular glaucoma, which begins about three months later. The relation between preexisting glaucoma and vein obstruction dictates a careful work-up in the opposite eye. Branch vein obstruction is much more common than central vein obstruction and usually involves the superior temporal vessel (two-thirds of cases) or the inferior temporal vessel (one-third of cases). The patient may describe acuity loss or distorted vision. If the macula is not involved, there may be no symptoms. The ophthalmoscopic picture is a segmental area of hemorrhages and exudates.

Flashes and floaters are common complaints of the elderly. They may represent only innocuous muscae volitantes, but also can be precursors of serious vitreoretinal disease. Floaters are usually vitreous opacities or aggregates: the closer they are to the retina, the more obvious the shadow they cast. When the pupil is small, as in reading outdoors, the opacity is more likely to block the light and become visible. Movement depends on the fluidity of the vitreous. Traction on the retina or bumping of detached vitreous against the retina causes flashes, often compared to lightning streaks. They differ from the scintillating scotomas of migraine, which are uninfluenced by eye movements. The incidence of retinal complications in patients complaining of flashes and floaters is 10 to 15 percent. It follows that separating the innocuous from the pathologic requires meticulous examination with the indirect ophthalmoscope, fundus biomicroscope, and perimeter.

Retinal detachment is a serious and complex disease that may occur with (rhegmatogenous) or without breaks. Most rhegmatogenous forms begin in the peripheral retina. Predisposing peripheral degenerations that may lead to holes are lattice degeneration, zonular traction tufts, and degenerative retinoschisis. The retinal break connects the vitreous cavity to the subretinal space. Symptoms include blurred vision, flashes, floaters, and a curtain of visual loss corresponding to the detached area. Ophthalmoscopy reveals the typical gray membrane with folds or bulla when highly elevated. Aphakia and myopia predispose to retinal detachment, probably on the basis of vitreous detachment and traction. The importance of identifying and localizing breaks is that these are surgically treatable lesions. An adhesive chorioretinitis surrounding the break is created by heat, cold, or photocoagulation to reduce the risk of fluid undermining the retina.

In general, untreated rhegmatogenous detachments are progressive and spread from ora to disc. They usually have regular convex borders with pigment lines at stationary edges. In contrast, nonrhegmatogenous detachments tend to be confined to either the peripheral or central fundus, with irregular, sometimes concave borders and no pigment lines. Peripheral cystoid degeneration has a characteristic stipled appearance and does not progress. Retinoschisis tends to be circular, without folds, and does not undulate with movement. Areas of retinal edema are shallow, nonprogressive, with irregular borders that gradually regress. Exudative detachments from tumors and inflammation show gravitation of fluid, fluid shifts, and an bulous configuration. Tractional detachments occur in proliferative diabetic retinopathy, lattice degeneration, chorioretinitis, trauma, aphakia, and following the use of strong miotics. The combination of rhegmatogenous and traction detachments may result in massive vitreous retraction with a crumpled retina and star folds. Complications of surgical repair of retinal detachment include uveitis, glaucoma, cataracts, hazy media, preretinal membranes, and refractive changes.

Preretinal macular gliosis is a disorder of older eyes characterized by a membrane on the surface of the retina. There may be preexisting retinal disease, or the condition may be primary. The ophthalmoscope reveals traction lines, vascular tortuosity, and a cellophane appearance. Posterior vitreous detachment is common. The pathology is migration of glial cells through breaks in the internal limiting membrane. The usual predisposing causes of preretinal membranes are retinal detachment, diabetic retinopathy, retinal vein obstruction, inflammation, and photocoagulation.

Diseases of the Optic Nerve

Diseases of the optic nerve may be inflammatory, compressive, vascular, infiltrative, degenerative, toxic, or traumatic.

Inflammation of the optic nerve, characterized by hyperemia, edema, and cells in the vitreous, may accompany any inflammatory process of the retina. When inflammation affects the nerve head, the term papillitis expresses the ophthalmoscopic appearance. If the retro-ocular portion of the nerve is involved, the disc appears normal, and diagnosis depends on acuity, fields, pupil signs, and color or brightness comparison. The differential diagnosis of papillitis includes edema, high refractive errors, drusen, tilted-disc syndrome, myelinated nerve fibers, and preretinal gliosis. Although demyelinating diseases rarely start in later life, the residua of previous episodes may be visible as optic atrophy.

Disc edema, as contrasted to papilledema, is the result of local ocular disease. There is progressive visual loss, an afferent pupillary sign, color defects, and field changes if conduction is compromised. Disc edema can be unilateral, whereas edema from raised intracranial pressure is always bilateral, although it may be asymmetric (for example, if there is prior optic atrophy on one side). Unilateral disc edema may be found in orbital disease, optic nerve tumors, uveitis, periphlebitis, intraocular tumors, papillitis, occlusive disease of retinal veins, hypotension following intraocular surgery, drusen, ischemic neuropathies, and accelerated hypertension. The pathophysiology may involve neural elements (axon transport block), neuroglial elements (for example, drusen), and vascular components (for example, central retinal vein obstruction or ischemic neuropathies). Fluorescein angiography and ultrasonography can be helpful in the differential diagnosis. Papilledema is discussed under neuro-ophthalmic disorders.

Low-tension glaucoma refers to a disorder characterized by normal intraocular pressures, normal diurnal pressure curves, and normal tonography, yet complicated by progressive glaucomatous-type field loss and disc cupping. The mechanism apparently is some imbalance in ocular pulse volume and systemic blood pressure. The disease is difficult to treat and may involve central fixation much earlier than ordinary open angle glaucoma. A more common disorder of the optic nerve—characterized by pathologic cupping and sector field defects, but which is not progressive—is shock optic neuropathy. The mechanism is some hemodynamic crisis such as cardiac failure or acute blood loss in an older patient. Overcontrol of hypertension may result in decreased perfusion pressure and nerve damage.

Ischemic optic neuropathy is primarily a disease of the elderly, with a peak incidence in the sixth decade. There is sudden loss of vision in one eye and practically no visual recovery. The ophthalmoscope reveals a pallid disc edema. Perimetry shows a typical altitudinal defect, although isolated central scotomas are also found. The nerve gradually becomes atrophic. A recurrent attack in the same eye is very rare, but months to years later a similar, often symmetrical attack occurs in the opposite eye. The second eye may be involved in one-third of cases, and in one-half of these within 6 months. Disc edema in the second eye, coupled with atrophy in the other, may be confused with a Foster-Kennedy syndrome. The pathology is an ischemic infarction of the prelaminar portion of the optic nerve. Associated diseases commonly found in these patients include hypertension, diabetes, arteriosclerotic heart disease, and cerebrovascular disease, but the relation, if any, remains unclear. There is no satisfactory treatment for this disorder. The differential diagnosis includes mainly two other entities: hypertensive optic neuropathy and temporal arteritis, both of which are treatable. These are discussed under systemic disorders.

Toxic optic neuropathies present as painless, bilateral, progressive loss of visual acuity. Visual fields may show a central or caecocentral scotoma with sloping margins. Among the causes implicated are malnutrition, pernicious anemia, tobacco or alcohol toxicity, heavy metals, chemicals such as methanol and benzene, and assorted drugs (ethambutol, isoniazid, streptomycin, chloramphenicol, quinine, penicillamine, Antabuse, vitamin A excess, steroids, and cancer chemotherapy). The importance of recognizing these disorders is that the damage is potentially reversible if nutritional deficiencies are replaced or toxins removed.

Optic atrophy in the elderly entails a difficult differential diagnosis. Care must be taken not to call every pale disc an optic atrophy unless there is confirmatory acuity and visual field evidence. The most common cause is glaucoma, followed by vascular, demyelinating, compressive, and traumatic disorders. Drusen of the disc may give it a pale appearance.

Injuries to the optic nerve may occur at any age and can be direct or indirect. Direct injuries are caused by sharp instruments, missiles, avulsions, and fractures. Indirect injuries are generally the result of head trauma. Visual loss is immediate and often complete. Pupillary signs are positive. X-ray evidence is often nonconclusive. The mechanism of indirect injury is probably on a concussion basis, with contusion and edema of the nerve tissue, interruption of its vascular supply, or an actual tear.

Glaucoma

Glaucoma is a leading cause of blindness throughout the world. Since the incidence of elevated intraocular pressure and the susceptibility of optic nerve damage increases with age, early recognition is a fundamental responsibility in the care of the elderly.

Glaucoma refers to a group of diseases characterized by elevated intraocular pressure, which, if sustained, causes progressive optic nerve damage. Two broad categories are recognized, based on whether the anterior chamber angle is open or narrow. In addition, glaucoma may be classified as primary or secondary. Primary glaucomas are probably genetically influenced, although the exact cause is unknown. Secondary glaucomas are the result of some prior or concurrent ocular abnormality or trauma. Secondary glaucomas may have open angles (as in steroid-induced pressure rise) or closed angles (for example, those induced by a swollen cataractous lens). Space precludes discussion of these many entities which encompass a vast and detailed literature. This section is limited to primary open angle glaucoma and, specifically, to its early recognition.

Patients with primary open angle glaucoma have no symptoms, and the condition is almost invariably discovered by checking intraocular tensions on routine examination. It is generally possible to distinguish three groups on the initial office visit: normal, glaucoma suspects, and those with definite glaucomatous disease. In the first group are those with normal discs, normal fields, and an intraocular tension under 21mm Hg. In the second group are those whose tension is above 21 mm Hg and who will therefore require further investigation. In the third group are those whose tension is obviously abnormal (say, over 30 mm Hg) or where the diagnosis is already established. The third group also includes those who have ophthalmoscopic or visual field changes consistent with glaucoma even though intraocular pressure appears to be within normal limits. Our emphasis will be on the second group.

At what pressure level does one become suspicious? Although there is no absolute value, 21 mm Hg applanation is widely accepted. After the sixth decade, 23 mm Hg might be considered the upper limit of normal. Care must be taken to avoid tonometric artifacts such as incomplete patient relaxation, incorrect instrument calibration, corneal edema, and postural effects.

What factors increase the risks of glaucoma? Several conditions are recognized as predisposing eyes to optic nerve damage: a family history of glaucoma, advanced age, myopia,

previous retinal vein occlusion, pressure rise induced by steroids, diabetes, pseudoexfoliation of the lens capsule, evidence of prior uveitis, albinism, postoperative complications such as vitreous loss, and vascular crises such as changes in blood pressure or blood volume.

How does one detect the earliest features of glaucomatous damage? The two primary techniques are ophthalmoscopy of the optic disc and perimetry. While optic disc cupping is highly correlated with field changes, the relation is by no means absolute. Older patients tend to demonstrate field loss before disc changes; hence, the two techniques complement each other. Moreover, field changes are unequivocal, whereas disc anomalies are more open to interpretation. Finally, ophthalmoscopy is objective, whereas perimetry is a psycho-physical measurement.

What are the earliest optic disc changes in glaucoma? The best way to detect early disc changes is with fundus biomicroscopy. The second best way is with the narrow beam of the direct ophthalmoscope. In evaluating appearance with respect to glaucoma, the most important factor is the size of the optic cup compared with the size of the entire nerve head (cup/disc ratio). This comparison is usually made in the horizontal meridian, although it can be made in any direction. Values exceeding 0.3 may be expected in 80 percent of normal eyes but in only 18 percent of normal eyes. An asymmetric cup/disc ratio found by comparing one eye to the other is also highly suspicious. Although the size of the cup can be defined by color change, the configuration is more important. These estimates should be made (and recorded) on every patient to gain familiarity with normal variations. The cup is usually centrally located; extension to the disc margin—especially above, below and temporally—is highly suspicious. The depth of the excavation will determine how much blood vessels are pushed aside (bayonet appearance) as they climb up the cup. Patients with such symptoms are likely to have advanced rather than early field defects. Small, flame-shaped hermorrhages may be found near or crossing the disc margin. Other patterns of abnormal cupping such as ovalization, saucerization, temporal unfolding, polar notching, and increased translucency of the neural rim have also been described. Glaucomatous changes must always be interpreted in light of many normal disc variations. A drawing or photograph is of great help in documenting progression.

What are the earliest field changes in glaucoma? The most important field defect seen in glaucoma is the nerve fiber bundle defect. This is not pathognomonic; ischemic neuropathies, branch vessel occlusion, neuritis, drusen, and even chiasmal lesions can produce arcuate field defects. In early stages, nerve fiber damage can cause small paracentral defects, arcuate scotomas; later, nasal steps and sector-shaped defects. These lesions are best demonstrated by tangent screen examination with emphasis on the innermost 30 degrees. In advanced glaucoma, the perimeter can record progressive overall concentric contraction, which eventually results in a temporal island of vision and culminates in total blindness. Automated instruments can be programmed to search for early features of glaucoma, but they require an alert and cooperative patient. These desirable characteristics are not always available in the older population.

Eyes that have suspicious pressures but no field or disc defect always present a challenge. One must balance potential visual damage months or years down the line, with the inconvenience, side effects, and expense of lifelong treatment. Obviously, the higher the pressure, the greater the risk of eventual damage. In the context of this chapter, moreover, the older the patient, the greater the risk.

Age-Related Ocular Disease: Systemic Aspects

To the poet, the eyes are the windows of the soul, but to the physician—whatever the specialty—the eyes provide a glimpse into the state of general health or disease. A corollary is that when the eye specialist refers a patient to a medical colleague, the latter naturally assumes that purely ocular disease has been ruled out. Thus, the neurologist, asked to evaluate a patient with suspected optic neuropathy, is likely to proceed on the basis that visual loss is not caused by amblyopia, refractive error, or macular disease.

Arteriosclerosis

The cardiovascular system undergoes significant changes with age. Cardiac output decreases almost linearly after the third decade. Systolic blood pressure rises because of loss of recoil of larger arteries; diastolic pressure rises because of increased peripheral resistance. Arterial walls undergo a symmetrical increase in intimal thickness. Lipid infiltration—mainly cholesterol ester and phospholipid—progressively increases with age, even in the absence of disease. These diffuse age changes differ from the focal raised fibromuscular plaques that characterize atherosclerosis. Atherosclerosis involves mainly the intimal layers of major vessels, including coronary and cerebral arteries. Arteriolosclerosis is characterized by hyaline and degenerative changes in the media and intima of small arteries and arterioles, usually the result of hypertension. In severe hypertension, there may be actual necrosis of the vessel wall. Arteriosclerosis is a generic term for thickening or hardening of any arterial wall.

The most significant effect of arteriosclerosis is narrowing of the vascular lumen, thus reducing blood flow to the tissues (ischemia). In addition to arteriosclerosis, narrowing or obstruction can result from thrombosis, embolism, spasm, inflammation, or mechanical compression. Thrombosis refers to an intraluminal obstruction formed from elements of circulating blood; an embolus is an abnormal mass of undissolved material carried in the bloodstream. The main factors in thrombosis are changes in the vessel wall, blood stasis, and altered blood coagulability. Emboli may be atheromatous plaques, detached thrombi, tumor cells, fat, gas, or foreign bodies. Spasm is rare, except in severe hypertension. Inflammatory obstruction is exemplified by syphilis and polyarteritis. Mechanical compression might be caused by tumors, hematomas, and displaced bone fractures. Unlike arterial thrombosis, which often is based on atherosclerosis, venous thrombosis is usually precipitated by blood stasis and, in the case of retinal veins, compression by a crossing artery.

Normal retinal vessels are actually invisible; what is seen ophthalmoscopically are blood columns. When the walls become opacified—usually by arteriolosclerosis—there is a change in color, and stripelike densities may appear along the vessel surface. Colors have been compared to copper or, in more advanced stages, to silver wire. These changes do not imply vascular obstruction, which is more closely related to the width of the light reflex along the surface of the blood column. In contrast, yellowish stripes along the sides of a vessel—called perivascular sheathing— are due to exudation into the surrounding spaces. Perivascular sheathing is characteristically seen along veins in papilledema and along arteries in hypertension. Sclerosis may also result in generalized narrowing, so the normal two-to-three ratio of arteries to veins is altered.

The retinal arteries lie mainly in the nerve fiber and ganglion cell layer. At its entrance within the nerve, the central artery has several layers of smooth muscle; this decreases to two or three at the equator. An anatomic peculiarity is that arteries and veins share a common adventitial coat; hence, one can be compressed by the other (arteriovenous nicking). Branch retinal vein obstruction is most commonly due to this mechanism, and it increases in frequency with age. More rarely, occlusion is the result of stagnation and primary thrombus formation or of intrinsic venous disease. In the acute stage, the ophthalmoscopic picture has been described as if one had stroked the involved retinal area with red paint because of the massive hemorrhages. In the chronic stage, one sees retinal edema, serous detachment, vessel collaterals, exudates, microaneurysms, and neovascularization. Visual loss is due to macular edema and vitreous hemorrhage. Central retinal vein occlusion has the same pathogenesis, but the entire retina is involved because of compression at the lamia cribrosa. Macular edema always occurs. The most serious complications are vitreous hemorrhage and neovascular glaucoma.

Branch retinal artery occlusion is usually the result of embolization. Cotton wool spots appear in the region of nonperfusion and may last for days or weeks. In hypertension, oclusion may be due to focal arteriolar necrosis. The occlusions seen in collagen diseases are probably on a hypertensive basis. Central retinal artery obstruction is usually due to atheromatous changes but may be caused by emboli or hemorrhages beneath the atheromas. Rarer causes are arteritis and trauma. The clinical picure is a white, edematous retina with a cherry red macular spot and narrowed arteries. The cherry red spot differs from lipoidoses, where the macula actually contains material deposited in ganglion cells. A wider area of perfusion may be observed with a patent cilioretinal artery. Central retinal artery occlusion causes total visual loss without recovery. The scotoma of branch artery occlusion is confined to the involved area. Involvement of the opposite eye, fortunately, is rare. Obstruction of small vessels behind the lamina cribrosa may give rise to ischemic optic neuropathy. Arcuate scotomas of vascular occlusion may be centered on the disc rather than on the macula, as they are in neurologic disorders.

Hypertension

Hypertension is a disorder characterised by sustained elevated blood pressure (arbitrarily defined as exceeding 160/95 mm Hg at rest). In most cases, the cause is unknown (essential hypertension). Hypertension is said to enter the accelerated phase when retinal hemorrhages and exudates develop—irrespective of the absolute blood pressure level, although this is often above 200/140 mm Hg. Age, race, sex, smoking, serum cholesterol levels, glucose intolerance, weight, and renal factors modify the prognosis for the disease. Young untreated hypertensives have a poorer life expectancy than the aged; conversely, accelerated artheriosclerosis invariably accompanies hypertension.

The ophthalmic manifestations of hypertension can be classified in various ways, the most popular of which is the Keith-Wagener. It recognizes four stages of progressive severity (see Table 11–1). In fact, there is probably a qualitative change between the early and later stages. Only about 1 percent of hypertensive patients develop the malignant phase; even with the advent of effective therapy, only half of these survive for more than 5 years.

Table 11–1
Keith-Wagener Classification of Hypertension

Grade 1 :	Mild narrowing or sclerosis of retinal vessels
Grade 2 :	Focal constrictions, arteriovenous nicking
Grade 3 :	Cotton wool spots, hemorrhages, retinal edema
Grade 4 :	Papilledema

The diagnosis of hypertension is made with a blood pressure cuff, not an ophthalmoscope. Nevertheless, fundus changes provide clues to severity and progression, particularly when the disease enters the accelerated stage. These include linear or flame-shaped hemorrhages, cotton wool spots, hard exudates, and blot hemorrhages. Of course, exudates and hemorrhages are found in diseases other than hypertension; hence, the association between these and general medical features, (for example, high blood pressure, dyspnea, proteinuria, and chest and cardiac findings) is crucial. Unusual but known mechanisms of hypertension must be ruled out (for example, pheochromocytoma, Cushing syndrome, renal disease, aldosternomism, oral contraceptives, and coarctation). "Unilateral" hypertension fundus changes may occur in patients with stenosis of the carotid system, which maintains lower pressures on that side.

The pathophysiology of vascular changes can be studied in experimental hypertension followed by fluorescein angiography. Recall that the retinal circulation is controlled by autoregulation, which permits a nearly constant blood flow over a wide range of perfusion pressures (that is, mean arterial pressure minus intraocular pressure). A rapid rise in arterial pressure causes vasoconstriction; the precapillary arterioles become occluded and eventually necrose. The vessel loses its ability to remain constricted, and a dilation and plasma leakage follow. Fluorescein demonstrates this breakdown of the blood-retinal barrier. Further leakage into the vessel wall causes capillary occlusion, retinal edema, cotton wool spots, and hemorrhages. The presence of arteriosclerosis modifies the response of retinal arterioles to pressure changes. This is probably the reason for focal constriction.

The malignant phase of hypertension is characterized by retinal and disc edema, in addition to exudates and hemorrhages. The pathology is fibrinoid necrosis of the arterioles. The patient may complain of headaches, shortness of breath, and blurred vision, and there may be signs and symptoms of renal failure. Papilledema is due to accumulated cotton wool spots at the disc rather than hypertensive encephalopathy, although axoplasmic transport block may occur in both. Prolonged disc edema may result in atrophy. Hypertensive optic neuropathy must be distinguished from ischemic neuropathy and the neuropathy associated with temporal arteritis.

Diabetes

The incidence of diabetes in the United States is estimated at almost 5 percent of the population. About three-fourths of the patients first diagnosed under age 29 eventually develop retinopathy. Retinopathy develops earlier in older patients. About 10 to 18 percent of those with retinopathy progress to the proliferative stage. Diabetes therefore is, or soon will be, the leading cause of blindness in the United States.

Diabetes is a disease that gets more complex with every advance in metabolic and biochemical research. For our purposes, it may be defined as a hormone-induced metabolic abnormality involving carbohydrate, fat, protein, and insulin utilization. Long-term complications are the result of microvascular lesions demonstrable by electron microscopy. The classic symptoms of diabetes are polyuria, polydipsia, and polyphagia. Weakness, weight loss, recurrent infections, ulceration of the extremities, and neuropathies are other features of progression. Two distinct forms of the disease are recognized: juvenile-onset (insulin dependent) and maturity onset (noninsulin dependent). Juvenile-onset diabetes can progress rapidly to ketoacidosis, lethargy, and coma. It is difficult to control, and death may result from cardiovascular or renal failure. However, juvenile-onset diabetes, which used to be the equivalent of a death sentence, is now well controlled by insulin and dietary management. Most juvenile diabetics survive to old age. Adult-onset diabetes can usually be managed by diet and oral hypoglycemic agents. For every symptomatic diabetic patient, however, there is probably another without symptoms but abnormal blood glucose tolerance (preclinical diabetes). Obesity, advancing age, and a family history of diabetes are predisposing factors.

Ophthalmic complications of diabetes are partly metabolic (crystalline lens swelling and cataracts), but mostly vascular (diabetic retinopathy). Although the vascular changes are mainly evident in the fundus, they also may involve conjunctiva, iris, choroid, ciliary body, and nerves (diabetic neuropathy). Diabetic fundus changes may be classified into background retinopathy (in which the pathology is essentially within the retina) and proliferative retinopathy (in which the changes extend over the retinal surface and into the vitreous).

Probably the earliest change in diabetic retinopathy is increased capillary permeability. This has beeen demonstrated by an elegant technique that measures small amounts of fluorescein in the vitreous. Leakage can be demonstrated within 6 months after onset, even in those without clinically recognizable retinopathy.

Although fundus changes in diabetes are not characteristic, they are generally so typical that the diagnosis can be suspected without difficulty. Mild background retinopathy is characterized by microaneurysms and punctate hemorrhages in the posterior pole, particularly in the region temporal to the macula. The arrangement is haphazard, but occasionally they border an area of soft exudate. Cotton wool spots gradually become more numerous but are less white and less opaque than those seen in hypertension. Microaneurysms are much more numerous than one suspects from ophthalmoscopic observation. This has been repeatedly demonstrated by fluorescein angiography. Microaneurysms are round, range in size from 15 to 50 μ, and vary in color from venous to arterial blood. Histopathologically they are seen chiefly on the venous side of the capillary and represent bulges due to a selective loss of mural pericytes. Some aneurysms become hyalinized, and their lumens are lined with degenerated endothelial cells. The cause remains unclear; weakness of the wall, traction, and abortive new vessel formation have all been postulated. Aneurysms differ from blot hemorrhages in that the latter are absorbed and disappear. Capillary closure with areas of nonperfusion persists after the associated cotton wool spot is absorbed. Shunt vessels, connecting arterioles to venules, appear. Damaged vessel walls take up fluorescein. Venous changes include dilatation, tortuosity, beading, and sheathing, and arteriosclerotic changes are accelerated. Hard exudates appear as yellow to white lesions that may coalesce or form a circinate or star pattern around the macula. The visual prognosis is poor if a ring is formed around the macula or hard exudates encroach on the fovea. Hard exudates may improve with time. The most common cause of poor vision, however, is macular edema. It tends to be symmetric, progressive, and surrounded by an area of nonperfusion larger than normal. Edema is the result of abnormal vascular permeability. If the site of leakage can be identified—and it is some distance from the fovea—photocoagulation may help. Long-standing edema, macular hemorrhage, holes or membranes have a poor outlook.

Proliferative diabetic retinopathy is characterized by the formation of new vessels, which may develop either on the disc or in the periphery. New disc vessels have a poorer prognosis, because they tend to bleed into the vitreous. The pathophysiology of new vessel formation is unknown, but ischemia and anoxia are undoubtedly major factors. The vessels are accompanied by a thin film of fibrous tissue that runs across the retinal surface and through the internal limiting membrane. Hemorrhage and retinal detachment result from vitreous contracture. This form of vitreous collapse differs from the normal aging process in being more gradual and incomplete. Traction and epiretinal membranes may respond to vitrectomy and retinal microsurgery, in which epiretinal membranes are actually peeled off the surface with specially designed instruments.

New iris vessels may involve the angle and produce neovascular glaucoma. The mechanism is unknown, is presumably anoxia, and the prognosis is poor. Other causes of neovascular glaucoma must be kept in mind; retinal vein occlusion, central retinal artery occlusion, malignant melanoma, and retinal detachment. Recurrent anterior chamber hemorrhages progressively compromise aqueous outflow. These eyes respond poorly to miotics, carbonic anhydrase inhibitors, or surgery. Laser photocoagulation holds some promise for controlling this serious disease.

Diabetic neuropathy may affect any part of the nervous system. It presents most commonly as a peripheral neuropathy. Symptoms are palsies, paresthesias, numbness, and pain. Diabetic neuropathy may involve any of the ocular motor nerves (painful ophthalmoplegia); hence, diplopia may be the presenting symptom. Pathologically, there is small vessel occlusion with local demyelination, but recovery within weeks to months is the rule. Aberrant regeneration does not occur, and the pupil is spared. Differential diagnosis includes trauma, tumor, aneurysm, migraine, and increased intracranial pressure. Decompensated strabismus is an unlikely cause.

Giant Cell Arteritis

Giant cell arteritis (temporal arteritis, cranial arteritis, polymyalgia rheumatica) is an inflammatory disease of arteries in older people. The etiology is unknown, but both humoral and cellular immune reactions to elastic arterial tissue have been postulated. Any large- or medium-sized artery may be involved, and there is a predilection for extracranial vessels. The peak incidence is in the 60- to 75-year range. Both sexes are affected, with a slight predominance in women. The disease is not rare; about 1.7 percent of 889 postmortem cases where temporal artery sections were taken. Familial associations are uncommon, but there is a geographic preference for northern climates. The condition is uncommon in blacks.

The importance of recognizing this disease is that it is potentially blinding for both eyes consecutively, it may be fatal, and treatment is available that may avoid these complications.

Systemic symptoms include headache; malaise; low-grade fever; scalp tenderness; jaw claudication; arthralgias and myalgias; anorexia; weight loss; depression; and tenderness of the course of the temporal arteries, which may feel thickened.

Ophthalmic findings include a sudden, transient loss of vision (amaurosis fugax) that may persist for minutes to hours. This may be followed by unilateral blindness, which may be partial or complete. The pathology is an ischemic optic neuropathy. The opposite eye may be involved within a week or months later. If untreated, 65 percent of patients develop bilateral disease, and almost one-third of these are totally blind. Ophthalmoplegia with ptosis or other extraocular muscle palsy occurs in 5 percent of the patients. More rarely, presenting findings are central artery occlusion or anterior segment ischemia with neovascular glaucoma. Ophthalmoscopy shows a pale (not hyperemic), swollen disc. Disc edema may be minimal, but the margins are blurred, and a few hemorrhages may be seen. The arterioles of the affected eye are narrowed and often show focal constrictions. The visual deficit is generally out of proportion to the mild disc changes. After about a week, disc edema disappears, and the optic nerve gradually becomes pale. The narrowed arteries persist, and no improvement in vision is to be expected.

The most significant laboratory findings are an elevated erythrocyte sedimentation rate—usually exceeding 50 mm per hour by the Westergren method—and a positive temporal artery biopsy. The histopathology shows the occluded lumen and multiple giant cells. Prompt recognition and initiation of steroid therapy may prevent loss of vision. If ischemia is complete, treatment may prevent loss of the opposite eye. The patient should be warned that treatment is not invariably effective. The management of this disease is best undertaken as a joint effort between ophthalmologist and internist.

Cranial arteritis should be distinguished from ischemic and hypertensive optic neuropathy. In classic ischemic neuropathy, no treatment is effective. In hypertensive neuropathy, reduction of blood pressure is indicated. Neither condition shows an elevated sedimentation rate, and both

tend to occur in a somewhat younger age group (late middle life). Low-tension glaucoma and shock optic neuropathy must also be kept in mind.

Transient Ischemic Attacks

Transient ischemic attacks are fleeting episodes of focal neurologic deficits lasting minutes to hours. An attack that lasts longer than 24 hours is treated as a completed stroke, and it is in the prevention of stroke that the recognition of transient attacks is important.

The pathogenesis of ischemic attacks is complex and varied. Causes might include stenosis of the carotid and vertebrobasilar systems, embolism (atheromatous, platelet, or myxomatous), decreased cardiac output (from failure, arrhythmias, dehydration, anemia, or overcontrol of hypertension), compression of vessels in the neck, hypoglycemia, hypercoagulation states, cranial arteritis, migraine, and reverse flow in cerebral vessels (for example, steal syndromes). Snapping mitral valve syndrome has recently been implicated as a source of emboli.

Clinical features depend on whether the carotid (anterior) or vertebrobasilar (posterior) distribution is involved. The importance of this differentiation is that carotid disease is potentially subject to surgical treatment, whereas the posterior distribution is usually not.

Signs and symptoms of carotid system disease include monoparesis, hemiparesis, hemiparesthesias, and contralateral visual loss. Vertebrobasilar diseases produce brain stem symptoms, including monoparesis, alternate-side paresis, facial numbness on one side and motor loss on the other, diplopia, dysarthria, vertigo, drop attacks, and dysphagia. Loss of consciousness, confusion, amnesia, and tonic-clonic activity are not usually due to transient ischemic attacks, and the practitioner should suspect mass lesions.

Examination might include testing the blood pressure in each arm, auscultation of carotids, determining the pulse rate, palpation of temporal arteries, taking the temperature of limbs, and looking for signs of congestive failure. Compression of neck vessels is never done as a provocative test. The laboratory work-up might include a complete blood count (CBC), urinalysis, electrocardiogram, serology, echocardiogram, lipid profile, sedimentation rate, glucose tolerance, chest X-ray for cardiac configuration, skull films, brain scan, and arteriography if the patient's condition permits.

Ophthalmic manifestations occur in 40 percent of patients with carotid disease and are the result of transient hypoxia of the retina rather than of the higher visual pathway. Monocular visual loss is therefore more common than transient episodes of hemianopia. Amaurosis fugax may be described by the patient as blur-outs, gray-outs, visual field contractions, a curtain or window shade phenomenon, or a cloud or mist in the field of vision. If one has a chance to observe the patient during the attack one may observe nonreactive pupils; narrowed retinal arteries; perhaps an embolus at the bifurcation of an artery; and, occasionally, a Horner syndrome. Cotton wool spots and hemorrhages are features of retinal ischemia. Two types of emboli are commonly seen: orange, scintillating cholesterol flakes (Hollenhorst's plaques) and dull white platelet emboli.

Ophthalmic signs of vertebrobasilar insufficiency may include transient visual loss, but this tends to be mild and is often unreported. Oculomotor palsies, including nystagmus, are important eye symptoms. Attacks may be precipitated by turning the head to one side or using one arm. Diplopia is uncommon with carotid insufficiency.

Ophthalmodynamometry is a noninvasive, but not totally innocuous, procedure. If performed incorrectly, it may result in severe ischemia or even central retinal artery occlusion. Several techniques are available: compression, suction, oculoplethysmography, Doppler flow sonography studies, and oculocerebrovasculometry. The principle involves elevation of intraocular pressure with a tension-recording instrument while observing the pulsation of the central retinal artery opthalmoscopically. Carotid stenosis must exceed 50 percent to become hemodynamically significant. Observation of diastolic pressure is safer than increasing tension to the point of total collapse of the artery. Diagnosis is based on noting a pressure difference of the two sides.

The significance of emboli in producing transient episodes of visual loss is apparently related to fragmentation and dissolution of plugs on the one hand and passage to smaller vessel branches on the other. Another mechanism appears to be a transient circulatory arrest within the eye followed by reactive vasodilation. In some cases, no emboli are found, and the mechanism may be transient optic nerve ischemia.

The time sequence has some diagnostic value. Vascular ischemic attacks last 5 to 15 minutes and are unilateral. Attacks lasting seconds, occurring in both eyes, and repeated many times during the day may be due to chronic papilledema. Migraine attacks may be accompanied by photopsias and headache and can last up to 30 minutes. Very short episodes that alternate from one eye to the other may be hysterical. In auscultating the carotid system, a pediatric bell endpiece should be placed over the angle of the jaw, the middle of the neck, and the heart. The absence of a bruit can mean either normal flow, les than 50 percent stenosis, or total stenosis.

Thyroid Ophthalmopathy

Thyroid opthalmopathy be discussed equally well under neuro-ophthalmic disorders, because eye manifestations are often independent of the endrocrine course, motility disorders are a common presenting complaint, and the chief visual risk of the disease is compression of the optic nerve.

Grave's disease may occur at any age but is most common in the fourth decade. It has a greater prevalence in women and in those who have other autoimmune disorders. The etiology is unknown; an imbalance in the homeostatic mechanism between thyroid secretion and tissue utilization is postulated, possibly because of the presence in plasma of an abnormal thyroid stimulator. Clinical manifestations of hyperthyroidism include goiter, weight loss, fine tremor, nervousness, excessive sweating and heat intolerance, palpitations, arrhythmias, tachycardia, and cardiac failure.

Ophthalmic features include a characteristic frightened appearance because of proptosis and lid retraction, lid lag on downgaze, infrequent blinking, convergence insufficiency, and restriction of ocular movements (exophthalmic opthalmoplegia). In rapidly progressive exophthalmos, there is chemosis, conjunctival injection, corneal exposure with ulceration, and optic nerve compression leading to atrophy. The proptosis is usually bilateral, but it may be unilateral. The differential diagnosis includes orbital masses, hemorrhage, vascular malfunctions, inflammation, uremia, and Cushing's syndrome. The pathology is characterized by an inflammatory infiltrate of orbital contents with water, connective tissue, lymphocytes, plasma cells, and mast cells. Infiltration of extraocular muscles may simulate tumors on computerized tomography and is responsible for the ophthalmoplegia. Neural and myopathic ophthalmoplegias may be confused with this. Lid retraction and lid lag are important signs and are attributed to excessive innervation of Müller's muscle. If the levator muscle actually is infiltrated, exposure keratopathy is possible. Bell's phenomenon therefore should be checked. Other causes of lid retraction are uncommon (aberrant third nerve regeneration, pineal tumors, myotonic dystrophy, and ptosis on the opposite side).

The most common motility disorder is a double elevator palsy (an old orbital floor fracture should be considered). Forced ductions may help identify mechanical restrictions. The most serious complication is optic nerve compression. Danger signals are a central scotoma, color defects, afferent pupil sign, and disc edema. Such findings require emergency decompression of the orbit to save vision.

The course of the disease is unpredictable; the ophthalmopathy may progress despite the resolution of hyperthyroidism, and radioiodine therapy may in fact aggravate it. After reaching a plateau, the eye findings may subside spontaneously, with variable recovery.

Neuro-ophthalmic Disorders
Neurologic diagnosis is thrice unique; it logically follows anatomy, requires minimal equipment, and demands the most systematized reasoning. A practical plan of examination consists of an appropriate history, a specific work-up, and pertinent laboratory tests. If a diagnosis is still found wanting, either Nature cures the patient, or autopsy reveals the exact pathology.

The history is fundamental, because many neurologic symptoms have no physical manifestations (for example, headache, pain, photopsias, parethesias, or obscurations). We must rely on patients to tel us what they see or feel, or, indeed, if they can see at all. Moreover, the history is not only a diagnostic, but a therapeutic, tool.

Diminished smell, hearing and sight contribute to sensory deprivation in the elderly. Hearing loss (presbycusis) increases with age and is usually sensorineural. Speech sounds become distorted and unintelligible, although patients know when they are being spoken to. People with hearing loss naturally must rely more on visual cues; then, concurrent visual impairment greatly compounds the sense of isolation.

Dizziness is a common complaint of older patients. True vertigo is characterized by a sensation of motion or rotation, either of self or the environment. It is often accompanied by nausea and blurred vision, hearing loss, tinnitus, and nystagmus, prehaps aggravated by head turning and upright posture. True vertigo should be differentiated from lightheadedness, faintness, nervousness, or spatial disorientation precipitated by new glasses. Labrynth disease is the most common cause of vertigo. Meniere's disease on the other hand is an endolymphatic hydrops characterized by vertigo, unilateral fluctuating senorineural deafness, and tinnitus. Toxic labyrinthitis may follow the use of drugs (streptomycin, sedatives, phenytoin, or diuretics), heavy metals, or alcohol. Common motion sickness may be precipitated by sudden movements of the head in the elderly. Lesions of the vestibular nuclei cause severe vertigo and may result from demyelinating disease, vascular insufficiency, tumors, and edema. Central vertigo is usually associated with headaches, diplopia, vomiting, and elevated intracranial pressure. Vertigo may be a prodrome of migraine, epilepsy, or transient ischemic attacks. Vertigo associated with facial, trigeminal, and auditory signs may be due to acoustic neuromas.

Trigeminal nerve disease can be caused by aneurysm; mass lesions; inflammation of the orbital apex, the superior orbital fissure, the cavernous sinus, or the gasserian ganglion outside the brain stem, or within the brain stem. The chief ocular sympton is corneal anesthesia. Local corneal anethesia also occurs with herpes simplex infection and following a variety of intraocular surgical procedures. The combination of facial nerve palsy, insufficient tear production, and corneal anesthesia is part of the cerebellopontile angle tumor syndrome. Trigeminal neuralgia is a disease of older people characterized by attacks of intense pain in the distribution of any of the three branches of the ganglion; its cause is unknown. Surgical relief may be complicated by corneal anesthesia. Neuroparalytic keratitis may result in perforation in a matter of days unless the cornea is properly protected.

Headaches are probably universal, but the patient who presents with headache as the chief complaint deserves special attention. Since physical signs are usually absent, a meticulous history is essential. The key question is, In what way are these headaches different from those you usually experience? Any headache of sudden onset, incapacitating severity, or increasing frequency or duration that is not relieved by previously successful therapy or that is accompanied by focal neurologic signs or mood changes should have an ophthalmic work-up, including pupil evaluation, intraocular tension, funduscopy, visual field, blood pressure, carotid auscultation, temporal artery palpation, and whatever laboratory tests are indicated by the examination. As a checklist, headaches may be conveniently classified as vascular (including migraine), muscle contraction, traction, inflammatory, and psychogenic (especially depression).

About 60 percent of patients with brain tumors complain of headaches. The pain may be dull, intermittent, and interrupt sleep. It is often made worse by factors that increase intracranial pressure (coughing, stooping, or straining). Mass lesions in the elderly may include abscess, aneurysm, and tumor. The tumors are frequently metastatic and may be symptomatic before the primary lesion. The diagnosis of mass lesions depends on correlating signs and symptoms with neuroradiologic findings. The most common symptoms are headache, seizures, personality changes, and motor and speech disturbances. Diagnosis has been markedly facilitated by computerized tomography (over 90 percent detection by this method). Angiography is indicated in planning surgery.

The chief ophthalmoscopic sign of increased intracranial pressure is papilledema. Its features include the loss of a previously noted venous pulse, hyperemia, blurring of the disc margin, venous congestion, peripapillary edema with concentric traction lines, and hemorrhages. Filling in of the physiological cup is not a reliable sign, and an enlargement of the blind spot is of no help except in following the course of the disease. In contrast to optic neuritis, the vision is generally good, there is no Marcus Gunn pupil, no inflammatory cells in the vitreous, and no pain upon eye movement. Color vision is not affected. Patients with increased intracranial pressure are often ill, with nausea, vomiting, headaches, and even fluctuating levels of consciousness. In chronic papilledema, there may be transient obscurations of vision. When conduction in the nerve is compromised, the signs and symptoms of neuritis appear. Funny-looking discs may be confused with papilledema. These include congenital anomalies, staphylomas, hyperopia, and optic never drusen. Drusen are often familial, are rare in blacks, and have an

incidence of almost 0.5 percent. Disc margins may be blurred, with a scalloped contour. Drusen tend toward a yellow translucent color and may be elevated several diopters. Buried drusen are invisible but become more superficial with age. Occasionally, they erode peripapillary capillaries (causing hemorrhages) or compress optic nerve fibers (causing atrophy). Optic nerve drusen can be associated with any ocular disease, including papilledema.

Perimetry plays a major role in neuro-ophthalmic diagnosis because of the long course of visual sensory fibers from one end of the skull to the other. The concept of the field as an island of vision in a sea of blindness is useful in understanding that the field can be approached from the side (kinetic perimetry) and from above (static perimetry). The use of targets of different sizes (or differing luminances and colors) is termed *quantitative perimetry*. The problem is that it also takes a quantity of time, but the temptation to omit or postpone the test must be resisted. As regards automated instruments, Traquair's admonition – that visual fields are tested by the perimetrist, not the perimeter – should be kept in mind. At least two isopters are always plotted to confirm validity and reliability. In many disorders, field defects are the only clue to the presence of disease. Unilateral field abnormalities suggest a careful search for defects in the "normal" eye, for bilaterality is not always symmetrical. A bilateral anomaly usually places the problem in the chiasma or beyond. Recall that lesions of the optic tract and anterior radiation tend to be incongruous, whereas posterior lesions are congruous; this rule is of no value once the hemianopia is complete.

Acquired diplopia is a serious, potentially life-threatening symptom in the elderly. The causes may be traumatic, infectious, vascular, metabolic, or neoplastic. In a certain proportion of cases, no cause can be discovered. True diplopia can be distinguished from monocular dipolopia by asking the patient to close one eye. Neural disorders can be differentiated from mechanical restrictions by forced duction tests; from myopathies by lack of innervational pattern; and from strabismus by history, old photographs, and presence of amblyopia. Diagnosis is based on accompanying features, and in this way the disease generally can be traced to the orbit, the obital apex, the cranial cavity, or the brain stem. For example, a painful sixth nerve palsy associated with a hearing loss on the same side may suggest Gradenigo syndrome or an angle tumor. Bilateral sixth nerve palsies with papilledema suggest intracranial pathology. Isolated fourth nerve palsies are often traumatic. Third nerve palsies may result from aneurysm, diabetes, migraine, and tumors. Aberrant regeneration is found after aneurysm and trauma, rarely with tumors, and never with infarcts or diabetes. Multinerve involvement is often neoplastic. Lesions of the base of the brain may show visual field defects or other signs of vascular insufficiency. Supranuclear palsies are characterized by disturbances of saccadic, pursuit, vergence, or vestibular eye movement systems; diplopia is rare. Brain stem lesions often involve adjacent nerves (facial, auditory, vestibular, or trigeminal), the pupils, and the medial longitudinal fasciculus. Unlike strabismus in the young, diagnosis is simplified by the absence of suppression, anomalous correspondence, and eccentric fixation. The work-up should include specification of the timing, direction, and magnitude of the deviation in different cardinal positions. Note head tilt, ptosis, proptosis, pupil involvement, visual field defects, lid retraction, papilledema, orbital and carotid bruits, tenderness of temporal arteries, facial and auditory nerve function, corneal sensation, mechanical restriction, periorbital anesthesia, nystagmus, blood pressure, and evidence of aberrant regeneration. Pertinent laboratory tests, in addition to radiologic investigations, might include blood sugar level, sedimentation rate, serology, and hematocrit. When indicated, Tensilon test, angiography, lumbar puncture, biopsy, and neurosurgical cconsultation are helpful.

Transient diplopia occurs in multiple sclerosis, vertebrobasilar insufficiency, epilipsey, myasthenia, parkinsonism, minor strokes, phoria decompensation, and intermittent squint. The presence of a head tilt means fusion is present in some directions of gaze. Mechanical mechanisms of diplopia have no neural pattern. Peripheral neuropathies may involve any nerve branch.

Involvement of the extrapyramidal system is commmon in the aged, evident as rigidity, hypokinesia, flexed posture, and tremor. The tremor exists at rest, is coarse, and is aggravated by voluntary movements and stress. In contrast, the tremor of parkinsonism exists at rest but subsides on willed movements. In its fully developed form, the clinical picture of paralysis agitans is highly characteristic: stooped posture, stiffness, slow movements, fixed facial expression, festinating gait, and no sensory changes. Postencephalitic parkinsonism may be indistinguishable from the primary disease. Drug-induced parkinsonism should be ruled out. Disturbances of vertical gaze and lid movement, oculogyric crises, and blepharospasm are the usual ophthalmic findings.

Myasthenia gravis is a muscular disease that can occur at any age and in both sexes. In males, the peak incidence is in the sixth and seventh decade. The mechanism appears to be an increase in circulating antibodies to acetylocholine receptors on an antoimmune basis. Pathologically, muscles are infiltrated with small, round cells. Ophthalmic findings occur early becasue of the high nerve-to-muscle ratio of extraocular muscles. Clinically, the onset is chronic, and often insidious. Bilateral ptosis or other extraocular muscle weakness occurs in 90 percent of cases. Weakness progresses with exercise or during the day. Pupils are never affected. Choking and food aspiration may be due to weakness of palatal muscles, and the voice may have a nasal quality. Infections, large meals, and alcohol aggravate the symptoms. The incidence of thyroid disease, arthritis, and cancer is higher in these patients. Diagnosis is based on the history and the improvement of muscle function with the edrophonium test.

Joint and muscular disease in the elderly frequently is treated with corticosteriods. Steroid-induced glaucoma and cataracts, therefore, deserve special mention. Tonometry will reveal a rise in pressure, and funduscopy may show disc changes. The crystalline lens often exhibits posterior capsular opacities, and the patient may complain of glare, halos, and monocular diplopia. A disproportionate loss of reading vision compared with distance vision can be misinterpreted as progressive presbyopia. Finally, the presenting complaint may be a red eye due to bacterial, fungal or hepetic infection exacerbated by steriods.

The clinical syndrome of dementia is characterized by deficits of memory, judgment, language, and other cognitive functions, as well as changes in personality and behavior. The causes are varied; some are treatable, such as drug reactions, metabolic dysfunctions, infections, trauma, nutritional deficiencies, or benign neoplasms. Unfortuately, the most frequent cases of dementia are progressive, despite symptomatic treatment. These include Alzheimer's disease and multi-infarct dementia. Alzheimer's disease is a senile dementia of unknown etiology; its diagnosis is based largely on exclusion. Current research focuses on correcting possible neurotransmitter imbalances and preserving the function of surviving neurons. Treatment is symptomatic. Multi-infarct dementia may occur after repeated cerebrovascular accidents, and the diagnosis is based on a history of recurrent strokes. Dementia must be differentiated from functional and emotional disturbances. Apathetic patients may fail to respond to questions regarding orientation in time, place, and events. Loss of remote memory carries a more grave prognosis than loss of recent memory. All organic brain syndromes have a functional overlay, because patients react emotionally when aware of intellectual deterioration.

Care of the Elderly: A Summary

Older people are more fragile than their younger counterparts. Relatively trivial breakdowns in homeostasis can have irreversible and fatal consequences. Nevertheless, clinicians are sometimes "turned off" by the elderly. Several reasons require careful, introspective analysis. First, the tradition of health care savors the instant gratification of rapid and complete cures. In diseases of old age, we must settle for short-term gains instead of long-term satisfaction. Second, clinicians may have difficulty extrapolating from their own anticipated reactions to the actual responses of the elderly. Habits and attitudes are more rigid; they tend to resist change and hold tenaciously to their limitations. Third, emotional response to physical illness in the elderly is often colored by fears of death, isolation, pain, and blindness. The therapeutic value of communicated understanding is lost if one provides reassurance on matters that the patient is not concerned about. Such failures can only be avoided by listening to the patient carefully. Fourth, depression is the most frequent functional psychiatric disorder of the elderly. It is hard to praise life when life abandons us. Depression, in contrast to grief reactions, is accompanied by diminished self-esteem and overwhelming guilt. It is difficult to empathize with depressed people because of their intense self-preoccupation. Fifth, hearing loss, slow reaction time, and apathy make examination more difficult. This may result in misinterpretations or even omitting important tests. The solution is to allow more time, and, if necessary, repeat the

office visit. Sixth, the elderly often misunderstand the proper use of medications or fail to comply with directions because of economic and transportation problems. One therefore should question patient about the use and abuse of drugs, especially when multiple prescriptions are involved (as they frequently are). Seventh, drug interactions and the prolonged use of sedatives, tranquilizers, or alcohol may not only produce organic syndromes, but change previously controlled diseases such as glaucoma and diabetes. Eighth, older people may ignore or suppress important symptoms either from fear, a sense of inevitability, or depressed responsiveness. Such symptoms must be actively sought to avoid their being overlooked. Ninth, loss of appetite, indifference, lack of companionship, and economic factors make the elderly the most common undernourished segment of the population. This can alter wound healing, predispose to infection, and modify expected responses to therapy. Tenth, the clinician should make sure that incentives and means are available for periodic reexaminations and follow-ups.

To acknowledge senescence, however, is not to predict senility, although the terms are often used interchangeably in clinical parlance. Intelligence, in fact, is seldom impaired, and learning ability, in the absence of disease, is undiminished. The person who is too old to learn was probably always too old to learn.

Because the number of elderly people is increasing, the prevalence of visual impairment is growing. The major challenge of the future is to balance the services the elderly need against the availability and appropriateness of the services they receive. The best must sometimes yield to the best obtainable, but excellence cannot be bought by expediency. The notion that health care can be provided to the elderly (or anyone else) only on the basis of cost effectiveness substitutes economic policy for clinical judgment, platitudes for empathy, and "cases" for patients. Demographic studies that focus exclusively on common disorders are of little help to the patient with a rare disease or the symptomatic patient with no disease. In a free society, the individual must always remain the end and not the means to a better future.

This chapter has, of necessity, emphasized the constraints of age; little was said of its possibilities. But there is health as well as disease, pleasure as well as pain, growth as well as decay, life as well as death. The rules for caring for the as well as pain, growth as well as decay, life as well as death. The rules for caring for the old, it seems to me, are also good rules for growing old: To do what we can, the best we can, while we can.

Suggested Readings

General Texts

Apple, D. J. *Clinicopathologic Correlation of Ocular Disease.* St. Louis: Mosby, 1978.

Duane, T. *Clinical Ophthalmology.* New York: Harper & Row, 1980.

Duke-Elder, S. *System of Ophtalmology.* 15 vols. St. Louis: Mosby, 1956–1976.

Harrison's Principles of Internal Medicine. New York: McGraw-Hill, 1980.

Havener, W. H. *Synopsis of Ophthalmology.* St. Louis: Mosby, 1979.

Newell, F. W. and J. T. Ernest. *Ophthalmology: Principles and Concepts.* St. Louis: Mosby, 1978.

Perkins, E. S., ed. *Sceintific Foundations of Ophthalmology.* Exeter, N. H.: Heinemann Ed., 1977.

Scheie, H. G. and D. M. Albert. *Textbook of Ophthalmology.* Philadelphia: Saunders, 1977.

Vaughan, D. and T. Asbury. *General Ophthalmology.* Los Altos, Calif.: Lange, 1980.

Special Texts

Beard, C. *Ptosis.* St. Louis: Mosby, 1976.

Blodi, F. C., et al. *Stereoscopic Manual of the Ocular Fundus in Local and Systemic Disease.* St. Louis: Mosby, 1964–1979.

Boniuk, M. *Ocular and Adnexal Tumors.* St. Louis: Mosby, 1964.

Cogan, D. G. *Ophthalmic Manifestations of Systemic Vascular Disease.* Philadelphia: Saunders, 1974

Cogan, D. G. *Neurology of Ocular Muscles.* Ann Arbor, Mich.: Thomas Press, 1978.

Fedukowicz, H. B. *External Infections of the Eye.* New York: Appleton-Century-Crofts, 1978.

Friedlaender, M. H. *Allergy and Immunology of the Eye.* New York: Harper & Row, 1979.

Gass, J. D. M. *Macular Diseases.* St. Louis: Mosby, 1977.

Goldberg, M. F. , and S. L. Fine, eds. *Symposium on Treatment of Diabetic Retinopathy.* No. 1890. Washington, D. C.: U.S. Department of Health, Education, and Welfare, 1968.

Harrington, D. O. *The Visual Fields.* St. Louis: Mosby, 1976.

Hogan, M. J., and L. E. Zimmerman. *Ophthalmic Pathology.* Philadelphia: Saunders, 1962.

Jaffe, N. S. *Cataract Surgery and Its Complications.* St. Louis: Mosby, 1976.

Jones, I. S. *Diseases of the Orbit.* New York: Harper & Row, 1979.

Keeney, A. H. *Ocular Examination.* St. Louis: Mosby, 1976.

Kolker, A. E., and J. Hetherington. *Becker-Shaffer's Diagnosis and Therapy of the Glaucomas.* St. Louis: Mosby, 1976.

L'Esperance, F. A. *Current Diagnosis and Management of Chorioretinal Diseases.* St. Louis: Mosby, 1977.

Mausolf, F. A., ed. *The Eye and Systemic Disease.* St. Louis: Mosby, 1975.

Micheals, D. D. *Visual Optics and Refraction.* St. Louis: Mosby, 1980.

Paton, D., and M. F. Goldberg. *Management of Ocular Injuries.* Philadelphia: Saunders, 1976.

Reese, A. B. *Tumors of the Eye.* New York: Harper & Row, 1976.

Reichel, W., ed. *Clinical Aspects of Aging.* Baltimore: Williams & Wilkins, 1978.

Runyun, T. E. *Concussive and Penetrating Injuries of the Globe and Optic Nerves.* St. Louis: Mosby, 1975.

Schatz, H., et al. *Interpretation of Fundus Fluorescein Angiography.* St. Louis: Mosby, 1978.

Sekuler, R., et al., eds. *Aging and Human Visual Function.* New York: Liss, 1982.

Steinberg, F. U., ed. *Cowdry's The Care of the Geriatric Patient.* St. Louis: Mosby, 1976.

Straatsma, B. R., et al., eds. *The Retina.* Berkeley: The University of California Press, 1970.

Tolentino, F. I., et al. *Vitreoretinal Disorders.* Philadelphia: Saunders, 1976.

Walsh, F. B., and W. F. Hoyt. *Clinical Neuro-ophthalmology.* Baltimore: Williams & Wilkins, 1969.

Wise, G. N. et al. *The Retinal Circulation.* New York: Harper & Row, 1971.

Yanoff, M., and B. S. Fine. *Ocular Pathology.* New York: Harper & Row, 1975.

Zinn, K. M., and M. F. Marmor. *The Retinal Pigment Epithelium.* Cambridge, Mass.: Harvard University Press, 1979.

Chapter 12

Oculomotor Signs of Pathology in the Elderly

David Pickwell

Anomalies of the oculomotor system that affect binocular vision in the elderly patient can require optometric care. In some cases, an anomaly also can be a sign that the patient would benefit from medical attention. It is in the interests of patients that practitioners be able to determine promptly when oculomotor problems are a sign of pathology and the cooperation of a medical practitioner is indicated. In some cases, the primary cause of the disturbance is such that referral to another practitioner is essential before any optometric care proceeds. This chapter is concerned with the differential diagnosis of optometric problems from medical problems in patients where an oculomotor anomaly is apparent.

Pathological Deviations

For the purposes of this chapter, those deviations that indicate the onset of an underlying cause requiring medical attention are referred to as *pathological deviations*. In very general terms, they have two main characteristics. First, the onset is comparatively sudden; second, the deviation and diplopia are usually noncomitant. That is not to say that all deviations with a sudden onset are necessarily pathological, nor is it true that all noncomitant deviations are a sign of active pathology. However, these two signs are usually present in pathological deviations, and when they occur, the possibility of pathology should be carefully explored.

A noncomitant deviation varies in angle in different parts of the motor field. The squint may be present when the eyes turn to look in one direction of gaze and absent in all other directions. In other cases, it is present in all directions of gaze but increases in angle when the eyes turn in one direction. Pathological deviations are usually accompanied by diplopia of sudden, recent onset, and are also noncomitant. In long-standing squint, the sensory adaptations of suppression and anomalous retinal correspondence will have intervened, so the patient is not disturbed by diplopia; the motor anomaly will be observable, but sensory adaptations will have alleviated the symptoms.

Investigation

Normally, a full routine optometric examination will proceed in each case, but particular attention will be given to these aspects outlined in the following sections.

History and Symptoms

From what has been said about the nature of pathological deviations, it can be seen that history and symptoms become an important aspect of the differential diagnosis. Patients with a dramatic onset of diplopia accompanied by other signs and symptoms of ill health present an obvious picture of suspected pathology. Indeed, it may be so obvious that the patient will consult a medical practitioner rather than an optometrist. It is the more insidious cases that require more care in evaluation. A recent onset of intermittent diplopia associated with headaches during reading could be due to a functional anomaly such as exophoria becoming decompensated with age. It also might be due to a fourth nerve palsy (Duke-Elder 1973, 714). Although the symptoms need careful evaluation, they must be considered together with the rest of the clinical investigation. The following symptoms are particularly important:

1. *Diplopia.* When diplopia is given as a symptom, the question of comitancy must be explored. The patient may be able to recog-

nize the variation in different parts of the motor field. In pathological deviations there is very frequently a vertical element, and sometimes a tilting of one image is reported. It will be appreciated that diplopia in pathological deviations is not usually associated with any particular use of the eyes, such as reading, but rather with a direction of gaze.

2. *Abnormal head posture.* The patient may be aware that a compensation for the diplopia can be made by holding the head in an abnormal position.

3. *Headache.* The underlying cause of the deviation may cause headaches; for example, it can be present in vascular disturbances, neoplasms, and so on. Other conditions are considered later in this chapter.

4. *General health.* A deterioration in general health may occur when the cause is a metabolic anomaly. The patient may report loss of weight, increased or decreased appetite, general fatigue, loss of muscular ability, tremor of limbs, breathlessness, and so on.

5. *Injury.* In the elderly, an accident such as a fall can be responsible for an intra-cranial injury that can lead to an oculomotor disturbance, even when the patient has thought it not serious enough to seek medical advice but considered that rest was all that was needed.

6. *History.* The history of the patient's ocular and vision health also will help. When there has been a long-standing squint, an elderly patient usually will know. However, it must not be assumed that when the patient has had a squint throughout life, pathology cannot also occur. When there is amblyopia, symptoms that are due to a pathological deviation can be lessened if the amblyopic eye is primarily affected and increased when it is the nonamblyopic eye.

Motility

Most pathological deviations are paralytic or paretic. The term *paretic* will be used here to indicate all ocular deviations that are caused by the malfunction of one or more of the extrinsic ocular muscles. Such deviations are noncomitant, and the motility test is therefore an important part of the investigation. The eye movements are observed as the eyes follow a fixation target moved in different directions of gaze in and beyond the limits of the binocular field of fixation.

A small light or penlight is a very suitable target for the patient to follow, and observation of the corneal reflex will assist precise judgment of the eye movements. The binocular field can be thought of as an area 50 cm (20 inches) square at a distance of 50 cm in front of the patient's face. If the fixation target is moved outside this area, fixation will not be possible with one of the two eyes, since the target always will be obscured by the patient's brow or nose for one eye. Any diplopia of the penlight target must occur within the area of the binocular motor field (some patients may report doubling of the general field outside this area, even when fixation of the penlight with one of the eyes has been lost). Patients are asked to follow the moving light outside the binocular field into the extremes of gaze. They are asked to report any doubling of the fixation light. The practitioner observes the eyes, noting whether both are following smoothly, whether there is a corresponding lid movement accompanying vertical eye movements, and whether there is a restriction or overshooting of one eye in a particular direction of gaze. In elderly patients, there is often a bilateral restriction, particularly upwards; that is, the eyes do not move as far as they do in younger patients. When the eyes follow the light out of the binocular part of the field, one eye will continue to fix the light, and the other normally will undertake movement similar in degree and direction. In noncomitant deviations, the patient may report diplopia in the binocular field, and the restriction of movement becomes more obvious to the practitioner as the fixation light moves toward the extremes of the monocular field of fixation.

In one simple and quick routine (Pickwell 1981), the penlight is first held centrally so that the eyes are in the primary position and fixation can be checked in both eyes. If the observer sits directly behind the light, the corneal reflections of the light should appear symmetrical in the pupils and slightly nasal for a normal angle kappa. The penlight is then moved downward and back to the horizontal center of the field on the median line. The lid signs can be checked when this is being done (to be discussed later). Then the light is moved into the right extreme of the top of the field and slowly across the upper part of the field to the extreme left. This horizontal movement is repeated across the horizontal center of the field and again at the lower extremities. The horizontal movement across the top of the field allows the actions of the elevator muscles to be checked. The movement across the center of the field allows any abnormality of the lateral and medial recti muscles to be detected, and the movement across the bottom of the field should reveal any anomalies of the depressors. If an abnormality is seen, the likely cause can be determined from an analysis of the restrictions with respect to the actions of the individual muscles (Pickwell 1974).

The medial and lateral recti muscles are simple adductors and abductors, respectively, so when the eyes move to the left or right across the center of the field, they do so mainly by the action of these four muscles (two in each orbit). Movements to the right should be executed by the right lateral rectus and left medial rectus. If the right eye does not move adequately in this direction, there probably is a lateral rectus (or sixth nerve) palsy.

In people with no paresis but normal binocular vision, the elevator muscles are the superior rectus and the inferior oblique in each orbit. Their anatomy is such that the line of action of these two muscles lies in two different vertical planes that intersect medially to the plane containing the center of rotation of the eye. This is shown in Figure 12–1, in which *ab* represents the plane containing the superior rectus and *cd* represents the plane containing the inferior oblique. The right eye is shown in the primary position. As the superior rectus muscle is attached to the eye slightly above the limbus at *a*, and its line of action is in a direction a little nasal to the center of rotation (*R*), it will have secondary actions of adduction and intorsion, as well as its primary action of elevation. The inferior oblique is attached to the back of the eye, and its line of pull passes under the eye and is again nasal to the center of rotation. From the primary position, therefore, its secondary functions—abduction and extorsion— will be opposed to those of the superior rectus, but its primary function will be elevation. The primary and secondary actions of these muscles can be seen to arise from the anatomical fact that their lines of actions pass medial to the eye's center of rotation.

Figure 12–2 shows the lines of pull as the eyes move across the top of the motor field. When the eye is turned out (abducted), elevation is maintained by the superior rectus, because in this position its line of pull will have been carried more nearly over the center of rotation. In this position it will have the greatest advantage as

Figure 12–1

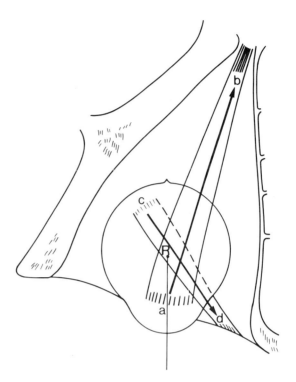

Patient's Right Orbit Showing the Planes of the Actions of the Superior Rectus (*ab*) and the Inferior Oblique (*cd*) Muscles Relative to the Eye's Center of Rotation (*R*).

an elevator. However, the inferior oblique will be pulling nearly at right angles to the line of sight, and therefore it will have little ability as an elevator in this position; it will have become primarily an extortor. It also can be seen from Figure 12–2 that when the eye turns inward (is adducted), the mechanical advantage of the superior rectus to maintain elevation of the eye will decline, and the inferior oblique will increase its ability to maintain elevation. Elevation is maintained by the superior rectus when the eye is turned out by both elevators when fixing directly above the primary position, and by the inferior oblique when turned in. In other words, one elevator gradually takes over from the other as the eye moves across the top of the motor field. (Pickwell 1974).

A similar analysis of the depressor muscles can be made. This is illustrated for normal binocular vision in Figure 12–3. Depression of the eyes is maintained by the inferior rectus when the eyes are turned outward, by both muscles when fixing in the median plane, and by the superior oblique when turned inward.

It follows from this that an inability of one eye to maintain elevation or depression when turned outward is most likely to be due to an anomaly of the superior or inferior rectus muscle. An inability to maintain elevation or depression when abducted is due to an anomaly of one of the oblique muscles. Difficulty in elevation or depression when fixing in the median plane is likely to indicate a malfunction of several muscles or some more general orbital anomaly.

The motility test is the only clinical method of detecting noncomitancy objectively in routine eye examination. Small deviations of an eye in a tertiary position are not easy to see. Observation of the corneal reflection makes them easier to detect. Also, the eye's position is compared with the lid positions. The lid openings are not symmetrical, but the position of one eye during dextroversion can be compared with the other eye on levoversion. Fortunately, underaction of a muscle often is accompanied by an overaction of the contralateral synergic muscle, and this exaggerates the angle and assists detection.

Patients with active pathology will nearly always have diplopia. The exception is when a pathological cause occurs in a patient who has had a long-standing squint, deep amblyopia in one eye, or both. Where there has been no previous squint, very small degrees of diplopia can be appreciated by the patient, making diagnosis more certain. The subjective analysis of the oculomotor deviation can be asisted by the use of red-green diplopia goggles.

The usual elderly patient suffering from

Figure 12-2

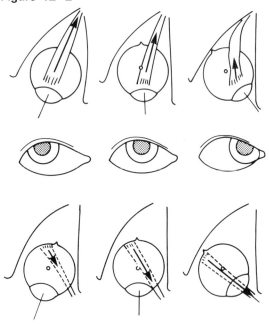

Actions of the Elevator Muscles, the Superior Rectus and the Inferior Oblique. (Left) The eye is in the abducted position. The upper figure shows the superior rectus pulling over the center of rotation and having its maximum elevating power with no secondary actions. The lower figure shows the inferior oblique pulling at an oblique angle to the visual line and having little power as an elevator, but greater secondary action. (Center) Both muscles are contributing to elevation. (Right) The eye is in the adducted position. The ability of the superior rectus to elevate the eye has declined in the upper figure. The lower figure shows the inferior oblique muscle in the position of maximum power as an elevator, with minimum secondary action.

Figure 12-3

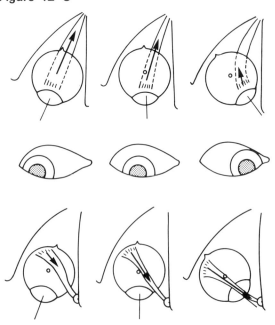

Relative Actions of the Inferior Rectus and Superior Oblique Muscles As the Eye Moves across the Bottom of the Motor Field in the Positions Shown (Center). The power of the inferior rectus to depress the eye is maximum when the eye is turned outward and the muscle pulls over the center of rotation, and minimum when the eye is turned inward (top). The lower figures show the increase of the power of the superior oblique to depress the eye as it moves in the same direction from the abducted to the adducted position.

sudden diplopia will be mentally alert and can readily appreciate small degrees of diplopia when wearing red-green goggles and also can appreciate and report changes in the magnitude of the diplopia as fixation is changed into the different fields of gaze. This subjective evaluation is more sensitive and quicker than the objective observation of restrictions in ocular movements when the patient is mentally alert. If the fixation target is a streak of light rather than just a spot, the patient can report whether the target tilts as the gaze is changed. This helps differentiate between an involvement of one of the oblique muscles and an involvement of one of the vertically acting recti. (The fixation light can be most easily changed to streak by using a Maddox rod before one eye instead of the red-green goggles.)

Where it is appropriate to monitor any change in a noncomitant deviation, a quantitative analysis can be made. All methods of recording the actual amount of noncomitancy rely on measurements of the subjective diplopia in different parts of the field. The Hess screen or one of its modifications is the most appropriate method for doing this.

Lid Signs
Abnormalities of the lids sometimes may indicate the presence of noncomitant deviations in elderly people. The width of the lid openings should be observed with the eyes in the primary position and during the motility test.

Lid Openings in the Primary Position. Compare the right and left palpebral fissures. The depth can be judged by comparing the amount of the limbus visible through the fissure. In elderly patients, less of the upper part of the limbus is seen with the eyes in the primary position. An abnormally wide fissure (Dalrymple's sign of thyrotoxicosis) may be accompanied by hypophoria or hypotropia, which increases on elevation of the eyes. A hypotropic position of one eye may be revealed by pseudoptosis; the upper lid is slightly lower as the eye is turned down. Ptosis may be a sign of third nerve palsy.

Lid Openings during the Motility Test. A failure of the upper lid to follow downward movements of the eyes (von Graefe's sign) also may be present in thyroid conditions.

Abnormal Head Postures
In elderly patients, a habitual abnormal head posture can be present in a number of circumstances, which vary from unilateral deafness to oculomotor anomalies. It is recently acquired abnormal head position that is significant in diagnosing paretic oculomotor conditions. Abnormal head postures also can be due to a recession of the near point of convergence, out-of-date spectacle corrections, or restrictions of the field of view in one or both eyes.

As a response to an oculomotor anomaly, an abnormal head posture is an attempt to compensate for the binocular vision difficulty by holding the head in a position that gives more comfortable single vision. It therefore indicates that binocular vision is possible in at least part of the motor field. It may be adopted in the early stages of a paresis, when there is still binocular vision in one direction of gaze. With other patients, no such compensation is possible, and diplopia is present in all directions from the dramatic onset of the disease. Sometimes an abnormal head posture will be adopted as the paresis diminishes. The patient may then cease to complain of diplopia.

Sometimes an abnormal head posture can be used to compensate for congenital conditions throughout life; in elderly patients, however, the head tends to straighten, and this gives rise to intermittent diplopia. Old photographs of the patient will show if there had been an abnormal head position for most of the patient's life. (Hugonnier and Hugonnier 1969, 281–283).

An unusual head position may be thought of as having one or more components:
1. *Facial turn to the left or right.* By itself, such a habitual turn may accompany an anomaly of a medial or lateral rectus muscle. For example, diplopia may be avoided in right lateral rectus palsy by turning the face to the right so that contraction of the right lateral rectus muscle is not necessary.
2. *Lowered or raised chin.* This may occur in the A or V syndromes, which are congenital deviations. A raising or lowering of the chin, however, may accompany other components of the abnormal head positions that are due to paresis.
3. *Head tilt.* If binocular vision is present in only part of the motor field, the head tilt may make it easier to avoid diplopia or extend the area of single vision. The head tilt usually is combined with a facial turn and a raised or

lowered chin. The direction of the tilt may be determined by the interests of leveling the diplopic images to assist fusion or by the attempt to compensate for the loss of cyclorotation of one eye if there is paresis of one of the oblique muscles.

Localization Disturbances

The localization of objects in space is determined by a combination of two visual mechanisms: sensory retinal localization and the motor system. The position of the image on the retina determines the direction in which it will be perceived (its visual location). Because the eyes and the head can move, the brain must take these movements into account in localizing objects in space. Disturbances of localization can occur in either the retinal or motor aspects of the combined system. Eccentric fixation will disturb the retinal system, and past pointing may occur. Also, if the eyes do not move correctly in response to the nerve impulses sent out from the brain, as in paretic squint, the motor system will be disturbed. The patient will not be able to locate things correctly and will have difficulty moving about. This will be more marked if the unaffected eye is covered or closed.

The past pointing test may be used to demonstrate these motor disturbances. It is applied monocularly to each eye in turn. The past pointing will be most marked in the eye with the affected muscles. The degree of past pointing will increase in the direction of gaze of the primary action of the affected muscle, and it will not occur in the opposite direction of gaze. The test can be made more effective by holding a card horizontally at the level of the patient's upper lip. A small object is placed on the far edge of the card, and the patient is asked to point with the finger under the card directly below where the object is perceived to be. The card occludes the patient's hand from view and insures that the location of the object is determined only by the motor system. The patient's head is kept still while the object is moved across the field, and the patient is required to locate it with the eyes in different directions of gaze.

External Examination and Ophthalmoscopy

The general appearance of the patient may show an obvious squint. Scars or asymmetries of the orbital region may indicate a previous injury. Eye signs of systemic disease may be present; for example, there may be exophthalmos, ciliary injection, or ptosis. The internal examination of the eyes also may reveal signs of vascular or metabolic disease, which may be accompanied by a noncomitant deviation and therefore help confirm the diagnosis that medical help is needed.

Evaluation

Having carried out full optometric examination that gives special emphasis to the aspects previously discussed, it is necessary to assess the results. No one clinical procedure will indicate in every case that a binocular vision anomaly involving the oculomotor system is pathological. In some cases it will be very easy to decide, but in others a careful evaluation of all the clinical findings will be necessary. The practitioner needs to look at all the results of all the tests undertaken and ask, "What does it all add up to?" A sudden onset of diplopia in elderly patients can have a number of nonpathological causes that have created the decompensation of the binocular vision. An adverse change in visual working conditions, the need for up-to-date spectacle correction, worry and anxiety, and old age itself all can cause a long-standing heterophoria to become decompensated. It would be wrong, however, to attribute all decompensated heterophoria to these causes without carefully considering the possibility of pathology.

Similarly, noncomitancy can be long-standing and not the result of active pathology. Where it exists, careful evaluation is required in the interests of the patients' getting the sort of care needed. A summary of the factors that will help assess noncomitancy deviations is given in Table 12–1.

Possible Causes of Binocular Pathology

In deciding if a patient with a noncomitant deviation requires immediate medical investigation, it is often helpful to be aware of the conditions that can cause ocular paresis and the other signs and symptoms that may accompany them. In the elderly patient, a very large number of conditions may have paretic deviations as part of their characteristics. These include infections of the nervous system, metabolic disorders, vascular lesions, neoplasms, and toxic conditions. Some of the conditions that most commonly occur with older patients and can present ocular palsy as an early sign follow. The signs and symptoms that also could be present in these conditions also are summarized, as these can

Table 12-1
Comparison of Long-standing Noncomitant Deviations
with Those of Likely Pathological Cause

Factor	Signs of Long-standing or Congenital Deviations	Signs of Deviations of Likely Pathological Cause
Diplopia	Unusual	Always present in at least one direction of gaze
Onset	Usually gradual; the patient may not know when	Sudden and distressing
Amblyopia	Often present	Very unlikely
Comitancy	Increases with time; becomes nearly comitant	Always noncomitant
Abnormal head posture	Slight, but persists on covering the paretic eye	More marked; patient aware of it; disappears on covering the paretic eye
Past pointing	Absent	Present
Other symptoms	Unlikely	May be present because of the primary cause

help diagnose the deviation as being of recent pathological cause. These conditions are also reviewed in other chapters.

Diabetes. A high percentage of ocular palsy is found in diabetic patients. It usually affects the third cranial nerve and sometimes may include pupillary anomalies. In older patients the onset is usually gradual.

In addition to the diplopia, general symptoms may include generalized headache, increased thirst and urination, increased appetite with loss of weight, constipation, and boils or other skin conditions. Where diabetes occurs in older patients, it is more frequent in overweight females.

Thyrotoxicosis. Thyrotoxicosis can occur with muscle palsy but without the exophthalmos. There usually is difficulty in elevation of the eyes, and more than one muscle is involved. A contracture of the inferior rectus is most frequent; this may give a clinical picture of a palsy of the superior rectus muscle.

General signs and symptoms may include exophthalmos (due to the enlargement of the muscle tissue in the orbit), von Graefe's sign, retraction of the upper lid, infrequent blinking, conjunctival injection, and vertical diplopia. It occurs more in older females and may be accompanied by increased appetite with loss of weight, clammy hands, and tremor of the outstreched hand and arm.

Hypertension. The chances of high blood pressure's being accompanied by ocular palsy increase with age as the blood supply to the cranial nerves becomes involved. Hypertension is the cause of about 10 percent of muscle palsy in older patients. There usually are fundus signs of the vascular changes. General symptoms may include headache that is present early in the day, dizziness, breathlessness, and ringing in the ears.

These are perhaps the three most common underlying causes of pathological deviations in elderly people. It must be remembered, however, that other conditions may give incomitant deviations. Another aspect that may help diagnosis is the recognition of particular palsies.

Fourth Nerve, or Superior Oblique Palsy.
Fourth nerve, or superior oblique palsy is most common as a congenital palsy or as a result of an accident, but it may occur after an intercranial vascular accident. Diplopia will be greatest when looking down and in or when reading.

Sixth Nerve, or Lateral Rectus, Palsy. The long intracranial nerve path of the sixth nerve makes it particularly susceptible to the sort of lesions that occur in later life. Because of the close association of the seventh cranial nerve in the midbrain, the facial muscles may also be involved.

Third Nerve Palsy, or Ophthalmoplegia. If the extrinsic ocular muscles are involved, the condition is known as *external ophthalmoplegia;* it is called *complete oculomotor palsy* if all are involved. Paresis of the ciliary muscles and sphincter of the iris is known as *internal ophthalmoplegia,* and when both internal and external muscles are affected, there is *total ophthalmoplegia.* In the latter case, there will be a divergent squint with the eyes slightly depressed, as well as a loss of accommodation and pupil action. Other accompanying symptoms can include headache, a tremor of contralateral limbs that is due to the involvement of the red nucleus where the third nerve fibers pass, and the other symptoms that may be present in diabetes.

Gaze Palsies. Gaze palsies occur because of lesions in the frontal motor center, gaze centers in the pons, or the interconnecting pathways. There is seldom diplopia, but the eyes move together in most directions of gaze. In one direction, however, the eyes cannot move reflexly to take up fixation, or more rarely, they cannot follow a moving target (pursuit palsy). In lateral gaze palsy, the two eyes do not move beyond the midline. In vertical gaze palsy, movements above the horizontal are restricted, or there is no movement at all; rarely, there is no downward movement.

Reporting and Referral

It is first essential to decide if the oculomotor anomaly is likely to have a contributory cause that requires medical attention. From the discussion so far, it is clear that the clinical procedures, the history, and the symptoms may cause the practitioner to suspect that pathology is present. Further questions of the patient may reveal signs and symptoms of general bodily conditions that the patient has not previously mentioned. This is particulary true in the early stages when intermittent diplopia is the patient's main reason for consultation, and the other symptoms have not yet become a very major cause of concern to the patient. In such cases, the patient may have a heterophoria rather than an actual squint. However, during the examination it may be found that the binocular vision is very unstable and likely to break down into a squint if some slight impediment is applied. For example, a septum that dissociates the center of the field, as in the Turville infinity balance method, sometimes will cause binocular vision to break down. Fixation disparity may be present and may increase if the patient's eyes are not in the primary position. The patient can be asked to report any fixation disparity with a Disparometer or Mallett Fixation Disparity unit with the head in the primary position and then with the head tilted so that the eyes are moved into a tertiary position relative to the orbits. Another useful procedure is to repeat the cover test with the eyes looking in different directions of gaze. A failure of the normal heterophoria recovery movement in one direction of gaze can give a useful indication of noncomitant heterophoria. However, it must be remembered that if this test is applied while the patient is wearing a correction for anisometropia, the differential prismatic effect will change the apparent degree of heterophoria, but not just in one direction of gaze.

If a pathological cause is suspected, referral needs to be considered, along with whether to refer the patient to a general medical practitioner, an ophthalmologist, or a neurologist. If the patient is under the care of a general physician, a report of the optometrist's examination should go to him or her, particularly when the coordination of the patient's health care is being undertaken through such a general medical practitioner, as is the case in many countries. The report should include the diagnosis made or suspected, and the ocular signs and symptoms that have led to this conclusion. This will enable the doctor to know where to begin the medical investigation or whether to refer the patient on to a specialist colleague. When a vascular accident or other urgent problem is apparent, the patient should be referred straight to the appropriate specialist and a copy of the report sent to the general practitioner.

Patients with general bodily conditions also may require optometric care of some kind. Usually, elderly patients require at least a pair of reading glasses. These may require some prism relief in the case of small or intermittent deviations. However, this may be only a temporary measure, as the primary condition may inprove; as the condition responds to treatment or to time, it is to be hoped that the binocular problem also will be alleviated. When optometric treatment of any kind is given or considered, it is useful to mention this in the report to the medical advisor.

In some cases, the patient's general condition may already be receiving medical attention. For example, this is often the case with vascular conditions in elderly patients. Where this is the case, the optometric care usually can proceed and the ocular deviation be reported to the medical practitioner so that this development can be taken into account in the general health care of the patient. This is particularly true of those cases in which the binocular anomaly is in its early stages. As mentioned earlier, other cases are more likely to have a dramatic onset of diplopia and other marked symptoms of the primary condition, which takes them to a medical practitioner in the first place rather than to the optometrist.

The possibility of detecting a pathological deviation in its early stages should be a primary concern of optometrists in respect to elderly patients with heterophoria or intermittent squint. This possibility must always be kept in mind, and the optometric examination must include the necessary clinical procedures to diagnose deviations with a primary cause that indicates the patient requires medical attention.

References

Duke-Elder, Sir Stewart. *System of Ophthalmology:* 6. Ocular Motility and Strambismus. London: Kimpton, 1973.

Hugonnier, R. and S. C. Hugonnier. *Strabismus, Heterophoria and Ocular Motor Paralysis.* Translated by S. Veronneau-Troutman. St. Louis: Mosby, 1969.

Pickwell, L. D. "Analysing Eye Movements." *Australian Journal of Optometry,* May 1974, 154–158.

Pickwell, L. D. "Incomitant Deviations: 2." *Optician,* April 24, 1981, 11–15.

Suggested Readings

Ball, G. V. *Symptoms in Eye Examination.* London: Butterworth Scientific, 1982.

Burian, H. M., and G. K. von Noorden. *Binocular Vision and Ocular Motility.* St. Louis: Mosby, 1974.

Moses, R. A. *Adlers's Physiology of the Eye: Clinical Application.* St. Louis: Mosby, 1981.

Pickwell, L. D. "Basic Clinical Concepts in Binocular Vision: Incomitant Deviations." *Optician,* March 27, April 24, May 22, June 26, 1981.

Chapter 13

Ocular Pharmacologic Aspects of Aging

Jule Griebrok Jose

Because of physiological or anatomic changes or disease states that accompany aging, drugs may produce different effects on an older than a younger population. The effects of some drugs are potentiated, and the effects of others are lessened with age; drug side effects also may be enhanced in older individuals. The eye care practitioner must consider these effects in deciding which drugs to use for a given patient. In addition, the medications the elderly patient already is using may interfere with or potentiate the actions of ocular pharmaceuticals. In some cases, ocular pharmaceuticals may potentiate the action of systemic medications, resulting in side effects such as palpations or hemorrhages. Practitioners thus must take a careful case history to avoid rare, but potentially significant, drug interactions. They also must be wary of ocular effects that may accompany the use of either ocular or systemic pharmaceuticals so that they can prevent their occurrence or progression.

This chapter will first discuss the factors that determine which diagnostic ophthalmic agents to select in examining the eye of the aging patient. This discussion will be limited to mydriatics. Topical anesthetics will not be discussed in a separate section, because the effects they produce in the older patient are not substantially different from their effects on the young. The practitioner, however, should be aware of the need for anesthetics in examining the elderly, with whom tonometry is an essential component of the routine yearly examination. Also, older persons are more likely to have narrow angles; this necessitates gonioscopic examination of the angles, a procedure that also requires corneal anesthesia.

Side effects of anesthetics frequently include stinging and vasodilation. Edema and epithelial staining also may occur, especially after tonometry is performed. Occasionally, patients will demonstrate a local ocular allergic reaction to an anesthetic. For all patients, it is important to record which anesthetic was applied, so another can be substituted at future visits should a local allergic response occur. It is also wise to note the allergy in the patient's record so that this will not be overlooked. A systemic allergic reaction is not likely to occur following the application of topical anesthetics. Nonetheless, the practitioner is cautioned against using topical anesthetics with patients who have experienced allergic reactions to systemic anesthetics.

The chapter also will consider ocular over-the-counter agents that are frequently used by older persons and then will discuss some of the more common and significant ocular side effects of both ophthalmic and systemic medications frequently used by the elderly.

Selection of the Diagnostic Agent

Dilated fundus examinations are an integral part of a thorough examination of the eye of the aging patient. When the eyes are to be dilated, patients may feel more comfortable after the examination if they have been advised *in advance* to bring along a friend to drive them home from the appointment. Patients may be bothered in the daytime by photophobia and distortions and at night, by the streaked optical image of streetlights or oncoming headlights. These effects may make patients very nervous, which the thoughtful practitioner should keep in mind for older patients whose reflexes already may be reduced.

Before an appropriate dilating agent can be selected, a careful case history is required. It is necessary to determine whether the patient has any systemic disease or is taking any medication that might influence the activity of, or be affected by, the diagnostic drug. Systemic diseases of particular concern with respect to diagnostic agents are cardiovascular disease and diabetes. Glaucoma and narrow angles are the most significant ocular conditions in determining the selection of the dilating agent. Under some circumstances, the latter condition may preclude dilation.

Anticholinergics

When the aging eye is to be dilated, a weak anticholinergic generally will be chosen for several reasons. First, even the weakest anticholinergics are effective, producing sufficient dilation to provide a very adequate view of the peripheral fundus in most patients. In addition, because they block the sphincter muscle, the pupil cannot constrict to the bright light of diagnostic instruments. Generally, this factor makes using anticholinergics an absolute requirement when fundus photographs are to be taken. Also, for any patient reporting symptoms such as floaters, flashing lights, reduced or distorted vision, altered color vision, or visual field losses, a widely dilated pupil is required to facilitate examination of the lens, the macula, and the peripheral fundus. This will necessitate the use of an anticholinergic mydriatic to dilate the pupil, particularly if the peripheral fundus is to be observed.

Furthermore, anticholinergic agents rarely produce significant systemic or ocular toxicity. Although several of the stronger anticholinergic drugs have been found to increase intraocular pressure, the amount of elevation generally is small. Homatropine (5 percent) was found to increase intraocular pressure by 3 mm Hg in 73 percent of a group of known open angle glaucoma patients (Christensen and Pearce 1963). A much higher elevation in pressure was reported by Harris (1968), who found an average increase of 10 mm Hg following the application of potent cycloplegic agents (1 percent cyclopentolate, 1 percent atropine, or 5 percent homatropine). He observed significant pressure elevation in 23 percent of the open angle glaucoma patients tested, contrasted with an incidence of 2 percent in patients not known to have glaucoma. These pressure elevations produced by the potent cycloplegics were observed approximately 40 minutes after application of the drug.

Harris also suggested that intraocular pressure measurements taken before and after the application of potent cycloplegics could be used as a diagnostic aid for patients with borderline elevations of intraocular pressure. Patients demonstrating pressure increases of 6 mm Hg or more would be viewed as possibly having open angle glaucoma.

Interestingly, Harris (1968) additionally found that intraocular pressure was not elevated by anticholinergics possessing weak cycloplegic action. For example, neither 0.5 percent tropicamide nor 0.2 percent cyclopentolate hydrochloride (Cyclogyl) elevated intraocular pressure in the 23 percent of the population that responded with pressure increases to the more potent anticholinergic agents. At a concentration of 0.2 percent, cyclopentolate has little cycloplegic action. Because these measurements were taken on patients under treatment for glaucoma, they also imply that 0.5 percent tropicamide would not interfere with pressure control in patients undergoing therapy with miotics. The results further support the hypothesis that miotics reduce intraocular pressure because of their effects on the ciliary body rather than because of any effect on pupil size.

One ophthalmologist (Lowe 1966) has suggested that anticholinergics, although potent, are much less likely to produce a pharmocologically irreversible angle closure than adrenergics; thus, he suggested that they would be preferable for use in dilating the pupil of eyes with suspiciously narrow angles. Many ophthalmologists disagree very strongly with this and believe it is always much easier to counteract an angle closure induced by adrenergics than one induced by anticholinergics. The argument as to which is easiest to counteract is not resolved by the literature. However, no matter which dilating agent is used, dilating the eye with a narrow angle potentially can induce an angle closure that requires surgical intervention.

Of the anticholinergics available, tropicamide is the fastest acting (which is convenient for the practitioner) and has the shortest duration (which is desirable for the patient). It also produces the least systemic or ocular toxicity and is the easiest anticholinergic to overcome in the event of precipitation of angle closure. Thus, tropicamide (0.5 percent) is clearly the anticholinergic dilating agent of choice, particularly in an older population in whom cycloplegia is obviously unnecessary.

Sympathomimetics

Dilation of the pupil with sympathomimetics offers a major advantage for the patient in that the sphincter is not blocked, so the pupil constricts to, and the patient is not bothered by, bright light. They also have an advantage over some anticholinergics in that adrenergics do not elevate intraocular pressure in open angle patients. In fact, they commonly reduce intraocular pressure (Lee 1958), so they can be used with confidence to dilate the pupils of patients on miotic therapy (Havener 1978).

Unfortunately, the source of their advantages for the patient produces disadvantages for the practitioner. They are far less effective mydriatics inasmuch as the pupil can constrict to the bright light of an ophthalmoscope. Pupil dilation is sometimes only a few millimeters, so adrenergics typically are inadequate when the retinal periphery is to be examined. The practitioner also must take their slow onset of action (about 50 minutes) into account and plan the examination accordingly. The practitioner also should keep the slow onset in mind and resist the temptation to give unnecessary repeated applications of these pressor substances.

In combination with anticholinergic drugs, adrenergics can produce greater dilation than either type of drug would produce if used alone. This increases the ability to examine the periphery and makes the adrenergics a valuable adjunct for retinal photography.

Adrenergics tend to produce a mid-dilated rather than a fully dilated pupil. If aqueous humor builds up behind an iris in mid-dilation, the iris can bulge into the chamber and block off the angle. This type of angle block may be more difficult to reverse than an angle block induced by anticholinergics (Gartner and Billet 1957; Lowe 1966). It is suggested that the iris enters into a tonic state as a consequence of the tug-of-war set up between the adrenergic effect on the dilator and the cholinergic effect on the sphincter (Lowe 1966). The ability of these drugs to resist the constrictor effect of miotics can result in an iris locked in mid-dilation and iris bombé. Angle closure induced by adrenergics is very difficult to reverse with pharmaceuticals. Generally, surgical intervention is required (Gartner and Billet 1957; Lowe 1966). Thus, although many practitioners recommend the use of adrenergics to dilate suspiciously narrow angles because of the ease with which these drugs are counteracted in most patients, those who use them must be aware of the possibility of setting up a pharmacologically irreversible angle closure. They therefore must be prepared to rush the patient to surgical intervention should the need arise.

Becker et al. (1959) found that 10 percent phenylephrine hydrochloride does not interfere with aqueous outflow in patients on miotic therapy for glaucoma, and therefore it can be used to dilate their pupils. However, the fact that phenylephrine can counteract miosis induced by cholinergic drugs demonstrates the difficulty of the reverse situation: attempting to overcome phenylephrine-induced mydriasis with even the most potent miotics (for example, echothiophate iodide). This again emphasizes the need for caution in using adrenergics to dilate eyes with very narrow angles.

These drugs, however, can be used with confidence in the open angle glaucoma patient (Havener 1978), in whom they do not alter aqueous outflow (Becker et al. 1959). Most studies also have found a reduction in intraocular pressure in glaucoma patients upon the application of phenylephrine (Becker et al. 1959; Lee 1958). This effect can have diagnostic value in the glaucoma suspect, since intraocular pressure generally drops very little in normal patients but may drop 10 mm Hg or more in the glaucomatous eye after the application of an adrenergic drug (Lee 1958). A drop in intraocular pressure, therefore, would add to the suspicion of glaucoma. However, failure of an adrenergic to cause a drop in a suspiciously high pressure does not rule out glaucoma.

Sympathomimetic agents repeatedly have been reported to cause systemic side effects, particularly cardiovascular problems. Among those reported are hypertensive crises with cerebral hemorrhages, arrhythmias, and cardiac arrest (Fraunfelder and Scafidi 1978). These effects have occurred in patients with increased susceptibility to adrenergics—for example, patients with diabetes or cardiovascular disease or patients taking guanethidine, monoamine oxidase inhibitors, beta-blockers, or tricyclic antidepressants (Kim, Stevenson, and Mathewson 1978).

Cardiovascular side effects are not typically induced in normal, healthy adults (Brown, Brown, and Spaeth 1980), and the significant systemic side effects that have been reported have occurred only secondary to the use of repeated applications of 10 percent phenylephrine. Effects have not been reported following the use of 2.5 percent phenylephrine or of 1 percent hydroxyamphetamine hydrobromide (Paredrine). Of the two, hydroxyamphetamine would be expected to be less likely to produce systemic effects, since it has an indirect mechanism of action that depends on the release of the body's own neurotransmitter stores to produce adrenergic effects. Phenylephrine, in contrast, acts directly on the adrenergic neuron in the same fashion as the normal neurotransmitter; therefore, it can produce an effect greater than that of the normal body stores.

Unfortunately, hydroxyamphetamine appears to have a much reduced effect in dilating the pupils of older persons as compared with young persons. The converse is true for phenylephrine; young persons respond poorly to 2.5 percent phenylephrine, whereas older persons respond with clinically useful mydriasis (Borthe and Davanger 1971; Korczyn, Laor, and Nemet 1976; Salminen, Aaltonen, and Jantti 1980). One study on an older population found that the degree of dilation induced by 2.5 percent phenylephrine was no different than that induced by 10 percent phenylephrine, although the rate was somewhat slower at 2.5 percent (Salminen, Aaltonen, and Jantti 1980).

Another study found that phenylephrine could induce as much mydriasis as that induced by cyclopentolate hydrochloride (Cyclogyl) in older patients (Borthe and Davanger 1971). Therefore, 2.5 percent phenylephrine should be considered a very useful drug for the elderly patient. Presumably, this low concentration should be easier to counteract than the 10 percent concentration in the event of an angle closure. This represents a dramatic change from the situation in the young eye. It has been suggested that the tonus of both the dilator and the sphincter muscles is decreased with age; therefore, augmentation of the dilator tonus by the application of phenylephrine induces better mydriasis in the older eye, because it is not counteracted by the strong tonus of the aged sphincter (Borthe and Davanger 1971).

Because of its indirect mechanism of action, hydroxyamphetamine can be predicted to have a significantly reduced effect on patients taking drugs such as guanethidine, which reduce the amount of neurotransmitter in the terminus. In contrast, it would have dramatically increased effects on patients taking drugs such as monoamine oxidase inhibitors, which increase neuro-

transmitter stores. Because of the risk of hypertensive crisis, hydroxyamphetamine should never be used for patients taking monoamine oxidase inhibitors. These include, but are not limited to, pargyline hydrochloride (Eutonyl), phenelzine sulfate (Nardil), and tranylcypromine sulfate (Parnate). Fortunately, these drugs are rarely used. A hydroxyamphetamine-like effect is produced by tyramine, an amine naturally occurring in many common foods. Taking monoamine oxidase inhibitors and eating tyramine-containing foods can result in hypertensive crisis and death (Goodman and Gilman 1980, 183).

Summary of Diagnostic Agents

The practitioner is likely to find 0.5 percent tropicamide generally the most useful drug for mydriasis in the aging patient. Its speed of onset and good dilation (even in bright light) make it very valuable for the routine case in a busy practice. A second drug that has considerable application in an older population is 2.5 percent phenylephrine. For an eye with elevated pressure or a patient under therapy for open angle glaucoma, phenylephrine is probably the dilator of choice, but it must be used with discretion for patients with known cardiovascular problems or diabetes. It should be avoided for patients taking guanethidine, monoamine oxidase inhibitors, beta-blockers, or tricyclic antidepressants. Multiple applications of 10 percent phenylephrine in rapid succession are contraindicated.

Empirical clinical "wisdom" and the literature conflict over whether tropicamide or phenylephrine is the most appropriate choice for dilating the eye of the patient with a suspiciously narrow angle. Therefore, the practitioner cannot be advised to use one or the other for all patients with narrow angles whose eyes require dilation. Suffice it to say that either drug can induce angle closure. Where angles are dangerously narrow but dilation is required, the practitioner should dilate only one eye at a time to avoid the precipitation of binocular angle closure.

The practitioner is strongly advised against routinely putting pilocarpine into a dilated eye. Although this has been considered a preventive measure against angle closure, the weight of evidence suggests that the application of a miotic following a mydriatic is far more likely to precipitate angle closure than merely allowing the pupil to return to its normal size without adding a constricting agent. Evidence for this is the fact that the combination of dilating plus constricting drops has been used as an effective experimental tool to induce angle closure attacks in eyes that do not exhibit angle closure when the dilating drop is used alone (Mapstone 1974). The theory behind this effect is discussed by Meyers (1976).

In the rare event that an angle closure attack should occur, 1 drop of pilocarpine (2 percent) can be administered every 5 to 10 minutes for three to four applications. Thereafter, the drops should not be applied more than once every 1 to 2 hours because of the risk of systemic toxicity from the pilocarpine. The noninvolved eye should be treated one time only to prevent its closure.

Another method of relieving a closed angle that has met with some clinical success is to apply force repeatedly to the cornea. This is done, for example, with a gonioprism or the Goldmann tonometer tip. Moderate force is applied for several seconds and then released for several seconds. This process is repeated over 4 to 5 minutes, during which the pressure also is evaluated. This method seems to work best if the attack is caught early. It must be remembered that the reversal of pressure in this manner is only temporary, and surgery probably will be required. The technique is discussed by Anderson (1979).

Over-the-Counter Agents
Two major types of over-the-counter ophthalmic agents may be valuable to the aging person: ocular lubricants and decongestants. Lubricants commonly are needed by older people, who frequently have problems with dry eyes precipitated by an age-related decrease in tear production (Henderson and Prough 1950). An age-related decrease in tear turnover also occurs (Fraunfelder 1976b). The elderly patient commonly develops associated problems, including burning or itching of the eyes or a dry, sandy feeling in the eyes. In addition, the practitioner is likely to see punctate staining in the lower half of the cornea. Tear break-up time is reduced, and there is a positive Schirmer test. Dellen and an abnormal tear meniscus also may be observed.

It is important to recognize that excessive tearing may be a sign of dry eyes. This seems contradictory unless it is recognized that the irritation of a dry eye can produce reflex tearing. Thus, if there is no other obvious cause of tearing such as a blocked punctum or severe ectropion, the patient may well be suffering from dry eyes

and benefit from the use of ocular lubricants.

The primary ingredient of most artificial tears is a viscosity builder such as hydroxymethyl cellulose. These agents slow tear movement and thus hold the tears in the eye. Generally, artificial tears are hypertonic solutions. A major exception to this is Hypotears, an isotonic solution developed for the treatment of keratoconjunctivitis sicca. Patients with this disease were found to have very hypertonic tears (Gilbard, Ferris, and Santamaria 1978), a condition that was hypothesized to pull liquid from the cornea and thus to increase irritation. Consequently, Hypotears (Cooper Vision) was developed with what the manufacturers have called a "tonicity adjuster" to keep tear osmolarity low. Although this product will not benefit all patients with dry eyes, it is worth remembering it as an alternative to the majority of artificial tear preparations. The practitioner may wish to provide a sample of both hypertonic and isotonic artificial tears so that the patient can decide which is best.

A fairly new product for use by patients with dry eyes is Lacrisert (Merck, Sharp, and Dohme). This is not yet an over-the-counter preparation—not because of any inherent danger from the medication itself, but because the manufacturer felt the patient needed detailed instruction in handling the applicator. Lacrisert is a small, compressed rod of hydroxypropyl cellulose that dissolves slowly when placed in the lower culde-sac of the eye. Thus, it obviates the need for constant reapplications of eye drops. The cellulose derivative increases the viscosity of the tears and slows their outflow from the eye. However, the rod provides no moisture, so patients with a reduced aqueous component of tears may require the application of both the Lacrisert and an additional tear substitute.

Exposure keratitis may occur more frequently in an elderly population than a younger because of reduced tear production and loosening of the eyelid skin. If corneal staining is isolated to the palpebral opening, it is likely that the patient is sleeping with the eyes slightly open. Patients may or may not complain of irritation, but they should be treated in any case so that the problem does not worsen. Two over-the-counter ointments are very effective for treating this condition. Either Duratears (Alcon) or Lacrilube (Allergan), applied just prior to bedtime, will prevent drying out of the tears and cornea during sleep. These drugs are less desirable for daytime use, because they blur vision. Patients may benefit from the additional application of an aqueous ocular lubricant during the day. The patient should return to the practitioner in a week to 10 days, by which time the condition should be significantly improved. The patient should continue to use the lubricant periodically to prevent recurrence of the staining.

Ocular decongestants may provide symptomatic relief for patients with dry, irritated eyes or ocular allergies. Some caution is prudent in advising older patients to use such medications. The major serious ocular side effect that may occur is precipitation of angle closure. All patients with narrow angles must be advised of the nature of the condition and be educated about the ocular and systemic symptoms so they can seek medical attention should such an attack occur. The eye care practitioner should inform the patient about signs and symptoms such as halos, red eyes, hazy corneas, nausea, and vomiting. These patients should be advised to use medications with mydriatic side effects cautiously and should be made aware that many pharmaceuticals have this side effect. This does not mean that they must consider such medications absolutely contraindicated, because not every narrow angle will close. Instead, they should know the risks and what to do should a reaction occur.

Patients who are under treatment for open angle glaucoma will be aware of their ocular condition and think they must avoid all over-the-counter medications containing a warning against use by persons with glaucoma. This is ironic, since many of these contain adrenergic agents that might favorably affect intraocular pressure.

The concentration of the active compound in most ocular over-the-counter preparations is unlikely to produce systemic effects in the elderly patient.

Caution is perhaps prudent, however, in advising their indiscriminate use by patients with known cardiovascular disease. Topical adrenergics are contraindicated for patients taking monoamine oxidase inhibitors (Fraunfelder 1976a). They should probably also be avoided by patients taking guanethidine, which makes the adrenergic synapse more sensitive to direct-acting compounds (Kim, Stevenson, and Mathewson 1978). The occasional use of 1 drop of a topical decongestant is unlikely to increase systemic blood pressure significantly, even for patients with cardiovascular disease. If a patient

is heavily or chronically medicated, however, it is advisable to consult the physician regarding the wisdom of encouraging the regular use of vasopressor compounds.

Ocular Side Effects

The side effects of most drugs are not peculiar to the elderly. However, some drugs are more commonly used by older patients, so side effects from them will occur more commonly in the elderly. Several of these already have been discussed in this chapter. Although it is impossible to discuss the side effects of all drugs that an elderly population of patients might be taking, a few additional drugs should be mentioned. For further information, the practitioner can consult the *Physician's Desk Reference* (Oradell, N.J.: Medical Economics Co., published yearly) or the excellent and easily usable *Drug-Induced Ocular Side Effects and Drug Interactions* (Fraunfelder 1976a).

Among the most important of these drugs are the corticosteroids, which can be used to treat inflammatory conditions, including rheumatoid arthritis. They can play a dramatic and crucial role in preventing tissue destruction and scarring because of their potent anti-inflammatory actions. Unfortunately, they also have a pronounced tendency to induce very serious ocular side effects, whether given topically or systemically.

One side effect that commonly occurs following topical steroid use is a marked elevation in intraocular pressure. Pressure elevation can occur at any age, but the magnitude of the effect is greater in older persons (Armaly 1963). Corticosteroids can reduce facility of outflow from the eye, producing a condition resembling open angle glaucoma. Cupping and irreversible field loss also can occur. The effect is genetically determined, with one-third of the population being very susceptible to steroid-induced pressure elevation (Becker and Hahn 1964). Pressure is also more likely to increase for patients with glaucoma, narrow or heavily pigmented angles, diabetes, or high myopia (greater than 5.00D). Pressure is less likely to be elevated as a consequence of systemic steroid use. Two topically used steroids, flurometholone and medrysone, have a reduced tendency to elevate intraocular pressure, perhaps because of reduced ocular permeability (Fairbairn and Thorson 1971). These drugs are preferred when patients must use steroids over prolonged periods to treat inflammatory conditions of the external eye. Any patients chronically using steroids should have their intraocular pressure monitored at regular intervals.

Other effects of steroids include reduced wound healing and increased susceptibility to infection (Brown, Bloomfield, and Pearce 1974). Patients with soft contact lenses seem especially susceptible to ocular infection when using steroids. It is recommended that soft contact lens wear be discontinued during corticosteroid therapy. If that is not possible, it is essential to monitor the patient closely for the presence of infection, especially fungal or herpes infections.

Systemic corticosteroid use only occasionally has been associated with elevated intraocular pressure. However, prolonged systemic use frequently has been associated with the development of posterior subcapsular cataracts (Oglesby et al. 1961a, 1961b; Sundmark 1966). Interestingly, topical use only rarely has been associated with cataract formation (Burde and Becker 1970; Cronin 1964). The development of corticosteroid-related cataracts is both dose and time dependent. Eleven percent of patients taking less than 10 mg per day of prednisone developed posterior subcapsular cataracts after 1 to 4 years of therapy. In contrast, 80 percent of those taking more than 15 mg per day developed cataracts (Oglesby et al. 1961a, 1961b). The cataracts occasionally worsen even if therapy is stopped.

Another group of drugs that would be expected to induce a higher incidence of ocular side effects in an older than in a younger population are the cardiovascular drugs. Fortunately, most reported side effects are transitory and insignificant. One effect—lowering of intraocular pressure—might even be beneficial in some cases. Reduced intraocular pressure is a common side effect with cardiovascular drugs, for example, with methyldopa, guanethedine, reserpine, digitalis, and diuretics (Fraunfelder 1976a). The effect is usually very small. It is also possible for a sudden overcontrol of systemic hypertension to reduce ocular perfusion pressure. This could lead to a marked progression of visual field changes in previously controlled glaucoma patients.

Another commonly reported side effect of cardiovascular medications is various types of color vision changes. Drugs producing this effect include amyl nitrite, nitroglycerin, reserpine, hydralazine hydrochloride, pargyline hydrochloride, digitalis glycosides, and diuretics (Fraunfelder 1976a). Of these, only the color vision

changes induced by digitalis are significant, as they may indicate overdosage (Manninen 1974). Patients taking digitalis also may experience scintillating scotomas, which are additional signs of excessive dosage.

The diuretics as well as acetazolamide also may produce corneal drying and contact lens intolerance. They presumably have this effect as a consequence of the water loss they induce. Corneal drying also may become a problem with the systemic use of beta blockers to treat cardiovascular disease (Fraunfelder 1976a). A loss of corneal sensitivity also may occur with systemic use, but this and corneal drying are more likely to be a problem with the topical use of Timolol maleate for the treatment of glaucoma.

Upon its introduction, there was considerable enthusiasm for Timolol because of its apparently low incidence of side effects. However, with increased use, the incidence of side effects also has increased (McMahon, Shaffer, and Hoskins 1979; Wilson, Spaeth, and Poryzees 1980). Unfortunately, its pressure-lowering effects may regress after many months' use. In addition to corneal problems, Timolol also produces a number of systemic effects, including central nervous system effects (depression, weakness, disorientation, and memory loss), cardiovascular problems (bradycardia, arrythmia, heart failure, hypotension, and syncope) and respiratory problems (dyspnea, airway obstruction, and respiratory failure; McMahon, Shaffer, and Hoskins 1979; van Buskirk 1980).

Several other antiglaucoma medications can produce side effects that may become significant if allowed to progress. Epinephrine, for example, causes maculopathy when used topically in treating aphakics for glaucoma. Visual loss is reversible if detected early, although recovery may require up to 6 months (Havener 1978). However, if undetected, permanent visual loss can occur. Thus, it is critical for those fitting aphakic lenses to be aware of this side effect and not discount visual loss as being due to senile macular degeneration or to problems with aphakic lenses (Havener 1978).

Adrenergics may cause the release of iris pigment into the anterior chamber, which may be mistaken for iritis (Aggarwal and Beveridge 1971). This response to adrenergics occurs primarily in older patients and is suggested to be a senile change (Mitsui and Takagi 1961). The use of topical epinephrine—especially old, discolored solutions (Krejci and Harrison 1969)—

can produce pigmentary changes in the cornea (Donaldson 1967; Reinecke and Kuwabara 1963) and conjunctiva (Corwin and Spencer 1963). On more than one occasion this has resulted in enucleation because the pigment was mistaken for a malignant melanoma (Ferry and Zimmerman 1964; McCarthy and LeBlanc 1976).

Miotics used in glaucoma therapy also produce ocular or visual changes. All miotics reduce the amount of light reaching the retina, which may decrease visual acuity, especially at night. This can produce spurious results when visual fields are tested, because the reduced intensity of the test object will decrease the apparent size of the isopters in the visual fields. The practitioner may be led to think that glaucomatous field losses have progressed and discourage cataract extraction. Therefore, it is recommended that visual field tests be repeated soon after the initiation of miotic therapy to establish a baseline field assessment under miosis (Havener 1978).

Evidence also seems conclusive that anticholinesterases used in glaucoma therapy induce cataracts (Axelsson and Holmberg 1966; deRoetth 1966; Shaffer and Hetherington 1966). These are seen as anterior vacuoles that may increase even if treatment is discontinued. In one study, this type of vacuolization was found in 51 percent of anticholinesterase-treated eyes as compared with 16 percent of pilocarpine-treated eyes and 15 percent of nonglaucomatous eyes (Shaffer and Hetherington 1966). These drugs are nonetheless valuable in recalcitrant cases and certainly in aphakics.

Finally, analgesics, a type of drug commonly used by the elderly, are worthy of mention not because of their side effects, but because of the frequency of their use. Side effects rarely have been reported following aspirin use, but they include allergic conjunctivitis, retinal hemorrhages, edema, and toxic amblyopia (Fraunfelder 1976a). The rarity of the reports makes it difficult to implicate aspirin definitively as the causative agent. Ocular side effects are more likely to occur and tend to be more serious with less commonly used analgesics; phenylbutazone, for example, produces considerable toxicity in as many as 30 percent of those under treatment (Fraunfelder 1976a). Visual disturbances also are reported frequently in persons taking ibuprofin (Motrin; Fraunfelder 1976a). These analgesics are much less commonly used, yet much more likely to produce significant ocular side effects, than is aspirin. Cotlier and Sharma

(1981) suggested that aspirin has a beneficial effect in the eye; their study found that the incidence of lens opacities was reduced in persons consuming large amounts of aspirin. This study was preliminary and should be viewed with considerable skepticism until more definitive studies have been performed.

References

Aggarwal, J. L., and B. Beveridge. "Liberation of Iris Pigment in the Anterior Chamber after Instillation of 10 Percent Phenylephrine Hydrochloride Solution." *British Journal of Ophthalmology* 55 (1971): 544–549.

Anderson, D. R. "Corneal Indentation to Relieve Acute Angle-Closure Glaucoma," *American Journal of Ophthalmology* 88 (1979): 1091–1093.

Armaly, M. F. "Effect of Corticosteroids on Intraocular Pressure." *Archives of Ophthalmology* 70 (1963): 482–491.

Axelsson, U. and A. Holmberg. "The Frequency of Cataract after Miotic Therapy." *Acta Ophtalmologica* 44 (1966): 421–429.

Becker, B.; T. Gage.; A. E. Kolker; and A. J. Gay. "The Effect of Phenylephrine Hydrochloride on the Miotic-Treated Eye." *American Journal of Ophthalmology* 48 (1959): 313–321.

Becker, B., and K. A. Hahn. "Topical Corticosteroids and Heredity in Primary Open Angle Glaucoma." *American Journal of Ophthalmology* 57 (1964): 543–551.

Borthe, A., and M. Davanger. "Mydriatics and Age." *Acta Ophthalmologica* 49 (1971): 380–387.

Brown, M. M.; G. C. Brown; and G. L. Spaeth. "Lack of Side Effects from Topically Administered 10% Phenylephrine Eyedrops." *Archives of Ophthalmology* 98 (1980): 487–489.

Brown, S. I.; S. Bloomfield; and D. B. Pearce. "Infections with the Therapeutic Soft Lens." *Archives of Ophthalmology* 91 (1974): 275–280.

Burde, R. M., and B. Becker. "Corticosteroid-Induced Glaucoma and Cataracts in Contact Lens Wearers." *Journal of the American Medical Association* 213 (1970): 2075–2077.

Christensen, R. E., and I. Pearce. "Homatropine Hydrobromide." *Archives of Ophthalmology* 70 (1963): 376–380.

Corwin, M. E., and W. H. Spencer. "Conjunctival Melanin Deposits." *Archives of Ophthalmology* 69 (1963): 317–321.

Cotlier, E., and Y. R. Sharma. "Aspirin and Senile Cataracts in Rheumatoid Arthritis." *Lancet* 1, no. 8215, (1981): 338–339.

Cronin, T. P. "Cataract with Topical Use of Corticosteroid and Idoxuridine." *Archives of Ophthalmology* 72 (1964): 198–199.

deRoetth, A., Jr. "Lens Opacities in Glaucoma Patients on Phospholine Iodide Therapy." *American Journal of Ophthalmology* 62 (1966): 619–628.

Donaldson, D. "Epinephrine Pigmentation of the Cornea." *Archives of Ophthalmology* 78 (1967): 74–75.

Fairbairn, W. D., and J. C. Thorson. "Fluorometholone: Antiinflammation and Intraocular Pressure Effects." *Archives of Ophthalmology* 86 (1971): 138–141.

Ferry, A. P., and L. E. Zimmerman. "Black Cornea: A Complication of Topical Use of Epinephrine." *American Journal of Ophthalmology* 58 (1964): 205–210.

Fraunfelder, F. T. *Drug-Induced Ocular Side Effects and Drug Interactions.* Philadelphia: Lea and Febiger, 1976. (a)

Fraunfelder, F. T. "Extraocular Fluid Dynamics: How Best to Apply Topical Ocular Medication." *Transactions of the American Ophthalmological Society* 74 (1976): 457–487. (b)

Fraunfelder, F. T., and F. A. Scafidi. "Possible Adverse Effects from Topical Ocular 10% Phenylephrine." *American Journal of Ophthalmology* 85 (1978): 447–453.

Gartner, S., and E. Billet. "Mydriatic Glaucoma," *American Journal of Ophthalmology* 43 (1957): 975–976.

Gilbard, J. P.; R. L. Ferris; and J. Santamaria. "Osmolarity of Tear Microvolumes in Keratoconjunctivitis Sicca." *American Journal of Ophthalmology* 96 (1978): 677–691.

Goodman, L. S., and A. Gilman. *The Pharmacological Basis of Therapeutics.* New York: Macmillan, 1980.

Harris, L. S. "Cycloplegic-Induced Intraocular Pressure Elevations: A Study of Normal and Open-Angle Glaucomatous Eyes." *Archives of Ophthalmology* 79 (1968): 243–246.

Havener, W. T. *Ocular Pharmacology.* St. Louis: Mosby, 1978.

Henderson, J. W., and W. A. Prough. "Influence of Age and Sex on Flow of Tears." *Archives of Ophthalmology* 43 (1950): 224–231.

Kim, J. M.; C. E. Stevenson; and H. S. Mathewson. "Hypertensive Reactions to Phenylephrine Eyedrops in Patients with Sympathetic Denervation." *American Journal of Ophthalmology* 85 (1978): 862–868.

Korczyn, A. D.; N. Laor; P. Nemet. "Sympathetic Pupillary Tone in Old Age." *Archives of Ophthalmology* 94 (1976): 1905–1906.

Krejci, L., and R. Harrison. "Corneal Pigment Deposits from Topically Administered Epinephrine." *Archives of Ophthalmology* 82 (1969): 836–839.

Lee, P. "Influence of Epinephrine and Phenylephrine on Intraocular Pressure." *Archives of Ophthalmology* 60 (1958): 863–867.

Lowe, R. F. "Angle Closure, Pupil Dilation and Pupil Block." *British Journal of Ophthalmology* 50 (1966): 385–389.

McCarthy, R. W., and R. LeBlanc. "A Black Cornea Secondary to Topical Epinephrine." *Canadian Journal of Ophthalmology* 11 (1976): 336–340.

McMahon, C. D.; R. N. Shaffer and H. D. Hoskins, Jr. "Adverse Effects Experienced by Patients Taking Timolol." *American Journal of Ophthalmology* 88 (1979): 736–738.

Manninen, V. "Impaired Color Vision in Diagnosis of Digitalis Intoxication." *British Medical Journal* 4 (1974): 653–654.

Mapstone, R. "Precipitation of Angle Closure." *British Journal of Ophthalmology* 58 (1974): 46–54.

Meyers, H. "Clinical and Theoretical Considerations of a Patient with Narrow Angles and Shallow Anterior Chambers." *Journal of the American Optometric Association* 47 (1976): 723–728.

Mitsui, Y. and Y. Takagi. "Nature of Aqueous Floaters Due to Sympathomimetic Mydriatics." *Archives of Ophthalmology* 65 (1961): 626–631.

Oglesby, R.; R. Black; L. von Sallmann; and J. Bunim. "Cataracts in Rheumatoid Arthritis Patients Treated with Corticosteroids." *Archives of Ophthalmology* 66 (1961): 519–523. (a)

Oglesby, R.; R. Black; L. von Sallmann; and J. Bunim. "Cataracts in Patients with Rheumatoid Arthritis Treated with Corticosteroids." *Archives of Ophthalmology* 66 (1961): 625–630. (b)

Reinecke, R. D., and T. Kuwabara. "Corneal Deposits Secondary to Topical Epinephrine." *Archives of Ophthalmology* 70 (1963): 170–172.

Salminen, L.; H. Aaltonen; and V. Jantti. "Mydriatic Effect of Low Dose Phenylephrine." *Ophthalmic Research* 12 (1980): 235–239.

Shaffer, R. N., and J. Hetherington, Jr. "Anticholinesterase Drugs and Cataracts." *American Journal of Ophthalmology* 62 (1966): 613–618.

Sundmark, E. "The Cataract-Inducing Effect of Systemic Corticosteroid Therapy." *Acta Ophthalmologica* 44 (1966): 291–297.

van Buskirk, E. M. "Adverse Reactions from Timolol Administration." *Ophthalmology* 87 (1980): 447–450.

Wilson, R. P.; G. L. Spaeth; and E. Poryzees. "The Place of Timolol in the Practice of Ophthalmology." *Ophthalmology* 87 (1980): 451–454.

Chapter 14

The Optometic Examination of the Elderly Patient

Ian L. Bailey

The elderly are a special group within optometry's patient population. Many of their visual characteristics and their varied needs make them different from the younger segments of the clinical population. This chapter will focus on the special considerations commonly required in the provision of vision care for the older patient. It is inevitable that a chapter such as this will be laden with generalizations, since it emphasizes features that may be relatively common in the elderly even though they are by no means universal within, or unique to, this group.

Visual needs are often changed by retirement or by changes in life-style imposed by physical or sensory limitations acquired through aging. Aging brings inevitable changes to the visual system, such as loss of accommodation, reduced transmittance of the ocular media, and pupillary miosis. The visual system also tends to be affected by ocular pathologies, the most notable of which are age-related maculopathy, cataracts, glaucoma, and retinopathies. Changes in visual needs and normal and pathological changes in the visual system create a wide diversity of special clinical problems. The clinician becomes obliged to apply special emphases and techniques, and special optical treatment or other rehabilitative attention often is essential.

It is the diversity of vision needs and characteristics that most distinguishes the elderly from the rest of the patient population. Therefore, when dealing with elderly patients, practitioners must use more imagination and flexibility in structuring the examination and treatment to suit these diverse individual needs.

Case History

The goal of all case history taking is to obtain an understanding of the patient's problems and needs. The case history shapes the sequence and emphasis of examination and assessment procedures, the design of treatment programs, and the presentation of recommendations and advice. The rapport developed in the case history interview can be a most crucial factor in determining the success of any treatment that may follow. The optometrist must develop and display a genuine strong concern for the patient's expressed problems and needs and periodically remind the patient that it is his or her needs that are motivating the investigative procedures and treatment considerations.

The patient's demands should be given some overt attention, but the optometrist should remain conscious of the possibility of an unspoken hidden agenda that might be harbored by either the patient or the optometrist. It can be useful for the clinician to mentally take stock and ask three questions: (1) What does this patient want? (2) What, in my opinion, does this patient need? and (3) What is the real reason for the patient's being here today? These three questions sometimes will give rise to the same answer; especially in the elderly, however, differences in answers can be most important in decision making and presentation.

The case history should begin with the patient's being asked to identify the main visual problem or problems. The optometrist should encourage a full elaboration of the present complaint by asking questions motivated by a genuine curiosity and a desire to fully understand the patient's problem. After the major presenting complaint has been adequately explored, the patient should be asked if there are other problems, and each of these should be pursued in turn. Some elderly patients, especially those who are lonely or have some doubts about their self-worth, may relish being the focus of attention, and the interview might become quite diverted. The clinician should be sensitive and tolerant toward such digressions.

When the patient exhausts the self-generated list of problems, some important topics should be raised, if they have not been covered already. These areas can be divided into four categories:

1. *Distance vision.* Patients should be asked about the adequacy of their distance vision for particular tasks, among which are recognizing faces, watching television or movies, driving, and reading street signs. Reactions to different illumination conditions may be included here.

2. *Near vision.* Reading is typically the most important near vision task. The optometrist should establish whether the patient can satisfactorily read books and magazines, private and business correspondence, and labels and price tags. Other near vision tasks such as handicrafts, maintenance chores, self-grooming tasks, and food preparation also usually warrant attention.

3. *Ocular and general health history.* Current and previous ocular health and general health conditions or treatment should be investigated. The clinician should determine whether the patient is currently taking any medication, and if so, consider any possible side effects. The patient's experience with glasses or other optical aids should be investigated, and any problems or shortcomings of previous optical treatment should be identified. When there has been some loss of vision, the pattern of development of the loss should be established. The patient's perception of the cause, as well as the prognosis of the underlying condition, should be discussed.

4. *Life-style.* With aging, particularly aging accompanied by loss of vision, there may be some major changes in the activities of daily life. The living environment may change; interests, aspirations, and habits may be altered; the capacity for independent travel and independent home management may be curtailed; and dependence on relatives, friends, or rehabilitation personnel may develop. The practitioner should be alert to such changes, as they can significantly influence the needs of the patient.

Aging patients often have special fears and prejudices that require consideration. Most people have some fear of vision loss accompanying their advancing years. This fear becomes heightened when contemporaries suffer vision loss or begin to require attention or treatment for cataracts, maculopathy, or glaucoma. It is not uncommon for older patients to strongly fear impending blindness or serious vision loss, but they rarely admit this fear. The optometrist therefore should be careful to "read between the lines" during the history taking and identify such fears.

Incurring a partial or total vision loss inevitably is an emotionally traumatic experience for the individual concerned. Following the initial shock, a sequence of emotional reactions can involve depression, anxiety, disbelief, grief, denial, and anger. In time, however, the individual's emotional state stabilizes. Optometrists dealing with patients who have a recently acquired loss of vision should be aware of the probability of changing emotional attitudes. The finalization of prescribing decisions often must be delayed until the patient comes to reasonable terms with the visual limitations.

Patients who already have some loss of vision commonly fear that total blindness or substantially worse vision is inevitable. The practitioner should encourage the patient to discuss these fears. Often associated with the fear of blindness is a concern that some abuse of the eyes in the past will soon produce dreaded injurious consequences. Excessive reading, excessive fine work, poor illumination, wearing glasses, failure to wear glasses, wearing the wrong glasses, sitting too close to the television, using fluorescent lamps, or watching color television all can be believed to ruin vision, and such beliefs are most well developed in the elderly. Patients with these concerns should be given appropriate advice and reassurance. Patients who have already suffered some vision loss are particularly likely to be influenced by erroneous but commonly held beliefs that may lead them to expect a dismal visual future. Furthermore, a low-vision patient may proudly claim great virtue and restraint because he or she does not sit too close to the television, does not read any more than is essential, and does not use strong light, when in fact the avoided behaviors pose no threat to remaining vision and could provide the means for a broader and more enjoyable range of activities. Thus, optometrists should take special care to counsel their elderly patients about their future eye care needs and the prognosis for changes in their vision to insure that they really understand the status of their own vision.

With retirement, interests and priorities often change. Especially if there is some age-related disability, elderly people often curtail their social, vocational, and recreational activities. Withdrawal from social and other pleasurable activities can be passive and unconscious. It is important for the optometrist to understand the patient's range of daily visual activities. When there has been some vision loss, the extent to which the vision loss is restricting current activities or aspirations should be determined. A most useful approach is to ask patients to describe their typical daily activities. Ask what they do from the time they get out of bed in the morning until they retire at night. Such questioning often reveals the range of visual demands and, when there is restricted vision, often indicates the extent to which people are modifying their lives because of vision difficulties. The frustration and regret associated with a vision loss is often revealed by the question, What things could you do when you had good vision that you cannot do now?

In bringing the introductory interview to a close, the careful optometrist will summarize the priorities for the examination process that is to follow: "So, if I understand things correctly, the most important thing for us to concentrate on is your reading, especially for those bank statements. And we should thoroughly check the health of your eyes. Is this right?"

It can be reassuring to remind the patient that mutually agreed upon goals have been established and that these goals motivate all the examination procedures. Advising the patient of the purpose of various tests and relating them to the patient's symptoms emphasizes the clinician's concern and develops a stronger spirit of participation in the patient.

Ocular Health Examination

A thorough inspection of the external and internal aspects of the eyes using appropriate instrumentation is especially important in elderly patients. Statistically, they are much more likely to have significant ocular pathological conditions or ocular signs of general health disorders.

The inspection of the interior of the eye can become more difficult than usual because of small pupils and lack of media clarity. Unless contraindicated, the pupils should be dilated to facilitate the examination. If pupillary dilation is to be used, however, it is best to postpone the instillation of the mydriatic and the full ocular inspection until after the visual capacity has been tested. When ophthalmoscopy remains difficult, easier observation is possible using small-diameter illumination beams, observing from as close as possible, and perhaps reducing the illumination level. The examination of the eyelid, conjunctiva, cornea, anterior chamber, and iris requires special attention in elderly patients because of the relatively high prevalence of aging changes affecting these tissues.

During the examination of the eyes, the optometrist should explain what is being done. Older patients are almost invariably aware of cataracts and glaucoma, and they should be reminded that these and other ocular diseases are being given close consideration. They should be fully and clearly advised of the state of their own ocular health. This not only is part of the clinician's basic responsibility, but also reinforces the message that regular eye examinations are most important to older individuals. The details of discussions about ocular disease will vary according to the patient, the examiner, and their previous interactions. Even though the examiner can grow tired of giving essentially the same routine explanations to patient after patient, this responsibility should not be neglected or conveniently curtailed.

Refraction

Objective Refraction

Retinoscopy can be more difficult on older patients because of small pupils and media irregularities and opacities. However, it remains an important technique, and the examiner should make every effort to obtain a retinoscopic estimate of refractive error. When retinoscopy becomes unusually difficult, however, the clinician should be prepared to vary technique. Moving to closer-than-usual observation distances or moving off axis may provide an "easier" retinoscopic reflex; Mehr and Freid (1975) describe this as *radical retinoscopy*. Of course, closer working distances demand a change in the power allowance for working distance. Furthermore, moving off axis may produce some inaccuracy in both the spherical and astigmatic components, so this procedure is used only when axial viewing does not provide an adequate reflex.

When there is substantial lenticular irregularity in spoke patterns, it may be impossible to obtain consistent or accurate results, because the apparent movement of the reflected light seems to be fragmented (moving in different directions or at different speeds). In these circumstances, a spot retinoscope may prove to be more useful than a streak retinoscope.

Objective optometers depend on light being reflected from the retina. Again, the small pupils and media opacities commonly found in older patients often cause less reliable results. Sometimes no result at all can be obtained.

Keratometry to estimate total astigmatism becomes more important when retinoscopy or objective optometer measurement fails. A record of corneal curvature is useful in quantifying any future changes.

Patients with low vision are often unable to make accurate judgments in subjective refraction procedures. Thus, it may be necessary to rely more than usual on objective refraction results.

Subjective Refraction

Subjective refraction often requires more time with older patients than younger ones. Their sensitivity to blur may be reduced because of small pupils or because of media or retinal changes that affect visual discrimination. It becomes difficult for them to judge changes of image clarity in response to small refractive changes. Slower presentation of alternatives and sometimes repeated presentations can become necessary. However, older patients, lacking accommodation, do have a stable refractive state, which enhances the reliability of refractive error measurement.

When visual acuity is expected to be normal or near normal, a phoropter and the usual range of refractive techniques may be employed. The bichrome (or duochrome) test, which is sometimes unreliable in younger patients, can be a more reliable test in older individuals. Again, small pupils make it difficult for the patient to discriminate the relative clarity of the red and green targets. Lenticular changes may cause the brightness of the green background to be reduced more than the red. It should be emphasized that clarity of the letters is the criterion rather than the brightness of the red or green background.

When the observation distance is 4 m or closer, an appropriate dioptric allowance (obtained by reducing the refractive correction by +0.25D for a 4-m distance) should be made if clearest distance vision is being sought. With older patients the binocular balancing of the spherical refraction becomes easy because of the stability of the accommodative state. Standard binocular balancing techniques may be used.

Astigmatism may be determined using crossed-cylinder techniques; the clock dial or related techniques also may be used. In the presence of media irregularities, however, the crossed-cylinder method is preferred. Clock dial, sunburst, paraboline, Humphrey, and similar techniques involving judgment of the clarity of lines in particular orientations all can produce anomalous results when there are refractive irregularities in the media. Similarly, the stenopaic slit method for determining astigmatism is contraindicated for patients with lens or corneal irregularities.

Refraction of Patients with Low Vision

Patients with low vision often require different refraction techniques. The phoropter should not be used. Patients should be free to move their heads and eyes to any preferred positions; they should not be artificially shielded from the ambient illumination; their eye movements and eye position should be observable by the clinician; and they should be aware that improvements achieved are due to simple lenses rather than the magic box that the phoropter might represent.

Trial lenses supported either in trial frames or in lens clips attached to the patient's current glasses should be used. However, trial frames tend to be clumsy, requiring repeated readjustment and repositioning. Furthermore, the vertex distance they provide is often larger than the eventual spectacle-lens vertex distance. These factors all become more bothersome when the refractive error is large. In general, therefore, trial lens clips (Halberg, Bernell, Jannelli, or Bommarito clips) that attach to existing glasses are easier to use. With trial lens clips used over the patient's current glasses, the frame usually sits securely, the lenses have a more appropriate vertex distance and pantoscopic tilt, and this together enables a more accurate determination of the required refractive correction.

Working over the current glasses, the optometrist typically has to use only relatively low-powered lenses. This is useful, as low-powered lenses are easier to insert and remove from trial lens mountings and are usually available in finer steps of power.

Astigmatism usually can be measured more accurately when trial lens clips are being used. For either retinoscopic or subjective determination of astigmatism, the clinician at first should completely ignore any astigmatic correction that may be in the old glasses. The astigmatic component of the over-refraction is determined as though it were completely independent. There is no need for the axis and power of the overcorrecting cylinder to bear any relationship to the cylinder present in the glasses over which the refraction is being performed.

When the overrefraction has been completed, the glasses—with lens clips and trial lenses still attached—are taken to a focimeter, and the back vertex power of the combination is measured. This gives the total power required to optimally correct the refractive error. For example, a patient may be wearing a correction of 0.00DS ∽ − 4.50 DC × 35, and the over-refraction in the trial lens clips may be +0.75DS ∽ − 1.25DC × 160. The examiner could do laborious calculations to determine the resultant power, but it is far simpler to measure the back vertex power of the combination with the focimeter. The resultant power will be found to be 0.00DS ∽ − 4.25DC × 27. This method is particularly valuable when the lens power is large.

In any new glasses, the pantoscopic tilt of the lenses and the vertical positioning of the optical centers probably will be quite similar to those in the existing glasses. Any power errors that may have resulted from the aberrational effects created by tilt and position of the lens will be compensated for by the overrefraction, and a more appropriate refractive correction determination will be obtained.

Patients with low vision are often less sensitive to refractive changes. In general, the poorer the acuity, the poorer the sensitivity to change. However, this is far from being a universal rule. Sometimes patients with visual acuities of 20/500 will be able to respond reliably to 0.50D of change, and patients with 20/60 acuity may not be able to respond to 1.50 or 2.00D of change. It is best for the clinician to begin the refraction with an open mind and wait for the patient's responses to reveal individual sensitivity to blur.

Refracting a low-vision patient begins with directing the patient's attention to visual acuity chart letters at (or close to) the patient's limit of resolution. Initially, the steps of dioptric power should be large enough to allow the patient to recognize changes in clarity easily.

Holding a plus lens in one hand and a minus lens of equal power in the other (say, +6.00 and −6.00D), the optometrist may ask the patient to make judgments involving 6.00 of change (+6.00D to plano or −6.00D). When using hand-held lenses, it is often advisable to fabricate the plano presentation by holding lenses of equal and opposite power together rather than using no lens at all. Some patients have already decided whether or not they want a change of correction, and this can influence their response to "with" to "without" comparisons.

Once the patient can make confident responses to dioptric changes, the size of the changes should be systematically reduced in the process of pursuing the refractive error. When large steps of dioptric power are being used, the clinician may be guided by the strength of the patient's response. This may be revealed by the patient's choice of words, tone of voice, or quickness of response. For example, upon the introduction of a +6.00D lens, the patient might respond, "That's blurry." Upon switching to the −6.00D lens, the patient says, "That's much worse." To a plano presentation (+6.00D with −6.00D), the patient responds, "That's better," and upon returning to the +6.00 lens, the patient says, "That's a little blurry again." From this sequence, the examiner has learned that plus is strongly preferred to minus and that there is a consistent but mild preference for 0.00 over +6.00D. It appears the refractive error is positive—closer to 0.00 than +6.00, but not very close to 0.00D, since there was such a strong difference between +6.00 and −6.00D. At this stage, a reasonable guess at the spherical refraction error would be in the range of +1.50 to +2.25D. It can also be argued that the patient can discriminate dioptric changes of at least ±3.00D.

The spherical refraction process continues making use of bracketing, going from an excess of plus to an excess of minus. It is finalized when changing from plus to minus in the finest discriminable step elicits a response indicating that both presentations appear slightly but equally blurred.

On completing the spherical power determination, the optometrist can begin the astigmatic determination with some knowledge of the patient's responsiveness to refractive blur. This knowledge can guide the practitioner in choosing the power of the Jackson cross-cylinder that is to be used. In a general optometric office, ±0.25 and a ±0.75D hand-held cross-cylinder should be available. The lower-power cross-cylinder is useful for normal patients, and the ±0.75D cross-cylinder will be strong enough for the majority of low-vision patients with poorer discrimination. The test target observed during the Jackson cross-cylinder refraction is usually a selected letter or letters on the Snellen chart at or close to the limit of the patient's acuity. Remember that the flip cross-cylinder test works best when the spherical equivalence of the test lens combinations is kept constant.

After the astigmatism has been measured, it is prudent to check the spherical component. If any significant change is necessary, the power of the cylindrical correction should be rechecked.

Visual Acuity Measurement

Visual acuity measurement requires a little more care in elderly patients than in younger ones. Older patients are more affected by test illumination and the distribution of light within the luminous environment. Thus, more care than usual should be taken to insure that the chart illumination is at a standard level (80 to 320 candelas per square meter) and that troublesome glare sources are eliminated from the field of view. Illumination conditions may need to be changed while visual acuity is being measured. Because older patients are more likely to acquire changes in their vision, for reference purposes it is important that the best practical measure of visual acuity be made.

When visual acuity is reduced, nonstandard techniques become necessary. Projector charts, which are suitable for the measurement of normal visual acuity, should not be used for low-vision patients. Most do not provide the contrast or adjustability in range of luminance that is available with printed cardboard or transilluminated charts. Also, projector charts lack flexibility to extend the range in order to measure poorer acuities. In contrast, with printed charts it is usually easy to alter the observation distance over a wide range.

For all visual acuity measurement, it is wise to record acuity by giving partial credit for rows that were only partially read correctly (20/20 − 2, or 20/15 + 1, and so forth). Optometrists who do not always use the same chart should always make note of the chart that was used.

Visual Acuity Measurement in Low-Vision Patients

Chart design can influence the visual acuity score, and this can become most important when there is disturbed macular function. The number of letters per row and the relative spacing between letters and between rows can cause substantial variations in visual acuity scores. Many low-vision patients require a reduced observation distance, and the practitioner should be aware that changing observation distances can influence the acuity scores obtained.

First, scaling may change. Many charts have a size sequence of 200, 100, 80, 60, 50, and so forth. At 20 feet an acuity of 20/200 might be recorded, indicating that the patient read the 200-foot symbols but failed to read the 100-foot symbols. On changing to a 10-foot observation distance, it may at first be anticipated that the acuity score will be 10/100. Consistency with the 20-foot measurement only requires that the acuity be at least 10/100, but not as good as 10/50. Thus, the acuity score could be recorded as 10/100, 10/80, or 10/60 and still be consistent with the 20/200 finding. Only when the chart follows a logarithmic (or constant-proportion) size progression can this scaling problem be avoided.

Second, changing to a closer observation distance often alters the nature of the task at threshold. The number of letters per row may increase, or the relative spacing between optotypes may change. With macular dysfunction, contour interaction becomes much more important than usual, and increasing the number of letters per row or reducing spacing can significantly reduce the acuity that can be achieved. A patient who reads a single 20/200 letter with ease might not be able to read any of three closely spaced letters on a 100-foot row when the viewing distance has been changed to 10 feet.

Visual acuity scores will be more valid and more impervious to change with changing observation distance if the task is made essentially the same at each size level. This requires that almost equally legible symbols be used, that there be the same number of symbols in each row, that the spacing between symbols and between rows be proportional to symbol size, and that size follow a geometric (or logarithmic or common-multiplier) progression. Bailey-Lovie charts and their derivatives follow these principles (Bailey and Lovie 1976; Ferris et al. 1982).

Bailey-Lovie charts were designed to avoid problems encountered in low-vision work. Their size range extends from 200- to 15-foot symbols. With the chart as close as two feet, acuities of 2/200 (equivalent to 20/2000) may be measured. The Feinbloom Visual Acuity Chart is a popular chart designed for low-vision work. The size progression is irregular, and there is wide variation in spacing and in the number of symbols at the different size levels. Nevertheless, the Feinbloom chart does have attractive features: the size range extends to 700-foot symbols, symbol size progresses in relatively small (albeit irregular) steps, and the page-turning mode of presentation can be psychologically encouraging to patients who have become accustomed to reading very few letters correctly when tested on more common charts. The Feinbloom chart also uses numbers rather than letters. Although these numbers may not be uniformly legible, they can be useful to patients who are not familiar or facile with the English alphabet.

Low-vision patients may have their visual acuity significantly altered by relatively minor changes in illumination. Thus, recommended procedure is to make the first measurement of acuity at the standard or customary illumination level. Then, referring the patient to the smallest letters that can be read, ask if there is any change when illumination is increased or decreased. When externally illuminated cardboard charts are being used, the illuminance may be controlled by moving the luminaire closer to the chart or by turning off other room lighting and moving the luminaire away from the chart or shielding it in some convenient manner.

When there is macular dysfunction, it can be informative to note the manner in which the patient reads the chart. Many patients perform much better when reading letters at the start or the end of rows and perform poorly when attempting to read more central letters. This usually indicates problems from central scotomas and may lead the clinician to expect some limitation of the patient's potential to read efficiently. When there is evidence or suspicion of macular disturbance, it can be useful to direct the patient to fixate above, below, to the right of, or to the left of a row of letters that has been found to be difficult. Any reported changes in visibility can indicate whether eccentric viewing strategies may facilitate reading the chart.

Assessment of Near Vision

Some aspects of the near vision assessment become much easier with elderly patients. Because these patients lack accommodation, their working distance becomes highly predictable from the power of the addition being used. The range of clear near vision depends on pupil diameter and the size of the test target detail. With newsprint or something similar as the target, the range of clear vision is often measured to be about 1.00D. With charts having a size range that goes smaller than the patient's resolution limit, and provided the patient always looks at the smallest print that can just be read, the range of clearest vision is often found to be reduced to about 0.25D.

For patients with normal distance visual acuity, an equivalent near vision performance usually will be achieved. On rare occasions, near visual acuity may be significantly worse if there are central lenticular opacities that have a more harmful effect on vision when the pupil constricts in response to viewing near objects. Even more rarely, acuity can improve at near distances because of peripheral opacities' being rendered less important by pupillary constriction.

The quantity and quality of illumination should be optimized, and elderly patients generally should be given advice on how to arrange their lighting for prolonged near visual tasks. An adjustable lamp with an incandescent (60- or 100-watt) bulb provides an almost universally useful means of controlling the task illumination. The task illuminance can be increased by moving the lamp closer to the material, and the bulb or bright spots from the reflector of the lamp should not be directly visible to the patient.

The most appropriate near vision addition can be determined in various ways, but it is the desired viewing distance that dominates the decision for the typical elderly patient. A variety of methods may be used to determine the power of the addition; the range of clear vision, biochrome, or cross-cylinder at near techniques all can work satisfactorily on older patients. After the clinician has determined the power of the required addition while using test charts at the desired working distance, performance should be tested using magazines, newspapers, bank statements, or whatever, represents the patient's most common or most important near vision tasks.

Given a particular visual acuity, the size of resolvable detail is determined by the working distance. If patients request clearer vision than they obtain with their present glasses even though the present glasses are in correct focus for the desired working distance, the clinician must increase the addition, thereby simultaneously reducing the working distance. More exotic optical devices also can be considered.

If a change in the power of the addition is to be considered, the clinician should be conscious of the magnitude of resolution improvement that can be expected. Almost all distance visual acuity charts use a size progression ratio of about 5:4 in the region of 20/20 (50, 40, 30, 25, 20, 15). Changing viewing distance by a 5:4 ratio (50 cm to 40 cm, 40 cm to 32 cm, and so forth) should proportionally increase resolution capacity equivalent to one line of improvement. Since dioptric power is inversely proportional to viewing distance, the addition must be increased by a ratio of 5:4 to achieve improvements that may be thought of as "one line." Thus, 1.50, 2.00, 2.50, 3.25, 4.00, and 5.00D is a series of lens powers in which each step represents about one line of acuity improvement. Note the close similarity between the numbers in this sequence and the size progression in the 20/20 region of the distance visual acuity chart. With this sequence as a reference, the clinician can deduce that a patient with a +2.50D addition will get only a marginal improvement (one-third of a line) by having the addition increased to +2.75D. A +3.25D addition is required to provide a resolution improvement that could be described as "one full line."

Optometrists usually measure and record the near visual acuity. The near visual acuity record should specify both the observation distance and the size of the smallest print that may be read. It is preferable to specify print size in M units or points. M units express the distance in meters at which the lowercase letters subtend 5 minutes of arc. Points indicate print size according to the units used by printers and typesetters. It is common (albeit inappropriate) to express print size as a reduced Snellen equivalent, a fraction that expresses the equivalent distance visual acuity required to read that particular print when it is viewed from 40 cm. This method becomes clearly inappropriate when the viewing distance is other than 40 cm. It is confusing and inaccurate to record *20/20 at 30 cm,* since this expression, as it is most commonly used, is intended to indicate that the visual acuity is in fact less than equivalent to 20/20.

Print that is truly equivalent to 20/20 at 40 cm can be said to be 0.40 M units in size. Using the M unit notation, near visual acuity can be expressed as a true Snellen fraction. Print that is 0.40 M (20/20 at 40 cm) viewed at 40 cm would demand an acuity of 0.40/0.40 M; if the same print were just legible at 30 cm, the acuity would be 0.30/0.40 M. The M unit system is far more appropriate and more consistent with the methods traditionally used to measure distance visual acuity. Fortunately, the Jaeger system is becoming less commonly used, as its lack of standardization is becoming well known.

In patients with normal or near-normal vision there is usually fairly close concordance between the near and distance visual acuities. The visual task for the near visual acuity measurement usually involves reading typeset print, which is more complex than reading the fairly widely spaced letters found on the distance visual acuity charts. Such differences in complexity do not have much influence on acuity scores in the normally sighted. In patients with disturbed macular function, however, task complexity can cause major inconsistencies in acuity scores. It is quite common for patients with macular degeneration to have a near or reading acuity score that is twofold or worse than the distance letter chart acuity.

Near visual acuity measurements with reading charts often serve as a basis for determining the magnification that a low-vision patient might require to satisfactorily perform a complex task at near. Distance visual acuity measurements taken with letter charts are much less reliable for this purpose.

Many satisfactory reading charts are available for testing normally sighted patients. Reading charts with larger size ranges and more systematic design features have been designed by Bailey and Lovie (1980), Keeler (1956), and Sloan (1959).

Assessment of Binocular Vision

As patients grow older, they are more likely to develop some occular motor difficulties because of changes affecting the neuromuscular mechanisms and the structural tissues around the eyes. In examining binocular coordination, care should be taken to observe the version movements of the eyes as they move in the six cardinal eye-movement directions (right, left, up and right, down and right, up and left, and down and left). A relative lagging of one eye indicates an oculomotor dysfunction that warrants a more detailed evaluation of the noncomitancy.

The cover test should be carefully and routinely performed at distance and near for older patients. Older patients lack accommodation and have no stimulus to accommodative convergence; thus, they show more exophoria at near. Vertical deviations are also more common in the elderly. Phorias or tropias should be measured at both distance and near using loose prisms. When large near exophoria is found, the strength of the fusional vergence mechanism can be judged by the facility and speed with which the patient makes vergence eye movements to obtain fusion when a base-out prism (say, $10\triangle$ diopters) is introduced before one eye. Poor fusion responses tend to indicate a need for prescribing prisms.

Although it is common practice to measure the near phoria with the test target close to eye level, it is more appropriate to have the target lower so that downgaze is required. This is more representative of the habitual reading eye posture, particularly if the patient holds or touches the near fixation target.

A variety of subjective tests are available for measuring heterophoria in younger patients, and these often provide different measures of the heterophoria. However, there is more consistency in the older patients because of their lack of accommodation, so the choice of method used to measure heterophoria becomes less important.

When there is a potentially significant heterophoria, the optometrist must decide if prism is to be prescribed, and if so, how much. There are many reasonable approaches to these decisions (see Chapter 21). Fixation disparity, rules involving fusional reserves, and rules based on phoria magnitude can all be useful in indicating how much prism should be prescribed. It can be prudent to check the advantage obtained from the prism by introducing the prism of the indicated power and orientation and asking the patient to report on the clarity or ease of vision while observing fine print. The prism is then removed and reintroduced after a pause, but with the base direction changed 180 degrees. If a patient with exophoria does not prefer base-in to base-out prisms, judged by changes in clarity or by relative difficulty in adapting to the change, the decision to prescribe prisms should be carefully reconsidered. With vertical prism, the prism power magnitudes are usually smaller, and it may be more convenient to make this kind

of change by keeping the prism in the same orientation but transferring it to the other eye, changing from 2 BUR to 2 BUL and so on.

Anisometropia creates special problems, especially relating to vertical phorias. Younger anisometropes can tilt their heads forward or back as needed to achieve viewing through the optical centers of the lenses and thus avoid differential prismatic effects. Older patients wearing bifocals must move their eyes in downgaze to view through the bifocal segment when they read.

When patients are already wearing a bifocal correction for anisometropia, decision making is easier. Unless there has been a substantial change in refractive error, the patient's need for vertical prismatic correction can be tested at distance and at near using methods such as those already described using the patient's old glasses. Patients with anisometropia often exhibit significant vertical heterophoria at near, but they will lack symptoms and will not show any strong preference for having the correcting prism in place. Each case should be considered individually. When the anisometropia is newly acquired—perhaps because of a myopic shift in one eye—symptoms and adaptation difficulties are more likely. Some practitioners prefer to prescribe some overall vertical prism to minimize such vertical phoria problems at near. Others choose to prescribe bifocals with no special prism compensation but may warn the patient of possible symptoms and adaptation difficulties; this strategy avoids prescribing special prism until it has been demonstrated that the patient has failed to adapt.

The remedies for the bifocal problems in anisometropia problems are to use slab-off or other prism-controlled bifocals, executive bifocals where there is no prism present at the dividing line, Franklin split-lens bifocals, or assymetrical bifocal segments (Ultex in one eye and flat-top in the other); or to revert to separate distance and reading glasses. Fresnel press-on prism can be cut so they are confined to the bifocal segment region. Although they are not often used as a permanent solution, they can be useful in investigating the potential value of a prismatic correction in the bifocal segments.

Several tests can determine whether a patient truly does have binocular vision in a particular situation. Good stereo-acuity, the ability to see both monocular targets on a fixation disparity test, and fusion with the Worth four-dot test are acceptable standard criteria. The simple bar-reading test is sometimes overlooked; holding a pen midway between the eyes and the page of print should not obscure any print if simultaneous binocular vision is present.

Visual Field Measurement

Visual field losses are more common in elderly patients than in younger ones. Field defects may come from chorioretinal pathology, glaucoma, optic atrophies, and intracranial disorders. When measuring visual fields, the clinician should be conscious of the purpose of conducting the test:

1. Is it to screen for otherwise unsuspected pathological conditions?
2. Is it to seek evidence that will confirm the presence of an already suspected pathological condition?
3. Is it to monitor the progress of a previously identified field defect?
4. Is it to evaluate the impact that the field loss already known to be present will have on the person's ability to function?

The test parameters (target size and luminance, as well as background luminance) and strategies for presentation will vary accordingly. See Anderson (1982) and Bedwell (1982) in the Suggested Readings list at the end of this Chapter for more information on visual fields testing.

For screening, test spots should be just comfortably detectable, and a systematic broad search should be made of the whole visual field. For confirming tentative diagnoses, the test targets should be just detectable—and only just detectable—in the region where the field defect is most likely to occur. The test target presentations should be largely confined to this region of the visual field, and the motion of dynamic targets should be such that the direction is at right angles to the probable border of the scotoma.

To monitor the progression of visual field defects, the stimulus condition must be as similar as possible to those used previously. Again, any target motion should be orthogonal to the known border of the scotoma.

For functional evaluation of the visual fields, binocular observation should be permitted. Relatively easy to see targets should be used.

Automatic or semiautomatic visual field screeners have become more popular over the last decade. These instruments present static targets in a controlled and repeatable manner. In general, they eliminate many of the problems associated with technique and bias that can so easily contaminate the results with the traditional, operator-controlled, dynamic target tests. The automated field screeners are available in tangent screen and bowl perimeter form. Several have been subjected to studies that establish norms and recommend the stimulus variables most suitable for different age groups. The popularity of automated screeners may grow further, but the tangent screen and bowl perimeter will remain very important to clinical practice.

Low-vision patients may have some special problems associated with visual field measurement. Central fixation, which is often a problem, can sometimes be overcome by providing a cross target centered on the fixation point. Elastic cord, masking tape, or even chalk may be used on the tangent screen to provide a cross through the central point. The patient is instructed to look toward the center of the cross, even though he or she may not see the actual intersection. Flashing the target can make it easier for the patient to maintain central fixation, because patients are less tempted to move their eyes to check on the presence of the target if it is flashing.

Functional visual field testing is important in low-vision patients. Whenever frank scotomas are found on the tangent screen or bowl perimeter, a much coarser test of functional detection ability should be made using larger and more visible targets. A hand or piece of writing paper used as a target against a black screen can establish whether the scotoma is truly absolute.

The Amsler grid can be a most useful test of central visual function, characterizing disturbances of central vision. Patients may report absences, fading, or distortion in parts of the grid pattern while they maintain fixation on its center. When patients report observable changes, the practitioner may gain insights into the nature of the visual disturbance and perhaps may be better able to predict or understand the patients' functional difficulties. Sometimes a patient will not recognize scotomas, as "filling in" seems to occur. Indeed, the normal physiological blind spot usually cannot be observed on Amsler grid patterns. Visual disturbances reported on the Amsler grid test are useful. When no visual disturbance is observed by the patient, however, no definite conclusion should be made about the presence or absence of scotomas.

Color Vision Testing

The purpose of testing color vision is twofold. First, the identification of color vision anomalies can assist in the diagnosis or detection of pathological changes in the visual system. Second, altered color vision can cause some difficulties with color discrimination tasks, and the possibility of such functional difficulties should be discussed with the patient.

Color vision usually changes as the patient ages because of yellowing of the crystalline lens and physiological and pathological changes in the macular region. Such defects tend to be tritanopic, the most obvious manifestation's being a reduction of discrimination in the blue and blue-green regions of the spectrum.

The test of choice for the routine assessment of color vision in older patients is the Farnsworth Panel D-15 test, in which 15 colored chips are arranged so that they appear to be in order according to chromatic similarity. Patients having normal aging changes affecting their color vision typically make only a few small-magnitude errors of the tritanopic type. When there is retinal pathology, however, the number and magnitude of the errors in arranging the D-15 targets become greater. In cases of substantial retinal pathology, the magnitude of errors in arranging the D-15 test targets becomes large, and the pattern of the errors is more random (see Chapter 10).

Other Tests of Ocular or Visual Function

Tonometry should be performed routinely on older patients because of the higher incidence of raised intraocular pressure and glaucoma.

A variety of tests of visual function can be useful in identifying the presence of ocular pathologies and predicting or explaining functional difficulties resulting from pathological changes. Tests of contrast sensitivity range from acuity testing with low-contrast charts to tests related to the detection of variable-contrast gratings on charts or video display screens. Glare sensitivity, which is more of a problem in the elderly than in younger people, can be tested by measuring reductions in acuity provoked by the presence of a paracentral glare source. Dark adaptation can be measured with sophisticated instrumentation, or functional estimates can be made of the patient's relative ability to detect large objects in very dim illumination. Differential diagnosis of pathological conditions may be facilitated by the use of electroretinograms, electro-oculograms, fluorescein angiography, measurement of responsiveness to flicker, special tests of color vision function, and visually evoked cortical potentials (see Chapter 15).

Prescribing Spectacles for the Normally Sighted

Most older patients require optical correction for both distance and near vision tasks. Driving, watching television and movies, spectating at public events, and referring to distant informational signs make good distance vision important to most individuals. At near, tasks ranging from writing and reading personal and business correspondence; reading labels on foods and medicines; reading price tags; reading directories; and recreational or educational reading of books, newspapers, and magazines are all part of regular daily life for most people. It is clearly desirable for most people to have easy access to clear distance and near vision.

Bifocals, trifocals, or progressive addition lenses are worn by older patients. Small in number are the emmetropes who do not need distance glasses, myopes who do not need vision glasses, and the people who choose to use single vision glasses and change their spectacles whenever they change from distance to near viewing.

In considering trifocals, the starting point is usually the questions, What is the person's range of clear near vision with the most appropriate reading glasses? and Are there important intermediate distance tasks that will not be seen with adequate clarity if simple bifocals are used? Trifocals almost invariably have an intermediate segment that is half the power of the stronger reading segment.

Progressive addition lenses have two benefits. One is that they are cosmetically preferable for people who do not like the appearance of the dividing line of the standard bifocal or trifocal segments. The other benefit is that progressive addition lenses provide a channel of progressively increasing power between the distance viewing point and the near viewing point. In effect, this provides a continuous sequence of focus for all possible intermediate distances. Objects at intermediate distances will be seen clearly when the head and eyes are positioned so that the most appropriate portion of the lens is being used. The patient will experience some diminished clarity and some spatial distortion when viewing through the areas in the lower half of the lens that are outside the channel of progressive power change. Many patients are not bothered by this, whereas others find it annoying and distracting.

The size and position of bifocal or trifocal segments should be chosen to suit the patient's functional needs and particular wishes. The width of the field of clear near vision, prismatic jump, and chromatic effects can influence the recommendations made.

Older patients are more likely to have ametropias of high magnitude. In progressive myopia, the magnitude of refractive error can continue to increase throughout life. Fairly large myopic shifts can occur from changes in the crystalline lens. On the other end of the scale, many older patients become highly hyperopic following cataract extraction.

High refractive errors require special consideration. When performing the refraction, care should be taken to insure that the vertex distance and pantoscopic angle of the lenses being worn are similar to those expected to be present in any new glasses that might be worn in the future.

The position of the optical centers relative to the patient's pupil can become much more significant when lens powers exceed about 8.00 D. The basic principle guiding lens positioning is that the optic axis of the lens should point toward the center of rotation of the eye. Lens designers assume this when they select lens parameters to avoid aberrational effects. The center of rotation is typically about 27 mm behind the spectacle plane.

It follows that pantoscopic tilt of the spectacle plane is a key factor in determining the vertical placement of the optical centers. The greater the pantoscopic angle, the lower the centers. A simple method for measuring pantoscopic tilt is to take a protractor with a plumb line (or a straightened paper clip) attached to its center. The base of this protractor can be held so that it is against or parallel to the spectacle plane. With the patient's head in its natural or habitual posture, the plumb line will indicate the most usual pantoscopic tilt. To compensate for the effects of pantoscopic tilt, the optical centers should be made lower than the center of the pupils by 1 mm for each 2 degrees of pantoscopic tilt. Ten degrees of pantoscopic tilt is quite common, and for this, the height of the optical centers should be 5 mm below to pupil center, which is about level with the corneal limbus. The

correctness of the optical alignment can be verified by having the patient tilt his or her head back while fixating a bright light at an appropriate distance. The optometrist, with the eye close to the light, should observe the reflex from the cornea in line with those from the lens surfaces (see Chapter 17).

Aphakic spectacle corrections often require special lens design considerations. Bifocals, and rarely trifocals, become virtually essential. The prescribing practitioner is obliged to consider a number of lens design options. For example, should the lens material be plastic to minimize weight, glass because of its scratch resistance, or higher-index glass to minimize thickness? If aspheric lens surfaces are to be used, the purpose may be to enhance appearance by reducing thickness and sagittal depth, or to provide imagery of better quality when viewing through more peripheral regions of the lens. Some aspheric lenses available today have been designed primarily to achieve a better cosmetic appearance. Other are designed to minimize aberrational effect; in general, this kind is a little less effective in minimizing thickness. The responsible optometrist stays abreast of developments in lens design and is prepared to consider the weight, appearance, durability, and aberrations of the lenses. Of course, many of the problems associated with spectacle lenses of higher power can be avoided or minimized by the use of contact lenses.

Prescribing for Low-Vision Patients

Most elderly patients with low vision can benefit from optical aids to enhance their visual performance. The optimal aid or aids for individual patients depend on the range and relative importance of the visual tasks they wish to perform, their vision characteristics, and their psychological attitudes toward their disability and the use of optical aids. Patients who need low-vision aids usually need more than one special optical aid. In prescribing optical aids, magnification is usually the first optical parameter considered. The field of view, distribution of image quality, image brightness, adjustability of focus, appearance, portability, convenience, cost, working distance, and maintenance requirements are other factors that enter the decision-making process. It is convenient to consider optical low-vision aids under three headings: (1) magnifiers for distance vision (telescopes), (2) magnifiers for near vision, and (3) nonmagnifying aids to vision (see Chapter 22).

Magnification for Distance Vision: Telescopes

Telescopes are commonly used by low-vision patients to enhance the resolution of signs, distant faces, television, movies, or other visual displays and scenery. Many elderly patients with low vision need to travel independently; if their vision is not adequate for driving, however, they may have to rely on public transportation. Dependence on public transportation, in turn, necessitates reading bus numbers, street signs, and traffic signals

Prescribing a telescope (or telescopes) for a low-vision patient involves both determining the required magnification and selecting an appropriate telescope.

Achieving the Required Acuity. The determination of the required telescope magnification is straightforward. The clinician determines visual acuity with best spectacle correction and estimates the resolution performance required to meet the patient's specific needs. Most commonly, an acuity performance of 20/30 to 20/40 is set as a practical and useful goal, but higher resolution is sometimes sought. When acuity is poor, the goal may be reduced to about 20/60. If acceptable telescopes do not improve visual acuity to 20/80, the value of a telescope prescription becomes questionable.

Calculating the required magnification is simple; it is a matter of ratios. For example, a patient with a visual acuity of 20/200 who wishes to read bus numbers might require 6× magnification to reach about a 20/30 level of performance.

Most low-vision patients do obtain the expected improvement in resolution. Exceptions may occur when using charts on which the task is made more difficult (more letters, closer spacing, or both for the smaller letters). In these cases the improvement may be less than simple theory predicts. The optometrist should verify that the patient does in fact obtain the expected visual acuity with the magnification originally predicted. Occasionally some modification of the magnification value will be necessary.

Certain techniques are important when testing patient performance with telescopes, especially with elderly patients. For best vision, the telescope must be properly focused. The greater the magnification, the more critical this becomes. If the patient has only a small refractive error, the clinician may focus the telescope for his or her own eye, observing from the correct viewing distance. Only small focus adjustments then should be required of the patient. When patients have higher refractive error, the clinician may use a trial lens to simulate the patient's refractive error and again adjust the telescope. Thus, for a 6.00 D myope, the clinician would hold a +6.00 D lens between the telescope eyepiece and his or her own eye (or glasses, if worn) and, being careful to be at the correct observation distance, focus to obtain clearest vision. The telescope should then be close to correct adjustment for the patient. Remember that adjustments that increase the telescope length add plus power to correct hyperopic refractive errors or to focus for closer viewing distances. Shortening the telescope length adds minus power.

Many telescopes of 6× or greater magnification do not provide enough focusing range to enable a focus for 20- or 10-foot distances. Should there be an insufficient range of focus, the clinician can effectively simulate optical infinity by moving the chart to 4 M (12.5 ft) and then holding a +0.25D trial lens against the objective of the telescope. A chart observation distance of 2 m with +0.50D lens in front of the telescope achieves the same effect.

It is necessary to insure in-focus vision when determining whether or not the patient achieves the resolution goal sought. The clinician should always verify that the telescope prescribed does indeed focus at the distance required. The patient's actual working distance should be established in the field or alternatively simulated in the office or local environment. The patient's observation distance may be 30 feet (say, a lecture theater) or 8 feet (an overhead menu at a fast-food restaurant); whatever this observation distance is, however, it should be simulated, and the clinician should check that the telescope's focusing range is adequate.

When more than one viewing distance is required, it may be necessary to prescribe a removable lens cap of appropriate power to achieve the change in focus. A series of monocular telescopes with a very wide focusing range (the Walters telescopes) recently has become available and has had a wide acceptance in the low-vision clinical community.

Another important optical parameter is the

exit pupil of the telescope, which defines the size of the beam of rays that can emerge from the telescope. The exit pupil almost invariably can be calculated by dividing the diameter of the objective lens by the magnification of the telescope. Thus, an 8 × 20 telescope has an 8 × magnification and a 20-mm objective lens diameter; the exit pupil size is 20 ÷ 8, or 2.5 mm. An 8 × 40 telescope has a 40-mm objective and thus has a 5-mm exit pupil. Telescopes of 4 × 20, 6 × 30, 8 × 40, and 10 × 50 all have 5-mm exit pupils.

The exit pupil can determine image brightness. If the exit beam is smaller than the eye pupil diameter, the image brightness is reduced as though the eye pupil had constricted to become the same size as the exit pupil of the telescope. An 8 × 20 telescope with a 2.5-mm exit pupil used by an eye with a 5-mm pupil will cause a fourfold decrease in retinal image illuminance. The effective diameter of the pupil is reduced by a factor of 2, so the effective area is reduced by a factor of 4. If the exit beam of the telescope is larger in diameter than the eye pupil, the image brightness should not be reduced except for the loss by reflectance and absorption. Lens coatings can reduce this kind of light loss.

This discussion of image brightness and telescopes applies to the observation of most objects. Different arguments and conclusions apply to the observation of stars, because the size of the retinal images of point sources is not affected by the magnification of the telescope.

Telescopes with smaller exit beams are generally more difficult to use, especially if the patient is inexperienced or has unsteady hands. It is more difficult to maintain a small exit beam in alignment with the eye pupil.

Older patients who have difficulty using telescopes to view the visual acuity chart are helped if the magnification is lower, the exit pupil is larger, or the field of view is larger. Sometimes it is necessary to develop the patient's skills gradually by beginning with telescopes of lower magnification. Patients with alignment difficulties can be assisted by reducing the room lighting and increasing the illumination on the chart. Then, if the telescope is not properly aligned, the exit beam will be visible as it illuminates the iris, sclera, or eyelids. The patient can be guided so that the exit beam enters his or her pupil. Even when the telescope is aligned, it may be necessary for the clinician to continue to help maintain alignment and guide the focus adjustment. In general, older patients need significantly more training and guidance to become proficient in using telescopes.

Selecting a Telescope. Once it has been verified that a patient can achieve the desired visual acuity with the use of a telescope of a particular magnification, the clinician must select the type of telescope that produces the required magnification and most conveniently satisfies the patient's needs. The telescope prescribed may be monocular or binocular. Binocular telescopes tend to be preferred when the visual acuity is similar for the two eyes. Some patients find binocular telescopes easier to hold, as the two eyecups can touch the eyebrows and provide some support or tactile feedback to help the patient maintain proper alignment. However, binocular telescopes are bulky and heavy, which detracts from their portability and comfort.

Patients who use telescopes to assist in their independent travel abilities usually prefer telescopes that are light in weight, concealable, easily carried in pocket or purse, and easy to use. Wrist straps, neck cords, or small finger ring mountings may help keep the telescope easily accessible for use as needed. Difficulties in holding a higher powered telescope with adequate steadiness can sometimes be reduced or eliminated by the use of a tripod, monopod, or other supporting structure.

Telescopes mounted in a spectacle frame or similar mounting have their advantages. They can prove most useful when observation with the telescope is for protracted periods (for example, when watching sporting events, stage presentations, or movies). Ready-made sports glasses, which are a pair of adjustable telescopes mounted in a spectacle-style frame, can be relatively inexpensive. Hook-on monocular telescopes can be attached to existing distance spectacles, thereby simultaneously correcting the refractive error and providing magnification.

Patients often request a spectacle-mounted system for viewing television. Generally, it is better to have the patient move closer to the television. Because telescopes restrict the field of view, in many television-viewing situations telescopes might not allow the patient to see the whole screen at one time. Many older patients resist sitting close to the television, as they believe it is harmful to the eyes.

Bioptic telescopes are spectacle-mounted telescope systems that are arranged to enable an easy transition from viewing through the telescope portion to viewing through the lens in which the telescope is mounted. These systems are more commonly prescribed for younger adults, but some older patients benefit from them. Bioptic telescopes can be used in driving, permitting the wearer quick access to telescope viewing for short-term observation of signs and traffic signals. Many state departments of motor vehicles permit driving with bioptic telescopes provided that the usual visual standard is met when the wearer observes through the telescope, and vision through the nontelescope section must be of a particular standard. Drivers wearing bioptic telescopes may have some general or individual restrictions on their driver's licenses. Older patients who use a bioptic telescope system for driving often want a bifocal addition for viewing the speedometer and other gauges and displays.

Spectacle-mounted bioptic telescope systems are available in magnifications up to 8 ×, but 3 × and 4 × seem to be most useful. The small field and difficulties with steadiness and with aiming the telescope make the stronger bioptic telescopes harder to use.

Older patients, who are often self-conscious about their visual handicap, may be reluctant to even consider the use of a telescope. Most patients whose visual acuity is 20/60 or poorer should be given information about telescopes so they can understand their potential advantages. Encouraging patients to borrow a telescope for use at home for a week or so can produce some appreciation of the benefits and may change attitudes about telescopes.

Magnification for Near Vision

Optical magnification to provide low-vision patients with assistance for near vision tasks can be considered in six categories: high-addition reading glasses, hand-held magnifying glasses, stand magnifiers, head-mounted loupes, near vision telescopes, and videomagnifiers and projection magnifiers.

There are three basic steps in prescribing a magnifier to provide a level of resolution that will meet the patient's visual needs: (1) determining the magnification or power required; (2) deciding what kind of magnifier (hand-held, stand, and so forth) would be most appropriate; and (3) given the magnification demand and the kind of magnifier, determining which of the available models has the best combination of features to satisfy the patient's requirements.

Determining Magnification Requirements. Magnification for near vision can be a difficult topic to discuss, because there are many conflicting definitions of *magnification*. To illustrate the difficulty, a 5.00D lens held at a full arm's length might produce an apparent magnification of 5 × and the resolution could be 2 × better than that obtained with a previous 2.50D addition that gave clear vision at 40 cm, yet the manufacturer may have this magnifier labeled 2.25 ×; to cap it all, the clinician may recall a simple formula ($M = F/4$) suggesting that the magnification should be 1.25 ×. The word *magnification* implies a comparison and demands the question, Compared with what? Because there are several alternative answers to this question, there are several alternative definitions of *magnification,* and it is not always clear which definition is most appropriate (as the example illustrates).

Much of the potential confusion surrounding the definition of *magnification* can be avoided if we simply refer to the equivalent dioptric power of the magnification system being used. Systems with the same equivalent dioptric power all provide the same resolution capacity for a given patient. For example, a presbyopic patient would obtain the same resolution with each of the following:

- A +12.00D spectacle addition.

- A +12.00D hand-held magnifier, regardless of how far it is held from the eye.

- A 3 × telescope with a reading cap of 4.00D on the objective.

- A 2.50D spectacle addition separated from a +17.00D stand magnifier lens by a distance of 17.5 cm.

- A closed circuit television giving a 6 times enlargement when it is being observed from 50 cm (using a +2.00D addition).

Each provides an equivalent viewing power of 12.00D so each affords the same resolution. It is assumed that the patient will arrange the task to insure an in-focus image in each case. In any evaluation of near vision performance, the patient should wear the appropriate addition and hold the test material so that it is in sharpest focus.

Determining the Power Required. Although it is possible to use distance visual acuity in estimating how much dioptric power is required to enable a patient to read print of a certain size, this is not the surest approach. Letter charts used for distance vision and reading cards used for near vision present tasks of quite different complexity; there is no strong concordance between letter chart acuity and reading chart acuity, especially when there are macular disturbances. Presbyopic patients almost invariably have a reading correction, and the most convenient and appropriate way to begin the power determination is to measure the patients' reading acuity while they use their existing reading correction. For example, a patient might have eyeglasses that incorporate a +3.00D addition, and holding the test card at 33 cm, this patient might be able to read 2.5-M print (which could, on some charts, be labeled *20 points* or *20/125.*).

The power required to reach a resolution goal then can be determined by simple ratios or proportions. For example, it might be decided that the patient should be able to read material of newsprint size (1-M, 8 points, or 20/50 in size). Whatever units are used, it can easily be seen that a 2.5× improvement in resolution is required. Since resolution at near is proportional to lens power, the lens power will need to be increased by the same factor of 2.5. This means that the addition must be increased from 3.00 to 7.50D. If the 7.50D dioptric power is to be given in spectacle form, the viewing distance (being inversely proportional to the addition) will change from 33 to 13 cm, which again represents a ratio of 2.5. The clinician should then verify that the patient does in fact achieve satisfactory reading of the 1-M print (8 points or 20/50) that had been set as the goal. This is usually done in spectacle format with a trial frame or trial lens clip.

When working over existing bifocals, the lens clip might not allow full access to the bifocal portion of the lens. In such a case, the lens clip can be raised so that only the distance portion of the lens is being used, and the full required addition can be introduced into the lens clip. Special care must be taken to insure that an appropriate working distance is being used, as some older people strongly resist working at close distances.

Selecting the Magnifying Aid. Once the dioptric power that will give the desired reading resolution performance has been determined, the optometrist must decide which of the various aids should be used to provide the required power.

Spectacle lens corrections afford the widest fields of view, leave both hands free to support or manipulate task materials, are convenient to carry, and are relatively inconspicuous. Their disadvantage is the close working distance they may impose. If a spectacle prescription is to be issued, the lens form must be considered. Will it be single vision lenses, bifocals in a usual configuration, bifocals with high placement of the segments, special series lenses, or aspheric lenses? Binocularity issues should be addressed. If binocular vision is to be achieved (it is usually achievable if addition powers are +10.00D or less), the prism or decentration must be considered. Fonda (1981) recommends as a rule of thumb that 2 mm of total decentration be given for each diopter of addition power. Thus, there should be 8 mm of total decentration for a 4.00D addition, 16 mm for an 8.00D addition, and so on. This method provides a small net amount of base-in prism.

Many patients with low vision must perform near vision tasks monocularly, either because there is substantial inequality between the two eyes or because the required lens powers are too high. Even though the other eye might not be used during the main reading tasks, some attention should be given to whether it should be totally occluded or blocked with a frosted lens, or whether some lens should be worn in front of that eye. Perhaps a simple balance lens will be indicated, but often monovision possibilities should be considered. It may be useful to have a single vision lens before the poorer eye to give in-focus distance viewing or to provide an intermediate or near vision focus. A bifocal or trifocal lens before the poorer eye might best satisfy the patient's overall visual needs and convenience.

Hand-held magnifiers have as their main advantage the adjustability of working distance. In one extreme, the patient can hold the magnifying glass in the spectacle plane, in which case the reading material will need to be in the appropriate focal plane. At the other end of the scale, the magnifier may be held at a full arm's length; again, the test card will need to be in the proper focal plane. The further the lens is held from the eye, the smaller the field of view. Provided patients are using their distance glasses, the resolution will be determinable directly from the equivalent power of the hand-held magnifying lens. Bifocal wearers should not view through their bifocal segments unless the magnifier is being held close (that is, closer than one of its focal lengths) to the spectacle lens. Holding the magnifier against the reading addition in spectacles effectively provides the sum of the two powers. The combination will then act as a strong spectacle lens.

Hand-held magnifiers provide portability and flexibility. They are ideally suited for looking at price tags, reading maps, and checking labels on containers in a store.

Stand magnifiers, which are usually used for reading tasks, are particularly helpful to elderly patients, since hand steadiness is not very important. If strong dioptric powers are required, and even if there are no hand steadiness problems, stand magnifiers provide a level of easy and reliable control not attainable with spectacles or hand-held magnifiers. For reading tasks of limited duration (examples are reading telephone books and television schedules, checking bills, and reading greeting cards), stand magnifiers can be of most value. Some even incorporate a light to illuminate the task. Stand magnifiers may be somewhat bulky and therefore less convenient to carry, and the working situation becomes much more rigidly defined.

The optometrist must understand a few basic optical principles in order to prescribe stand magnifiers intelligently. First, fixed-focus stand magnifiers produce images that are relatively close to the lens of the magnifier. Rarely is the image farther than 50 cm behind the magnifying lens, and most image locations are in the range 3 to 40 cm behind the lens surface. Consequently, presbyopic patients must wear a reading correction to obtain a clear view of the image. The image location and the power of the spectacle addition determine the separation required between the magnifier and the spectacles. If the image of the magnifier is 10 cm below its surface and the patient is focused for 40 cm because of a +2.50D reading addition, the required separation is 30 cm. Had the spectacle addition been 5.00D, the required separation would have been 10 cm. The clinician should know the image location for the stand magnifier being used.

The second basic optical principle to be understood is that the image produced by the stand magnifier is larger than the original object. The net effect of the magnifier is to produce an image that is both larger and more remote than the original object. The power of the magnifier lens and the object-lens separation determine the size of the image. The enlargement (which may unambiguously be called the *transverse magnification*) is constant and should be known to the clinician, since it influences the final resolution.

Third, when the patient uses the spectacle addition to view the enlarged image formed by the magnifier, the total dioptric power of the system can be obtained from multiplying the power of the addition (or the accommodation demand) by the magnitude of the enlargement (or the transverse magnification). If the transverse magnification provided by the stand magnifier is 4 × and the patient is able to view the image clearly while using a 3.00D addition, the equivalent power of the combination is 4 × 3.00D, or 12.00D. This permits prediction of the resolution the patient will be able to achieve.

The following demonstrates some of the important considerations that should be made when using stand magnifiers. Two widely used stand magnifiers made by Combined Optical Industries Ltd. are considered here:

Name	COIL 5428	COIL 5123
Labeled power	+20.00D	+28.00D
True power	+17.00D	+24.00D
Image position	12.5 cm	27.5 cm
Transverse magnification	3.0 ×	7.5 ×

Consider a patient who can just read 3-M print at 40 cm with a 2.50D addition. With these glasses in place, this patient should position the spectacles 27.5 cm from the COIL 5428 so that this separation and the image distance total 40 cm. Similarly, the required separation from the COIL 5123 is 12.5 cm.

The equivalent power achieved when using the COIL 5428 is 3 × 2.50D, or 7.50D. This is a threefold increase; now the smallest print legible should be three times smaller, that is, 1 M. For the COIL 5123, the final power is 7.5 × 2.50D, or 18.75D. The resolution will have improved by a factor of 7.5, so 0.40-M print should be legible.

If the addition were changed to 3.00D, the required separations would change to 21 cm for the COIL 5428 and 6 cm for the COIL 5123. The respective total equivalent powers achieved would be 9.00 and 22.50D. The resolution limits would then become 0.83 M (from 3 M × [2.5/9]) and 0.33 M (from 3 M × [2.5/22.5]).

Unfortunately, manufacturers specify neither image location nor transverse magnification; even their nominal lens powers or magnfication ratings often defy logic or understanding. However, there are simple in-office methods for measuring these key optical parameters (Bailey 1981a, 1981b, 1981c).

Head-mounted loupes are positive-powered lenses that are mounted so they sit in front of the spectacle plane. They are mainly used for manipulative tasks. A wide variety of such devices is available. Some are single lenses that attach to the spectacle frame or spectacle lens, and the lens generally is mounted on a pivoting bracket that allows the lens to be conveniently removed or inserted into the line of vision. These provide monocular viewing, and lens powers usually range from 10.00D up to about 30.00D. Binocular loupes, which are available in powers up to about 10.00 or 12.00D, usually incorporate some prism or decentration to facilitate convergence. Some binocular loupe systems attach to spectacles, but most are mounted on a headband that positions the lens bracket 2 cm or so in front of the spectacle plane. Many can be flipped up and down as needed. Another potential advantage of head-mounted loupes is that the mounting of the lenses an inch away from the spectacles means the task may be moved 1 inch farther away from the face. For some manipulative tasks, this change in viewing distance will be useful.

Near vision telescopes (sometimes called *telemicroscopes*) are not so commonly prescribed for older patients, but their distinct advantages sometimes make them essential. Near vision telescopes are called for when a certain level of dioptric power is required to achieve a given resolution goal but the patient is compelled to have a long working distance and unrestricted or bimanual access to the task. Performing surgery and viewing computer terminals are two tasks for which near vision telescopes are often prescribed, but they can be valuable for less unusual tasks. The advantage of near vision telescopes is the increased working distance, but this must be balanced against the principal disadvantage, the reduced field of view. The depth of focus is also quite small, so the working distance must be accurately maintained.

Near vision telescopes can be created most simply by adding a lens cap to the objective lens of a distance telescope. The equivalent power of the system achieved by this combination can be computed easily; it is simply the telescope magnification multiplied by the power of the addition. For example, a system made from placing a 4.00D lens cap on the front of a 2.5 × telescope will have an equivalent power of 10.00D. It will provide the same resolution as any other 10.00D system. The working distance, however, will be 25 cm, because this is determined by the power of the addition. Other 10.00D near vision telescope systems could be created by combining a 2.00D cap and a 5 × telescope (working distance = 50 cm), a 3.00D cap and a 3.3 × telescope (working distance = 33 cm), a 5.00D cap and a 2.0 × telescope (working distance = 20 cm), or many other combinations. Resolution and working distance are the prime parameters to be considered.

Videomagnifiers and projection magnifiers produce enlarged images on a screen. Closed circuit television systems use electronics to achieve the enlargement, whereas projector systems enlarge with optics. Videomagnifiers offer some special additional advantages over optical systems. There is usually easy reversal of contrast, a wide range of magnification is usually available, and masks and border enhancement can be created electronically to improve visual performance. Because such high transverse magnification or enlargement ratios can be achieved, it is usually possible for patients to read the videomagnifier display from a comfortable viewing position.

The equivalent dioptric power effect achieved with a videomagifier can be calculated by multiplying the transverse magnification by the dioptric viewing distance. For older patients, the dioptric viewing distance is typically close to the power of the reading addition of their general-purpose bifocals. A patient with a 2.50D addition, for example, viewing from 40 cm an image that is three times larger than the original, will have a system with a 7.50D equivalent viewing power. If testing with spectacle lenses had previously indicated that a patient required a +12.00D system to achieve a resolution goal and the patient was wearing a +3.00D addition bifocal, the videomagnifier should be arranged to give 4 × magnification.

Rarely do optical magnifiers used in low vision provide dioptric powers greater than 50, but most videomagnifier systems can easily provide 100.00D or more (for example, a 3.00D addition and a 30 × enlargement) without imposing extreme constraints on comfort or potential efficiency. Because videomagnifiers can provide such high magnification while allowing comfortable viewing postures, reading comfort and endurance are the main benefits provided by these systems. Low-vision patients with a moderate to substantial loss of vision who need to read for long periods or need very high magnification should be considered possible candidates for videomagnifier systems.

For all near vision magnification systems, care should be taken to adjust the illumination to suit the patients' needs. Most older low-vision patients require more illumination than usual, but they are more susceptible to glare. Consequently, more than the usual attention should be paid to positioning the luminaire and the task material so that potentially troublesome glare is avoided.

A device that has proved useful for glare control is the typoscope, or reading mask. This is a black card with a rectangluar aperture that is usually made large enough to accommodate three lines of one-column-width print. The typoscope can enhance reading acuity and comfort by reducing glare from white paper close to the immediate fixation point. This device also serves as a line guide and helps patients with field defects to maintain their place when reading.

Yellow filters are also found to be beneficial by some patients, who report that they make vision apparently clearer and more comfortable. Illumination control by varying the quantity and quality of the task and ambient lighting, as well as by the use of the typoscope and yellow filters, should all be routinely included in the assessment of the patient's near vision magnification.

Nonmagnifying Aids to Vision
Contact lenses can offer special advantages to low-vision patients. They can substantially reduce the effect of corneal irregularities that are due to corneal or anterior eye scarring or other causes. When the corneal distortion is more pronounced, soft contact lenses are not as effective, since some of the corneal distortion may be translated to the front surface of the lens. Hard lenses can be more effective in nullifying the optical effect of distortion, but they are more likely to cause potentially troublesome pressure spots on the distorted cornea. The other major

optical benefit of contact lenses is that they substantially reduce aberration and prismatic effects that can produce vision difficulties with the use of stronger spectacle lenses. Because the contact lenses move with the eye, the visual axis of the eye is always close to the optic axis of the correcting lens; this means that peripheral aberration problems are eliminated or at least greatly reduced. Differential prismatic effects that occur with spectacle corrections for anisometropia are much better controlled with contact lenses. Aphakic patients often experience perceptual and depth judgment difficulties when they are introduced to spectacle corrections, and they may be bothered by the field restriction and the jack-in-the-box effect created by the high plus spectacle lens. These effects are avoided or minimized by using contact lenses.

Filters also can be beneficial to many elderly patients. For reasons that are not fully understood, many patients with retinal disorders and some with cataracts report seeing better when yellow filters or some other "minus blue" filter is worn (see Chapter 10). Older patients, especially those with visual disorders, tend to be more sensitive to very bright light; thus, sunglass filters (sometimes very dense ones) are often required. The approach to prescribing tints is largely empirical. Decisions are based on reported symptoms and the patient's expressed perception of the effect of the filters.

Visual field defects accompanying pathological changes can produce functional difficulties for patients, especially in mobility tasks. Three kinds of optical devices can help patients with particular kinds of visual field defects: reversed telescopes, hemianopic mirrors, and partial prisms.

Reversed telescopes can be useful for patients who have developed a concentric loss of visual field such as occurs in advanced retinitis pigmentosa or glaucoma. Reversed telescopes obviously reduce visual acuity, but they can provide an enlarged visual field. Most patients who use reversed telescopes only do so for navigational purposes, and then only when the local environment contains repetitive or potentially confusing details. An example of such a situation is an intersection at which many roads or paths meet. Most reversed telescopes are hand held and are of a moderate range of magnification (3 to 6 ×).

Hemianopic mirrors can help patients with homonymous hemianopia. A mirror is mounted on the nasal eyewire of the spectacles in front of the eye that is on the same side as the field loss. The mirror is angled so that it is about 10 degrees with respect to the primary line of sight; it is about 20 to 40 mm in width. For a patient with a right homonymous hemianopia, therefore, the mirror would be mounted on the nasal portion of the right eyewire and angled slightly toward the right eye. By reflection, this mirror will present part of the right-hand field of view to the right eye. This segment from the blind field will appear to the right eye to be reversed and unstable, and it will be projected so that it seems to be superimposed on the left-hand field. The purpose of the mirror is to provide some awareness of events and hazards on the blind side. The patient must learn not to give close attention to detail seen in the mirror. When the patient becomes aware of an object or event deserving attention, the head should be turned so that the full inspection and any decision making is made with the benefit of direct vision. Only a small minority of hemianopic patients have mirrors prescribed, but optometrists nevertheless should consider them for each hemianopic patient.

Partial prisms are the third kind of optical device prescribed to help patients with field problems. Their main use is in hemianopias, but they can also be useful when there has been a concentric loss of visual field. Partial prisms are usually Fresnel membrane prisms of high deviation (20 to 30Δ) that are placed on the lens so that they are totally within the blind field when the patient looks straight ahead. The base direction of the prism is always away from the primary line of sight. When the patient makes an eye movement toward a blind part of the field, the prism will be encountered after a certain degree of deviation.

The prism optically shifts things in from the periphery. This means that smaller eye movements will be required to view more peripheral objects on the blind side. Expressed another way, an eye movement of a given magnitude allows the patient to see further to the periphery when viewing through the prism. The prism creates a blind spot, and the patient may be distracted by apparent jumping or disappearance of objects when eye movements traverse the edge of the prism. The prisms are placed so they will remain within the patient's blind field most of the time when relatively normal, small-magnitude eye movements are being made. When the patient wants to inspect more peripheral regions, large

eye movements are called for; these are supplemented by the effect of the prism.

A fairly typical configuration of the partial prisms for a right hemianope would be a 30Δ base-out prism mounted on the right lens so that it covers the full vertical height of the lens beginning at a point about 6 mm to the right of the primary viewing point. On the left lens there would be a much smaller area of prism (30Δ base in), and again the vertical edge of the prism would be about 6 mm from the primary viewing point. Because Fresnel membrane prisms can be removed and replaced easily, it is not difficult or expensive to experiment with this kind of correction.

Training in the Use of Optical Aids

Adaptation, practice, and training are often necessary if patients are to receive maximum benefit from their low-vision aids. Many aids demand that new skills be learned. Older patients are generally less able to adapt, and they require more training. For example, structured, guided practice in techniques for sighting and focusing with telescopes can be vital to success. Furthermore, it is often useful to give initial training with telescopes that have lower magnification and larger exit pupils, since these are easier to use.

A variety of skills may need to be developed for reading; these include positioning the head, the eyes, the aid, and the material to achieve clear focus and then making the required relative movements to enable the most fluent reading. Sometimes only brief instruction is needed, whereas other situations may require training and supervision.

Many low-vision patients have central scotomas, and their visual performance and efficiency may improve if they can learn eccentric viewing strategies. Similarly, many patients may need training in more efficient scanning and search techniques.

It is a good policy to insure that a patient is able to use any optical aid with reasonable proficiency before it is issued. Training the patient in the most efficient use of an aid or the eyes can be the key to success for many patients.

Advice and Recommendations

When all the clinical data has been collected, the optometrist should pause and take stock. Has all the relevant information been uncovered? Again, the following question would be asked: What does the patient really want? What do I want the patient to have? Really, why did the patient come to see me?

The clinician should decide on the treatment options and then consciously consider the strategy for presenting recommendations and advice. For example, should others be present when the advice is given, and to what extent should they be involved? What issues need to be given strongest emphasis, and what should be sidestepped or downplayed? How strongly should the treatment recommendations be advocated? What does the patient really need to know? What will the patient like to hear, and what will not be accepted easily?

The advice and recommendations the optometrist submits to elderly patients need not be confined to optical and visual matters. As a health care practitioner, the optometrist has a responsibility to the patient's general health, and any need for rehabilitative attention that may contribute to the patient's overall well-being should be discussed. The optometrist can be a critical link in the health care chain, taking the initiative in directing patients toward appropriate and broadly based care for their health and well-being.

Optometrists should remain well informed about the availability of health care and other support and social services available in the local community. In particular, the optometrist should maintain contacts with the medical community and rehabilitation counselors or social workers, as well as be familiar with the activities and services of organizations serving the visually handicapped or senior citizens.

References

Bailey, I. L. "Locating the Image in Stand Magnifiers." *Optometric Monthly* 71, no. 6 (1981): 22–24. (a)

Bailey, I. L. "The Use of Fixed-Focus Stand Magnifiers." *Optometric Monthly* 71, no. 8 (1981): 37–39. (b)

Bailey, I. L. "Verifying Near Vision Magnifiers," *Optometric Monthly* 72 (1981): 34–38. (c)

Bailey, I. L. and J. E. Lovie. "New Design Principles for Visual Acuity Letter Charts." *American Journal of Optometry and Physiological Optics* 53 (1976): 740–745.

Bailey, I. L., and J. E. Lovie. "The Design and Use of a New Near-Vision Chart." *American Journal of Optometry and Physiological Optics* 57 (1980): 378–387.

Ferris, L.; A. Kassoff; G. H. Bresnick; and I. L. Bailey. "New Visual Acuity Charts for Research Purposes." *American Journal of Ophthalmology* 94 (1982): 91–96.

Fonda, G. E. *Management of Low Vision.* New York: Thieme-Stratton, 1981.

Keeler, C. H. "On Visual Aids for the Partially Sighted." *Transactions of the Ophthalmological Societies of the United Kingdom* 76 (1956): 605–614.

Mehr, E. B., and A. N. Freid. *Low Vision Care.* Chicago: Professional Press, 1975.

Sloan, L. L. "New Test Charts for the Measurement of Visual Acuity at Far and Near Distances." *American Journal of Ophthalmology* 48 (1959): 807–813.

Suggested Readings

Anderson, D. R. *Testing the Field of Vision.* St. Louis: Mosby, 1982.

Bailey, I. L. "The Aged Blind." *Australian Journal of Optometry* 58 (1975): 31–39.

Bailey, I. L. "Telescopes: Their Use in Low Vision." *Optometric Monthly* 69 (1978): 634–638.

Bedwell, C. H. *Visual Fields.* London: Butterworth, 1982.

Borish, I. W.; S. A. Hitzeman; and K. E. Brookman. "Double Masked Study of Progressive Addition Lenses." *Journal of the American Optometric Association* 51 (1980): 933–943.

Faye, E. E. *The Low Vision Patient.* New York: Grune and Stratton, 1970.

Faye, E. E. *Clinical Low Vision,* 2nd ed. Boston: Little, Brown, 1984.

Hirsch, M. J., and R. E. Wick. *Vision of the Aging Patient.* Philadelphia: Chilton, 1960.

Jose, R. T. *Understanding Low Vision.* New York: American Foundation for the Blind, 1983.

Kitchin, J. E., and I. L. Bailey. "Task Complexity and Visual Acuity in Senile Macular Degeneration." *Australian Journal of Optometry* 63 (1981): 235–242.

Lederer, J. "The Effects of Age on Visual Functioning." *Australian Journal of Science* 32 (1969): 79–86.

Lovie-Kitchin, J. E.; E. J. Farmer; and K. J. Bowman. *Senile Macular Degeneration.* Brisbane, Australia: Queensland Institute of Technology, 1982.

Morgan, M. W. *The Optics of Ophthalmic Lenses.* Chicago: Professional Press, 1978.

Rosenbloom, A. A. "Low Vision." In *Principles and Practice of Ophthalmology,* eds. G. Peyman, D. Sanders, and M. F. Goldberg. Philadelphia: Saunders, 1980, pp. 241–277.

Rosenbloom, A. A. "Care of Elderly People with Low Vision." *Visual Impairment and Blindness,* June 1982, pp. 209–212.

Sekuler, R.; D. Kline; and K. Dismukes. *Aging and Human Visual Function.* New York: Allan R. Liss, 1982.

Sloan, L. L. *Reading Aids for the Partially Sighted.* Baltimore: Williams and Wilkins, 1977.

Weale, R. A. *The Aging Eye.* London: Lewis, 1963.

Weale, R. A. *A Biography of the Eye: Development, Growth, Age.* London: Lewis, 1982.

Chapter 15

Introduction to Special Tests for the Assessment of Vision in Elderly Patients

J. Randall Pitman
Robert L. Yolton

The need for electrodiagnostic, angiographic, psychophysical, and other special testing procedures arises when conventional testing cannot provide adequate assessment of a patient's visual system. For example, special testing is particularly useful for elderly patients, in part because conventional testing can be hampered by the presence of media opacities (Hirose 1977). Conventional evaluations of elderly patients also can be difficult if the patient is unable to respond reliably or give valid information when tested subjectively. Special testing can overcome problems such as these and thus be very useful in confirming tentative diagnoses or quantitatively monitoring the progression of known diseases in the elderly.

To properly utilize special tests, ophthalmic practitioners must not only realize when such testing would be beneficial for patients; they also must be able to select the appropriate test or tests and properly interpret the results. In addition, practitioners should be able to describe the general testing procedures to their patients so as to alleviate their fears and prepare them for testing (which may appear somewhat threatening).

Based on these considerations, this chapter presents to the general ophthalmic practitioner

a practical guide for special testing.* It is designed to answer pertinent questions without getting into the intimate details of how to conduct the special tests (for example, how to place electrodes on the patient). Detailed information regarding these procedures can readily be found in the references cited throughout the chapter, as well as in general references such as Carr and Siegal (1982).

Ordering the Appropriate Test

Once it has been determined that conventional testing is inadequate or inappropriate for a patient, the selection of the special test or tests to be conducted should be made by first determining which aspect or aspects of the patient's visual system need to be assessed. To aid in this process, Figure 15–1 presents a flow chart showing a logical sequence to follow when considering referral for special testing. As indicated, the special tests considered in this chapter fall into two categories: (1) tests of retinal/ocular integrity and (2) tests of the integrity of the entire visual pathway.

If pathology is suspected in the globe or retina, consideration should be given to ordering electroretinography (EGR), electro-oculography (EOG), fluorescein angiography, or ultrasonography tests. The question then arises as to which of these tests is most appropriate; the answer, of course, depends on the patient. If the patient has reasonably clear ocular media, any or all of the tests may be used, with the most appropriate one's depending on the specific aspect of the

---

*In preparing this chapter, the authors have assumed that the general ophthalmic practitioner does not have access to the often-expensive instrumentation required to perform special tests, but that special testing can be obtained from laboratories or consultants in the area. In this way, special ophthalmic tests are analogous to X rays or blood and laboratory tests that are available on order.

system to be tested. Ultrasonography evaluates structural integrity; fluorescein angiography evaluates vascular integrity; EOG evaluates primarily the retinal pigment epithelium (RPE); flash ERG evaluates the inner and outer layers of the retina; and pattern ERG evaluates ganglion cell function. If the patient has difficulty with steady fixation or has poor saccadic movement, the EOG probably would be inappropriate, since reliable results depend on such skills. Likewise, if the patient has ocular media opacities sufficient to bar fundus photography or prevent

fixation, fluorescein angiography and EOG should not be ordered.

In cases where the patient's problems suggest the use of special testing procedures, but there is no specific reason to suspect that the problems are confined to the retina, one of the subjective tests for the whole visual system can be used. If the patient has clear media and is responsive to subjective testing, the test of choice probably would be perimetry, dark adaptometry, or contrast sensitivity, depending on the symptoms. Perimetry is a powerful subjective test that can

Figure 15-1

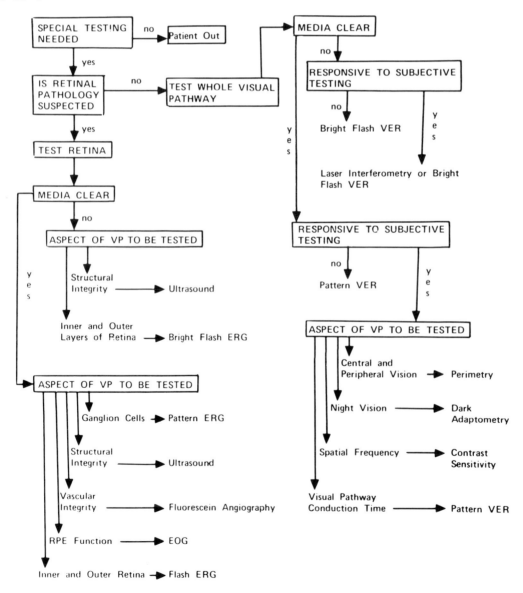

Flowchart Suggesting a Logical Sequence for Determining a Special Test or Tests Appropriate to Order for a Particular Patient. The chart branches at the top into two general categories: retinal testing on the left and whole visual system testing on the right.

be used for assessing pathology of neurological origin. Dark adaptometry is called for in cases of night vision difficulties, and contrast sensitivity is in order for those mysterious complaints of 20/20 vision that "just does not seem quite right" to the patient. For elderly patients with opaque media who respond well to subjective testing, interferometry, in which stimulus gratings are created on the retina via a laser, can be used for determining the patency of the visual system.

When the validity of the patient's verbal responses cannot be trusted, the most commonly used whole visual system objective test is the visual evoked response (VER), in which signals from the visual cortex are recorded and analyzed.

Thus, the specific choice of a test (or tests) depends on at least three important factors: (1) the pattern of the patient's signs and symptoms, (2) the aspect or aspects of the visual system to be tested, and (3) the validity of the patient's subjective responses. By considering these factors, appropriate special tests can be ordered to determine the nature of a suspected pathology, follow the course of a known pathology, or rule out the presence of pathology.

Tests of Retinal Integrity

First to be considered are those tests that give a specific indication of retinal integrity: ERG, EOG, fluorescein angiography, and ultrasonography. Special testing for retinal function is especially beneficial for patients with ocular opacities who are being considered for surgery.

Electroretinography

The electroretinogram (ERG) is an electrodiagnostic test designed to record the electrical potentials that arise from the retina in response to a flash of light (flash ERG) or to a patterned stimulus (pattern ERG).* Flash ERG provides an objective indication of overall retinal function; by using exceptionally bright flashes, it can be used to assess the retina in elderly patients who have media opacities.

Principles: Flash ERG. The flash ERG is a summed electrical response from cells across the entire retina. The ERG can be divided into a

number of components, of which the a and b waves are most commonly measured clinically (Figure 15–2). The a wave is a small negative voltage (referenced to the cornea) primarily generated by retinal photoreceptors; the b wave is a larger cornea-positive voltage generated by cells in the inner nuclear layer. Ganglion cells and the optic nerve fiber layer do not appear to contribute to the flash ERG response (Galloway 1975; Gouras 1970).

Recording Methods. The ERG is representative of several electrodiagnostic tests inasmuch as recording an ERG involves certain procedures common to most of these tests. These basic procedures include (1) presenting a stimulus to the patient, (2) detecting an electrical response from the patient via surface contact electrodes, (3) amplifying the electrical response, and (4) displaying and/or recording the amplified electrical signal.

In the case of the ERG, the patient usually is stimulated with diffuse strobe flashes presented in a Ganzfeld (a diffusing sphere into which the patient's head is partially placed; see Figure 15–3). Appropriate equipment can vary the duration, wavelength, and frequency of the light flashes presented in the Ganzfeld.

The patient's response is detected by a contact lens electrode placed on the dilated and anesthetized eye, as well as skin electrodes placed elsewhere on the body (typically near the lateral canthus and on an earlobe). Signals from the electrodes are differentially amplified and displayed on an oscilloscope.

The contact lens electrode is sometimes a problem for elderly patients, who may have fragile ocular tissues. They may suffer a brief period of discomfort, including stinging, tearing, and injection following the procedure. However, these symptoms are generally minimal and usually last only a few hours.

Interpretation of Results. The ERG can be evaluated by comparing the amplitude and latency of the a and b wave components with expected values, with values from the other eye, or with both. Typical ERGs show b wave amplitudes of roughly 0.5 mV, whereas a wave amplitudes are about 25 percent of those for the b wave. Latencies of the a wave are typically about 0.05 second and, with the b wave peaking at about 0.1 to 0.2 second (Berson 1981).

*Note that the abbbreviation *ERG* stands for both *electroretinography* (the production and study of the retinogram) and *electroretinogram* (the recorded electrical effect).

Figure 15-2

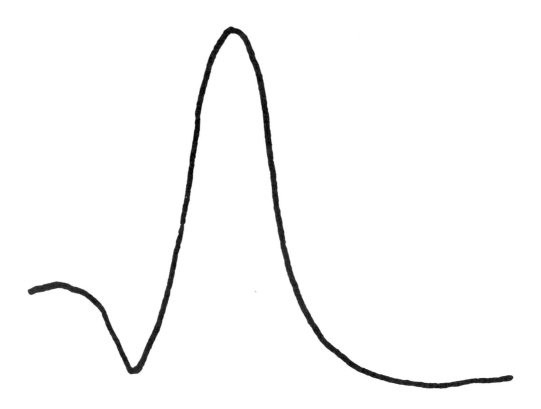

Schematic Representation of the Flash ERG Wave form. The *a* wave is the initial downward (negative) deflection in the trace, and the *b* wave is the larger positive deflection.

Abnormal ERG responses can be caused by retinal disruptions such as large chorioretinal scars, detached retinas, and media opacities. A patient with cataracts, but normal retinas, would be expected to have small-amplitude ERGs with corresponding long latencies (because of light absorbance and scatter by the lens), but the presence of retinopathies, detachments, or both would result in reduced-amplitude ERGs with normal component latencies (Gouras 1970).

In patients with clear media, ERG *a* wave amplitudes and latencies are not significantly correlated with age (Weleber 1981), but several studies have indicated that *b* wave amplitudes decrease with increasing age, especially after age 50 or 60 (Armington 1974; Krill 1972; Weleber 1981; Zollman et al. 1978). This decrease is more evident when the intensity of the stimulus is increased (Weleber 1981). In contrast, assuming that the ocular media remains clear, ERG *b* wave latency does not change with age. However, as media transparency decreases,

the stimulus intensity at the retina also decreases, causing a corresponding increase in latency and decrease in amplitude of all portions of the ERG wave form.

Bright-Flash ERG. For many elderly patients, the typical strobe stimulus (Grass Model PS22) must be replaced with an even brighter strobe to insure penetration of media opacities. Any response at all to this "brightflash" indicates a functioning (but not necessarily perfect) retina. If the patient is contemplating surgical removal of cataracts or other media opacities, the presence or absence of the bright-flash ERG response can be used in making a prognosis for visual rehabilitation (Fuller, Knighton, and Machemer 1975).

As a word of caution, the ERG is a summed response from the whole retina, so the loss of a small but critical area, such as the fovea, usually would not be detected. Therefore, any predictions of postsurgical *acuity* based on ERG data alone

Figure 15-3

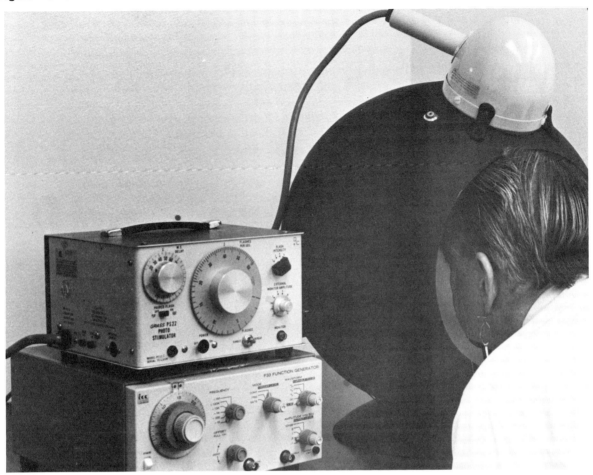

Patient Presented with a Uniformly Diffused Strobe Stimulus Using a Ganzfeld Dome during ERG Recording

are tenuous. The value of the bright-flash ERG is that it gives a gross indication of retinal integrity. For a person virtually blind because of media opacities, some useful vision could be restored through surgery even in the absence of a functioning macula. The bright-flash ERG, if recordable, gives reasonable hope of at least partial sight. A nonrecordable bright-flash ERG is not as conclusive. Again, because of the mass-response nature of the test, large portions of the retina may be damaged—thus producing no ERG—and yet the foveal region still may be functional. Because of this possibility, a nonrecordable bright-flash ERG should be followed up with other tests, such as a bright-flash VER or laser interferometry, to assess central visual function.

Additional Applications for the ERG.
Recently it has been shown that ERG responses also can be elicited by using a constant-luminance patterned stimulus, such as a grating,

which may be focused on specific parts of the retina. Using this stimulus, the ERG is produced primarily by ganglion cells (which do not contribute significantly to the flash ERG). Pattern ERGs have been used to assess ganglion cell damage that is due to temporary occlusion of the retinal artery, retrobulbar optic neuritis, and certain other diseases (Fiorentini et al. 1981). The objective nature of the pattern ERG makes it a powerful diagnostic tool for use with elderly patients, and when coupled with a laser-generated stimulus (see the section on laser interferometry), it can be used with patients who have opaque media.

The analysis of pattern ERGs is more complex than the analysis of flash ERGs, because computer averaging and processing of the pattern ERGs usually is required, and an electrode that does not interfere with the eye's optics must be used. Thus, pattern ERG recording is not yet readily available as a referral procedure except at teaching institutions or selected clinics.

Since it has distinctive dark- and light-adapted responses, the ERG also can be used to differentiate rod and cone degenerations. However, these more-involved test procedures usually are not applicable to the elderly patient, since hereditary degenerations typically manifest themselves relatively early in life and are well documented by the time the patient reaches old age. For the interested reader, a review of ERG testing for receptor degenerations is available (Gouras 1970).

Electro-oculography

Electro-oculography is another electrodiagnostic test of retinal integrity. It is particularly suited for testing the status of the pigment epithelium, but it evaluates certain other parts of the retina as well. It is, like the ERG, a mass cell response, and therefore it generally does not allow fine discriminations to be made about the functional status of small retinal areas. It is less difficult to conduct than the ERG, because a contact lens electrode is not used; however, EOG testing does require a reasonable degree of patient competence, since targets must be fixated accurately (Doft, Burns, and Elsner 1982).

Principles. In the resting (dark-adapted) state, there is normally about a 6 mV difference in electrical potential between the cornea (which is positive) and the back of the eye. This "standing potential"–which is produced largely by pigment epithelial cells–varies with time in the dark, so a minimal value is reached 5 to 10 minutes after the lights are extinguished.

When the lights are turned on again, the potential increases for about 5 to 10 minutes until a peak is reached. This increase is mediated by light's striking the receptor cells and probably also involves activity of cells in the middle retinal layers.

Methods. Following dilation of the irises, five skin electrodes are attached to the patient–one at each canthus and a reference electrode at a remote location, usually the earlobe. The patient is asked to alternate fixation between two target lights 30 degrees apart. This produces an oscillating voltage at the electrodes, which is then amplified and displayed on an oscilloscope or chart recorder. This voltage is recorded for about 15 minutes in the dark, then for 15 minutes in the light. Figure 15–4 shows a schematic

representation of an EOG trace with the light peak and the dark trough indicated (to be explained in the following section).

Interpretation of Results. It is known that the magnitude of the EOG depends on the state of the eye's light/dark adaptation. By dividing the maximum potential recorded during light adaptation (the light peak) by the minimum standing potential found during dark adaptation (the dark trough), a ratio called the Arden index (AI) can be calculated. It is this value that is commonly used as a clinical indicator of eye health.

Arden and Barrada (1962) found a significant negative correlation between age and the AI in normal subjects. For normal patients less than 50 years old, Krill (1972) found that an AI less than 2.0 was abnormal; in subjects over 50 years old, a ratio of less than 1.85 was abnormal. Zollman et al. (1978) also reported decreases in the AI with age among the normal subjects; their average index was 2.20 for patients aged 20 to 35 and 1.95 for patients aged 60 to 80.

An abnormal AI (lower than what is expected for the patient's age) indicates widespread dysfunction of the retinal pigment epithelium or other retinal elements. This may be caused by a number of conditions, including malignant melanoma of the choroid (Jones et al. 1981; Staman et al. 1980), retinal detachment, acute disseminated choroiditis, vascular insufficiency, and hypertensive retinopathy (Arden, Barrada, and Kelsey 1962).

Occasionally it is of interest to determine whether asymptomatic elderly family members are carriers of hereditary diseases. Electro-oculograms provide unique information regarding genetic traits for vitelliform macular dystrophy, because patients who carry this trait (as well as those who manifest the disease) have abnormal EOGs (Berson 1981).

As has been stated, the EOG is somewhat limited in its use, because it requires relatively accurate fixation. However, it does provide an objective assessment of retinal integrity and can be critical for diagnosing certain pathologies–especially those involving the pigment epithelium.

Fluorescein Angiography

Fluorescein angiography is a special photographic technique that can be used to evaluate the vascular integrity of the choroid and retina (Behrendt 1981). Referral for angiography has

Figure 15–4

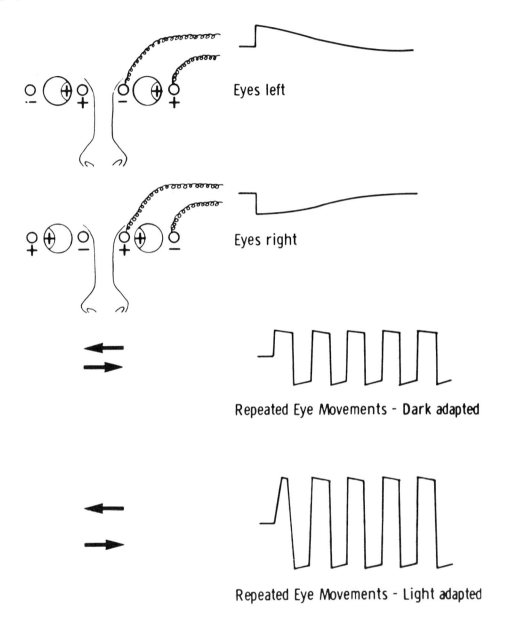

Eyes left

Eyes right

Repeated Eye Movements - Dark adapted

Repeated Eye Movements - Light adapted

Eye Movements as Indicated by the Arrows Produce an Alternating Voltage at the EOG electrodes. The amplitude of the voltage alternations is smaller in the dark (dark trough) and larger in the light (light peak).
Source: Reprinted with permission from N. R. Galloway. *Ophthalmic Electrodiagnosis.* Eastbourne, East Sussex, England: Saunders, 1975, p.23.

been suggested for patients with diabetic retinopathy, histoplasmosis, suspected malignancies, macular degeneration, disc edema, reduced visual acuity of unknown etiology, any area of retinal edema where the cause is not apparent, ischemia, and occlusion (Alexander, Sherman, and Horn 1979). These conditions are important to detect not only because of their vision-threatening consequences, but also because they may indicate similar problems occurring in other parts of the brain.

Principles and Methods. Fluorescein angiography involves taking a rapid sequence of photographs starting about 8 seconds after the injection of 500 mg of dye into the patient's hand or arm vein. As the fluorescein passes through the fundus vasculature, it is excited by flashes of light (485 to 500 nm), which cause it to emit yellow-green light (525 to 530 nm). Filters in the fundus camera select for this yellow-green light, and photographs of the fluorescing vasculature against a dark background are produced. Several such photographs are taken in seconds, allowing the examiner to observe the progressive filling and draining of the choroidal and retinal vessels (which usually takes less than 10 seconds).

The testing process is contraindicated for patients showing allergic or adverse reactions to fluorescein (about 0.6 percent, according to Stein and Parker 1971) and for those who are unable to achieve a minimum degree of fixation. Also, the photographs require a series of reasonably bright flashes delivered through the dilated pupil, and this can be uncomfortable for many patients.

Interpretation of Results. Several features of the vascular system may be studied in the angiography photographs. Disruptions in the normal laminar flow of blood in the vessels (especially the veins) can be detected; this turbulence often signals partial obstructions. The photographs also may show that some areas have more fluorescein than normal or hold the dye after it has been cleared from the rest of the retina. This suggests edema, neovascularization, hemorrhage, or decreased retinal pigment. Other areas may have less fluorescein than normal, suggesting ischemia and occlusion.

There is a negative correlation between age and the rate of filling for the retinal arteries, optic disc, and peripapillary choroid. Elderly patients typically have a slow filling rate for these tissues (Schwartz and Kern 1980), which can be interpreted as hypofluorescence if appropriate age-adjusted norms are not used. Such norms are most often developed by individual clinics and typically are based on experience rather than on published standards.

Ocular Ultrasonography

Ocular ultrasonography provides an objective assessment of the gross structural integrity of the eye. Its chief advantage over conventional techniques is that it can "see" beyond media opacities and give an indication of intraocular status. Among the pathologies that ophthalmic ultrasonography can detect and help to differentially diagnose are vitreous and subretinal hemorrhages, vitreal membranes, retinal and choroidal detachments, foreign bodies, malignant melanomas, metastatic carcinomas, hemangiomas, senile macular choroidal degeneration,

and a number of other orbital and/or ocular conditions (Coleman 1977; Coleman and Abramson 1981; Coleman and Dallow 1981b; Coleman, Lizzi, and Jack 1977; Hassani and Bard 1977; Hodes 1976; Tani, Buettner, and Robertson 1980).

Elderly patients may express concern about possible side effects associated with the use of ultrasound. Although ultrasound is potentially hazardous, average diagnostic ophthalmic ultrasound power levels are several orders of magnitude below the 2,000 to 3,000 mW/cm² required to produce pain and tissue damage. Recognized authorities in the field agree that there is now no evidence of damage caused by power levels used in diagnostic ultrasonography. However, possible cumulative effects of ultrasonic radiation have not been investigated thoroughly (Coleman, Lizzi, and Jack 1977; Posakony 1969).

Principles. Ultrasound is high-frequency sound above the range of human hearing (above 20 kHz). When ultrasound crosses a boundary between two heterogeneous tissues, some of the waves are reflected. The time it takes for this echo to return to a detector is recorded; knowing the velocity of sound in the particular ocular media involved makes it possible to calculate the distance to the reflecting boundary.

Two types of scanning techniques—A-scan and B-scan—are commonly used and yield different types of information (Coleman and Dallow 1981a). A-scan ultrasonography provides a linear representation of the eye; that is, it shows the location of tissue boundaries that would be encountered if a linear object—for example, a needle—were pierced through the eye. Typically, this information is displayed as a series of "spikes" on a time (distance) line trace on an oscilloscope. Interpretation of these spikes can allow fine discriminations between tissue types to be made and can provide distance measurements between intraocular structures.

B-scan ultrasonography provides a two-dimensional view of the eye analogous to a histological cross section. This gives a more picture-like representation of the eye and is very useful for detecting hemorrhages, tumors, and detachments. A combination of A-scan and B-scan often is used to make fine differential diagnoses of suspected pathologies.

Methods. Two general types of transducers have been developed for use with ultrasound.

Since ultrasound does not propagate well in air, one type makes direct skin contact through the closed eyelid, and the other type uses water as a contact medium. The more elaborate ultrasonography instruments can make equally spaced B-scans across the eye to provide a comprehensive series of cross sections. These are usually displayed on a cathode-ray tube and may be computer enhanced and photographed for permanent records.

Interpretation of Results. Interpretation of ultrasonography data largely involves detecting abnormal structures in the eye or orbit or determining that normal structures are displaced from their appropriate locations. Using B-Scan, structures can be viewed in relation to the rest of the eye; tumors, foreign bodies, and blood clots readily can be located. By comparing data to that from the other eye or to norms (which are often clinical impressions based on experience), tissue displacements also can be detected. Such displacements may indicate the presence of tumors, hemorrhages, or detachments.

A-scan often is used in making precise determinations of intraocular distances. Beyond detecting abnormal displacements of tissue, these distances (for example, from the cornea to the retina) have value in predicting the required power of an intraocular replacement lens.

Because of its noninvasive nature, ultrasonography can be used by various health care professionals. As computer enhancement and imaging procedures develop, this test will provide even more valuable information about orbital and ocular structures.

Tests of Whole System Integrity

If a problem is suspected in the visual system beyond the level of the retina, one of the whole system tests can be ordered. Several tests are available, including the VER, which provides an objective indication of macular function up to the level of the visual cortex. In addition, dark adaptometry, contrast sensitivity testing, and perimetry allow subjective testing of other important visual functions.

Visual Evoked Response

The VER is an electrical potential generated primarily by neurons in the visual cortex that represent the foveal region (Regan 1972). Among the applications for VERs in elderly patients are (1) noninvasive detection of optic neuritis, (2)

assessment of visual system patency, (3) preoperative prediction of postoperative visual acuity for patients with opaque media, (4) objective determination of visual acuity and refractive error, (5) objective color vision testing, and (6) objective visual field estimates (Sherman 1979; Sokol 1976). The VER recording is noninvasive, nonpainful, and requires only a minimal level of patient cooperation; this makes it possible to obtain recordings from nearly every type of patient.

Principles. Visual stimuli—either flashes of diffuse light or patterns—elicit cortical responses that can be detected via scalp electrodes placed over the occipital region of the brain. However, the VER itself is of such a small magnitude (about 5 μv) as compared with the normal electroencephalographic (EEG) "noise" (about 30 μv) that it must be specially processed before it can be analyzed. This processing is typically accomplished by using a computer that takes several samples of the VER and ensemble averages them. The result is a reduction in the amplitude of the EEG noise that accompanies the VER.

There are two major types of VER stimulus systems in current use: transient displays (in which a single, discrete change in the visual stimulus produces the response) and steady-state displays (in which the VER is produced by some continuous change in stimulus luminance, pattern, color, and so on).

The transient VER wave form has several deflections (Figure 15–5), the most clinically useful of which is the positive deflection that occurs 150 to 200 msec after the stimulus. Two characteristics of this wave—its latency (the time from stimulus presentation to peak response) and its amplitude—are of diagnostic importance.

The steady-state VER, as was mentioned, is elicited by a continuously changing stimulus such as a phase-reversing checkerboard pattern. The continuous VER that is produced is ensemble averaged to enhance the VER "signal" amplitude and reduce the EEG noise, and this results in a roughly sinusoidal VER wave form. Further computer analysis, using the fast Fourier Transform (FFT), often is performed in order to eliminate more noise. The amplitude and latency of the VER then can be measured and used in a fashion similar to corresponding data from transient stimulus presentations.

Figure 15–5

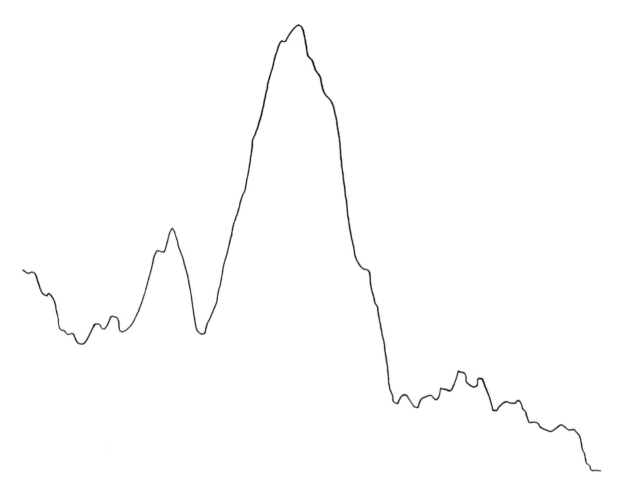

Transient VER Wave Form.

Methods. Typically, VER recording involves the attachment of at least three electrodes to the head (one on the occipital pole and one on each ear). The patient is placed in a darkened room and presented with a visual stimulus such as a bright light flash or a phase-reversing checkerboard pattern. Following computer processing, VER records are displayed on chart recorders or oscilloscopes and can be retained for reference. The recording procedure can take 20 minutes to an hour to complete, depending on the tests to be conducted.

Interpretation of Results. The VER latencies are indicators of the transmission time between stimulus presentation and visual response at the cortex. Normal latency values depend somewhat on the stimulus being presented and usually decrease as intensity increases. Thus, each laboratory establishes its own norms on a popu-

lation of subjects who are presumably free from disease, and individual patient data usually are reported as deviations from these norms. An increase in the latency of the VER is often regarded as an indication of optic neuritis, which may be due to a demyelinating disease such as multiple sclerosis (Asselman, Chadwick, and Marsden 1975). However, since latencies normally increase with the age of the patient (Celesia and Daly 1977), evaluations of latencies should be made with respect to appropriate age norms.

Theoretically, VER amplitude data can be used for several purposes. Since VERs represent primarily foveal region activity, they are especially useful for testing the patency of central vision from the retina to the cortex (Vance and Jones 1980). For elderly patients with media opacities, very bright or transscleral light flashes can be used to produce VERs (Rubin and Dawson

1978; Thompson and Harding 1978). A recordable bright-flash or transscleral VER can be a sign of potentially usable central vision, even in patients who have nonrecordable bright-flash ERGs.

When patterned stimuli are used, maximum VER amplitudes are obtained when the observer "sees" the pattern most clearly. This makes it possible to determine the patient's refractive error by simply changing lenses until the VER is maximized. Conversely, acuity can be determined by reducing the size of the elements (checks) in a checkerboard until the pattern no longer produces a VER (that is, when the pattern cannot be differentiated from a uniform field).

Other applications of the VER include the assessment of hereditary or acquired color vision losses, in which two-color checkerboards are presented (Kinney and McKay 1974), as well as the assessment of large field losses, in which stimuli are presented at various locations in the visual field (Cappin and Nissim 1975; Wolfe 1979). Neither of these procedures is totally successful with all patients, and data from VER field testing should be interpreted with particular caution if less than full-quadrant field losses are suspected (Regan and Milner 1978).

In summary, whereas VER latency data are fairly reliable and have been shown to be sensitive indicators of optic neuritis (Asselman, Chadwick, and Marsden 1975), VER amplitudes are quite variable, thus limiting the usefulness of procedures that depend on these measurements (Van Brocklin et al. 1979). VER recording, however, is the best currently available objective means of determining the patency of central vision from the retina to the visual cortex; as such, it can be a powerful diagnostic tool, especially for the noncommunicative elderly patient.

Laser Interferometry

Ophthalmic laser interferometry is a process in which low-power, coherent light beams (lasers) produce visible interference patterns directly on the retina (Green 1981). Since this process is relatively independent of the optics of the eye, it is possible to produce interference patterns with fine or gross detail even in eyes with media opacities or large refractive errors. Thus, interferometry provides a subjective means for determining the visual acuity that a patient could achieve if such problems could be eliminated. The process is not harmful (light power levels do not exceed normal daylight levels) and is especially useful for elderly patients for whom there is some question regarding whether they would benefit from cataract surgery. Totally accurate fixation is not required, since the pattern covers a relatively large retinal area, and the patient would be expected to use the part of the retina providing the maximum acuity. However, for the test to be conducted properly, the patient must be reliably responsive (unless interferometry is coupled with an objective assessment technique such as the VER; see Arden and Sheorey 1977).

Principles. Interference patterns occur when two coherent beams of light interact. In simple terms, the two beams can be thought of as alternately reinforcing (causing bright bands) and canceling each other (causing dark bands). If the ocular media are clear and homogenous, the bands thus formed are very uniform. As opacities are introduced, disruption of the pattern occurs; however, it is still possible to produce perceptible interference bands through formidably dense media. Presumably, there are enough minute spaces in such media to allow sufficient unscattered light to enter the eye to produce the patterns (Green 1970).

Methods. Commercial laser interferometers are available as attachments to certain slit lamps (Richter and Sherman 1979). Prior to testing, the patient generally is given a mydriatic to allow more light to enter the eye. Then interference bands are produced on the retina and made progressively closer together (finer) until any further reduction makes individual bands indistinguishable. This provides a measure of the best visual acuity for the patient.

The procedure may be complicated somewhat by extraneous patterns that are introduced in the presence of media opacities. These extraneous patterns sometimes may confuse elderly patients, making it necessary to help them understand which patterns they should attend to. To assure that the patient is indeed responding to the correct stimulus, an indication of the orientation of the interference bands is solicited. The band orientation is randomly varied throughout the test, and failure to indicate the proper orientation is analogous to missing a letter in Snellen acuity testing.

Interpretation of Results and Application. Recent studies show that in normal populations there is a high correlation between visual acuities obtained with laser interferometry and Snellen acuities (Green and Cohen 1971). Likewise, in a study of 150 patients (163 eyes) with cataracts complicated by retinal pathology, preoperative predictions of visual acuity agreed very well with postoperative acuities in 140 eyes (86 percent). Of the remaining 23 eyes, 21 had better postoperative acuity than expected, and 2 had unexpectedly low acuities, apparently because of pathological changes that occurred between preoperative and postoperative testing (Cohen 1976).

Laser interferometry testing is especially recommended for patients with moderate opacities and suspected macular changes, which together can result in moderately reduced visual acuity (about 20/80). For these patients laser interferometry is valuable, because it can differentiate between acuity losses that are due to media opacities and acuity losses that are due to retinal degeneration.

Dark Adaptometry
Dark adaptometry is a psychophysical method for determining the light sensitivity threshold as a function of time in the dark. Normal ranges have been established for the commonly used test equipment (Goldmann-Weekers Adaptometer made by Haag-Streit), and deviations from these norms can validate patient complaints of night vision difficulties.

Including the initial preadaptation phases, dark adaptometry usually takes at least 30 minutes to perform and requires attentiveness on the part of the patient, as well as the ability to make timely responses. Some elderly patients may find the process excessively fatiguing, and others may have difficulty concentrating on the test. These factors make it important for the clinician to exercise reasonable care in the referral of patients. Older people should be advised to get adequate rest before the procedure to increase their alertness and endurance.

Principles. A curve showing the change in light sensitivity as a function of time for a normal person is shown in Figure 15–6. There are two parts of the dark adaptation curve: the upper arm corresponds to the cone system, which is the dominant system for the first few minutes in the dark. (During this time the rod system has not yet recovered enough sensitivity to match that of the cones.) As dark adaptation progresses,

the cones become more sensitive until, after about 5 minutes, they reach a plateau. At this time a transition takes place (called the rod-cone break), after which the rods become more sensitive than the cones; overall sensitivity increases again until a final plateau is reached after approximately 20 to 30 minutes of dark adaptation.

Dark adaptometry data provide measurements of four important variables: (1) the time it takes for the rod-cone break to occur, (2) the cone threshold, (3) the rod threshold, and (4) the time to reach the final rod threshold. As aging occurs, the dark adaptation curve changes steadily, with the threshold for both rods and cones increasing. The time to the rod-cone break, however, remains constant (Pitts 1982).

Note that the ordinate scale in Figure 15–6 is in log units of light intensity. Thus, it can be seen that a small change in the patient's threshold corresponds to a marked change in intensity of the test light. Gunkel and Gouras (1963) showed that an average increase in threshold of 0.5 log units occurs between the ages of 20 and 80 years (using a white stimulus). This means that a white threshold stimulus for an 80-year-old is about three times as intense as it is for a 20-year-old.

The color of the stimulus can dramatically change the results of dark adaptometry, especially if the stimulus is at the blue end of the spectrum. For a violet stimulus, the change in the threshold of 1.8 log units between the ages of 20 and 80 years is apparently due to changes in the aging lens (Gunkel and Gouras 1963). Figure 15–7 shows the relationship between visual thresholds for various colors of stimuli and age.

Methods. Dark adaptometry procedures vary slightly, depending on the clinic and the apparatus used; however, the basics are similar especially if the standard equipment (a Goldmann-Weekers Darkadaptometer) is used. The patient often is given a mydriatic and then adapted for a fixed amount of time to a light of a standard luminance (typically, 5 minutes to a light of 1,400 to 2,100 apostilbs). The adaptation light is then extinguished, and the patient is asked to respond when he or she sees a test light that is gradually increased in intensity. As soon as the test light becomes visible, the patient responds, and the threshold is recorded as a function of time since the adaptation light was

Figure 15-6

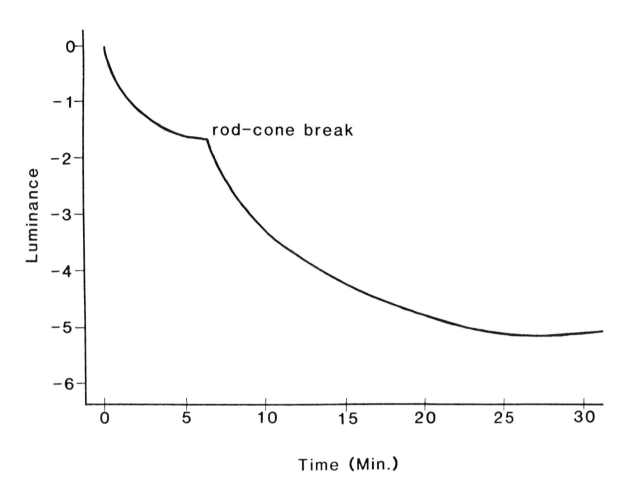

Dark Adaptation Curve Showing Light Sensitivity as a Function of Time in the Dark for a Normal Person.

extinguished. The procedure is repeated until no further decreases in threshold are found (usually about 20 to 30 minutes).

Interpretation of Results. The elderly patient who complains of night vision difficulties may or may not be experiencing normal changes that occur with aging. Possible "abnormal" causes of night vision problems in the elderly include media opacities, vitamin A deficiencies, and other metabolic difficulties. Assuming that the ocular media are clear, dark adaptometry is a method by which normal age-related changes can be distinguished from abnormal changes that may require treatment. In addition, patients who show substantial, non-treatable decreases in sensitivity can be counseled to avoid night driving and to take other appropriate steps

to avoid situations that require optimum performance in dim environments.

Contrast Sensitivity
A visual scene can be considered to be a complex amalgam of light and dark bands. These bands, or gratings, can have different spatial frequencies (the number of bands or cycles per degree of visual angle), contrasts (the ratio of the brightness of the light and dark bands), and orientations in space. Tests of Snellen acuity evaluate only sensitivity to high spatial frequencies, but most visual scenes contain low and midrange spatial frequencies, as well as high frequencies.

Loss of contrast sensitivity in the middle- and low-frequency ranges can be bewildering to the patient, as well as to the optometrist.

Figure 15-7

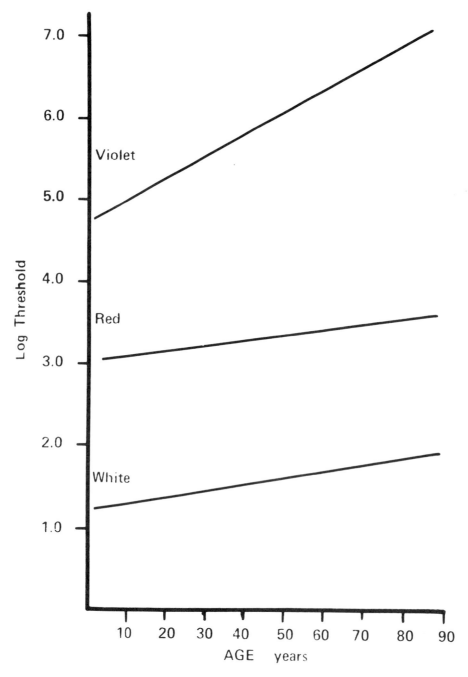

Relationship between Age and the Absolute Thresholds for Violet, Red, and White Test Lights. Note that as age increases, so does the threshold—especially for the violet stimulus. Source: Adapted with permission from R. D. Gunkel and P. Gouras, "Changes in Scotopic Visual Thresholds with Age." *Archives of Ophthalmology* 69 (1963): 5.

Visual acuity may be correctable to 20/20 but the patient may complain that "things just don't look right." Before dismissing this complaint as unimportant or "psychological," contrast sensitivity testing should be ordered, especially since decreased contrast sensitivity at various spatial frequencies has been shown to result from glaucoma, optic neuritis, cataracts, macular pathologies, and other abnormalities (Arden 1978; Arden and Gucukoglu 1978; Arden and Jacobson

1978; Arundale 1978; Lund and Lennerstrand 1981; Sjostrand and Frisen 1977; Weatherhead 1980).

The testing itself can take less than 10 minutes using Arden photographic plates (Arden 1978) or electronically produced stimuli (for example, Nicolet CS2000), but testing requires a cooperative and responsive patient. Of special importance when dealing with elderly patients is the fact that contrast sensitivity changes with age; thus, once again, appropriate norms must be used to evaluate data from these patients.

Methods. The contrast sensitivity function is obtained by presenting the patient with a series of grating patterns of different spatial frequencies. For each spatial frequency, the contrast of the pattern can be increased from subthreshold levels until the patient says, "I see the pattern," which determines the threshold. The results of these determinations then can be graphed, as Figure 15–8 shows, to form a contrast sensitivity function.

Contrast sensitivity data can be made more meaningful to ophthalmic practitioners if they are used to produce a visuogram (analogous to an audiogram). As Figure 15–9 shows, in a visuogram, the patient's response at each frequency is compared with the population norm (Bodis-Wollner 1980).

Figure 15–8

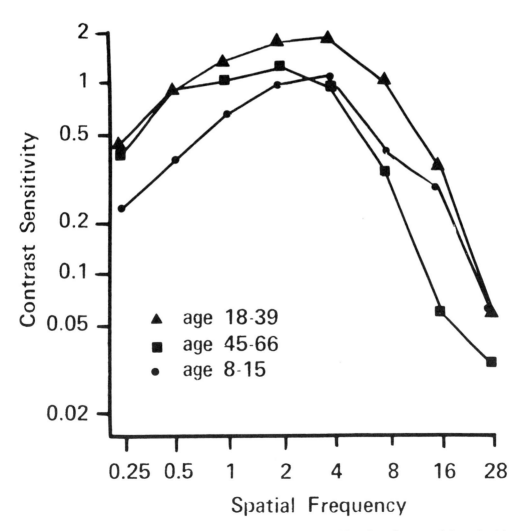

Normal Contrast Sensitivity Function. Note the changes associated with aging. Source: Adapted with permission from K. Arundale. "An Investigation into the Variation of Human Contrast Sensitivity with Age and Pathology." *British Journal of Ophthalmology* 62 (1978): 214.

Figure 15-9

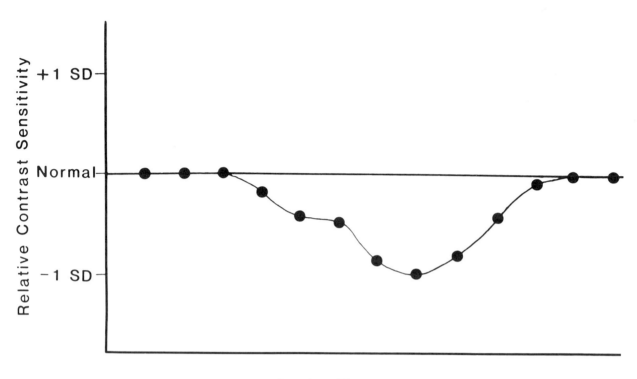

Contrast Sensitivity Data Represented by a Visuogram in which Patient's Data Are Expressed as Deviations from Normal Values. Y-axis coordinates represent plus and minus one standard deviation (SD) from the population norm. Plus indicates above-normal and minus indicates below-normal (reduced) contrast sensitivity. The patient whose data are shown has a selective loss in midrange spatial frequency contrast sensitivity.

Interpretation of Results. As indicated earlier, Snellen visual acuity is an indicator of high spatial frequency sensitivity; consequently, a loss in this part of the spatial frequency spectrum corresponds to a loss of visual acuity. Less easy to understand are the consequences of low- or midrange-frequency losses. Patients having such losses describe the sensation as being like looking through a fog or looking at a "washed out" visual scene. Figure 15–10 is an attempt at visualizing high-frequency loss (a) and low frequency loss (c), as compared with normal frequency sensitivity (b). The scene as a normal person would see it (b) contains low, medium, and high spatial frequencies. High-frequency loss (a) results in a loss of detail vision. Low-frequency loss (c) is more difficult to explain; fine details stand out, but the general shapes of large objects are lost.

Early investigations of contrast sensitivity showed little or no change with age (Arden 1978;

Arden and Jacobson 1978), but more recent investigations indicate that normal variations of the contrast sensitivity function do occur with age (Arundale 1978; Derefeldt, Lennerstrand, and Lundh 1979; Sekuler and Hutman 1980; Sekuler, Owsley, and Hutman 1982; Skalka 1980). These reports all indicate a lessening of contrast sensitivity with increasing age; however, the amount of change and the frequencies at which it occurs vary with the investigator, the apparatus used, and the testing conditions.

In summary, the available literature suggests that contrast sensitivity testing has the potential for becoming a very useful clinical tool. At present, however, the techniques for clinical assessment of contrast sensitivity are just emerging, and in some ways, it is not yet a definitive diagnostic procedure. It does, however, give some information to practitioners about the nature of patients' complaints, especially if 20/20 patients have difficulty in describing their

Figure 15–10

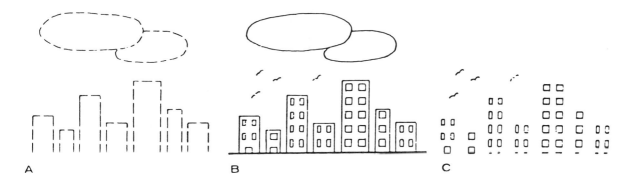

A   B   C

How High and Low Spatial Frequency Losses Affect the Perception of a City Scene. (a) A loss of high frequencies: details are missing, and the buildings and clouds are seen as gross shapes without sharp edges (dashed lines). (b) A full range of spatial frequencies is used to reproduce buildings, clouds, and birds. The general shape of the buildings and clouds (but not their edges) represent low frequencies, and the windows and birds represent high frequencies. (c) A loss of low frequencies: the details are preserved, but the overall outline of the clouds and buildings is lost. Source: Courtesy of Jurgen Meyer-Arendt, M. D., Ph.D.

problems and yet insist that "something just is not quite right with my eyes." For these patients, contrast sensitivity testing may reveal a midrange or low spatial frequency loss, but the cause of that loss would need further exploration.

Perimetry

Perimetric assessment of visual fields is often an important diagnostic procedure, especially for elderly patients whose conditions suggest glaucoma, strokes, or central nervous system lesions. Field-testing equipment ranges from the simple use of the examiner's fingers in confrontation testing to the use of complex computer-assisted devices available on a referral basis.

Principles and Methods. Perimetry can be divided into several categories based on the portion of the visual field being tested and on the nature of the test stimulus being presented. Perimeters of the bowl type are commonly used to test the entire field; the central 30 degrees can be tested with a tangent screen; and the macular region can be explored further with the Amsler grid. Testing with the Amsler grid is especially important for elderly patients, because it can reveal metamorphopsia, which can be an early sign of senile macular degeneration. Detection of this problem is especially important, since some types now can be successfully treated with laser photocoagulation (Macular Photocoagulation Study Group 1982).

Based on the nature of the stimulus presented

to the patient, field testing also can be divided into kinetic and static perimetry. Kinetic perimetry uses a moving stimulus of a constant size, color, and luminance. By determining the boundaries of the visual field in which a particular target can be seen, an isopter can be plotted. By using different target sizes or colors, several isopters can be plotted, and a contour map of the island of vision can be created (Harrington 1981). Tangent screens and Goldmann perimeters use the kinetic principle.

Static perimetry, in contrast, uses immobile targets. Several points of the visual field are selected, in which the stimulus is simply turned on and off. Typically, the stimulus presentation begins with a very low intensity that then is increased until the patient signals that he or she sees the light. Thresholds measured along various meridians can be plotted to provide cross sections of the island of vision. The Tubinger perimeter as well as a number of automated and computer-assisted devices (for example, the Fieldmaster), use the principle of static perimetry (Schindler and McCrary 1981). With the use of these computerized devices, perimetry is becoming a technicians's task in many practices. However, to completely define the defects uncovered by turnkey, computerized perimeters, the visual field ultimately must be analyzed with Goldmann perimetry, the tangent screen, or both (Harrington 1981).*

*The one current exception to this general statement appears to be the Octopus perimeter system (Gloor, Schmied, and

Static perimetry is generally considered to be more reliable than kinetic perimetry (Harrington 1981). Another advantage of static perimetry is that retinal edema can be detected at an early stage by measuring and comparing visual fields obtained under mesopic and photopic conditions; kinetic perimetry is not as sensitive an indicator of these subtle retinal changes (Greve, Bos, and Bakker 1976).

When considering the various options for perimetry referral of elderly patients, it must be realized that automated visual field testers may not work well with many elderly patients, because computers tend to be inflexible and unresponsive to the special needs of the older person. Elderly patients may be slow responders and may fatigue easily, requiring sensitivity, flexibility, and innovation on the part of the perimetrist (Goodlow 1981). Thus, when ordering field testing, it would be well not to specify the exact instrumentation to be used (thus allowing the perimetrist more flexibility), but rather to indicate the purpose of the testing and the general nature of the defect to be explored. In this way, the perimetrist will be able to deal creatively with the special needs of the elderly patient and obtain the best visual field information possible.

Interpretation of Results. The normal visual field shrinks with age, apparently in a continuous process starting in youth and proceeding on through senescence (Drance, Berry, and Hughes 1967). Until about age 50, the visual field size decreases slowly; after 60 years, however, shrinkage becomes much more apparent, particularly in the temporal fields (Wolf and Nadroski 1971). The changes may be due to yellowing of the lens, changes in positions of the upper lids and/or the globe, neuroretinal decay, and artifacts that are due to delays in reaction time (Drance, Berry, and Hughes 1967).

Normal changes must be considered when evaluating perimetry data from elderly patients. In addition, consideration should be given to the transparency (or lack of transparency) of the patient's ocular media. To aid in making the

subtle distinction between cataractous visual field changes and those caused by other pathological conditions such as glaucoma, Radius (1978) determined threshold isopters for five standard test stimuli in 148 eyes with varying degrees of cataractous lens changes. By correlating visual acuity with standard isopters (obtained with the Goldmann perimeter), Radius constructed a series of expected visual fields for patients with cataracts. By using these norms, it may be possible to detect subtle field changes that are due to complicating pathologies in elderly patients with cataracts.

Conclusions

Special testing procedures offer the ophthalmic practitioner the opportunity to gain diagnostic insight beyond that afforded by conventional techniques. Difficulties that are frequently encountered among elderly patients, such as media opacities and communication difficulties, often can be overcome by ordering appropriate special tests.

To select appropriate tests for elderly patients, their particular needs must be considered carefully. Subjective special tests such as perimetry, contrast sensitivity, and dark adaptometry depend on the ability of the patient to respond in a timely and reliable fashion. Certain objective tests also have special requirements; the EOG, for example, requires adequate fixation ability and relatively reliable eye movements. If there is some doubt as to the appropriateness of a particular test, consultation should be made with the laboratory or technician performing the test or tests.

Interpretation of the test results is perhaps the most critical area. The visual systems of elderly patients have undergone natural aging changes, and this makes it necessary to compare test results with population norms specific for the patients' ages.

Previous sections indicated changes that can be expected with aging, but the actual values that should be considered normal for a particular age group often depend on the specific clinic in which the test is performed. This is particularly true with electrodiagnostic testing. Each clinic tends to have its own particular testing routine and apparatus, and small differences can affect test values significantly. Therefore, the optometrist should consult with the particular clinic and inquire about the age norms that have been established in that clinic.

Fassler 1980). Studies have shown that this computer-assisted system is more sensitive in detecting field loss than manual perimetry in about 80 percent of glaucomatous eyes that were examined (Harrington 1981, 25). This expensive, elaborate system takes a minimum of 17 minutes to examine each eye, which is comparable to the time it takes for a well-done Goldmann field examination (Harrington 1981, 26).

If the clinic has no norms for elderly patients, data must be interpreted with caution.

With the appropriate use of special tests, ophthalmic practitioners can monitor and manage pathological cases more effectively, offer their elderly patients superior counseling regarding contemplated surgery for media opacity removal, and provide elderly patients who have special needs with a more extensive assessment of their visual health and function.

References

Alexander, A.; J. Sherman; and D. Horn. "Fundus Fluorescein Angiography: A Summary of Theoretical Concepts and Clinical Applications." *Journal of the American Optometric Association* 50, no. 1 (1979): 53–63.

Arden, G. B. "The Importance of Measuring Contrast Sensitivity in Cases of Visual Disturbance." *British Journal of Ophthalmology* 62 (1978): 198–209.

Arden, G. B., and A. Barrada. "Analysis of the Electro-oculograms of a Series of Normal Subjects." *British Journal of Ophthalmology* 46 (1962): 468–482.

Arden, G. B.; A. Barrada; and J. H. Kelsey. "New Clinical Test of Retinal Function Based upon the Standing Potential of the Eye." *British Journal of Ophthalmology* 46 (1962): 449–467.

Arden, G. B., and A. G. Gucukoglu. "Grating Test of Contrast Sensitivity in Patients with Retrobulbar Neuritis." *Archives of Ophthalmology* 96 (1978): 1626–1629.

Arden, G. B., and J. J. Jacobson. "A Simple Grating Test for Contrast Sensitivity: Preliminary Results Indicate Value in Screening for Glaucoma. *Investigative Ophthalmology* 17, no. 1 (1978): 23–32.

Arden, G. B., and U. B. Sheorey. "The Assessment of Visual Function in Patients with Opacities: A New Evoked Potential Method Using a Laser Interferometer." In *Visual Evoked Potentials in Man: New Developments*, ed. J. E. Desmedt. Oxford: Clarendon Press, 1977.

Armington, J. C. *The Electroretinogram.* New York: Academic Press, 1974.

Arundale, K. "An Investigation into the Variation of Human Contrast Sensitivity with Age and Pathology." *British Journal of Ophthalmology* 62 (1978): 213–215.

Asselman, P.; D. W. Chadwick; and C. D. Marsden. "Visual Evoked Responses in the Diagnosis and Management of Patients Suspected of Multiple Sclerosis." *Brain* 98 (1975): 261–282.

Behrendt, T. "Fluorescein Angiography." In *Clinical Ophthalmology*, Vol. 3, ed. T. D. Duane. New York: Harper & Row, 1981, chap. 4.

Berson, E. L. "Electrical Phenomena in the Retina." In *Adler's Physiology of the Eye: Clinical Application,* ed. R. A. Moses. St. Louis: Mosby, 1981.

Bodis-Wollner, I. "Detection of Visual Defects Using the Contrast Sensitivity Function." In *Electophysiology and Psychophysics: Their Use in Ophthalmic Diagnosis,* ed. S. Sokol. Boston: Little, Brown, 1980.

Cappin, J. M., and S. Nissim. "Visual Evoked Responses in the Assessment of Field Defects in Glaucoma." *Archives of Ophthalmology* 93 (1975): 9–18.

Carr, R. E., and I. M. Siegal. *Visual Electrodiagnostic Testing.*

Baltimore: Williams & Wilkins, 1982.

Celesia G. G., and R. F. Daly. "Effects of Aging on Visual Evoked Responses." *Archives of Neurology* 34 (1977): 403–407.

Cohen, M. M. "Laser Interferometry: Evaluation of Potential Visual Acuity in the Presence of Cataracts." *Annals of Ophthalmology* 8, no. 7 (1976): 845–849.

Coleman, D. J. "Ultrasonic Evaluation of the Vitreous." In *Vitreous Surgery and Advances in Fundus Diagnosis and Treatment.* ed. H. M. Freeman, T. Hirose, and C. L. Schepens. New York: Appleton-Century-Crofts, 1977.

Coleman, D. J., and D. H. Abramson. "Ocular Ultrasonography." In *Clinical Ophthalmology*, Vol. 2, ed. T. D. Duane. New York: Harper & Row, 1981, chap. 26.

Coleman, D. J., and R. L. Dallow. "Introduction to Ophthalmic Ultrasonography." In *Clinical Ophthalmology*, Vol. 2, ed. T. D. Duane. New York: Harper & Row, 1981, chap. 25. (a)

Coleman, D. J., and R. L. Dallow. "Orbital Ultrasonography." In *Clinical Ophthalmology*, Vol. 2, ed. T. D. Duane. New York: Harper & Row, 1981, chap. 27. (b)

Coleman, D. J.; E. L. Lizzi; and R. L. Jack. *Ultrasonography of the Eye and Orbit.* Philadelphia: Lea and Febiger, 1977.

Derefeldt, G.; G. Lennerstrand; and B. Lundh. "Age Variations in Normal Human Contrast Sensitivity." *Acta Ophthalmologica* 57 (1979): 679–689.

Doft, B. H.; S. A. Burns; and A. Elsner. " The Inverse Electro-Oculogram." *British Journal of Ophthalmology* 62 (1982): 379–381.

Drance, S. M.; V. Berry; and A. Hughes. "Studies on the Effects of Age on the Central and Peripheral Isopters of the Visual Field in Normal Subjects." *American Journal of Ophthalmology* 63, no. 6 (1967):1667–1672.

Fiorentini, A.; L. Maffei; M. Pirchio; D. Spinelli; and V. Porciatti. "The ERG in Response to Alternating Gratings in Patients with Diseases of Peripheral Visual Pathway." *Investigative Ophthalmology* 21, no. 3 (1981): 490–493.

Fuller D. G.; R. W. Knighton; and R. Machemer. "Bright-Flash Electroretinography for the Evaluation of Eyes with Opaque Vitreous." *American Journal of Ophthalmology* 80, no. 2 (1975): 214–223.

Galloway, N. R. *Ophthalmic Electrodiagnosis.* Philadelphia: Saunders, 1975.

Gloor, B.; U. Schmied; and A. Fassler. "Changes of Glaucomatous Field Defects: Degree of Accuracy with the Automatic Perimeter Octopus." *International Ophthalmology* 3, no. 1 (1980): 5–10.

Goodlaw, E. I. " Assessing Field Defects of the Low-Vision Patient." *American Journal of Optometry and Physiological Optics* 58, no. 6 (1981): 486–490.

Gouras, P. "Electroretinography: Some Basic Principles." *Investigative Ophthalmology* 9, no. 8 (1970): 557–569.

Green, D. G. " Testing the Vision of Cataract Patients by Means of Laser-generated Interference Fringes." *Science* 168 (1970): 1240–1242.

Green, D. G. "Laser Devices in Measuring Visual Acuity." In *Clinical Ophthalmology*, Vol. 1, ed. T. D. Duane. New York: Harper & Row, 1981, chap. 66.

Green, D. G., and M. M. Cohen. "Laser Interferometry in the Evaluation of Potential Macular Function in the Presence of Opacities in The Ocular Media." *Transactions of the American Academy of Ophthalmology and Otolaryngology* 75, no. 1 (1971): 629–637.

Greve, E.; P. Bos; and D. Bakker. "Photopic and Mesopic Central Static Perimetry in Maculopathies and Central Neuropathies." *Documenta Ophthalmologica Proceedings* 14 (1976): 243–257.

Gunkel, R. D., and P. Gouras. "Changes in Scotopic Visual Thresholds with Age." *Archives of Ophthalmology* 69 (1963): 4–9.

Harrington, D. O. "*The Visual Fields: A Textbook and Atlas of Clinical Perimetry.* St. Louis: Mosby, 1981.

Hassani, S. N., and R. Bard. "Evaluating the Eye through Ultrasonography." *Geriatrics* 32, no. 10 (1977): 94–95, 99–101.

Hirose, T. "Evaluation of Retinal Function in the Presence of Vitreous Opacities." In *Vitreous Surgery and Advances in Fundus Diagnosis and Treatment.* ed. H. M. Freeman, T. Hirose, and C. L. Schepens. New York: Appleton-Century-Crofts, 1977.

Hodes, B. L. "Eye Disorders: Using Ultrasound in Ophthalmologic Diagnosis." *Postgraduate Medicine* 59, no. 4 (1976): 197–203.

Jones, R. M.; R. Klein; G. DeVenecia; and F. L. Myers. "Abnormal Electro-oculograms from Eyes with a Malignant Melanoma of the Choroid." *Investigative Ophthalmology* 20, no. 2 (1981): 276–279.

Kinney, J. S., and C. L. McKay. "Test of Color-Defective Vision Using the Visual Evoked Response." *Journal of the Optical Society of America* 64, no. 9 (1974): 1244–1250.

Krill, A. E. *Hereditary Retinal and Choroidal Diseases.* New York: Harper & Row, 1972.

Lundh, B. L., and G. Lennerstrand. "Eccentric Contrast Sensitivity Loss in Glaucoma." *Acta Ophthalmologica* 59 (1981): 21–23.

Macular Photocoagulation Study Group. "Argon Laser Photocoagulation for Senile Macular Degeneration: Results of a Randomized Clinical Trial." *Archives of Ophthalmology* 100 (1982): 912–918.

Pitts, D. G. "Dark Adaptation and Aging." *Journal of the American Optometric Association* 53, no. 1 (1982): 37–41.

Posakony, G. J. "Ultrasonic Transducers and Acoustic Waves." In *Ophthalmic Ultrasound: An International Symposium.* ed. K. A. Gitter. St. Louis: Mosby, 1969.

Radius, R. L. "Perimetry in Cataract Patients." *Archives of Ophthalmology* 96 (1978): 1574–1579.

Regan, D. *Evoked Potentials in Psychology, Sensory Physiology and Clinical Medicine.* London: Chapman and Hall, 1972.

Regan, D., and B. A. Milner. "Objective Perimetry by Evoked Potential Recording: Limitations." *Electroencephalography and Clinical Neurophysiology* 44 (1978): 393–397.

Richter, S. J., and J. Sherman. "Electro-oculography, Dark Adaptometry, and Laser Interferometry." *Journal of the American Optometric Association* 50 no. 1 (1979): 101–104.

Rubin, M. L., and W. W. Dawson. "The Transscleral VER: Prediction of Post-operative Acuity." *Investigative Ophthalmology* 17, no. 1 (1978): 71–77.

Schindler, S., and J. A. McCrary. "Automated Perimetry in Neurophthalmolgic Practice." *Annal of Ophthalmology* 13, no. 6 (1981): 691–697.

Schwartz, B., and J. Kern. "Age, Increased Ocular and Blood Pressures, and Retinal and Disc Fluorescein Angiogram." *Archives of Ophthalmology* 98 (1980): 1980–1986.

Sekuler, R., and L. P. Hutman. "Spatial Vision and Aging, 1: Contrast Sensitivity." *Journal of Gerontology* 35, no. 5 (1980): 692–699.

Sekuler R.; C. Owsley; and L. Hutman. "Assessing Spatial Vision of Older People." *American Journal of Optometry and Physiological Optics.* 59, no. 12 (1982): 961–968.

Sherman, J. "Visual Evoked Potential (VEP): Basic Concepts and Clinical Applications." *Journal of the American Optometric Association* 50, no. 1 (1979): 19–30.

Sjostrand, J., and L. Frisen. "Contrast Sensitivity in Macular Disease: A Preliminary Report." *Acta Ophthalmologica* 55 (1977): 507–512.

Skalka, H. W. "Effect of Age on Arden Grating Acuity." *British Journal of Ophthalmology* 64 (1980): 21–23.

Sokol, S. "Visually Evoked Potentials: Theory, Techniques and Clinical Applications." *Survey of Ophthalmology* 21, no. 1 (1976): 18–44.

Staman, J. A.; C. R. Fitzgerald; W. W. Dawson; M. C. Barris; and I. Hood. "The EOG and Choroidal Malignant Melanomas." *Documenta Ophthalmologica* 49 (1980): 201–209.

Stein, M. R., and C. W. Parker. "Reactions Following Intravenous Fluorescein." *American Journal of Ophthalmology* 75, no. 5 (1971): 861–868.

Tani, P. M.; H. Buettner; and D. M. Robertson. "Massive Vitreous Hemorrhage and Senile Macular Choroidal Degeneration." *American Journal of Ophthalmology* 90 (1980): 525–533.

Thompson, C. R. S., and G. F. A. Harding. "The Visual Evoked Potential in Patients with Cataracts." *Documenta Ophthalmologica Proceedings* 15 (1978): 193–201.

Van Brocklin, M. D.; R. R. Hirons; W. H. Langfield; and R. L. Yolton. "The Visual Evoked Response: Reliability Revisited." *Journal of the American Optometric Association* 50, no. 12 (1979): 1371–1379.

Vance, J. R., and R. Jones. "Central Visual Field Contributions to the Visual-Evoked Response." *American Journal of Optometry and Physiological Optics* 57, no. 4 (1980): 197–204.

Weatherhead, R. G. "Use of Arden Grating Test for Screening." *British Journal of Ophthalmology* 64 (1980): 591–596.

Weleber, R. G. "The Effect of Age on Human Cone and Rod Ganzfeld Electroretinograms." *Investigative Ophthalmology* 20, no. 3 (1981): 392–399.

Wolf, E., and A. S. Nadroski. " Extent of the Visual Field: Changes with Age and Oxygen Tension." *Archives of Ophthalmology* 86 (1971): 637–642.

Wolfe, P. "Utilizing the Visual Evoked Response (VER) for Visual Fields When Subjective Responses Are Not Attainable." *Journal of the American Optometric Association* 50, no. 1 (1979): 117–118.

Zollman, R.; L. Cary; S. Dippel; and R. L. Yolton. "The Effects of Patient Age on Electroretinogram and Electro-oculogram Signals." *Review of Optometry* 115, no. 1 (1978): 46–48.

Chapter 16

The Vision Care Professional and Institutional Settings

Lorraine G. Hiatt

The vision care professional working in an institution is dealing not with one client, but with several levels of professionals and decision makers. The successful treatment of individual needs often requires that the professional successfully work with administration, those involved with reimbursement, nurses, and possibly occupational therapists to maximize services to the individual. As a result of this groundwork, it may be efficient for the professional to provide services to a number of clients within the institutional facility. From the residents' point of view, the organizational and financial complexities of the institutional setting often stand between their needs and their treatment.

Ideally, one vision care professional should follow each person throughout life, providing necessary examinations and treatment. In practice this seldom happens. If older people receive treatment at all (and there is much evidence to suggest that people in institutions do not receive vision care), they typically encounter a vision care specialist who is new to them.

This chapter will outline some techniques for working with and through an institution to successfully serve the vision needs of the older person. By planning ahead and becoming well versed in institutional systems, the vision care professional may go a long way toward achieving a much-needed objective—meeting the vision needs of older people throughout life, including the time in institutional settings.

What Are Institutions?

The term *institution* used here refers to facilities where the predominant services are supervised by a licensed nurse, where nursing assistance is available 24 hours per day, and where the majority of residents (a term preferable to *patients*) are past age 60. In the United States, these institutions typically are called nursing homes, although most states distinguish between *skilled nursing homes* and *intermediate care nursing homes* on the subtle basis of the number of nursing supervisors and assistants available. Unlike hospitals, in nursing homes physicians typically have played a limited role in the daily routine and might visit a single patient as seldom as once a month or once every three months. Each state has its own regulations for the staffing and treatments that can be offered in nursing homes. The people served in nursing homes tend to have three or more chronic conditions, often affecting agility, sensory function, and mental clarity. In some communities, nursing homes are called *rest homes, geriatric centers, convalescent homes,* or *extended care facilities.* In Canada and Great Britain, they may be called *nursing homes* or *homes for the aged.* Typically, the average length of stay ranges from three to five years; however, as many as 25 percent of the people in some facilities stay for a much shorter time.

This discussion has left out apartments specially built for older people, as well as adult homes, where residents tend to be more mobile and able to go to a clinician's office for vision care.

Issues for the Vision Care Professional in Providing Services to Institutions

Vision care professionals need to discuss four major topics with the appropriate managers and staff of an institution:

1. *Policy.* Does the institution have a vision care policy?
2. *Cooperation.* What support or assistance

does the vision care professional need from the nursing, occupational therapy, or social work staff for the examinations and any necessary follow-up or referrals?

3. *Translation and transfer of diagnostic data.* How can the information collected by the vision care specialist be useful in working with the older person?

4. *Institutional program and design.* Will the institutional staff commit itself to working with the vision care professional on methods of (a) realizing the fullest potential of the residents' visual senses, (b) developing and offering ongoing educational programs, and (c) adopting appropriate environmental design amenities?

State of the Art: Vision Care in Institutions

The vision care of older people is often the exception rather than the practice (Cullinan 1979; Silver et al. 1978; *Vision and Aging* 1981; Woodruff and Pack 1980). Once they are in institutions, older people's evaluation of sensory functions appear to be superseded by other physical or mental considerations (Berkowitz et al. 1979). In one study, fewer than 5 percent of all institutionalized older people had had their vision evaluated during their institutional stay (Leslie and Greenberg 1974); in another, 81 percent had no previous record of eye care during an average of five years in an institution (Snyder, Pyrek and Smith 1976).

Despite the fact that countries like the United States currently have no regulations requiring vision screening of older people in institutions, available data indicate that people do benefit from examinations and treatment (Cullinan 1978a, 1979; Miller 1974; Snyder, Pyrek and Smith 1976).

In the few institutions that have provided facility-wide vision evaluations, follow-up has been characterized as incomplete or inadequate (Cohen 1969; Miller 1974; Milne and Williamson 1972; Newman 1977; Snyder, Pyrek and Smith 1976), often resulting in statistical summaries rather than appropriate optical aids or services.

Policies are weak with regard to more general vision needs of institutionalized older people as well (*Vision and Aging* 1981). In the United States, there are no requirements that institutions improve lighting, reduce glare, or offer available supplemental reading materials. However, research indicates that environmental amenities would maximize the residual vision of many older adults (Fozard 1981).

The lack of policy-inspired vision care seems to coincide with the older person's conception that "to use it is to lose it" (Cullinan 1979; Silver et al. 1978). Older people may give up, substituting social activities or even inactivity for close work in an effort to "save their sight."

Why Should Vision Care Be Brought to Institutions?

Should the vision care professional "bother" with people in institutions? Are they not too far gone? Whereas it is clear that all residents of a nursing home do not need evaluation and treatment, and all may not benefit from it, the tendency to write off nursing home patients is a gross error. There is clear evidence that the majority of people who receive vision treatment do benefit, even to the point of minimizing the effects of memory impairment (Snyder, Pyrek, and Smith 1976; Woodruff and Pack 1980). The greater the multiple handicap, the more significant vision becomes to self-reliance and independent living (Hiatt 1981a).

It has been estimated that in the United States, on any given day, approximately 4 percent of all elderly people are in nursing homes; this represents over one million people. However, during their life span, perhaps 48 percent of the elderly will receive long-term care in a nursing home or related facility. This implies that the institution may be a focal point of health care; there, professionals knowledgeable about a full range of individual abilities can jointly consider the interaction of vision with, for example, manual dexterity, hearing, mobility, mental status, communication, and long-term prognosis.

Older people in U.S. institutions are four times as likely to have vision impairments as those in households (Peterson and Kirchner 1980; *Vision and Aging* 1981). This suggests that the institutionalized population is not only in need of vision care, but that vision care may be a factor in reducing unnecessary nursing home placement.

Tapping the market of older people has not been easy for vision care professionals. Difficulties in working with institutions, travel, the availability of facilities, follow-through, and the complexity of reimbursement sometimes have been interpreted as a lack of interest. Added to that problem is the fact that older people and their families have not demanded services (Cullinan 1978b). The more the public becomes informed about aging and about the potential improvement available through vision care, the more the vision specialist is likely to hear more vocal demand for services within an institution.

Some of the key issues in serving people from nursing homes have been the lack of mobility, agility, and endurance of the older person. This has made office visits too taxing for many. Furthermore, difficulties in communication due to hearing impairments, aphasia, or attentional deficits may render the older person less responsive or more difficult to communicate with. Working on-site, with the assistance of institutional staff, may overcome many of these difficulties. Individual testimonials of professionals who have made the effort to work in nursing homes are interesting and very compelling (Cohen 1969; Cullinan 1978a; Leslie and Greenberg 1974; Newman 1977; Sartoris 1975; Woodruff and Pack 1980). There is satisfaction in facilitating close work or mobility for a person who thought these were long-gone skills.

There is increasing evidence, at least in the United States, of emerging economic incentives and third-party payments, if only on a state-by-state basis. The care of vision (and hearing) has not been reimbursed for the indigent in many parts of the world. However, as the benefits of care are more widely communicated and costs are more clearly defined, there probably will be payment for time spent in the care of older people (contact the American Optometric Association and the American Public Health Association Committee on Low Vision for current details).

Developing a Vision Care Policy

A vision care policy can awaken demand, as well as develop and describe services. It is a corporate statement about the importance of vision care and treatment. The policy should identify for staff, as well as older people, the types of services that constitute such treatment.

For many institutions, preparing such a statement will be very educational, allowing staff members to update their knowledge about vision and aging. Policy statements also may be useful in coordinating the terms used to describe people with varying degrees of vision loss, establishing adequate services, and lining up payment methods.

The vision care specialist may offer to take a leadership role or to serve as a consultant in the development of the policy statement. In any case, the specialist should be prepared to offer suggestions on the following:

1. Who should be examined? Are some of the older people too frail, ill, confused, or otherwise unlikely to benefit from vision care?
2. What should be evaluated and by what methods?
3. Who should be involved in making the evaluations? In working with older people prior to and following the examinations?
4. When should vision evaluations be made? Before or at admission? When health status changes? On an annual basis?
5. How can information be most meaningfully translated from the examination to the overall care plan developed for each person?
6. How will various procedures and services be paid for?

Roles of the Institutional Staff

The institution's staff may have skills and experience that can greatly facilitate both individual and group examinations. In one facilitywide vision evaluation of over 250 older people, the staff provided the services described in the following five sections (Snyder, Pyrek, and Smith 1976).

Planning. Nurse administrators planned an in-service education program—attended by vision care specialists—describing the examination procedures. (Some information was based on Jolicoeur 1970 and Pastalan 1976.) Since the permission of attending physicians was required to make these evaluations, they were also invited; general questions were answered. The seminar was adapted and repeated for older persons, interested family members, and staff members of other departments.

The institution's medical director, social worker, and vision care specialist collaborated on the drafting of a formal letter informing attending physicians of the proposed evaluations and requesting their permission. The institution's billing department mailed the letter in the monthly correspondence to physicians.

Scheduling. Nurses scheduled the older people for appointments, assigned nursing assistants to transport older persons to the examination area, and kept the flow of people constant and controlled.

Transfer, Communication, and Clinical Assistance. One nurse, who was experienced in orthopedics, was assigned to the examination room. She assisted with the necessary transfer of people (for example, from wheelchair to examining chair, or wheelchair to examining table). Because she knew the older people, she could ease the conversation and set an example for the vision care specialist regarding any special communication needs. This nurse also assisted with procedures such as use of drops.

Responding to and Referring Questions. Older people raised many questions following the examinations. Some were expressed while the doctor was present; others did not occur to residents until a day or two later. The staff members were encouraged to respond within their experience and to raise questions with the vision care specialist.

Follow-up. Follow-up was the shared responsibility of the vision care specialist, attending physician, nurse, and social worker. It was coordinated weekly (except in emergencies).

The following is a list of some of the follow-up tasks and the staff members involved. Note that volunteers also were used.

1. Obtaining optical aids (vision care specialists, occupational therapists, or both).
2. Training in and practicing the use of optical aids (occupational therapists).
3. Alerting the vision care specialist to problems in optical aids or other interventions as well as to changes in vision-related abilities (all staff, especially nurses, activities therapists, and occupational therapists).
4. Setting up small groups to help older people cope with diminished vision (social workers, occupational therapists, nursing assistants, and volunteers). For examples of group work, see Carroll (1978); Jolicoeur (1970); Kimbrough, Heubner, and Lowry (1976). For a discussion of self-help programs, see Hiatt et al. (1982).
5. Providing specific skill training in activities of daily living (occupational therapists). See Yeadon and Grayson (1979).
6. Teaching older people to keep their spectacles clean; assisting with cleaning and storage (nursing assistants).
7. Locating and arranging for related services, including large print matter, Talking Books, volunteer readers or writer, and communication aids (librarians, activities staff, and volunteers). See American Foundation for the Blind (1982); Hale (1979); Mellor (1981); Vision Foundation (1980).
8. Assisting individuals in appropriately using their vision, including eye-resting techniques (occupational therapists under the direction of vision care professionals). See Padula and McQueen (1982).

The institution's research department prepared data on the needs of the entire population, and a presentation was made to a committee of department heads (for the purpose of planning) and to staff and families (who were interested in the highlights and the recommendations of the vision specialist).

Translation of Clinical Data into Services and Design

The most challenging task in the evaluation process was the translation of specific clinical findings into practical information as requested by caregivers and older people themselves.

Older people living in institutions, unlike those living in their own households, are often not fully responsible for what they do or for the design of facilities. Therefore, findings from the examination will need to be translated quite specifically into items that the individual may accomplish and those that caregivers or management must deal with.

Table 16–1 summarizes information of practical interest to older people and their caregivers and may be used as a case-by-case discussion guide. Table 16–2 illustrates a sample charting format that staff members might use to keep track of clinical information in functional terms, and Table 16–3 is an example of such a chart filled out. Written forms of information are helpful in institutions where many caregivers are involved with the older person. Institutions often have a relatively high staff turnover rate, so recording practical information resulting from a vision examination will help offer continuity in care despite changes in caregivers. However, there is no substitute for face-to-face meetings, where staff from recreation, dietary, or nursing departments might meet with the vision care specialist to discuss ways in which their services should be tailored to maximize older people's residual vision. To present such information solely to nurses or managers is to deny the other departments and family members information essential to responding to individual needs. Meetings with staff and family members may be particularly important when older individuals

Table 16-1
Supplemental Information Needed from Vision Examinations
on Older People in Institutions: A Team Planning Guide

1. Near Vision
   - How would this affect the person's ability to read?
   - What are the implications for dining or self-feeding?
   - What are the implications for dressing, grooming, and personal hygiene? Raise similar questions with respect to the activities and preferences of the individual (playing table games, taking medications, and so on).

2. Far Vision
   - How does this influence the person's ability to recognize faces?
   - What are the implications for residents' finding their way to the bedroom, bathroom, dining room, nurses' station, front entry, and so on?
   - What does this mean about participation in large-group social events, films, chapel, and so on? How should the person be positioned or seated?
   - If residents watch television, will their viewing be affected?
   - Raise similar questions for the person's other indoor and outdoor interests.

3. Mobility
   - How might vision influence standing, walking, or wheeling?
   - Will the person's mobility be different during days or nights?
   - Might vision be a factor in disorientation? In wandering?
   - Consider the mobility implications of on-unit, off-unit, outdoor, and motor excursions. Integrate this with plans for physical therapy and exercise.

4. Fear, Security, Fire/Life Safety
   - Are any aspects of vision loss likely to contribute to fear (real, imagined, or hallucinated), anxieties, or depression? How should we be dealing with this (Burnside 1976; Jolicoeur 1970)?
   - Do any particular measures need to be taken to secure personal safety or security in terms of accidents, victimization, or vulnerability?
   - What are the implications of this condition for fire evacuation, training, precautions needed for icy conditions and thunder storms, bathing techniques, and nighttime care?

5. Sensitivities
   - What are the implications of the person's vision for glare sensitivity?
   - What effects have vision changes had on the person's ability to differentiate and name colors? To respond to color contrasts?
   - How has the person's peripheral vision been affected?
   - Is the person susceptible to distorted perceptions, mirages, or accidents resulting from differences in lighting levels? Can the person move and adjust easily between dark and bright areas, inside and out? What about sunlight?
   - Consider other sensitivities: drug/vision factors, lacrimation, and so on.

6. Special Implications of Eye Conditions, Diseases, or Related Topics
   - Do the residents understand their vision condition? How do they feel about changing the ways they do things or the optical aids they use? What are their reactions to any correction, follow-up, or surgical procedures?
   - How might other factors influence vision (stroke, vertigo, irregularities of eyelids, posture, musculoskeletal conditions, hearing, sensitivity to touch, and pain)?

Table 16–2
Prototypical Resident Chart on Functional Aspects of Vision

	Clinical Results	Patients' Knowledge Staff Approaches	Implications for Correction/Aids	Positioning	Activities/ Environment
Near Vision a. Reading b. Eating c. Dressing d.					
Far Vision a. Faces b. Find Room? c. Group Events d.					
Mobility					
Fear/Security/Protection					
Sensitive? a. Glare b. Color c. Peripheral d. Shadows/Transitions e.					
Special Conditions/ Other Impairments					

Name _____ Unit/Room _____ Date _____ By _____
I.D. _____   Follow-up _____

Table 16-3
Sample of Completed Resident Chart

	Clinical Results	Patients' Knowledge Staff Approaches	Implications for Correction/Aids	Positioning	Activities/ Environment
See M.D./O.D. report Near Vision					
a. Reading	Assistance needed.	Not sure. OT to speak with her by 11/1 about options.	Best correction as is; keep glasses clean of sweat and ointment!	Sees best in room w/book on table; needs to lean close for fine work.	Family to bring 3-way lamp; paper-backs easier. Try 1 course at a time.
b. Eating	Training needed.	Aides and dietary to work with her. OK by self. See▶			
c. Dressing	Some adaptation.		She's trying magnifier + light for bills.		Family got ting some larger closures.
d. Financial	Volunteer requested.	Trusted friend helps.			
Far Vision		Staff are aware she has difficulties at greater than 8 feet.	Dr. says not much more can be done.		
a. Faces	Staff to adjust.				
b. Find Room?	Training needed at night.	Knows when she has problems. Staff practice and learn cues with her. Activities will try having some slide shows; easier for her to see.			
c. Group Events	Some adaptation.			Seat at front, esp. for candle-light services.	
d. Chapel	Clergy to adjust.				
Mobility Unstable, walks on unit, wheels to dine. Wants to be able to go out with family.		PT meeting with orientation and mobility instructor from Lighthouse; start training next wk.	Possible that she can use her walker for both needs; PT and O&M to try this with her.	Combine walk'g on unit with wheeling to dining so she learns her way.	
Fear/Security/Protection	More info needed	Night staff think some of her night-mares may be from vis. Trying night light + TLC + talk.			Wants flash-light. Family agreed to supply. Lent her one in meantime.
Sensitive?					
a. Glare	Assistance needed.	She pointed problems out to us, is helping us help her.	Has sunglasses; noted on ward-robe that she should wear outside. Seat in shade or No. entry.	Has glare prob. for bingo in dining room. Staff will position her.	
b. Color	Referral.				
c. Peripheral					
d. Shadows/Transitions		Psych. to test 10/11.			
e.					
Special Conditions/ Other Impairments	More info needed	CVA, being observed for changing symptoms.			

Name __Della Woods (Mrs.)_____ Unit/Room __N-234__ Date 10/1/83 By __Barker, RN__
I.D. 000000001   Follow-up 10/11/83Smith/Peters

are less communicative because of physical or mental conditions.

Issues of Cost

In the United States, 75 percent of all geriatric institutions are operated on a private, for-profit basis. In Canada and Great Britain, the proportion of private facilities is smaller. In some instances, the sponsor may want information on the connection between vision care and profit expectations. Most will be interested in the costs of such services.

One U.S. institution costed out its examination, including estimates of staff time but excluding refraction. Screening each individual was estimated to cost U.S. $12.20 per person in 1975, which would be inflated to about U.S. $22.00 in 1983 (Snyder, Pyrek, and Smith 1976).

We know of no research that has looked at the overall personal and economic benefits of people's being able to feed themselves, find their own way, and in general be more comfortable and independent, yet these may be some of the by-products of vision evaluations, corrections, and follow-up care.

Institutional Design and the Visual Environment

The physical facilities may do little to support good vision care. Studies of facilities in the United States, Canada, and Great Britain have indicated that lighting is insufficient in most institutions to support close work activities of even the most visually able of older residents (Boyce 1980; Cullinan 1980a, 1980b; Hiatt 1980; Woodruff and Pack 1980). In many institutions, the best lighting seems to be in the hallways, and this is where older people are sometimes found reading (Berkowitz et al. 1979; Hiatt 1980b). Even nursing stations seem inadequately lighted.

Most facilities would benefit from a room-by-room and service-by-service design evaluation and improvement program, which would have the following goals:

1. Reduction of reflectance glare (Fozard 1981; Hiatt 1978, 1980b).
2. Improved lighting levels and lamp location in relation to tasks (Boyce 1980; Fozard 1981; Hiatt 1978, 1980b; Hughes and Neer 1980, Lefitt 1980).
3. More effective use of colors, including the following:
   a. Increased use of contrasting colors and materials (light against dark and dark against light) in order to increase visibility of significant features such as lettering on signs, food in dishes, or one step from the next (Braf 1974; Finch 1981; Fozard 1981; Genensky 1980; Hiatt 1980b, 1981b; Hiatt et al. 1982; Sekular and Hutman, 1980; Sicurella 1977; Wardell 1980).
   b. Less concern about the color per se than its effect on older people. The human lens yellows with age (Marsh 1980). Many institutions do not compensate for this, and they use a variety of soft or muted pastel colors that are difficult to distinguish. Administrators may not know that bright colors are also difficult to differentiate. They may need to be advised about using color contrasts in areas where openings or objects should be defined and using similar color combinations when they wish to make features recede from awareness. (See Hiatt 1981b.)
4. Simplification of patterns—particularly on floors, where patterns may look like objects or steps (Hiatt, 1980a).

Special Design Considerations

For more severely vision impaired older persons, the vision care specialist may want to advise special design considerations.

Territory. Visually impaired older people may require special assistance in the identification of their own possessions and area. In an institution, it may be particularly important to distinguish a predictable chair and seating area, to have a clear pathway through bedrooms, and be able to anticipate placement of personally stored possesions. See Roberts (1980) for further suggestions.

Tactile Signs and Braille. Braille signs may help those older people who have learned to read braille. However, this tends to be a very small minority (Berkowitz et al. 1979). Other forms of tactile signs, such as recessed-lettered signs, may be more useful to people unfamiliar with braille (Blasch and Hiatt 1983; Braf 1974; Wardell 1980). A key to the use of signs to help people find their way is often placement height; this should be based on the eye level of older people, who may be in wheelchairs (Blasch and Hiatt 1983). Lettering also needs to be sufficiently large—about 1½ inches high for signs the individual can read at a foot or more distance.

Organization and Predictability. Severely vision impaired people may be hampered in independent negotiation of the physical environment because of the inadvertent activities of staff, visitors, and other residents. Organizing pathways so they are clear (even of temporarily stored carts or cleaning equipment, or "wet floor" signs) and advising others of the importance of clear paths minimizes hazards.

Orientation and Wayfinding. *Orientation* refers to people's ability to be aware of their own location relative to the surroundings. *Wayfinding* is the ability to intentionally get from one place to another (Welsh and Blasch 1980). Whereas we typically would offer mobility training and actual practice to a younger, severely visually impaired person, such training is often overlooked for older people (Love 1982; Welch 1980). Since one sign of memory impairment is the tendency for a person to become lost, vision may be a major factor in unjust judgments of mental incompetence (Fozard 1981; Snyder, Pyrek, and Smith 1976).

The combination of minor to moderate vision impairments and minor to moderate memory impairments may render individuals confused about their whereabouts. Landmarks may be helpful, such as the placement of simple, three-dimensional, nameable objects at intersections and meaningful signs at choice points (Hiatt 1980a). Staff and family members should be encouraged to offer mobility and orientation practice in a nonjudgmental, nonthreatening way to familiarize individuals to their whereabouts.

Mobility. One of the greatest concerns of vision-impaired older people is a loss of mobility (Welsh 1980). Sometimes staff members respond to the vulnerability of older people to accidents—particularly falls—by restricting their freedom. Staff members may restrain people in chairs, rooms, or areas of a building. A preferable method of dealing with the risks might be to create areas that are safe for movement, to train staff and families on techniques for minimizing risks, and to improve design factors that may contribute to risks.

Older people tend to stoop forward when walking (Rodstein 1978). As a result, ramps may be hazards, and they are specially dangerous when they have no handrail or inadequate lighting. Other hazardous features for visually

impaired older people are chairs that are too deep or low, or that have legs that extend needlessly into a room; sharp furniture edges; poorly repaired handrails; and uneven flooring. With the combined effects of stooped posture and diminished vision, older people may be unaware of projecting features such as telephone booths, drinking fountains, or signs (American Association of Workers for the Blind 1977; Braf 1974; Duncan et al. 1977).

It is quite possible that if visual and environmental needs were more adequately met, we might be able to reduce the needs for institutionalization and apply some of these environmental interventions to people at home (Hiatt 1983).

Reactions to Institutional Life

For the uninitiated, visits to institutions may arouse curiosity, as well as pique emotions. There are remarkable differences even among the "good ones" and, paradoxically, a permeating sameness about institutional life.

After visits to a sample of 46, Hiatt reflected, "While we observed few abuses, we were overwhelmed by those suffering from boredom" (cited in Berkowitz et al. 1979). The fanfare associated with bingo games, birthday parties, and the accomplishments of a few often overshadow the inactivity of the majority.

Kindly staff may be uninformed about the rehabilitative potential of older people under their care. Added to that, geriatric programs often are managed according to the motives of their sponsors, who may be governmental agencies, nonprofit churches, or voluntary agencies and private entrepreneurs.

Facilities differ in their conceptual images of the potential of older people, often reflecting the differences in opinions of the medical community. The same type of individual may be involved in activities in one facility and sit, barely dressed, in another.

Frankly, it is easier on the professional to implement a vision care program in an organization that sees its objective as facilitating independence, even if the older people are unlikely to be discharged into the community. However, it also may be very satisfying to offer services in a resource-depleted institution, although the follow-up may be more difficult to accomplish because of the attitudes of the caregivers.

Of all the factors that influence the success of a vision care program, perhaps none is more significant than medications (Green 1978; Walker and Brodie 1980). Overmedication, mismatched medications, and inappropriate drugging are factors that may result in the perception that older people are confused, disabled, and even incompetent. It is critical to make the attempt at the outset to understand the actual pharmacologic policies and practices of the organization. If vision impairment is misdiagnosed as depression or memory impairment, drugs may be used when the difficulties could have been corrected by appropriate refraction and vision care.

Vision care specialists may want to group with others involved in gerontology or long-term care policies to keep abreast of the trends affecting institutions and to have an appropriate forum in which to raise questions about institutional practices.

Summary

This chapter has attempted to outline specific considerations in serving older people, as well as the importance of providing these services in the context of an institutional service delivery system. Improved services are possible within the next decade through the interest of clinicians and the involvement of professionals with the system of care, as well as the individual. One of our highest priorities must be to bring low-vision evaluation and follow-up to the full range of institutions.

What is needed now are examples that can be shared among professionals, greater attention to mechanisms for payment, and broadly based programs of education for professionals, as well as for older people themselves.

References

American Association of Workers for the Blind. *Guidelines: Architectural and Environmental Concerns of the Visually Impaired Person.* Fullerton, Calif.: American Association of Workers for the Blind, 1977.

American Foundation for the Blind. *Products for People with Vision Problems.* New York: American Foundation for the Blind, 1982.

Berkowitz, M.; L. G. Hiatt; P. de Toledo: J. Shapiro; and M. Lurie. *Reading with Print Limitations: The Role of Health Care Institutions in Satisfying the Reading Needs of Residents with Print Limitations.* Vol. 3. New York: American Foundation for the Blind, 1979.

Blasch, B., and L. G. Hiatt. *Orientation and Wayfinding.* Washington D.C.: U.S. Architectural and Transportation Barriers Compliance Board, 1983.

Boyce, P. "The Relationship between the Performance of Visual Tasks and Lighting Conditions." *Light for Low Vision,* ed. R. Greenhalgh. Proceedings of a symposium. London: University College, 1980.

Braf, P. G. *The Physical Environment and the Visually Impaired.* Bromma, Sweden: ICTA Information Centre, 1974, FACK, S-161 03.

Burnside, I. M. "The Special Senses and Sensory Deprivation." In *Nursing and the Aged,* ed. I. M. Burnside. New York: McGraw-Hill, 1976, pp. 380–395.

Carroll, K. ed. *Compensating for Sensory Loss.* Minneapolis: Ebenezer Society, 1978.

Cohen, J. "Geriatric Optometry in an Institutional Setting." *Journal of Optometry and Archives of American Academy of Optometry* 47 (1969): 1014–1020.

Cullinan, T. R. "Epidemiology of Visual Disability." *Transactions of the Ophthalmological Societies, United Kingdom* 98 (1978): 267–269. (a)

Cullinan, T. R. "Visually Disabled People at Home." *New Beacon* 63, no. 743 (1978): 57–59.

Cullinan, T. R. "Studies of Visually Disabled People in the Community." *Regional Review* 63 (Spring 1979): 21–25.

Cullinan, T. R. "Low Vision in Elderly People." In *Light for Low Vision,* ed. R. Greenhalgh. Proceedings of a symposium. London: University College, 1980, pp. 65–70. (a)

Cullinan, T. R. "Visual Disability and Home Lighting." *International Journal of Rehabilitation Research* 3, no. 3 (1980): 406–407.

Duncan, J.; C. Gish; M.E. Mulholland; and A. Townsend. *Environmental Modifications for the Visually Impaired: A Handbook.* New York: American Foundation for the Blind, 1977.

Finch, J. "Making Things Easier to See." *RP Newsletter* 8, no. 4 (1981): 2–4.

Fozard, J. L. "Person-Environment Relationships in Adulthood: Implications for Human Factors Engineering." *Human Factors* 23, no. 1 (1981): 7–28.

Genensky, S. "Architectural Barriers to the Partially Sighted—And Solutions." *Architectural Record* 167, no. 5 (1980): 65, 67.

Green, G. "The Politics of Psychoactive Drug Use in Old Age." *Gerontologist* 18, no. 6 (1978): 523–530.

Hale, G. *The Sourcebook for the Disabled.* New York: Bantam, 1979.

Hiatt, L. G. "Architecture for the Aged: Design for Living." *Inland Architect* 23 (1978): 6–17.

Hiatt, L. G. "Disorientation Is More Than a State of Mind." *Nursing Homes* 29, no. 4 (1980): 30–36. (a)

Hiatt, L. G. "Is Poor Light Dimming the Sight of Nursing Home Patients? Implications for Vision Screening and Care." *Nursing Homes* 29, no. 5 (1980): 32–41. (b)

Hiatt, L. G. "Aging and Disability." In *America's Retirement Population: Prospects, Planning and Policy,* eds. N. McClosky and E. Borgotta. Beverly Hills, Calif.: Sage, 1981, pp. 133–152. (a)

Hiatt, L. G. "Color and Care: The Selection and Use of Colors in Environments for Older People." *Nursing Homes* 30, no.3 (1981) 18–22. (b)

Hiatt L. G. "Environmental Design and the Frail Older Person at Home." *Pride Institute Journal of Long-Term Home Health Care* 2, no. 1 (1983): 13–22.

Hiatt L. G.: R. Brieff; J. Horwitz; and C. McQueen. *What Are Friends For? Self-Help Groups for Older Persons With Sensory Loss: The U.S.E. Program.* New York: American Foundation for the Blind, 1982.

Hughes, P. C., and R. M. Neer. "Lighting for the Elderly: A Psychobiological Approach to Lighting." *Human Factors* 23, no.1 (1980): 65–86.

Jolicoeur, R. M. *Caring for the Visually Impaired Older Person: A Practical Guide for Long-Term Care Facilities and Related Agencies.* Minneapolis: Minneapolis Society for the Blind, 1970.

Kimbrough, J. A.; K. Heubner; and L. Lowry. *Sensory Training: A Curriculum Guide.* Professional Series 2. Pittsburgh: Greater Pittsburgh Guild for the Blind, 1976.

Lefitt, J. "Lighting for the Elderly: An Optician's View." In *Light for Low Vision,* ed. R. Greenhalgh. Proceedings of a symposium. London: University College, 1980, pp. 55–61.

Leslie, W. J., and D. A. Greenberg. "A Survey and Proposal Concerning Visual Care at the Nursing Home Level." *Journal of the American Optometric Association* 45 (1974): 461–466.

Love, J. "Orientation and Mobility." *Journal of Visual Impairment and Blindness* 76, no. 2 (1982): 66–68.

Marsh, G. R. "Perceptual Changes with Age." In *Handbook of Geriatric Psychiatry,* eds. E. W. Busse and D. G. Blazer. New York: Van Nostrand, 1980, pp. 147–168.

Mellor, M. *Aids for the 80s: What They Are and What They Do.* New York: American Foundation for the Blind, 1981.

Miller, D. "Vision Screening and Hearing in the Elderly." *Eye, Ear, Nose and Throat Monthly* 53 (1974): 128–133.

Milne, J. S., and J. Williamson. " Visual Acuity in Older People." *Gerontologia Clinica* 14, no. 4 (1972): 249–256.

Newman, B. Y. "Vision Care in Nursing Homes." *California Optometrist* 3, no.9 (1977).

Padula, W., and C. McQueen. "Avoiding Eye Strain." In *What Are Friends For? Self-Help Groups for Older Persons With Sensory Loss: The U.S.E. Program,* eds. L. G. Hiatt, R. Brieff, J. Horwitz, and C. McQueen. New York: American Foundation for the Blind, 1982, pp. 70–72.

Pastalan, L. A. "Age-related Vision and Hearing Changes: An Empathic Approach." Ann Arbor: Print and Audiovisual Resources from the Institute of Gerontology at the University of Michigan, 1976. (Slides)

Peterson, R., and C. Kirchner. "Prevalence of Blindness and Visual Impairment among Institutional Residents." *Journal of Visual Impairment and Blindness* 74, no.8 (1980): 323–336.

Roberts, S. L. "Territoriality: Space and the Aged Patient in the Critical Care Unit." In *Psychosocial Nursing Care of the Aged,* 2d ed., ed. I. Burnside. New York: McGraw-Hill, 1980, pp. 195–210.

Rodstein, M. "Accidents among the Aged." In *Clinical Aspects of Aging,* ed. W. Reichil. Baltimore: Williams and Wilkins, 1978, pp. 499–513.

Sekular, R., and L. Hutman. "Spatial Vision and Aging: 1. Contrast Sensitivity." *Journal of Gerontology* 35, no.5 (1980): 692–699.

Sicurella, V. "Color Contrast as an Aid for Visually Impaired Persons." *Journal of Visual Impairment and Blindness* 71 (1977): 252–257.

Silver, J. H.; E. S. Gould; D. Irvine; and T. R. Cullinan. "Visual Acuity at Home and in Eye Clinics." *Transactions of the Ophthalmological Societies of the United Kingdom* 98, part 2 (1978): 252–257.

Snyder, L; J. Pyrek; and K. Smith. "Vision and Mental Function." *Gerontologist 16, no. 3 (1976): 491*–495.

Vision and Aging. Report of the Mini-Conference on Vision and Aging prepared for the 1981 White House Conference on Aging. Washington, D.C.: U.S. Government Printing Office, 1981. (Also available from the American Foundation for the Blind, New York City.)

Vision Foundation. *Coping with Sight Loss: The Vision Resource Book.* Newton, Mass.: Vision Foundation, 1980.

Walker, J. I. and II. K. H. Brodie. "Neuropharmacology of Aging." In *Handbook of Geriatric Psychiatry,* eds E. W. Busse and D. G. Blazer. New York: Van Nostrand Reinhold, 1980, pp. 102–124.

Wardell, K. T. "Environmental Modifications." In *Orientation and Mobility,* eds. R. L. Welsh and B. Blasch. New York: American Foundation for the Blind, 1980, pp. 477–525.

Welsh, R. L. "Older Persons." In *Foundations of Orientation and Mobility,* eds. R. L. Welsh and B. B. Blasch. New York: American Foundation for the Blind, 1980, pp. 420–427.

Welsh, R. L., and B. B. Blasch, eds. *Foundations of Orientation and Mobility.* New York: American Foundation for the Blind, 1980.

Woodruff, M. E., and G. A. Pack. "A Survey of the Prevalence of Vision Defects and Ocular Anomalies in 43 Ontario Residential and Nursing Homes." *Canadian Journal of Public Health,* 71 (1980): 413–423.

Yeadon, A., and D. Grayson, *Living with Impaired Vision: An Introduction.* New York: American Foundation for the Blind, 1979.

Chapter 17

Aphakia

E. Richard Tennant

In the United States alone, an estimated 400,000 people are made surgically aphakic each year by the removal of a cataractous crystalline lens (J. Morgan 1981). With the perfection of microsurgery and the increasing successful use of implants, surgery is often performed today before visual impairment becomes significant. More than ever before, the restoration of normal vision to aphakic patients is approaching reality. Spectacle lenses have been designed to correct the defects commonly found in high-powered lenses. Hard and soft contact lenses have been developed that offer the patient not only cosmetic advantages but many visual advantages as well. Today the vast majority of postcataract surgery patients become pseudophakes through the use of lens implants.

Optics of the Aphakic Eye

The aphakic eye is essentially a simple optical system comparable to a single refracting spherical surface. The principal planes, located in the normal eye behind the cornea and in front of the lens, move forward in the aphakic eye to occupy a position at the apex of the cornea. The nodal points—which in the normal eye are located toward the back portion of the crystalline lens— also move forward to occupy the position at the center of curvature of the single refracting spherical surface (the cornea). The visual axis approaches the optical axis. The reflection of a light directed toward the eye is no longer located on the nasal side of the cornea, but rather in its center. If the eye were previously emmetropic, the total refractivity of the aphakic eye would be that of the power of the cornea alone (approximately +43.00D).

If the radius of curvature of the cornea (r) is assumed to be 7.8 mm and the index of the

medium of the eye (n') 1.337, the power of the eye (F) is obtained using the formula for a single refracting surface (n is the index of air):

$$F = \frac{n' - n}{r} \times 1,000.$$

$$= \frac{1.337 - 1}{7.8} \times 1,000 = +43.21D.$$

When a correcting lens is placed in front of a single refracting surface (the aphakic eye), optical changes occur, which make this combination somewhat more complex. The principal points, which were located at the apex of the cornea, now move forward in front of the eye and, at the same time, reverse their position so that the second principal point is located in front of the first principal point. The nodal points remain within the eye, but closer to the cornea; they, too, change their position so that the second nodal point is now in front of the first nodal point.

The anterior principal focal length of the eye-lens measures approximately 21 mm, compared with 17 mm for the aphakic eye. Dividing the two focal lengths, or 21 ÷ 17, yields 1.235, or a change in magnification of near to 24 percent. The fact that the image in the eye-lens combination is some 24 percent larger creates the difficulties encountered in the spectacle lens correction and, to a lesser degree, in contact lenses correction. Even though the diameter of the entrance pupil in the eye-lens combination is larger, the increased focal length of the system leaves the relative aperture unchanged.

When the crystalline lens is removed, any facility of accommodation is lost. However, since most aphakic patients have been presbyopic for some time, this loss does not create a new handicap. If the iris is not involved in the surgery and the pupil remains round, a considerable depth of focus still will exist. If spectacle lenses are used to correct the aphakia, the consequent magnification helps increase the apparent depth of focus.

According to Roenne, the limits of the normal visual field for white objects are out, 93 degrees; in, 62 degrees; up, 76 degrees; and down, 69 degrees. The eye that before surgery had a normal visual field will be restricted by approximately 20 percent after surgery when spectacle lenses are used to give out, in, up, and down values of 74, 48, 61, and 55 degrees, respectively (Stimson 1979, 250). If the correction lens were placed some 10 mm in front of the eye, a 30-mm-diameter lens would fully satisfy the necessary size of the prescription area.

In addition to increased magnification (which also means that objects appear closer, thereby causing the new aphakic some space perception problems), there is distortion caused by the vertex distance's increasing from the optic axis toward the periphery of the lens. Magnification also causes a given retinal area to be covered by a smaller visible field, creating the effect of field constriction. The visual field is reduced by approximately 20 percent, and a blind wedge (ring scotoma) extends around the lens (Figure 17–1). Objects appear and disappear as they traverse this gap. Since the center of the entrance pupil and the center of rotation of the eye do not coincide, this ring scotoma shifts as the eye rotates and creates a moving (or roving) scotoma. Some objects, which may be visible in the periphery of the visual field with the eye in one position, disappear from view when the spectacle-corrected aphakic attempts to look directly at them. Other objects pop in and out of the field of view as the eye moves, creating what is sometimes referred to as the *jack-in-the-box* phenomenon.

Ring scotomas are especially annoying to patients viewing objects at intermediate distances. In addition, when patients view through peripheral portions of the lens, a disagreeable effect called "swim" is created because of distortion. This can be reduced by learning to move the head with the eyes fixed rather than by rotating the eyes behind the lens. In addition, diplopia is a serious problem encountered by an aphakic patient because of prismatic displacement induced by high-powered correction lenses.

Restoring Vision after Cataract Surgery
The objective of cataract surgery is to restore vision. The type of aphakia existing (unilateral

Figure 17–1

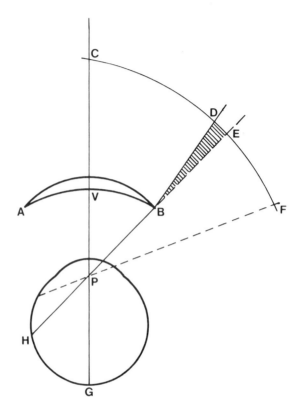

Ring Scotoma. P = entrance pupil, PV = 20 mm, AB (spectacle lens diameter) = 40 mm, CD = 37°, DBE (scotoma) = 9°, EPF = 25°, and GPH = 45°.

or bilateral) and the patient's age, health, and occupation are all factors to be considered in choosing the correctional approach. Since an ever-increasing number of patients are being fitted with intraocular lenses, correcting pseudophakes is becoming a common refractive procedure today. Where implants are not used, correction can be achieved with spectacle lenses, contact lenses, or a combination of both.

Unilateral aphakia is more difficult to manage than bilateral aphakia, since the successful combination of an aphakic and nonaphakic eye is not readily achieved. If the operated eye is the only one with useful vision, the approach is obvious. If, in contrast, the non-operated eye possesses useful vision, the practitioner must carefully consider the combination of both. If the nonaphakic eye has better corrected vision than the aphakic eye, the practitioner might prescribe for the nonaphakic eye and place a "balancing" lens before the aphakic eye. Patients often poorly tolerate a balancing spectacle lens over the dominant eye. Even when the acuity in the dominant eye is not as good as in the corrected aphakic eye, the patient prefers to use the dominant eye. Some patients learn to use each eye alternatively with surprisingly good results.

If both eyes have good vision when corrected, and if implants were not used, the only practical solution is to correct the aphakic eye with a contact lens. Do not assume that binocularity is automatically established by using contact lenses. If the aphakic eye was emmetropic before surgery, the correction with contact lenses would produce a size difference of 6 to 9 percent. This may prevent normal binocular vision and reduce stereo-acuity (Rosenbloom 1953).

A patient with bilateral aphakia usually can be fitted with either spectacles or contact lenses. Here, as before, the practitioner must perform a thorough refraction, fully realizing that motility imbalances and prismatic effects can induce difficulties for the patient. Correction for exophoria and vertical imbalances are frequently necessary. Contact lenses are much preferred in the correction of bilateral aphakia. However, older patients may find the insertion and removal of contact lenses more difficult, so spectacle lenses may be necessary. Even when a patient can learn to insert and remove the lenses, extended wear contact lenses are preferred, because the patient does not have to handle the lenses daily. Patients fitted with an intraocular lens in one eye and a contact lens in the other often prefer the intraocular lens over the contact lens eye (Michaels 1980, 604).

Examination and Correction of Aphakia

The ocular examination for aphakic patients follows a normal routine procedure. The fundus appears minified with the ophthalmoscope, and the examiner must study the background of the eye with great care. Ophthalmometry is important, since it provides a clue to the healing process of the cornea and is obviously important in fitting contact lenses. Retinoscopy is performed in the usual manner and subjectively confirmed and modified. Although it is possible to perform a satisfactory examination using a phoropter, it is better to use a pair of spectacles with +12.00D spherical lenses fitted properly to the face of the patient. Overrefracting devices (for example, Janelli and Whitney overrefraction devices and Halberg clips) into which lenses are placed are used to obtain both objective and subjective data.

Most major companies manufacturing cataract lenses make a trial set available to the practitioner (Figure 17–2). The examiner selects a pair of lenses with the same base curve as the final prescription and mounted in a frame with the proper interpupillary distance for the purpose of performing an overrefraction. In this manner the vertex distance, lens tilt, and base curves are controlled from the very beginning. After arriving at a final end point, the examiner merely needs to neutralize the combination with a Vertometer to obtain the final prescription.

Figure 17–2

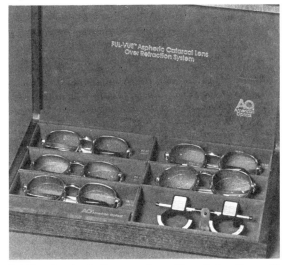

Ful-Vue Aspheric Cataract Lens Over Refraction with Whitney Overrefraction Device in Lower Right Corner. Source: Reprinted by permission of American Optical Corporation.

In adjusting the frame used for overrefraction, the examiner should place the spectacles as close to the eye as possible to reduce the magnification. Where overrefraction is not used but a trial frame or phoropter is employed, the practitioner must take into account such factors as vertex distance and lens effectivity.

Near point refraction depends on the viewing distance, available lighting, and contrast. The fact that magnification helps increase central acuity should be kept in mind. Problems frequently encountered with near vision are caused by the base-out effect of the distance prescription itself. Base-in prisms can be prescribed to overcome this difficulty and are incorporated automatically by some manufacturers in the bifocal addition (for example, the Freider Lens System). Sedentary patients are often well served by lenses that make the distance of acute vision 6 to 10 feet rather than the standard 20 feet. These patients may be able to read with such a distance correction by sliding the spectacles down their noses to increase the vertex distance and the "effective power" of the lens correction. If the patient has not used bifocals previously, separate distance and reading spectacles should be considered.

Cataract Spectacle Lens Design

The design of cataract spectacle lenses has improved considerably in the last decade because of the use of plastic aspheric lenses corrected for some combination of spherical aberration, curvature of field, marginal astigmatism, and distortion. All these aberrations cannot be fully and simultaneously corrected in a single spectacle lens, so each manufacturer chooses which to correct.

Modern plastic aspheric lenses are manufactured by casting the convex surface using aspheric glass molds. The concave surface is finished by the prescription laboratory, where a spherical surface is generated and polished. The power of the central area of the aspheric surface is usually referred to as the *base curve*.

It is not possible to correct all monochromatic aberrations in high-powered convex lenses by alterations of only two surfaces of a single lens, so lens designers must choose which aberration should be eliminated or minimized. By and large, two different approaches are used:

1. Establish a large field of view while maintaining good cosmetic appearance of both the lens and the patient's eye seen through the lens.
2. Establish a design that creates the best possible optical imagery through the lens periphery.

Lenses with the largest possible field of view usually have an almost flat back curvature and a front aspheric surface with a change in dioptric powers from the center to the periphery of between 2.00 and 5.00D. These lenses do not have the lenticular design effect of a central button surrounded by a flatter base. They are available with fewer base curves than are lenticular lenses (Fowler 1983).

The second design concentrates on maximum attainable acuity. These lenses are invariably of lenticular design with a rear surface of approximately −3.50D. Some have a certain degree of asphericity, but rarely more than 1.50 to 2.00D. They are available in a greater number of base curves than are the full-size lenses just mentioned. They have a smaller peripheral field, somewhat less distortion, and a greater amount of central magnification (Tennant 1983).

Summary of Available Lenses

The practitioner today can prescribe a number of well-designed cataract lenses according to the patient's needs (Atchison and Smith 1980, 1983, 1984; M. W. Morgan 1978). The following paragraphs give a brief description of a few of the available lenses, and Table 17–1 summarizes the

Table 17–1
Some Available Cataract Lenses

Company	Lens Name	Construction	Bifocal Style
American Optical	Ful-Vue aspheric cataract lens	Aspheric plastic	22-mm round top
Armorlite	OV-AL and Welsh Four-Drop Aspheric lens	Aspheric plastic Aspheric plastic	22-mm flat-top Round top
Cataract Lens Laboratory	Freider Lens System	Aspheric plastic full-field	25-mm flat top prism segment
Signet Optical	Hyperaspheric	Aspheric full-field plastic	22-mm flat top
Silor Optical	Super Modular Aspheric	Aspheric	Round top
Tech Optics	Volk conoid	Aspheric full-field glass	22-mm flat top
Universal Ophthalmics Laboratories	Unikat Uniphakic	Lenticular plastic Lenticular or full-size aspheric plastic	22-mm round top Round and flat top
Vision-Ease	Unilite Aspheric Lenticular	Aspheric	Flat top and 22-mm round top

Figure 17–3

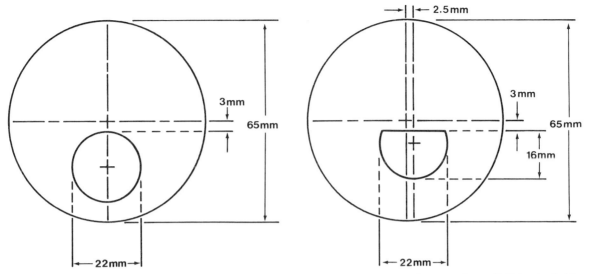

Full Field Lens System: Signet 22-mm Full Aspheric Round-Top Lens (Left) and Signet 22-mm Full Aspheric Flat-Top Lens (Right). Note drop and inset of segments.

information. Since this list is not inclusive and new designs appear and others are discontinued from time to time, the practitioner must keep abreast of the scientific and professional literature, as well as *Frames-Lenses Update,* which is published quarterly by Zulch and Zulch, Inc. (P.O. Box 4427, Sylmar, CA 91342).

The *Ful-Vue aspheric cataract lens* is manufactured by the American Optical Corporation. Its design objective is to reduce the aberration of oblique astigmatism and curvature of field for an eye rotation of at least 30 degrees from the center, as well as to provide increased correction of errors in the tangential meridian as compared with the sagittal meridian. It is constructed as a full field type of lens, thereby eliminating the concept of lenticular construction. It attempts to minimize the ring scotoma, as well as distortion. The manufacturer makes available to the practitioner a trial case of five pairs of spectacle lenses containing +12.00D lenses in various interpupillary distances together with a Whitney overrefraction device.

The Signet Optical Corporation manufactures the Hyperaspheric Lens, which incorporates a greater amount of asphericity as the base curves become progressively greater. The net clinical effect for the aphakic patient is an increased peripheral field. The recommended segment types for this lens are a round top of 22 mm and a segment placement of 2.0 mm below, as well as a flat top (22 mm × 16 mm) set 3.0 mm below and 2.5 mm in. The design of this lens was

stimulated by the early work of David Volk on the conoid lens. Volk claims that conoid cataract lenses minimize or eliminate many of the restrictions of the visual function of corrected aphakic patients. The greater the prescription power the patient requires, the greater the amount of asphericity that should be incorporated into the lens (see Figure 17–3).

Hyperasphericity in a single lens can be defined as the concentric arrangement of different spherical curves, each with a different radius of curvature. These different spherical front curves are smoothly joined and become flatter as they progress from the optical center toward the edge of the lens. A +12.00D front curve Hyperaspheric lens, for example, starts out with a +12.00D curve at the optical center and decreases to a +9.50D curve at the edge of the lens. The fitting guide provided for this lens stresses the importance of the vertex distance measurement, the proper pantoscopic tilt, and the necessary adjustment for alignment of the optical center with the patient's visual axis.

Another lens that falls into the general category of full-size aspheric lenses is the *Frieder Lens System.* Cataract Lens Laboratory, the manufacturer of this lens, has available a trial kit that consists of a number of eyeglasses of +12.00D, full-field, aspheric, single vision mounted lenses. The interpupillary distances vary from 60 to 68 mm and eye sizes vary from 50 to 54 mm. The Frieder Lens System has a bifocal containing a base-in prism segment.

(Figure 17–4).

The Armolite oval cataract lens, OV-AL, and the Welsh Four-Drop Aspheric Lens are plastic, aspheric, and lenticular; have a 22-mm flat-top bifocal; and are available in three base curves (Figure 17–5).

Signet also manufactures an aspheric lenticular lens, as well as a full aspheric and hyperspheric lens. These plastic lenses are available in single vision form as well as in flat- or round-top bifocals.

Vision-Ease manufactures an aspheric lenticular plastic lens that is also available in trifocal style. However, trifocal lenses are not recommended for aphakics, since the intermediate segment displaces the reading segment to the edge of the lens, thereby increasing the aberrations. In addition, the size of the field of view through a 7.0-mm segment is so small it is practically useless.

Tech Optics manufactures the Volk conoid aspheric full-field glass lens. This lens has, as mentioned earlier, a corrected curve bifocal.

The bifocal style best suited for aphakic prescriptions has not been clearly established, and various designs use both round and flat tops. None are aspheric in construction with the exception of the Volk conoid lens.

The Unikat round lens, which is frequently employed as a temporary lens, is made in a lenticular plastic design by Universal Ophthalmic Laboratories. The same company also manufactures the Uniphakic cataract lens, which is available in a lenticular or full-size aspheric plastic form.

An aspheric cataract lens manufactured by Silor Optical Company is the Super Modular Aspheric Lens. Its central area is ellipsoid with the same optical characteristics as the Silor aspheric lenticular lens with a diameter of 43.0 mm. The total lens has a diameter of 67.0 mm.

Cataract Contact Lens Design

Three varieties of contact lenses are available today for aphakic patients:
1. Rigid contact lenses—polymethyl methacrylate (PMMA) and gas permeable.
2. Soft contact lenses.
3. Extended wear contact lenses (hydrophilic, silicone, and silicone acrylate).

The patient with the ability to remove and insert contact lenses can wear single cut or lenticular lenses. Routine contact lens fitting procedures apply, and the use of a trial fitting set is recommended. Lenticular lenses can have an overall diameter of 10.5 to 8.6 mm, whereas single-cut lenses are about 8.2 to 6.8 mm in overall diameter. Gas-permeable lenses fit the aphakic patient well and permit satisfactory results. Since most patients wear spectacle lenses over their contact lenses, additional spherical and cylindrical lens power can be incorporated. Of course, the bifocal addition tends to make this type of fitting satisfactory to the patient.

Instruction on the insertion and removal of contact lenses can be enhanced through the use of proper illumination, mirrors that magnify, flip-up spectacles, and insertion and removal devices (DMV removers, vented hard lens removers, and soft lens remover/inserter).

Figure 17–4

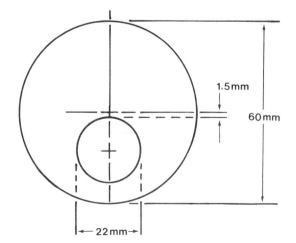

Frieder Full Field Aspheric Round-Top Lens (Left) and Full Field Aspheric Flat-Top Lens with Base-in Prism (Right)

Figure 17-5

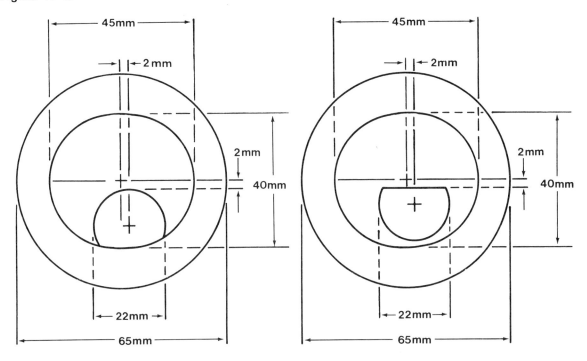

Armorlite OV-AL Round-Top Aspheric Lenticular Lens (Left) and Flat-Top Aspheric Lenticular Lens (Right)

For aged patients and those not capable of inserting and removing contact lenses, hydrophilic extended wear lenses are very useful. These lenses are available in aphakic lenticular form in comparably high dioptric powers. As with hard contact lenses, residual astigmatism can be corrected and bifocal power added by the use of conventional spectacle lenses. Hydrophilic lenses now available for extended wear include Permalens, Sauflon lens, Hydrocurve, and Hydrocurve II_{55}.

The EN-79 (lidofilcon B) and Bausch & Lomb Sauflon soft contact lenses for extended wear have a high water content with a resultant high oxygen transmissibility, a power range of +10.00 to +20.00D, and a wide selection of base curves and diameters.

The Permalens (manufactured by Cooper Laboratories) is fabricated of perfilcon A; its high percentage of water also permits a high degree of oxygen transmissibility. The Permalens covers the commonly found prescriptions of aphakic patients and has a sufficient range of base curves and lens diameters.

The ultrathin design of Hydrocurve II (manufactured by Barnes-Hind/Hydrocurve) provides maximum oxygen transmissibility and covers a refractive error of +10.00 to +20.00D.

This lens fits a wide range of corneal curvatures. Hydrocurve II, of bufilcon A, has a low (45 or 55 percent) water content and a thin design. It is a lathe-cut lens.

A careful schedule of follow-up visits is important during the early wearing period of hydrophilic lenses. Their fitting follows the same routine as for ordinary hydrophilic contact lenses, and the selection of the lens is based on the structural difference of higher water versus ultrathin design (Edmonds 1983).

Silicone acrylate contact lenses are now available for aphakic patients. This biologically inert material has been used for many years in medicine. It is less comfortable than hydroxyethyl-methacrylate (HEMA) because of its hydrophilic nature, but it is easier to adapt to than PMMA because of its high percentage of oxygen permeability. Under normal conditions silicone acrylate lenses undergo no dehydration. Corneal changes are rarely observed, and edema is infrequent. Some advantages of the silicone acrylate lens as compared with the hydrogel lens are better visual acuity, good oxygen permeability, durability, and corneal stability. Among the disadvantages are surface deposits, which may cause corneal abrasions.

Most practitioners feel that lens movement is

important to obtain optimum fit. Refractive astigmatism may be compensated for up to 0.75D and astigmatism of the cornea, up to 2.00D. In fitting silicone acrylate lenses, sodium fluorescein can be used without discoloration of the lens. The fact that some of these lenses can be used for extended wear indicates their stability and physiological integrity.

The practitioner must carefully supervise patients wearing extended wear aphakic lenses. Frequent evaluation and replacement of lenses as soon as they show wear, discoloration, or deposits that cannot be removed by normal cleaning procedures is advisable (see Chapter 19).

Intraocular Lenses

In the past decade the number of cataract extractions with intraocular lens implantation has grown dramatically as ophthalmologists have sought to improve the functional vision and quality of life of their patients. The use of intraocular lenses greatly reduces the magnification created by the correction of aphakia with spectacle lenses (25 to 35 percent) or even with contact lenses (8.0 to 12 percent). In addition, these lenses reduce aberrations and enlarge the field of vision. For all practical purposes, patients using lens implants may be called *pseudophakes.*

Three types of intraocular lenses are used, depending on how and where the implanted lens is fixated in the eye. Some lenses are implanted in the anterior chamber and fixated by the iris; some are anchored in the anterior chamber angle and fixated by the anterior angle; and some are implanted in the posterior chamber behind the iris (Nevyas 1983).

The basic design of all three types is very similar. All consist of a 5.0- or 6.0-mm optic portion made of PMMA; this is inserted so that the optical center of the lens coincides with the visual axis of the eye. Loops (haptics) attached to the lens to fixate it are also made of PMMA and are continuous with the optical portion of the lens in a rigid, one-piece construction. They also may be made of very thin, flexible polypropylene attached by heat fixation to channels on the optical part of the lens. Modern haptics are very thin (0.10 mm). The optical portions of the intraocular lenses are made by injection, compression, case molding, or lathe cutting.

In the iris-fixated lens, the loops float in front and behind the iris, which supports the lens. In some cases they are sutured to the iris. This type of lens frequently produces a squarish and somewhat fixed pupil.

The anterior chamber lens is placed into the anterior chamber, which is kept open with an air bubble of Healon, one of the basic components of the vitreous. The injection of this material into the anterior chamber during surgery protects the corneal endothelium from possible trauma. Whereas the anterior chamber lens can be used after an intracapsular cataract extraction (ICCE) or extracapsular cataract extraction (ECCE), posterior chamber fixation lenses can be used only after an ECCE. One of the advantages of the ECCE is that the clean posterior capsule protects the vitreous and, at the same time, avoids trauma to the ciliary body.

The majority of cataract cases lend themselves to lens implantation. Aphakic patients who have been unable to handle either contact lenses or spectacles in a satisfactory manner show good results after secondary implantations. Complications with intraocular lens implants occur in patients with major congenital malformations and chronic eye diseases such as glaucoma, chronic uveitis, and diabetic retinopathy.

Intraocular lenses are either plano convex or biconvex. To determine the power of an intraocular lens, the following parameters are used:

1. Axial length of the eye.
2. Anterior chamber depth.
3. Corneal curvature.

The axial length of the eye can be determined by A-scan ultrasonography. The anterior chamber depth is estimated using a slit lamp and the curvature of the cornea, by keratometry. The following equation gives the power of an infinitely thin intraocular lens in the aqueous humor:

$$F = \frac{1336\,(4r - a)}{(a - d)\,(4r - d)},$$

where F is the power of the intraocular lens, r is the radius of curvature of the anterior corneal surface (in millimeters), a is the anterior-posterior length of the eye (in millimeters), and d is the distance between the anterior corneal apex and the intraocular lens (in millimeters) (Michaels 1985, 510).

Considering the complications of aniseikonia, it is not always desirable to make the aphakic eye emmetropic. Instead, by considering the condition of the nonaphakic eye, the practitioner should use a power more suitable for an iseikonic correction. The existing aniseikonia can be reduced by making the nonaphakic eye hyperopic with a minus-powered contact lens and then correcting it with a spectacle lens. The practitioner also can correct the pseudophakic eye and use a minus spectacle to correct the myopia created. A rule of thumb used in calculating the aniseikonia reduction is that for every diopter of artificial hyperopia, the aniseikonia is decreased by approximately 3 percent.

Contact-Spectacle Lens Combination

As has already been stated, the correction of unilateral aphakia by spectacle lenses, contact lenses, or both creates more aniseikonia than is created by lens implants; it also requires much greater effort if binocular vision is to be obtained. Combining a contact lens and a spectacle lens to form a reversed Galilean telescope before the aphakic eye is a workable procedure with a very few selected patients. The contact lens is made relatively more convex, and the excess plus power is neutralized by excess minus power in a spectacle lens. For example, a minification of about 9 percent can be obtained by a vertex distance of 11 mm if the contact lens plus power is made 9.00D more than is required for the correction of the aphakia (Michaels 1985, 514).

Visual Adaptation
for Newly Corrected Aphakics

Except perhaps for pseudophakes, newly corrected monocular or binocular aphakic patients may require a period of adaptation before moving about freely and without conscious effort in a new visual world that may differ markedly from the presurgical world to which they had gradually adapted. Much more detail is usually visible, the apparent brightness is increased, and the size-distance relationship is usually markedly different. In addition, there is a significant increase in the intensity of light of short wavelengths, including the near ultraviolet light, reaching the retina. Consequently, all lens corrections should incorporate a tint that absorbs near ultraviolet light.

The adaptation to the sudden alteration in size-distance relationship takes time (Woods 1963). At first the patient may need to limit wearing the new correction to familiar surroundings, such as the home. A schedule of office visits for reevaluation and reassurance will give great comfort to the patient.

References

Atchison, D. A., and G. Smith. "Assessment of Aphakic Spectacle Lenses: High Power Flatback Lenses for the Correction of Aphakia." *Australian Journal of Optometry* 63 (1980): 258–263.

Atchison, D. A., and G. Smith. "Laboratory Evaluation of Commercial Aspheric Lenses." *American Journal of Optometry and Physiological Optics* 60 (1983): 598–615.

Atchison, D. A., and G. Smith. "Clinical Trial with Commercial Aspheric Aphakic Lenses." *American Journal of Optometry and Physiological Optics* 61 (1984): 566–575.

Edmonds, S. A., "Selection Grows as Technology Matures." *Review of Optometry* 120 (1983): 65–66.

Fowler, C. W. "Aspheric Spectacle Lens Designs for Aphakia." *Review of Optometry* 120 (1983): 737–740.

Michaels, D. D. *Visual Optics and Refraction.* 2nd ed. St. Louis: Mosby, 1980.

Michaels, D. D. *Visual Optics and Refraction,* 3rd ed. St. Louis: Mosby, 1985.

Morgan, J. *Cataracts and their Treatment.* Bryn Mawr, Penn.: Dorrance, 1981.

Morgan, M. W. *Optics of Ophthalmic Lenses.* Chicago: Professional Press, 1978, chap. 8–10.

Nevyas, H. J. "An Age-Old 'Cure' Gets Better." *Review of Optometry* 120 (1983): 58–62.

Rosenbloom, A. A. "The Correction of Unilateral Aphakia with Corneal Contact Lenses." *American Journal of Optometry and Physiological Optics* 30 (1953): 536–542.

Stimson, R. L. *Ophthalmic Dispensing.* 3rd ed. St. Louis: Mosby, 1979.

Tennant, E. R. "A New Look at an Old Standby." *Review of Optometry* 120 (1983): 66–74.

Woods, A. C. "The Adjustment to Aphakia." *American Journal of Ophthalmology* 55 (1963): 1268–1272.

Suggested Readings

Davis, J. K. "Problems and Compromises in the Design of Aspheric Cataract Lenses." *American Journal of Optometry and Archives of the American Academy of Optometry* 36 (1959): 279–288.

Feldman, G. I. "Fitting Soft Lenses." In *Refraction and Clinical Optics,* ed. A. Safir. New York: Harper & Row, 1980, pp. 279–288.

Grolman, B. *Ful-Vue Aspheric Cataract Lens.* Technical report, American Optical Co., Southbridge, Mass., 1980, pp. 1 –9.

Jaffe, N. S.; M. A. Galen; H. Hirschman; and H. M. Clayman. *Pseudophakos.* St. Louis: Mosby, 1978.

Michaels, D. "Spectacle Correction of Aphakia: How Aspheric Do They Need to Be?" *Ophthalmology* 85 (1978): 59–72.

Millodot, M. "Peripheral Refraction in Aphakic Eyes." *American Journal of Optometry and Physiological Optics* 61 (1984): 586–589.

Newell, F. N. *Ophthalmology: Principles and Concepts.* 5th ed. St. Louis: Mosby, 1982.

Safir A. *Refraction and Clinical Optics.* New York: Harper & Row, 1980.

Schechter, R. J. "Optics of Intraocular Lenses." In *Refraction and Clinical Optics,* ed. A. Safir. New York: Harper & Row, 1980, pp. 535–543.

Chapter 18

Fitting and Dispensing Spectacles for the Elderly Patient

Albert L. Pierce
Meredith W. Morgan

The relationship between the older patient and the vision care practitioner all too frequently is marred by frustration or despair. Dispensing procedures that would normally be successful often involve an endless series of office returns and complaints. The unique problems associated with the aged patient were well defined over two decades ago by Archer and Eakin (1960). Many of their suggested methods of treatment still are considered appropriate in dealing with the spectacle problems of today's older generation. However, technology and the development of new materials has advanced dramatically in this field during the past few years. This chapter will discuss methods for offering better care to the ever-increasing number of older patients.

The basic design of the traditional frame has changed very little during the past 50 years. Ever-changing fashion trends, of course, have profoundly influenced certain styling changes, and many of the extreme designs have negatively affected the comfort and fitting qualities of certain styles. Within variations, however, the basic geometric fitting principles have remained virtually unchanged. Today's contemporary frame styles still depend on the patient's nose for the prime support base; almost two-thirds of the entire spectacle weight is concentrated there. Most of the weight in the majority of cases is transferred directly to the sides of the nose through the contact pads of the bridge, and herein lies the fundamental problem for many aging patients. The temples also play an important stabilizing role to maintain control and positioning of the front section of the spectacles. The nose, however, remains the single most important area when fitting spectacles to the older patient.

Age-related Problems

In the professional care and treatment of the older patient, practitioners must remember they are seldom dealing with an amateur when it comes to wearing spectacles. Most elderly patients have worn a spectacle correction for many years. During a lifetime they have accumulated their full share of spectacle-related difficulties. Thus, they usually consider frame adjustment problems and occasional fitting difficulties as minor annoyances that are worth the benefits received. Through experience, these patients have usually developed a high degree of patience, tolerance, and understanding. Thus, to be plagued with additional spectacle problems during the later years of life is both ironic and sad.

Many older people develop an age-related physical impairment that interferes with the normal placement and wearing conditions of spectacles. The bony structure of the nose, which is the main support base for the spectacles, does not change with age, but the skin and connective tissue surrounding the nasal area do change. The parchmentlike skin often becomes extremely thin, fragile and loose. The gradual change in the skin's texture and its loss of resilience result in a weakened footing for the weight-bearing surfaces of the spectacles. The skin no longer can support the continual downward gravitational pull of the spectacles, so it folds and becomes irritated and painful.

Assuming the older patient is wearing a conventional spectacle frame, the following may result from an improperly fitting frame:

1. Simple contact dermatitis may cause increased redness that persists when the spectacles are removed.
2. The cutaneous or underlying tissue may

become irritated and infected.

3. Constant sagging and squeezing of the skin can affect the nasal arteries and veins.
4. Consequent tissue breakdown is often a contributing factor in certain forms of skin cancer.
5. The visual performance of the prescription may be affected because the lenses cannot be maintained in their proper position.

Treatment Plans

The aged patient, either because of mental impairment or a reluctance to complain, may ignore the resultant problem until it has advanced to a serious stage. Once the diagnosis has been made, the form of treatment, to a great extent, will depend on the circumstances and the severity of the conditions.

Throughout all forms of treatment, the plan must relieve the weight-bearing load of the spectacles. Abstinence from wearing all forms of spectacles would be a natural solution, but this is usually impossible, since the patient may not be able to go without spectacles during the recovery period. Reduced pressure at the weakened area of the nose will insure air circulation and promote healing of the abused skin tissue. The following represents a general approach to solving this problem:

1. Use temporary or permanent accessories of various kinds that can be applied quickly to the frame. Some available devices are shown in Figure 18–1.

Figure 18–1

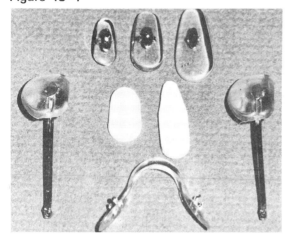

Attachments to Change the Weight-Bearing Surface of Frames: (Top) Pads of Different Sizes; (Center) Stick-on Cushions; (Right and Left Sides) Usden Crutch, and (Bottom) Flexit-Fit Bridge.

2. Modify the bridge contour, particularly in fixed-bridge frames.
3. Custom design and construct a frame that meets the specific requirements of a particular patient.

Adjustable Bridge Control Techniques

The vast majority of frames worn by the older population are equipped with some type of adjustable nose piece. Frequently, this causes problems when the nasal skin's natural resilience has deteriorated as a result of the aging process. The following information regarding adjustable nose pads may prove helpful in dealing with older patients who show the typical signs of an unsound resting base for the nose pads:

Foam stick-on nose pad cushions may ease the discomfort caused by a previously worn ill-fitting frame (Figure 18–2). However, they should never be used as a permanent means of correction, as the real reason for a fitting problem may be masked by the cushion pad itself.

Pad size, shape, and texture are very important. The patient's frame may have small, hard, plastic pads, which should always be replaced. The most suitable nose pad for the aged individual is a soft, flexible, polyvinyl pad. Its size depends on factors relating to the spectacle weight and the type of nose to be fitted. As a general rule, the fitter should use a pad size that will distribute the bearing load over as great an area as possible (Figure 18–3).

The Usden Crutch technique is recommended for extreme or advanced cases where the skin and tissue have become seriously damaged. If the skin shows signs of marked irritation or redness, complete rest from the irritating spectacles may be necessary to prevent further complications. Relief is possible through the use of the Usden Crutch, a device that easily attaches to the patient's spectacles. The simple attachment consists of two 1½-inch-long extension bars that are fastened to the underside of each temple hinge assembly. On the end of each bar is a large polyvinyl pad. By adjusting each of the bars, the pads can be positioned so as to rest on the cheek. This results in a slight vertical elevation of the entire front so that the regular nose pads will be clear of skin contact (Figure 18–4). The patient should be referred to a physician if the condition appears to be serious or if the inflammation does not show definite signs of improvement after a few days of Usden Crutch wear.

Figure 18-2

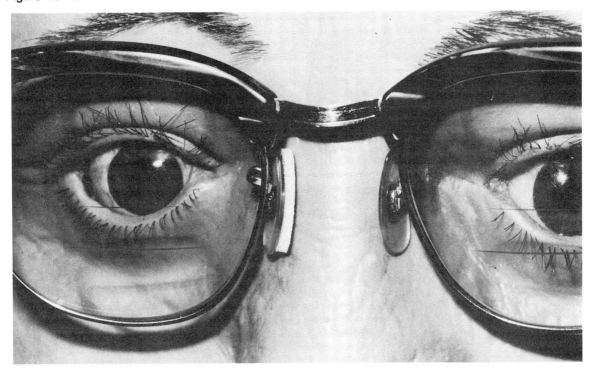

Stick-on Pad Cushion.

Figure 18-3

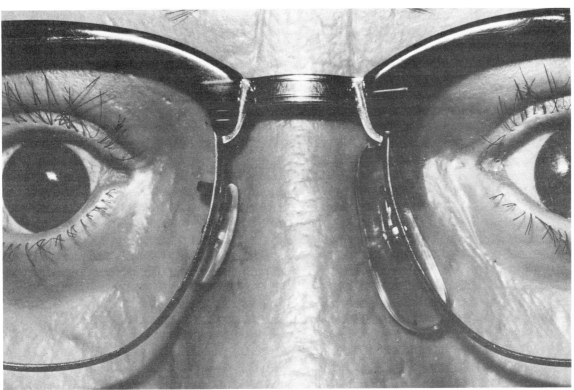

Jumbo Pad, Which Replaces Regular-Sized Pads.

Flexit-Fit bridges offer one of the best opportunities for increasing the weight-bearing surface of the spectacle load to an absolute maximum (Figure 18–5). The individual nose pads are replaced by a one-piece polyvinyl strap that forms a U-shaped bridge. When properly attached to the pad arms, the strap can be adjusted to allow major contact over the crest region rather than at the sides of the nose. Removing the weight from the sides and redirecting it to the more firm foundation of the nasal crest will lessen the strain on the worn and weakened side tissue.

Temple grips (Huggies) also act as temporary aids in fighting the effects of irritating spectacles. During the early stage of treatment, the general frame fit should be adjusted slightly on the loose side to avoid further complications. Temple grips slipped over the ends will prevent slippage and also add to overall comfort. Pad cushions and temple grips, however, never should be considered a "cure" for frame ailments. They never should act as a substitute for a well-fitted and properly adjusted frame.

Solid or Fixed Bridge Control Technique

Aside from the Usden Crutch, the most effective treatment for solid bridge fitting problems involves a molding treatment. Add-on foam cushions are seldom effective. Perhaps the best approach is one that uses a compound developed by the dental profession, Coe-Soft, a soft relining plastic that eases the discomfort caused by ill-fitting dentures.

When applied to the bridge area of a frame, Coe-Soft forms a soft, nonslip lining between the hard surfaces of the frame and the delicate tissue of the nose (Figure 18–6). Nontoxic and nonirritating, Coe-Soft offers one of the best and least expensive methods of controlling irritation resulting from this type of nose-fitting problem. The material bonds itself readily to all acetate or acrylic frame materials.

It is equally effective for adjustable pads when inner changeable polyvinyl pads are not available. Applied to the surface of hard plastic nose pads, it forms an outer layer of soft flexible plastic that molds itself to the exact contour of the nose. Additional uses for this versatile compound will be discussed later.

Altering the Basic Bridge Style: Saddle Conversion

When none of the temporary measures already discussed have completely solved the problems of the aged patient, one final treatment can be applied to the patient's saddle conversion. This technique alters the basic fitting arrangement

Figure 18–4

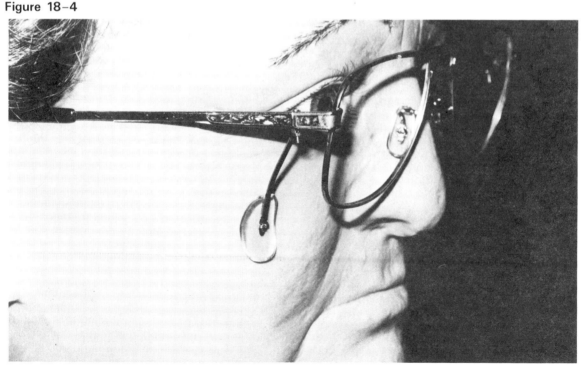

Usden Crutch in Place.

Figure 18-5

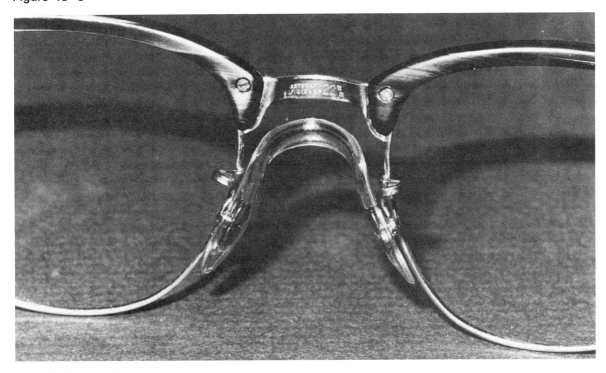

Flexit-Fit Bridge in Place.

Figure 18-6

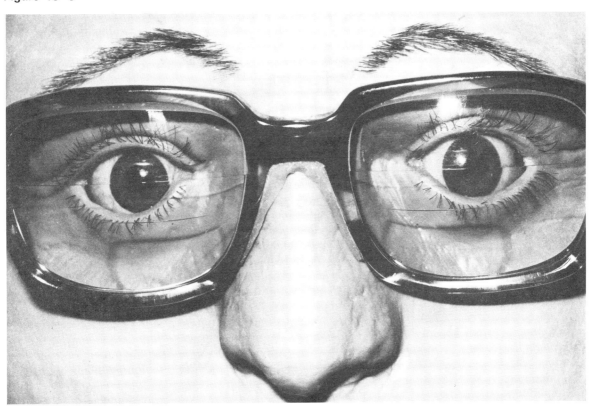

Re-formed Solid Bridge using Coe-Soft.

of the nose piece. A few years back, this technique was a difficult and time-consuming operation that required a considerable degree of skill and proficiency. Thanks to today's plastics, however, this technique now can be performed efficiently with only a minimum degree of technical ability.

Experience has proved that the nose crest of the aged individual is far more capable of supporting the weight of the spectacles than are the sides of the nose. This technique, therefore, changes the patient's bridge from a side-of-the-nose fitting position to an over-the-nose or saddle bridge fit.

Saddle Conversion for Adjustable-Pad Bridges. This technique used for adjustable-pad bridges takes advantage of the adjustable features of the bridge to form a new network for the saddle fit. This procedure may appear to be complicated, but after a few practice sessions with an old frame, all fears and hesitation will be dispelled quickly. The entire operation is an in-office procedure and requires no unusual equipment.

The steps in the procedure follow:

1. After the nose pads have been removed, each of the adjustable arms must be straightened and then rebent into a horizontal position. The ends of each pad arm should meet or overlap in the center of the bridge. This will form the rough network or inner reinforcing core for the construction of the plastic portion of the saddle bridge. The frame then should be placed on the patient's face. Adjustments to the metal core over the crest of the nose will regulate the frontal positioning of the spectacles. Exactness of the bridge fit is not important at this stage. Establishing the correct eyewire distance and the vertical positioning of the spectacle front are the two most important adjustments to be completed. (See Figure 18–7.)

2. Jet Acrylic, a dental plastic used in the restoration of teeth and denture materials, should be mixed and applied to the metal network of the newly formed bridge bar. A sufficient quantity of the plastic should be applied while the mixture has a soft, puttylike consistency. The saddle design can be shaped

Figure 18–7

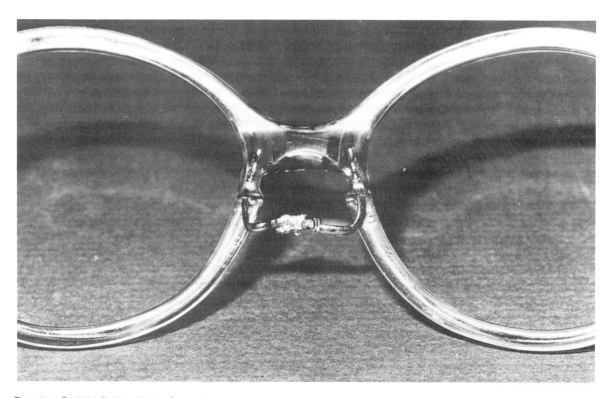

Forming Saddle Bridge from Guard Arms.

Figure 18-8

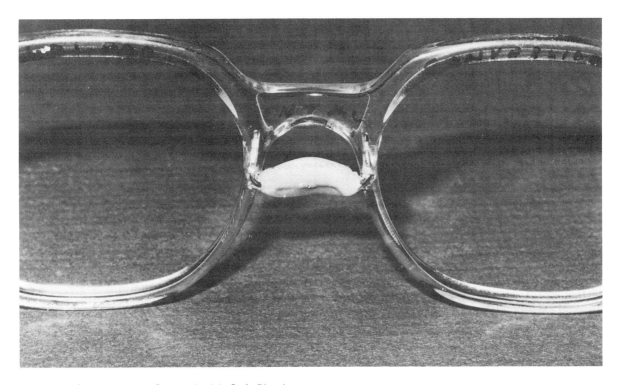

Re-formed Saddle Bridge Covered with Soft Plastic.

with the use of a small spatula. Continual applications of the mixing liquid will keep the material soft and pliable. After shaping the bridge, and while the material is still pliable, the frame should be placed carefully on the patient's face. The back side of the newly formed saddle should be lightly pressed against the face to mold the soft plastic to the shape of the nose. (A thin film of mineral oil applied to the nasal region prior to this step will prevent the skin from sticking to the soft plastic.) Within 10 minutes the material will begin to harden. The frame then should be removed from the face and placed in a container of warm water. After approximately 30 minutes the hardening process will be completed.

3. The final phase involves filing, sanding, and polishing to complete the saddle piece. Figure 18-8 shows the finished product.

Saddle Conversion for Nonadjustable Bridges. The same technique may be applied to all-plastic solid or fixed bridge designs. Since this type does not have the adjustable guard arms necessary to form the framework for the saddle

construction, the metal portion must be improvised. A metal pin must be implanted across the bridge area to form the reinforcing bar for the saddle. The procedure follows:

1. The frame is placed on the patient's face, and the bar and nose crest locations are marked. The correct placement of the saddle bar should raise the front high enough to allow minimal clearance at the normal nose pad contact area.

2. Two small holes (made with a size 50 twist drill) then are drilled into the nasal edge of each eyewire where the frame was marked. The metal part for the saddle can be fashioned from a large paper clip. The piece for the part should be cut long enough so it can be forced between the two opposing holes (Figure 18-9).

3. The procedure for finishing the plastic portion of the saddle will be the same as it was . for the adjustable-pad bridge saddle conversion technique.

Alternate Method of Saddle Construction. Frames also can be converted to a saddle fit arrangement by incorporating the natural bridge bar into the design. This technique is possible only when the frame bar is relatively close to the crest area of the nose. The conversion should not be attempted when the bar is more than a quarter inch above the crest position. This method follows:

1. Optyl plastic salvaged from a temple is ideal for the saddle piece construction. Since the usual wire found in other temple materials is absent, a small strip can be fashioned easily into the U-shaped design of the saddle.
2. Norland Optical Cement is an effective, slow-setting adhesive for bonding the Optyl plastic to the existing bridge bar. After the plastic strip has been heated and shaped so it will conform to the bone structure of the nose, it should be filed, sanded, and polished. The finished saddle piece is then lightly fastened to the regular bridge bar with a drop of any fast-setting cement. Complete bonding will be done with optical cement. The cement must be applied slowly while the frame is under an ultraviolet light source (the cement will harden only when it is exposed to ultraviolet light).

Adjustment of the Saddle Frame. To obtain the best results from these modification techniques, the spectacles must be refitted. The temples must be fitted correctly, since extra tightness in the temples no longer will be necessary after the saddle conversion. The frame will be more balanced and require only minimal temple pressure. The addition of Coe-Soft to the newly formed saddle bridge also will increase the comfort of the nose fit when the overall spectacle weight is excessive. Nonslip temple covers also should help older patients who are bothered with irritation or frame slippage.

Permanent Off-the-Nose Treatment Plans

It now must be obvious that coping with the spectacle problems of the aged patient presents a real professional challenge. Decisions about the best form of treatment must be made according to the circumstances surrounding each individual case. Often practitioners are reluctant to attempt some of the more advanced forms of treatment, and there is no question that a few of the techniques require considerable time and technical ability. Perhaps one of the most effec-

Figure 18-9

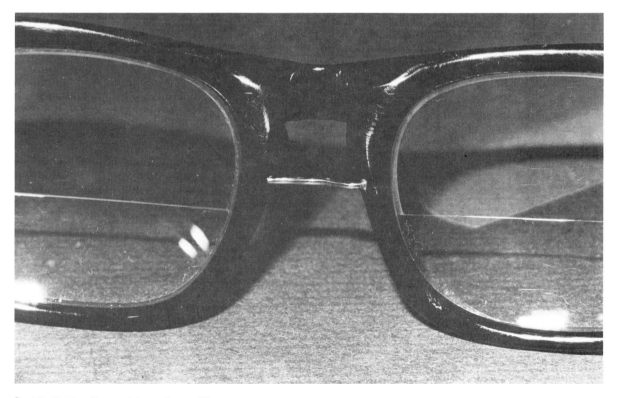

Saddle Bridge Formed from Paper Clip.

Figure 18-10

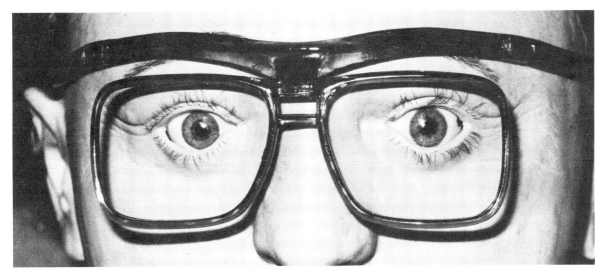

Astro-Spec.

tive and least involved solutions, then, might be to incorporate the patient's prescription in a spectacle frame that does not depend on the nose for support.

The Astro-Spec is a unique design that has contributed enormously to good vision care for the aged patient (Figure 18-10). It is strongly recommended for any case that requires absolute freedom from nasal contact. The principal component is a headband that uses the brow region of the face as the main support base. The narrow headband is flexible and therefore requires minimal side pressure to maintain correct positioning and to insure comfort. The detachable front section holding the lenses is hinged to the headband. This feature alone has certain advantages from an optical standpoint. For instance, the pantoscopic angle and multifocal positioning now are within the patient's control. The practitioner, however, should exercise discretion when prescribing this unusual and unorthodox device. It should be dispensed only to older patients who are capable of understanding the significant mechanical and optical innovations built into this different spectacle design. Patients who cannot understand or remember how to adjust the Astro-Spec may adjust it in such a way that the lens correction is not properly centered before the eyes and thus destroy the usefulness of the correction.

Criteria for Geriatric Spectacle Design

Failure will still occur despite the best efforts. Assuming that none of the treatment plans discussed so far have offered a workable solution to the problem, what is the next procedure? We must create an entirely new spectacle design. Having established the fact that the nose area is the primary area for concern, perhaps we might incorporate one of the special bridge innovations in the new design. What type of frame should be chosen? What about reducing weight? What type of lens material should we use, and how do we handle the safety aspect? These are only a few points to ponder. Although circumstances and conditions may alter certain design features, the following are suggested guidelines for solving this problem.

Frame Considerations

The frame should be strong, but lightweight. It should be no larger than absolutely necessary to accommodate the facial size. For centering purposes, the frame PD should be equal to the distance interpupillary separation. The bridge should be adjustable, with the DBL as small as possible. The temples should preferably be of a cable type, with covers over the mastoid ends. Finally, the frame style and color must be pleasing to the patient. One of the commercially available frames that can be altered to meet these criteria is the Rimway.

Lens Considerations

The lens material must be high quality, light in weight, and of an index that will afford good performance in all the prescription parameters. It must be ground to an absolute minimal edge or center thickness. The lenses must meet or surpass all the nationally recognized safety standards and must be capable of passing the FDA-required drop ball test. Finally, the lens surfaces must be coated with a high-quality, multilayer, antireflective, and protective coating.

Frame Modifications

When a frame has been selected, an empty frame of the correct size (with the DBL as small as possible) first should be tried on the patient. The adjustable pad arms should be spread to allow the bridge to rest on top of the nose at the general crest area. The top of eyewire should assume a position slightly lower than the brow. However, if the front appears too low in relation to the eyebrow, the pad arms should be bent into a linking arrangement as described earlier. This will correct the frontal placement. Dental acrylic is applied directly to the bridge bar or to the linkage of the pad arms to form the molded portion of the saddle arrangement. The pad arms can be severed from the front if they are not incorporated into the technique. Following completion of the acrylic mold, the empty frame should be placed on the patient's face to determine the vertical dimension of the shape and the multifocal height (Figure 18–11).

Special Lens Considerations

The choice of lens material to be used in the modified frame will be governed by a number of factors relating to the lens power and the type of frame selected. For example, in rimless frames, holes must be drilled for mounting, and fabricating regulations require plastic lenses. The average prescription (of a noncataract nature) for older patients is usually of a moderate spherocylinder plus power. Therefore, polycarbonate is the first choice. It has a higher index of refraction (1.586) than CR-39 (1.4885), which results in a slightly thinner lens (which reduces weight). Polycarbonate also is far superior to regular CR-39 in safety. The lens is virtually unbreakable, even when ground to a knife-edge thinness. Polycarbonate absorbs almost 100 percent of the ultraviolet radiation after coating (it screens 97 percent of the ultraviolet radiation up to 400 nm). Finally, mounting polycarbonate lenses to the frame allows the holes to be threaded; thus, the lenses are held tightly to the frame without the usual loosening effect.

In addition, the correction should be ground

Figure 18–11

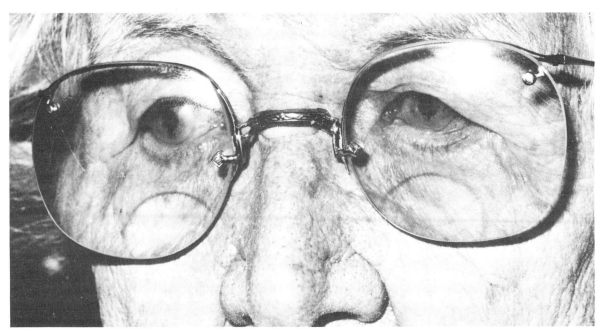

Saddle Bridge Formed by Cutting Off Guard Arms and Covering Remaining Bridge with Soft Plastic.

on the flattest base curve possible. Older patients, especially those who are hypermetropic, are seldom bothered by the spatial distortion induced by lenses with flat base curves. These lenses result in a reduction of magnification and an improved appearance.

General Lens Design Considerations for the Older Patient

For the older patient, the primary consideration in choosing a lens design and type is how well the patient was performing with the previous correction. Except for the dramatic change in vision that occurs with the onset of aphakia or the change in visual requirements that may occur at retirement, changes in both vision and visual requirements are very gradual in the healthy aging patient. Even at retirement the change may not be great, since among the active elderly, avocations already may be more important and demanding than vocations at the time of retirement.

Before changing the lens type or design from that previously worn, the optometrist must answer the following question: Are there any compelling reasons to change the type and design of the lenses that the patient is now wearing? As has already been mentioned, most elderly patients are experienced spectacle wearers, and unless there has been some significant change in the lens prescription or in the patient's visual requirements, the same type and design of lenses should be prescribed, providing performance was adequate. The optometrist must carefully question and listen to the expert, the elderly patient. Some of the factors that need to be considered are performance distances, desired visual field sizes, freedom of head and eye movements, acuity of vision required and desired, visual performance through the edges of the old lenses, weight of the old lenses and the new frame, and appearance. The primary considerations are the adequacy of the old lens design and type and the changes desired or needed.

Performance Distances. Patients must be questioned about working distances used and the need for visual performance at these distances. If a patient must perform well at various distances, multifocal lenses or progressive addition lenses should be considered (Borish, Hitzeman, and Brookman 1980; Schultz 1983). One of the few advantages that results from the miosis of aging is that the depth of field increases, which in a sense replaces lost accommodation.

Desired Visual Field Sizes. Patients also must be questioned about the usefulness of the size of field, particularly through the segments of their old lenses. If the field is too small, it may be made larger by increasing the segment size, reducing the vertex distance of the lenses, or increasing the working distance (reducing the power of the addition). Whether any of these solutions is possible must be determined for each patient. Fortunately, another advantage of aging miosis is an increase in the size of the field of view for segments of the same size and power.

The size of the field of view decreases, however, as the total power through the segment becomes more convex. For this reason, when the power of the distance correction is greater than +5.00D, great caution must be exercised in prescribing trifocals or multifocals. The intermediate field may be too small to be useful, and it displaces the near segment lower in the lens, where optical performance is poorer. Certainly trifocals are virtually useless in aphakic corrections of +10.00D or more.

Freedom of Head and Eye Movements. To view objects through specific regions of a lens, the head, the eyes, and the object of regard must be in a specific location in relation to one another. If the patient does not have good vertical movement of the head and eyes for any reason, placement of the segment becomes even more critical than it usually is. Lack of free head and eye movement may limit the effectiveness of trifocals, because the intermediate segment occupies space and forces the near segment to be placed lower in the lens. This also may limit the usefulness of progressive addition lenses, because the distance between the area of clear distance vision and clear near vision is fixed; the region of clear near vision may be too low in the lens for it to be usable by the patient for extended periods, as when reading. The limitation of head movement may be caused by a short neck or a lack of facility in adjusting the head, eyes, and object into the proper relationship. The optometrist should observe each patient in action to determine the extent and ease of head movement possible.

Acuity of Vision Required and Desired. The optometrist must determine the acuity required and desired by the patient for visual tasks. Sometimes these are not the same, since some individuals always want to see the "gnats eye," whereas others are happy if they can just recognize what they are looking at. Still others, because of their vocation or avocation, must be able to resolve critical detail and may be willing to adapt to a short viewing distance to achieve the necessary resolution (low-vision patients do this all the time).

Several aberrations, such as marginal astigmatism and chromatic dispersion, tend to destroy the ability of a lens to create sharp images. Both these aberrations increase as the visual angle increases toward the edge of the lens—particularly as the power of the lens increases, as the index of refraction increases, or as the ν value of the lens material decreases. Thus, if it is important to achieve really excellent resolution at near through a segment, the segment must be placed high in the lens, the proper base curve for minimum astigmatism should be chosen, and high-index lens materials should be avoided. Remember that as optical imagery by the lens is improved, the range of acceptable vision is increased.

Visual Performance through the Edges of the Old Lenses. Especially if the correction exceeds ±4.00 or ±5.00D, the optometrist should determine if the patient has noticed distortion or blurring through the edges of the old lenses. The patient can be instructed to look at the edge of a doorway monocularly while turning his or her head from left to right and back again. The patient then is asked to note whether the edge remains straight or becomes curved as the line of sight passes into the periphery of the lens. Likewise, the patient may be questioned about sharpness of vision. Some care should be exercised in subjective perception testing to avoid suggesting to older patients that they should see the doorway curved, the floor tilted, and so forth. In other words, the questions asked should not suggest the answers. Usually, the well-adapted spectacle wearer will not notice distortion but may notice a decrease in clarity. Some patients, however, do not adapt to distortion subjectively but avoid it by not using the edges of their lenses. If this is the case, the optometrist should consider the use of lenses of deeper base curve (Katz 1983; Morgan 1978).

Distortion may become especially annoying when high-index glass is used. To limit the marginal astigmatism and distortion to that present in crown glass lenses of the same power, high-index lenses must be made on steeper base curves; however, this tends to defeat the purpose for which the high-index glass was used in the first place. Jones (1980) has calculated that a +6.00D lens of crown glass with a back surface power of −4.00D has the same marginal astigmatism for a 30-degree eye rotation as a +6.00D lens with a −6.50D base curve made of glass of 1.700 index.

Weight of the Lenses. If patients complain that their old spectacles weigh too much and the optometrist wishes to avoid using the procedures described in the first half of this chapter, lenses made of CR-39 or polycarbonate should be considered. These should be geometrically centered in a frame of the smallest acceptable eyewire size and the lenses made as thin as possible. For lenses with between +5.00D and −5.00D power, high-index glass will not produce a lighter-weight lens, even though the lens is thinner. In powers outside this range, however, high-index lenses will be both thinner and lighter.

Weight is primarily a function of lens thickness and eye size (equivalent diameter). Jones (1980) has calculated that for a −6.00D lens with an equivalent diameter of 50 mm, a 10 percent increase in weight would result from any one of the following: (1) 10 percent increase in specific gravity (density), (2) a 1.00D increase in power, (3) as little as 0.25 mm increase in thickness, or (4) less than 1 mm increase in equivalent diameter.

Appearance. In general, aging patients have the same complaints about the appearance of their spectacles as do young patients, but they tend to be somewhat more philosophical and reticent about expressing their complaints. Many aging patients, furthermore, are willing to forget glamour for the sake of comfort. Nevertheless, the chief complaints about appearance are lack of style (usually too small), visible segments, edge thickness and internal reflections, too much lens bulge, and enlarged eyes with aphakic corrections.

Style, of course, is a matter of taste and advertising. It should be pointed out to the patient that sometimes comfort and good visual performance are not compatible with high style; choices must be made. One of the best choices is two pairs of spectacles: an everyday, at-home, comfortable, high-performance pair and a high-style, tolerable-performance pair.

Segments can be made virtually invisible by prescribing round-top, fused-segment bifocals made in light pink tinted glass with the surfaces coated. The other solution to this problem is to prescribe one of the progressive addition lenses.

Edge thickness in concave lenses can be reduced by making the lens smaller, thinner, or of higher-index glass. Frequently, only the latter is practical.

Lens bulge—that is how much the lenses protrude in front of the plane of the frame—is a function of the lens power, equivalent diameter, base curve, index of refraction, and thickness. Presumably, nothing can be done about lens power, and little can be done about reducing thickness below that required. However, the other factors can be controlled to some extent. Altering the base curve and the index of refraction may change the optical performance of the lens, as already described. However, the patient may not complain about, or even notice, a slight decrease in visual performance in the absence of a comparison standard. Also, some of the decreases in performance are very slight and can be appreciated only after very precise and careful determinations. One of the wonders of the world is the adaptability of the human sensory mechanisms.

Internal reflections and the visibility of the lenses can be reduced by antireflection coatings. This will not reduce the edge thickness nor the bulge, but it will make both less noticeable.

Little can be done about the magnification of the patient's eyes as seen through the lenses except to keep the vertex distance and the lens thickness to a minimum. Magnification is less noticeable when the power of the lens decreases gradually toward the periphery, as it does in some so-called full-field high-plus lenses.

High-index lenses deserve special mention. As the mean index of refraction goes up, the ν value decreases and dispersion increases. Patients may see colored fringes around some objects viewed through the edges of their lenses, or they may report a blurring of vision. As the index goes up, reflection from the surface increases, so the lenses become less transparent and more visible. Antireflecting coating is effective in eliminating this problem, and all high-index lenses should be coated as a matter of routine. The specific gravity of high-index glass is greater than that of plastic or crown glass. As a rule, only when

the lens power is greater than 5.00D will the decreased thickness result in a lighter lens.

Specific tradenames of lenses and glass have been avoided, because these change with time. The reader is urged to maintain a file of trade publications and journal articles to stay abreast of current developments (Bennett 1983).

References

Archer, J. E., and R. S. Eakin. "The Fitting and Adjusting of Spectacles for the Older Patient." In *Vision of the Aging Patient*, eds. M. J. Hirsch and R. E. Wick. Philadelphia: Chilton, 1960, pp. 202–213.

Bennett, I. "The Changing World of Lenses." *Optometric Management*, September 1983, pp. 29–50.

Borish, I., S. Hitzeman; and K. E. Brookman, "Double Blind Study of Progressive Addition Lenses." *Journal of the American Optometric Association* 51, no. 10 (1980): 933–943.

Jones, W. F. "High Index Glasses: The Manufacturer's View." *Manufacturing Optics International*, November 1980, pp. 33–36.

Katz, M. "Distortion by Ophthalmic Lenses Calculated at the Farpoint Sphere." *American Journal of Optometry and Physiological Optics* 60 (1983): 944–959.

Morgan, M. W. *The Optics of Ophthalmic Lenses*. Chicago: Professional Press, 1978, pp. 309–327.

Schultz, D. N. "Factors Influencing Patient Acceptance of Varilux-2 Lenses." *Journal of the American Optometric Association* 54, no. 6 (1983): 513–520.

Chapter 19

Contact Lenses and the Elderly Patient

A. J. Phillips

Contact lenses have long been regarded as cosmetic devices for young people. This was largely true until recent years; increasingly, though, this attitude is changing for the following reasons:

1. The population over retirement age is increasing.
2. One of the biggest barriers—the psychological acceptance of contact lenses by older people—is being broken down.
3. Both the manufacturing and fitting expertise related to bifocal contact lenses has improved significantly in recent years.
4. Clinical expertise and new technology have increased the number of conditions that can be treated or aided by contact lenses.
5. Wearers fitted in the 1960s and 1970s are now becoming presbyopic, thereby increasing the need for presbyopic help.

It is assumed that readers will have a reasonable knowledge and understanding of contact lens practice and fitting. This chapter, therefore, will provide information on dealing with the conditions and problems associated with the older patient. The fitting of conventional lens forms to older patients will not be discussed.

The general areas considered specific to the elderly patient are (1) presbyopia, (2) aphakia, and (3) therapeutic applications more likely to occur in the elderly. Each will be dealt with in turn. Psychological aspects of dealing with elderly patients will be incorporated into the general text.

I would like to express my sincere thanks to Professor Douglas Coster, head of the Eye Department, Flinders Medical Centre, Adelaide, South Australia, for his critical appraisal of this chapter. I also thank Eva Andrea for her excellent work in the typing and layout of the chapter.

Patient Selection

Patient selection is one of the most important factors in achieving success in contact lens wear, particularly for older patients. Motivation in this age group is often quite different than in the case of younger wearers. The younger wearer is usually motivated by cosmetic factors, with sportswear considerations a poor second. The older patient has a wider variety of motivating factors; optical reasons—particulaly aphakia—and medical needs take a much higher place. Some criteria may overrule others as to whether a patient is suitable or not. The vision care practitioner has to balance the optical or medical requirements of patients against their motivation, temperament, physical disability, degree of activity, and handling difficulties.

As a general rule, the younger group of older patients probably will do better with a corneal-type lens. The older group, in contrast, is more likely to have handling problems or difficulty in even seeing a lens; therefore, perhaps this group is better suited to extended wear lenses.

Many older patients may have been advised by an ophthalmic surgeon to get contact lenses, and these patients may have little idea of what a contact lens is, let alone the pros and cons of the various lens types. The practitioner must take great care in explaining to the patient exactly what is involved in care, handling, cost, and professional visits. If the patient is very elderly, it is helpful to have a spouse, son, or daughter present both at this discussion and at least the first few visits to insure that advice and instruction are fully understood and can be reinforced.

Anatomic and Physiological Changes

General changes in the older eye are dealt with in Chapter 10. However, the contact lens fitter should bear in mind from the outset the following changes relevant to prospective contact lens wearers.

Lids. General loss of elastic tissue in the orbicularis oculi causes a gradual loss of tonus. This has the advantage of reducing the wearer's awareness of hard lenses, but it creates difficulty in lens removal by the normal "stare-pull-and-blink" method (to be discussed later in the chapter). In addition, blatant ectropion, entropion, and trichiasis are found among elderly patients and should be noted.

Tear Flow. Tear flow tends to be reduced slightly throughout life. However, many elderly patients show a particularly reduced tear flow often associated with the rheumatic-arthritic group of conditions such as Sjögren syndrome. The measurement of tear flow is described later and is an important aspect of the pre-examination routine of elderly patients. Older patients also tend to show a lower tear pH (Koetting and Andrews 1979).

Conjunctiva. Slit lamp examination of the conjunctiva will determine whether it is thickened and insensitive because of previous infection. Large pingueculae can physically lift the lids away from full contact with the cornea, creating a mildly desiccated area in the 3 and 9 o'clock areas. The palpebral conjunctiva may show "concretions," which may require excision prior to lens fitting if they are marked or numerous.

Corneas. Older patients tend to show flatter corneas. Perhaps because of the larger surface area or greater lid movement associated with the looser lids of older patients, those with complaints of dry eyes tend to have significantly flatter corneas and more acidic tears than the others. Such patients are more likely to show deposits on soft contact lenses.

Because of the effect of cataract surgery—the most common ophthalmic surgical procedure—the apex of aphakic patients generally is displaced slightly below the visual axis. Allowance therefore may have to be made, since the K (keratometer) reading could be slightly flatter than the true corneal apex value. This may explain low-riding lenses and create problems when associated with large pupils or superior iridectomy enlargements. The epithelial thickness is slightly thinner after corneal surgery. Cataract surgery also tends to flatten the vertical corneal meridian and steepen the horizontal meridian.

Cataract extraction also frequently changes the innervation level of the cornea. Researchers have established that in the human aphakic the corneal response to hypoxia is reduced by an average of 30 to 50 percent; epithelial oxygen uptake, by approximately 15 percent; corneal sensitivity, by 85 percent; and endothelial cell density, by 15 to 20 percent (Holden, Mertz, and Guillon 1980; Holden and Zantos 1981; Mertz and Holden 1981; Vannas et al. 1979; Zantos and Holden 1981; and Zantos, Holden and Pye 1980). The reduction of sensitivity and edema response partially explains why the aphakic patent is more tolerant of contact lens wear.

Presbyopic Patients

The largest proportion of older prospective contact lens wearers are presbyopes. As the current generation of contact lens wearers ages, the demand for presbyopic corrections is increasing. This has been greatly encouraged in recent years as manufacturing expertise and the choice of corrections available to the practitioner have increased.

The simplest method of correcting presbyopia is, of course, ordinary reading spectacles over the distance contact lens correction. Bifocals have the advantage that any residual astigmatic error can be incorporated into the distance portion. However, for many patients who wear contact lenses, a return to any form of spectacle correction is unacceptable.

Monovision Technique

The monovision technique involves correcting one eye for distance vision and the other, for near vision. Although it has been used for many years by some practitioners, others have been concerned about the possible loss of stereopsis. Nevertheless, in the author's experience, the method has worked very well for some patients when certain guidelines have been met.

In most cases the dominant eye should be corrected for distance vision and the nondominant, for near. This may be reversed if the patient's job involves prolonged close work. The dominant eye may be selected by any of the well-known methods (for example, pointing, hollow cone, and so on). The *full* reading correction must be given to the nondominant eye. Although a reduced addition will reduce distance blur from this eye, it also causes confusion to the wearer in knowing which eye to use for near vision. Provided the addition is not too high (and the method works best for patients requiring low- to medium-strength additions) the power of hard or gas-permeable lenses can be reduced by the laboratory or practitioner back to the distance correction so that the lens is not wasted if not tolerated by the patient. In general, patients either adapt to the monovision technique fairly quickly (within 1 to 2 weeks) or not at all.

The philosophy of monovision must be discussed with patients before starting. Some patients require reassurance that no damage to their sight will occur. The likelihood of the need for supplementary spectacles, as will be described, also should be emphasized to prevent later misunderstanding.

Monovision should not be used for patients requiring long periods of critical distance vision, but it is useful for patients who do casual reading. Shopkeepers who need to look at situations such as high shelves and people in similar situations also find the technique valuable. A fairly high proportion of monovision wearers require overcorrecting spectacles for either distance, near, or both for certain situations, such as driving.

Bifocal Hard Contact Lenses

Bifocal hard contact lenses utilize either the simultaneous vision (bivision) or alternating vision technique.

Simultaneous Vision Technique. Generally, simultaneous vision bifocal hard lenses have a small, central distance portion surrounded by a circular near area and are known as back surface concentric bifocals. Thus, the patient sees both distance and near in focus at the same time and has to learn to switch concentration from one to the other as needed. This process is aided by the slight upward movement of the lens on the downward gaze during reading.

The lenses must be fitted so they center well and have the minimum amount of movement acceptable to the practitioner and patient. This can be done by fitting the lenses larger, steeper, or thinner than usual. All three methods can result in an uncomfortable lens, so considerable care is required in fitting and manufacture. Such lenses often need to be fenestrated or manufactured from gas-permeable material. A lens that rides up very slightly is preferable to one the ettles slightly below center, since this make

near vision more difficult.

The diameter of the distance portion depends mainly on the pupil diameter. Generally, the optic diameter is slightly less than three- quarters of the pupil diameter in low illumination (for example, 2.80 mm for a 4.00 mm pupil and 2.10 mm for a 3.00 mm pupil). The diameter of the distance portion can vary according to the patient's visual requirements; for example, a patient with a minimal near vision requirement may be fitted with a larger-than-average distance portion.

Although simultaneous vision lenses are fitted infrequently in conventional hard lens form nowadays, they can be very useful when the prism-ballasted type (to be discussed) has been found unsatisfactory because of a very loose lower lid. Furthermore, they have become more popular recently in soft lens bifocal designs, where lens movement is often minimal.

Dow-Corning recently produced a multifocal aspheric gas-permeable bifocal that operates on the simultaneous vision principle: the Silcon VFL lens. It has a standard size of 9.2 mm diameter, 7.1 to 7.9 mm base curves, and a power range from +20.00 to −20.00D.

The main disadvantage of these methods of presbyopic correction is the slight blur noticed around objects, particularly when the pupil is dilated at night; this can cause great problems for some patients. Similarly, the lens design is not ideal for patients who normally have large pupil diameters or people whose pupils have been enlarged surgically.

Alternating Vision Technique. Alternating vision bifocal hard lenses may be divided into two general groups: front surface concentric bifocals and fused bifocals. As its name would suggest, front surface concentric bifocals have a central distance portion on the front surface that is surrounded by an annular reading area (Figure 19–1). The base curve diameter should be as large as possible and the intermediate and peripheral curves sufficiently flat to allow a moderate amount of lens movement. The diameter of the distance portion must be measured carefully. If it is too large (or the lens is fitted too tightly), the lens will not be able to move sufficiently to allow the patient to look through the near portion. If the diameter of the distance portion is too small, the patient will have a noticeable blur surrounding distance objects; this can become annoying when the lens moves during blinking. The diameter of the distance portion should not be smaller than the pupil size in a normal artificially lit room. If the pupil is larger than 5 mm, it is preferable to fit these lenses by the simultaneous vision method; with smaller pupils, however, the lenses normally are fitted using the alternating vision principle.

Figure 19–1

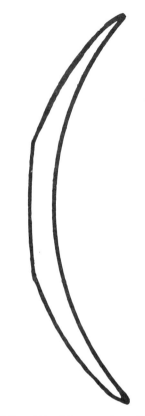

Concentric Bifocal Hard Contact Lens Shown in Cross Section

The base optic radius (BOR) is determined by the flattest K reading. If the BOR is flatter than this, the lens may ride slightly high on the cornea so that the distance portion is displaced upward. Conversely, if the BOR is made too steep, the lens may remain in a central position; thus, the patient will have difficulty getting the lens to move in order to use the near portion.

An increase in the power of the addition sometimes is required when there is a slight negative tears lens on the front surface. In such cases, fused bifocals are useful. Fused bifocals are now made in a variety of shapes and sizes. The most popular are the D and curved D segments (see Figure 19–2). These designs aim to minimize

"jump" when the wearer transfers gaze from one portion of the lens to the other. The aim of the up-curved top and Pan-O-Site (Fused Kontact, Chicago) designs is to insure that the center of the segment top is always in the same position in relation to the pupil if the lens swings slightly in a pendulum fashion on the eye (Goldberg 1969). The disadvantage of this type of segment is the possibility of slight peripheral blur at the sides during distance vision.

The portion of the edge just below the segment is extremely important. This part of the lens is pushed upward by the lower lid when the wearer looks down to read. Positive lenses obviously create the biggest problem: how to increase the lower edge thickness without increasing the overall thickness and weight more than absolutely essential. Except lenses for patients with very tight lower lids, most positive lenses are better made in a decentered convex carrier lenticular form (Figure 19–3). This keeps the weight down but increases the lower edge thickness.

For most fused lenses, prism ballast of 1.5Δ is adequte for lens orientation. For negative lenses above -4.00D, however, this should be gradually increased up to 4Δ to provide effective ballasting. The lower edge of the lens often is truncated to further aid lens orientation and lower lid support, especially if the patient has a high lower lid. In such cases the lower edge should not be thinned and should be polished minimally to prevent the lens's slipping under the lower lid on infraversion movements and thereby preventing use of the reading portion. The lower truncated edge also should be slightly curved to match the shape of the lower lid. Truncation or increased truncation also may be used to lower a near (reading) portion that partially centers in front of the pupil on distance gaze (Figure 19–4).

Before the segment position is measured, the normal head position should be ascertained. One method is to stand patients in front of a mirror and ask them to turn their head away several times, each time returning to look straight ahead at their own image. By standing behind them, it is possible for the fitter to note whether the head position is natural, as well as the relationship of each pupil to the bottom lid. If the patient then freezes in the habitual position, the fitter can step in front and measure the height of the pupil margins above the bottom lid margins. The patient's head then should be returned to duplicate this position and measure-

Figure 19-2

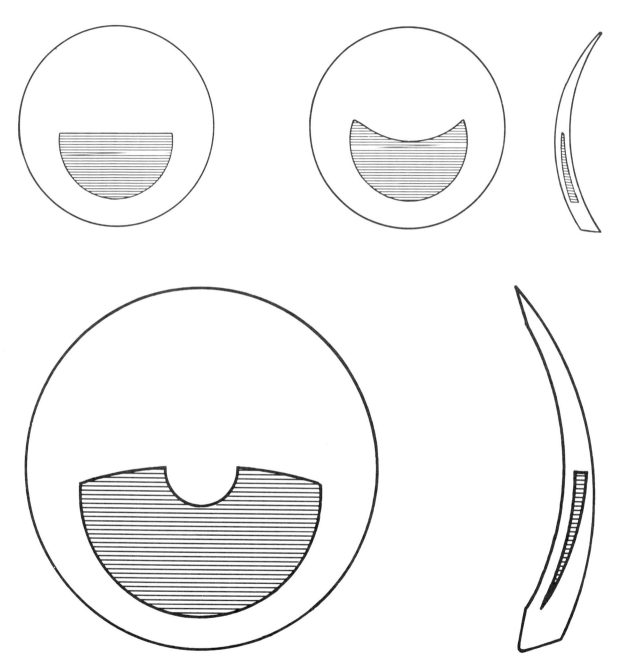

(Top, Left to Right) Fused Straight Top D Segment Contact Lens, Curved Top D Segment Contact Lens, and Cross Section of Curved D Lens (Bottom) Pan-O-Site Bifocal

ment when the fitter measures the segment position as follows.

The height of the segment above the lower edge of the lens should be ordered as high as possible without affecting the distance vision. This reduces the amount by which the lens has to rise to allow good near vision. It has been found in practice that the top of the segment can be one-quarter of the pupil diameter above the lower edge of the pupil without causing visual annoyance. Ideally, trial lenses should be used for this very important measurement; where possible, they should be supplemented by external eye photography with a fine-line scale held in

Figure 19–3

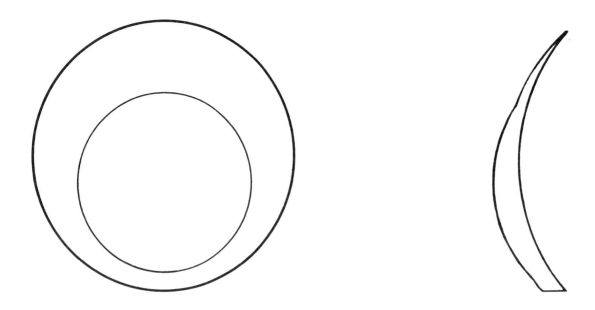

Decentered Convex Carrier Lenticular Positive-powered Bifocal Contact Lens (Reading Segment Not Shown)

Figure 19–4

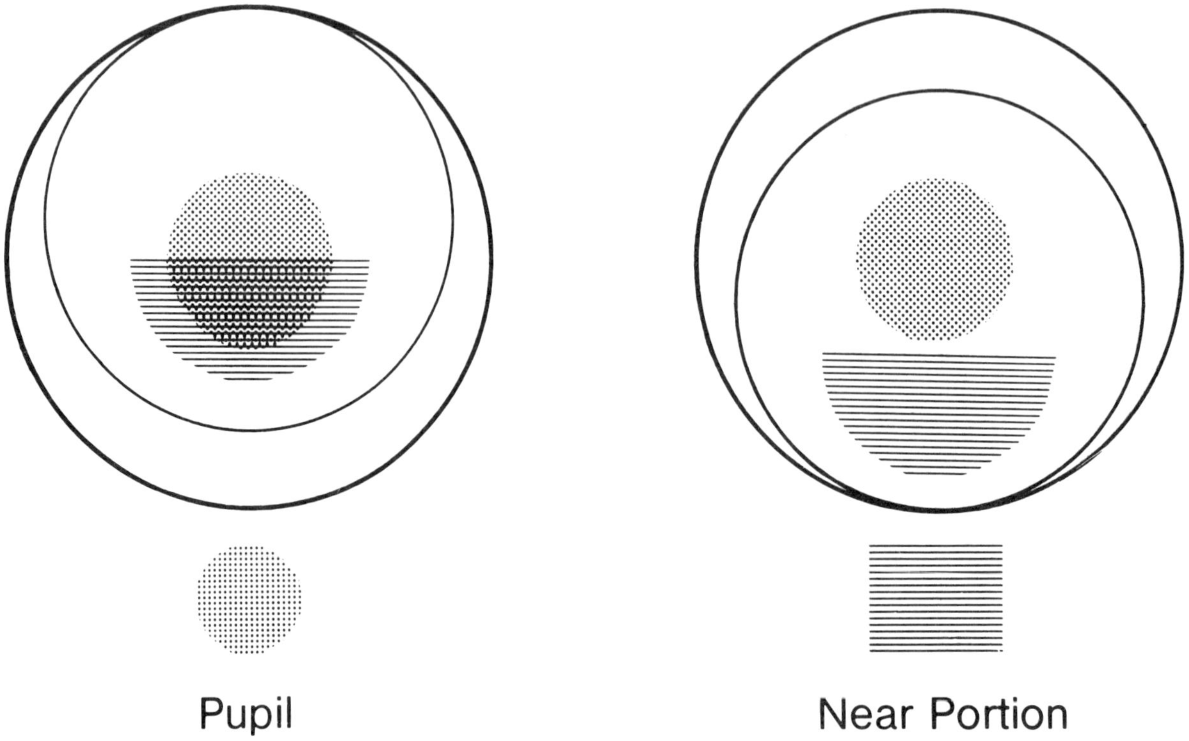

Pupil   Near Portion

Centering of a Fused Bifocal Hard Lens Generally Seen in Practice: In a Depressed Gaze for Near Vision (Left) and In a Straight-Ahead Gaze for Distance Vision (Right) approximately the same place as the iris or a measuring eyepiece in the slit lamp biomicroscope.

In addition to the information needed to order a single vision lens, the practitioner also will need to specify the following: (1) the near addition, (2) the size and shape of the segment, (3) the height of the segment above the lower edge of the lens, (4) the amount of prism ballast and thickness of the lower edge, and (5) the vertical overall size.

Trifocal and Multifocal Hard Contact Lenses

El Hage (1976) described a corneal lens having an entirely aspherical back surface with three possible variations of asphericity. The peripheral flattening of the back surface provides a continuously variable near addition. Because of the rapid degree of flattening, the posterior optical radius of the lens should be fitted approximately 0.20 to 0.25 mm steeper than the flattest K reading. To provide the maximum near addition, the greatest degree of peripheral flattening or asphericity must be used; this can result in a lens that is too mobile (and, hence, fluctuating vision) even though fitted centrally steeper than the cornea. In general, though, the results with the lens are reported to be good. Dow-Corning recently has produced an aspheric multifocal of silicon that minimizes the physiological problems of the steeper-fitting lenses necessary in this design. Because the amount of addition available at near is limited, aspheric lens designs should be ordered with the maximum plus power possible in the distance correction.

Fused trifocals are also available in the D segment design. Because each area, of necessity, is very small, the theoretical upper limit of pupil diameter is around 4.0 mm. The thickness of the segment also should be kept as thin as possible to reduce annoying reflections from the two segment tops. Alternatively, two front curves can be cut over a single segment to minimize these reflections and provide a trifocal effect.

Bifocal Soft Contact Lenses

Bifocal soft contact lenses have been produced in both the alternating and simultaneous vision designs. Table 19–1 summarizes the types discussed here. The Bi-Soft (Ciba Vision Care) bifocal is of concentric simultaneous vision design aided by the normal slight lens lag on downward gaze. Although it suffers from the general disadvantages of simultaneous vision lenses mentioned earlier, the lens has the advantages of comfort due to the thin edge and a good physiological response because of the thin center thickness (0.07 mm at −3.00D and 0.12 mm at +3.00D). The lens is available in a 13.8 mm overall diameter; three base curves; and four additions of +1.50, +2.00, +2.50, and +3.00D. The power range is +6.00D to −6.00D in 0.25D steps. The distance optic zone diameter is small; thus, the design works best for patients with small pupils.

Refraction always should be done in normal room lighting to prevent interference from the reading zone in the case of dilated pupils. The pinhole effect of the small distance area often results in more minus or less plus power than expected. Correspondingly, the addition power will have to be increased to compensate. Care should be taken that the patient does not either keep accepting more and more minus for distance vision or more and more plus for reading and eventually read through the distance portion. Although theoretically the Bi-Soft is an alternating vision lens, in practice the lens centers very well and therefore most likely functions as a simultaneous vision lens. Many practitioners find that it provides good near vision but slightly poor distance vision (Jurkus 1983).

The Bausch and Lomb Soflens Progressive Add No. 1 (PA1) bifocal is a modification of the conventional concentric design that provides a gradual change from the central distance portion to the reading portion in the midperiphery. The lens, in fact, functions on the simultaneous vision principle, and movement of only a fraction of a millimeter increases the effective addition power. Therefore, the lens functions as a multifocal lens in any direction of gaze movement, with no doubling or image jump. The lens is available in a 13.5 mm overall diameter and a single nominal addition power of +1.50D. The lens is of "thin" design (0.08 to 0.15 mm thickness for all minus powers and 0.15 to 0.21 mm thickness for the plus power range). The back vertex range is +6.00 to −6.00D. The front optical zone is 9.00 mm.

Patients fitted with this lens ideally would have reading addition requirements between +0.75 and +1.75D. The first trial lens should be selected by adding between −0.50 and −1.00D to the patient's spherical equivalent to compensate for the temporal lens decentration commonly found with spin-cast lenses that results

Table 19–1

Bifocal Soft Contact Lenses

Name	Laboratory	Base Curve (mm)	Distance Power (D)	Addition (D)	Diameter (mm)	Design
Progressive Add No. 1 (PA1)	Bausch & Lomb	Aspheric	+6.00 to −6.00	+1.50	13.5	Aspheric
Bi-Soft	Ciba Vision Care	8.3, 8.6 (and 8.9 in plus only)	+6.00 to −6.00	+1.50, +2.00, +2.50, +3.00	13.8	Concentric
Bal-Focal	Salvatori	8.4, 8.7	+5.00 to −5.00	+1.50, +2.00, +2.50	13.5, 14.0	Tapered negative carrier ballasted; concentric
Trufocal	Wesley-Jessen	8.3, 8.6, 9.0	+4.50 to −4.50	+1.00 to +2.75 in +0.25 steps	14.5	Crescent segment, prism ballasted
Softsite	Paris	8.9, 9.2	+2.00 to −4.00	+1.50, +2.00, +2.50	13.0, 13.5	Crescent segment, prism ballasted, truncated

in the patient's looking through a more positive-powered zone. The optimum distance acuity is obtained by overrefraction. Occasionally a compromise between distance and near acuities is necessary. The main problem with this design is the lens decentration and the consequent visual compromise and flare at night.

The limited single addition can be adapted for higher additions by overplussing the non-dominant eye (or the eye usually used for near vision); alternatively, the nondominant eye can be fitted with a single vision reading-powered lens and the other eye, a bifocal lens. This modified monovision approach still allows intermediate vision and greater binocularity at near than the conventional monovision technique.

In the solid, alternating vision design the lens is usually prism ballasted and truncated, and the bifocal is worked on the front surface. As the top of the segment cannot be seen when the lens is on the eye, one British-designed lens has two small indicator lines, 1.50 mm in length, engraved on the lens to enable easy practitioner location (R. L. Bifocal, Madden Lenses Ltd.).

The Sof-Form Bal-Focal (Salvatori Ophthalmics) is a ballasted lens design available in two overall diameters of 13.5 and 14.0 mm.

The distance zone diameter is 4.0 mm and the total optic zone diameter, 8.3 mm. Two base curves are available (8.4 and 8.7 mm) with a power range of +5.00 to −5.00D and three addition powers of +1.50, +2.00, and +2.50D.

The manufacturers recommend the smaller-diameter lens for vertical palpebral apertures under 10 mm or where the distance portion centers above the pupil and vice versa. Patients with pupil diameters between 2.5 and 4.5 mm only are generally considered suitable. In contrast with previously discussed lenses, this lens design has no prism ballast or truncation. Instead, a "bal-flange" construction stabilizes the lens for translation to occur. This construction is a modified −18.00D lenticulated carrier thinned at the superior portion of the lens to allow for minimal center thickness but still provide lens stability.

The Wesley-Jessen Trufocal has a prism-ballasted, truncated upsweep design, (see Figure 19–5). The lens is available in back vertex powers of +4.50 to −4.50D with addition powers of +1.00 to +2.75D in +0.25D steps. The lens is 38 percent water. Its overall diameter is 14.5 mm with a 1 mm truncation and three base curves of 8.30, 8.60, and 9.0 mm.

Figure 19-5

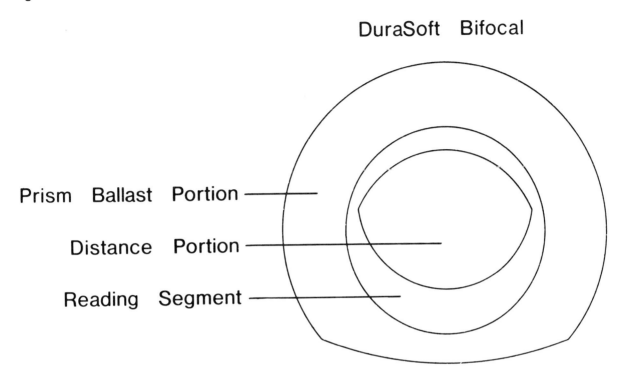

DuraSoft Bifocal

Prism Ballast Portion ——

Distance Portion ——

Reading Segment ——

Trufocal Soft Contact Lens (Wesley-Jessen)

Lens translation is the principle for the performance of this lens design. The lifting power of the upper lid holds up the lens on distance viewing, and the lower lid acts as a stop for the lens on downward gaze. The lens is not permitted to move downward, the cornea is allowed to turn behind the lens, and the pupillary axis passes from the distance to the near portion of the lens. The base-down prism and truncation helps supply a ledge to stop at the lower lid.

The Paris Softsite bifocal is an upsweep segmented design with 1Δ of prism ballast and a slight truncation. The distance power is +2.00 to −4.00D. Two diameters, 13.0 and 13.5 mm, are available; two base curves, 8.9 and 9.2 mm; and a large distance optic zone 6.00 mm in diameter. This latter property makes the lens very useful for patients with large pupils, but occasionally vertical diplopia can result. Three additions are currently available: +1.50, +2.00 and +2.50D. This lens, like the Wesley-Jessen lens, functions by the translation principle; the lens is fitted as flat as possible to enhance the movement. A retinoscope can determine the segment position in relation to the pupil. If there is a position problem, the manufacturer can adjust the seg-

ment height in the lens.

The possible problems with the prism-ballasted lens in hydrophilic form spring from the difficulties in keeping the lens from becoming excessively thick and heavy and thereby creating discomfort or long-term anoxia problems. Also, whereas vertical movement is normally required for prism-ballasted lenses to function properly, hydrophilic lenses are usually more comfortable and successful when this movement is minimal.

Bifocal Summary

The fitting of hard or soft bifocal contact lenses requires patience and skill. It should not be attempted by the novice practitioner. There are many pitfalls even for the skilled practitioner, and a one-third to one-half success rate would be considered acceptable, if not good. Patients, therefore, must be warned of this from the onset, particularly with regard to the fees and time involved should the fitting not be successful. Nevertheless, when the fitting is successful, the rewards in terms of patient satisfaction are very gratifying.

Aphakia and Extended Wear Contact Lenses

Aphakia is the major reason elderly people need extended wear contact lenses (See chapter 17). Aphakic patients who might be considered suitable candidates for extended wear lenses include the following:

1. Those who have a physical disablement, such as arthritis or Parkinson's disease, that would prevent them from inserting and removing a daily wear lens.
2. Monocular aphakics who have sufficient residual vision in the phakic eye to obtain an optical benefit from the binocular vision afforded by a contact lens but sufficiently poor vision to make the handling of a daily wear lens difficult.
3. Intraocular lens candidates who did not have a lens implanted during surgery because of contraindications such as endothelial damage.
4. Patients who are aphakic in one eye and have an intraocular lens implant in the other. These could use extended wear lenses as a trial before undergoing the surgical procedure for a secondary implant. Such a trial is preferable to the risk of the secondary implantation.
5. Patients with poor facilities or ability for lens disinfection.
6. Patients with reduced macular function for whom the additional restriction of the visual field afforded by aphakic spectacles creates problems.

Many different forms of extended wear lenses now exist throughout the world. Space does not permit more than a brief summary of the most well known ones. These will be described later as examples from which the reader should be able to deduce (with the help of laboratory manuals) routines and techniques applicable to most other lens forms.

Intraocular Lenses or Extended Wear Contact Lenses?

Although the decision between intraocular lenses and extended wear contact lenses ultimately will be made by the surgeon, of course, patients may ask optometrists to discuss or explain the advantages and disadvantages of the two modes of aphakic correction. Basically, an extended wear contact lens has the following advantages over an intraocular lens:

1. A contact lens is probably safer than an intraocular lens, because it easily can be removed and refitted at a later date.
2. An extended wear lens usually can be used when an intraocular lens is contraindicated (for example, with reduced corneal endothelial function or corneal damage).
3. Extended wear lenses can prevent the need for secondary intraocular lens insertion or keratophakia—both relatively high risk procedures.
4. The power of the contact lens can be changed easily to give the desired spherical equivalent.
5. Intraocular complications rarely develop with extended wear lens use.
6. Patients with long life expectancies may be fitted more safely with contact lenses than intraocular lenses, since the long-term effects of intraocular lenses over many years remain unknown.

There are some advantages of an intraocular over an extended wear lens, however, if no operation or postoperative complications develop from lens implantation:

1. Although the intraocular lens is more expensive initially, its lower ongoing costs make it less expensive in the long term.
2. The intraocular lens is significantly more convenient for the patient.
3. The intraocular lens may provide more stable vision (but not better stereoscopic acuity).
4. The intraocular lens may be more successful for patients with external ocular problems such as blepharitis, eyelid abnormalities, and dry eyes.

Most patients fitted with a successful intraocular lens in one eye and a contact lens in the other prefer the intraocular lens. However, a survey carried out at Flinders Medical Centre, Adelaide, South Australia, showed equally good results for the two types of correction on Visual Disability Scale scores. Both types of lenses performed better than the spectacle correction.

Initial Examination

The beginning of this chapter discussed the importance of patient selection. In general, the main motivating factors for extended wear are optical or medical, and these should be balanced against a patient's own desire for lenses, temperament, physical disability, degree of activity, and potential handling ability. In general, extended wear lens patients should have the following characteristics:

1. Sufficient mental alertness to clearly understand the concept, care, and potential problems involved in extended lens wear.
2. Ideally, the capability of handling the lenses themselves or a spouse, relative, or friend residing nearby.
3. No anterior segment pathology. Although at higher risk, these patients sometimes may be included with careful planning.
4. Normal tear flow. Keratitis sicca is a relative contraindication, but the frequent instillation of artificial tears may allow patients to successfully wear the lenses. The risk, however, in such cases is the decreased lysozyme component and the resultant risk of infection.
5. Normal intraocular pressures. Placing an extended wear lens on the eye slows down the oxygen supply to a cornea that might already be taxed by an elevation of intraocular pressure. Even mild cases of ocular hypertension, therefore, should be approached with great care.
6. Ready availability and easy access for aftercare and any emergency treatment. This should include access to a hospital with ophthalmological expertise.
7. No previous history of problems such as edema or deposits with daily wear soft lenses.
8. Normal lid margin function. Chronic blepharitis of almost any cause greatly limits the success rate of extended wear lenses. Often, prescribing systemic tetracycline (250 mg twice daily), antibiotic lid ointments at bedtime, and daily lid scrubs using dampened cotton wool buds can control posterior blepharitis with inflammation of the meibomian glands. Similarly, many patients with chronic dermatitis such as acne rosacea will have limited success unless the condition is carefully controlled.
9. Normal endothelial function. Patients who have had unplanned vitreous loss with marginal corneal decompensation may not wear the lenses successfully. Similarly, patients who exhibit cornea guttata may be at high risk.
10. No unplanned or filtering blebs. Not only do these areas displace lenses, but the risk of irritating the blebs with subsequent infection lead most authorities to reject such patients for extended wear.

Following the initial discussion with the patient, careful refraction and calculation of ocular refraction should be carried out. The normal relationship of corneal to refractive cylinders following keratometry should be noted, and acuities should be recorded. Ophthalmoscopy and slit lamp biomicroscopy should reveal none of the contraindications just listed. In addition, the presence of residual sutures should be noted, along with the placement of any cataract incision and the vascular pattern around suture scars. Great care should be shown if the vascular pattern extends further than the suture scar line. Tear flow may be measured using conventional Schirmer or break-up time (BUT) methods. Apposition of the puncta to the globe should be noted and the lid margins and conjunctiva carefully examined for abnormalities. Intraocular pressure and visual fields should be recorded for future reference.

Fitting Routine

The materials generally used in extended wear fitting are of higher water content and take longer to equilibrate on the cornea than the thinner materials of lower water content. Ideally, therefore, the initial fitting should be done in the morning; this enables examination of both the fitting and initial response of the eye after 4 to 8 hours. If possible, patients should be taught how to handle the lenses and be given an emergency telephone number if maintaining extended wear. They then should be examined the next morning while they are wearing the lenses. If the practitioner possesses a pachymeter, corneal thickness readings can be compared with the prefitting values.

For a typical daily wear soft lens, the cornea will have thickened by the normal 3 percent on waking; this will settle to about 2 percent during the day with the lens in place. In extended wear, the waking figure is around 12 to 14 percent and reduces to about 4 to 6 percent during waking hours. The cornea appears to be able to reduce its overnight edema by about 8 percent (Holden 1983). Overnight thickness increases of greater than 15 percent or daytime reductions of less than 7 to 8 percent should be regarded as contraindications for extended wear. As the lens will partially dehydrate overnight, the fitting will appear slightly tight upon waking and soon thereafter. The practitioner should bear this in mind when assessing the fitting and general response of the eye, along with the acuity and subjective symptoms.

Signs of obvious endothelial striae or blebs, edema greater than that previously discussed, epithelial staining more than a mild superficial punctate keratitis, marked perilimbal injection, or subjective discomfort all may be contraindications unless some change in fitting is indicated. In the latter case the eye should be reexamined 24 hours later with the new lens in place.

Provided the acuity is reasonable, small lens power changes can be ignored until full settling has taken place by the next appointment. It usually is helpful to overestimate the positive power of aphakic lenses before putting a lens on the eye, even after allowances for vertex distance have been made. Fatt (1983) pointed out that hydrogel lenses typically lose 10 to 15 percent of their total water content during wear. This, in turn, reduces the positive power of the lens, sometimes by as much as 2.00 to 3.00D

Patients with compromised corneas or any other physiological or pathological complication should not immediately begin extended wear; they should build up their wearing time to waking hours only prior to an ocular examination. Only then should they begin extended wear, and careful monitoring must still be maintained.

The patient is next examined one week later. A full history and overrefraction should be carried out. Most elderly patients will need bifocals prescribed for near vision, and any cylindrical correction can be usefully incorporated into the distance portion. Prescribing a maximum plus correction in order to require a negative cylinder spectacle overrefraction will aid intermediate vision without the spectacles if the residual astigmatism is not too great. In cases of monocular aphakia where there is reasonable vision in the other eye, the lens power should be selected to give an overrefractive correction approximately similar to this other eye. Although large differences occasionally are tolerated, anisometropia of more than approximately 2.00 to 3.00D may give rise to symptoms of aniseikonia.

Careful evaluation of the fitting should show good centration; no accumulation of postlens debris; adequate lens movement; and no signs of limbal compression or blurred vision between blinking, which indicates a tightly fitting lens. This should be strongly avoided in extended wear. Slit lamp examination should show no epithelial staining, minimal striae and endothelial bleb formation, and minimal limbal injection. Edema may be expected to peak at one week. It will subside slowly over the next few weeks, leveling at about 4 percent more than the normal with current-generation lenses. Keratometry generally will show little change; any edema is usually across the whole cornea, and the thickness increase thereby produced changes the curvature uniformly.

By one month the eye should be quiet and settled. The patient should have no awareness of the lens. The acuity with any overrefractive correction worn should approximate the spectacle acuity, although it is often one line worse. Provided no adverse subjective or objective reaction is present, the patient can be examined every three to four months thereafter.

Extended Wear Contact Lens Selection

The goal of extended wear is clear, comfortable vision without adverse ocular side effects. To reduce complications, it is extremely important that extended wear lenses not disrupt corneal physiology. It has been well established that the cornea becomes edematous when the oxygen level available to it falls below a critical level. Polse and Mandell (1971) established this level to be between 1.5 and 2.5 percent, or 11.4 and 19.0 mm Hg minimum oxygen tension. Hill and Carney (1976) suggest that a 10 percent level would permit a favorable margin of safety for normal corneal metabolism.

Lens design for extended wear, therefore, has emphasized the importance of oxygen transmissibility. Oxygen transmissibility of hydrophilic soft contact lenses is directly proportional to their water content and inversely proportional to their thickness. In designing an optimum hydrogel extended wear lens, the gain in oxygen transmission must be balanced with the increased fragility and flexibility and the decreased stability and tensile strength that occur when water content is increased and center thickness is decreased. Thus, as the power increases with the Hydrocurve II lens, for example, the oxygen transmission goes down. With other lenses—Permalens, for example—this problem has been reduced by reducing the size of the front optic as the power increases. However, the thinner, stronger material may be preferred either because it is easier for the patient to handle, because it is less vulnerable to tearing, or because the larger optic is necessary due to a decentered or enlarged pupil following surgery. Alternatively, one lens form may be selected because the power is outside the range produced by another manufacturer. The following summary of the commonly available aphakic lenses can help practitioners select the most appropriate lens type for each particular patient.

Hydrocurve II. Hydrocurve II (Barnes-Hind/Revlon) lenses are fabricated from bufilcon A, a terpolymer containing largely hydroxyethylmethacrylate (HEMA) plus acrylamide in water contents of 45 and 55 percent. The lenses are made of minimal thickness and are designed to improve the oxygen permeability normally associated with materials of higher water content. The 55 percent material is used for aphakic extended wear lenses.

The range of parameters for Hydrocurve II lenses follows:

Back Vertex Power (D)	Base Curve (mm)	Diameter (mm)	Center Thickness (mm)	Front Optic Diameter (mm)
+7.25 to +20.00	8.5	14.0	0.29 (+10.0)	
	8.8	14.5	0.32 (+12.0)	
	9.2	15.5	0.35 (+14.0)	8.5
	9.5	16.0		
	9.8	16.0	0.39 (+16.0)	
			0.43 (+18.0)	
			0.48 (+20.0)	

The 14.0 and 14.5 mm diameter lenses are used for the majority of eyes; the 15.5 and 16.0 mm lenses are used for large or flat corneas or where centration is a problem. Normally, the 8.5 mm radius lens is used for corneas steeper than 7.9 mm (42.00D) and the 8.8 mm radius, for flatter corneas.

Permalens. The Permalens (Cooper Laboratories) is lathed from the polymer perfilcon A, a terpolymer of 2-HEMA vinylpyrrolidone and methacrylic acid. It contains approximately 71 percent water by weight at 38°C. The lens may be chemically or thermally disinfected, although repeated heating causes lens browning, a problem common to nearly all materials containing N-vinylpyrrolidone.

For most corneas the 8.6/14.5 mm is the most commonly fitted; the 8.3/14.5 mm, 8.3/14.0 mm, and 8.0/14.0 mm being used for progressively steeper, smaller corneas. Conversely, the 8.9/14.5 mm lens is used for larger, flatter corneas or where greater lens movement is required.

The parameters available in the aphakic range follow:

Back Vertex Power (D)	Base Curve (mm)	Diameter (mm)	Center Thickness (mm)	Front Optic Diameter (mm)
+10.00 to +20.00 in 0.50D steps	8.0	14.0	0.39 mm (at +10.00D) to 0.43 mm (at +14.00D and above)	7.7 (at +10.00D)
	8.3	14.0		7.5 (at +12.00D)
	8.3	14.5		7.2 (at +14.00D)
	8.6	14.5		6.8 (at +16.00D)
	8.9	14.5		6.0 (at +20.00D)

Sauflon PW and Bausch & Lomb CW 79. The Sauflon PW lens is made of lidofilcon B, a copolymer of methylmethacrylate and N-vinyl 2-pyrrolidone with a water content of 79 percent at 38°C. The Bausch & Lomb CW 79 lens is similar to the Sauflon PW material, but the manufacturers claim improvements including reduced lens susceptibility to heat discoloration in thermal disinfection.

The following parameters are available:

Back Vertex Power (D)	Base Curve (mm)	Diameter (mm)	Center Thickness (mm)	Front Optic Diameter (mm)
+10.00 to +20.00 in 0.50D steps	8.1		0.49 to 0.79	
	8.4	14.4		8.0
	8.7			

By comparison, the Bausch & Lomb daily wear aphakic H series lenses (38 percent water content) have the following parameters:

Back Vertex Power (D)	Base Curve (mm)	Diameter (mm)	Center Thickness (mm)	Front Optic Diameter (mm)
+6.50 to +20.00 in 0.50D steps	8.1 (H3)	13.5 (H3)	0.53 (H3)	9.0 (H3)
	8.9 (H4)	14.5 (H4)	0.50 (H4)	9.0 (H4)

Silsoft. Silsoft (Dow-Corning) lenses are made from elastofilcon A, a specially formulated 100 percent silicone polymer. The claimed advantages of the Silsoft lenses are oxygen permeability, durability of the wettable surface, ease of handling, enhanced visual performance, ability to use fluorescein to assess fitting, durability and mechanical strength, and physical stability. The lenses are made by precision molding under high temperature and pressure. Their power, base curve, and lot number then are engraved on the lenses using laser technology. The back surface has three curves, and the front surface is lenticulated.

The following lens parameters are available:

Back Vertex Power (D)	Base Curve (mm)	Diameter (mm)	Center Thickness (mm)	Front Optic Diameter (mm)
+7.00 to +32.00	7.3			
	7.5			
	7.7			
	7.9	11.3 and 12.5	0.35 (at +14.00D)	Approximately 8.0 mm
	8.1			
	8.3			
	8.5			

Unlike natural silicon, the finished Silsoft lens surface is wettable. This is an integral property of the material and is not due to a surface coating. However, the lens wettability is reduced slightly if it is stored dry; therefore, it should be stored in one of the recommended solutions (for example, Barnes-Hind Softmate or Soft-Therm) and a surfactant daily cleaner and proteolytic enzyme should be used as needed. However, some authorities feel that any form of cleaning likely to remove or damage the treated surface layer of the lens and recommend no cleaning beyond rinsing with the storage solution upon removal from the eye. The lenses may be chemically or thermally disinfected.

The Silsoft lens should be fitted to give minimal apical clearance, light intermediate bearing, and moderate edge lift. The lens generally is fitted on K. It is most important to achieve both an adequate fluorescein pattern and adequate lens movement of 1 to 2 mm on blinking.

The general subjective reaction to Silsoft lenses is between that of conventional hard and soft lenses, so a definite adaptation period is necessary. Greater-than-normal edge standoff will exacerbate lens awareness, whereas too close an edge will result in a tightly fitting lens.

Softcon. The Softcon (American Optical) lens is of vifilcon A, a copolymer of 2-HEMA and povidone. It is lathe cut and has a water content of 55 percent. The following parameters are available:

Back Vertex Power (D)	Base Curve (mm)	Diameter (mm)	Center Thickness (mm)	Front Optic Diameter (mm)
+8.00 to +18.00	7.8	13.5	Maximum of 0.64 mm	
	8.1	14.0		7.3 mm
	8.4	14.5		
	8.7			

The most commonly used lens for the aphakic eye is the 8.4/14.0 mm. Approximately 20 to 30 minutes should be allowed for lens settling. There should then be correct centration around the limbus and 1.0 to 1.5 mm of lens movement on vertical gaze. If this is not achieved, the lens fitting should be amended in the usual ways.

The lens may be disinfected by either chemical or thermal methods, although repeated use of the latter method causes discoloration of the lens material.

TC 75. The TC 75 (Trans Canada Contact Lens Ltd.) lens is a lathe-cut lens of the copolymer of HEMA and methacrylic acid. The water content varies from 68 to 75 percent. The following parameters are available:

Back Vertex Power (D)	Base Curve (mm)	Diameter (mm)	Center Thickness (mm)	Front Optic Diameter (mm)
Up to +20.00	7.8	13.0	0.435 (at +10.00D) to 0.49 (at +13.00D and above	10.36 (at +10.00D) to 6.00 (at +20.00D)
	8.1	13.5		
	8.4	14.0		
	8.7	14.5		
	9.0			

The 8.4/14.0 mm and 8.7/14.5 mm are the most commonly used aphakic parameters. After 20 to 30 minutes of settling, a correctly fitted lens should show good centration; stable acuity; and, ideally, 0.5 to 1.0 mm of movement upon vertical gaze.

Patient Instruction

Whenever possible, patients should be instructed to remove, insert, and clean their lenses themselves (Figure 19–6). In certain cases these procedures may best be done by a spouse, son, or daughter, but any relative helping should live near the patient. Instructions should be given both orally and in printed form. The spouse, son, or daughter should be present where feasible.

Lens handling often can be a major stumbling block. Often the problem is simply seeing the lens. To solve this problem, ordinary reading spectacles can be worn up to the time of lens insertion. Some patients find that when inserting the first lens, it helps to use reading spectacles that have had one lens and lower rim removed. In most cases a magnifying (concave) mirror is adequate, particularly an illuminated makeup mirror (see Figure 19–7). The table and mirror used for insertion practice should be kept fairly high, as most elderly patients find bending

Figure 19-6

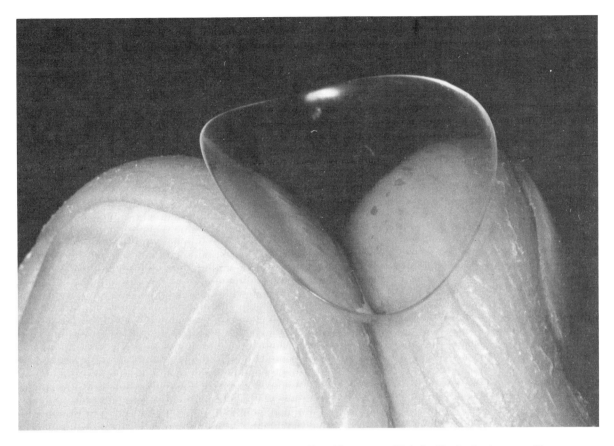

In Handling Aphakic Lenses, Balance the Lens across Two Fingers or Slightly Pinch the Lens as Shown

difficult. A towel placed over the lap is useful in case lenses are dropped. Patients always should check their own acuity after insertion, as elderly patients (particularly the aphakic group) often have little lid or corneal sensation to confirm the presence of a lens.

The following special advice should be given to the elderly extended wear lens patient:

1. Emergency telephone numbers should be given, including that of the nearest hospital eye department for use when the practitioner is unobtainable.
2. Provide specific instructions to report immediately if symptoms of pain, persistent discomfort, red eye, foggy vision, or white spots on the cornea that do not move on blinking are noticed (see the example in Figure 19-8).
3. Warn the patient that slight fluctuation of vision may occur toward the end of the day.
4. Tell the patient that the lids may be slightly encrusted upon waking.
5. Explain that slight foggy vision on waking

may occur.
6. Have the patient check his or her vision on waking (that is, check for lens presence) and then use an in-eye cleaner (to be discussed) or eye wash.
7. Explain necessary care in handling an ejected, dehydrated lens.
8. Warn of the risk of occasional diplopia if vision is being restored in one eye after a long period of nonuse.

Cleaning Solutions

Lenses of higher water content used on a daily wear basis lead to more solution preservative reaction than normal. However, if they are used intermittently, as in extended wear, solution reactions are seen infrequently. Only one range of solutions is produced largely for extended wear lens use: the Mira-range by Cooper. This consists of the following solutions:

1. *MiraSoak.* This contains chlorhexidine, 0.008 percent; and ethylenediamine tetraacetate (EDTA), 0.1 percent.

Figure 19-7

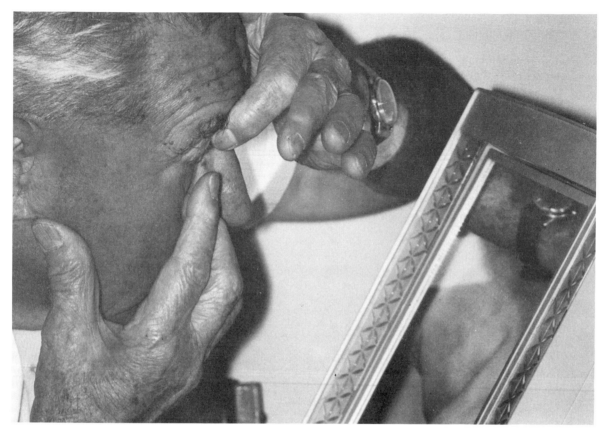

Illuminated Concave Makeup Mirror Used for Patient Insertion of Contact Lens

2. *MiraSol.* This contains sodium and potassium borate, 0.8 percent; thimerosal, 0.001 percent; EDTA, 0.1 percent; sorbic acid, 0.1 percent; sodium borate, 0.22 percent; and poloxamer 407, 1.0 percent.
3. *MiraFlow.* This contains 20 percent isopropyl alcohol plus two surfactants with no preservatives.
4. *Clerz.* This contains sodium and potassium borate, 0.8 percent; EDTA, 0.1 percent; sorbic acid, 0.1 percent; sodium borate, 0.22 percent; and poloxamer 407, 1.0 percent.

Clerz has been found very useful in reducing lens deposits without the patient's having to remove the lens from the eye. This is achieved by the surfactant and the slight hypertonicity of the solution, which withdraws surface contaminants from the lens by osmotic pressure. This latter property helps reduce morning edema if used upon waking. Also, the dehydrating of the front lens surface may effectively flatten the fitting slightly and temporarily increase lens movement, thereby reducing

retrolens contaminants. Kersley and Kerr (1981) have found a significant improvement in deposit reduction by instructing patients to use an eyebath containing fresh unpreserved saline (from packets) each morning upon waking. Keates (personal communication, 1980) recommends the use of an alkaline eyewash (to be discussed in "Red Eye Reaction").

Boiling lenses in saline can be a safe method of disinfection. However, because of the N-vinyl 2-pyrrolidone contained in nearly all extended wear materials, lenses will discolor increasingly with each cycle. This does not appear to affect the physiological properties of the lens, but the lens appearance may be psychologically unacceptable to the patient. The effect of heat disinfection on lens deposits is more important, since extended wear lenses usually have more surface contamination than regularly cleaned daily wear lenses. Problems from denatured protein therefore will be exacerbated by thermal disinfection, and this will cause marked difficulties in the patient prone to heavy lens deposition.

Figure 19-8

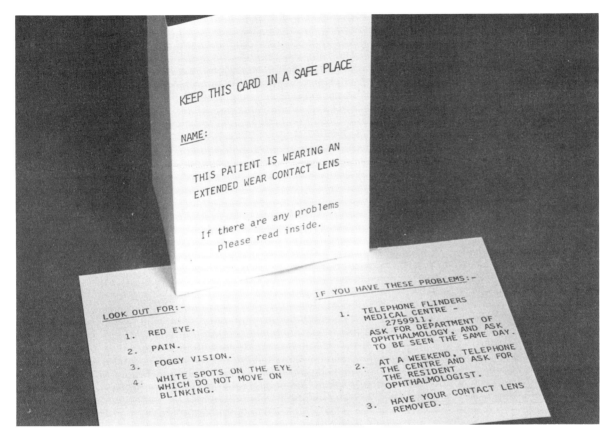

Warning Card Issued to Extended Lens Wearers by Flinders Medical Centre, Adelaide, South Australia

Other solutions particularly suitable for the extended wear lens patient are hydrogen peroxide methods such as the American Optical Lensept/Lensrins system. Because of its oxidizing process, this method not only acts as an effective disinfecting technique, but also breaks down lens deposits and minimizes lens discoloration. The Softab method of Contact Lens Manufacturing uses sodium dichloroisocyanurate, which breaks down in saline to release 3 ppm free chlorine. This acts in a way similar to the hydrogen peroxide method (oxidizing action), but it is perhaps less effective. However, it has the advantage of being a one-step method, unlike the hydrogen peroxide methods, which almost invariably require a neutralization step.

As stated earlier, in practice almost any solution intended for use with hydrogel lenses can be used safely with extended wear lenses. The infrequent use of the storage solution does not allow buildup within the lens structure, so solution sensitivity rarely occurs.

Aftercare

Specific pathological and other complications occur with extended wear lenses. Ruben (1976) listed the following pathological complications:
1. Neovascularization.
2. Edema.
3. Anterior uveitis.
4. Follicular conjunctivitis.
5. Keratoconjunctivitis.
6. Chronic superficial keratopathy.
7. Stromal lysis with marginal degeneration.
8. Hypertrophic epithelial reaction.
9. Corneal abscess.

Ruben (1977) also stated that infection occurred in 8 percent of extended wear lens wearers with preexisting ocular disease, 4.1 percent of cosmetic wearers of extended wear lenses, and 30 percent of aphakic patients who wear extended wear lenses. The major problems that occur with extended wear lenses, therefore, may be summarized as *infection* and *neovascularization*. Other general problems that occur are described in the following paragraphs.

Lens Displacement. Most extended wear lens patients rarely lose lenses through spontaneous ejection, but some lose large numbers. Often they are unaware when this happens, although it is most likely during the night or on first waking, while the lens is partially dehydrated. Some patients find it helpful to wear an eyepatch during the night for the first few weeks.

Breakage. Breakage rarely occurs while the lens is on the eye; it usually occurs during cleaning. The lack of tactile sensitivity in most elderly patients makes delicate lens handling and cleaning difficult. During cleaning, the finger-palm method is best avoided; the lens should be supported on the tip of one finger and massaged with the cleaner using a finger from the other hand. The lens then is everted to clean the other surface.

Deposits. Deposits are the major reason for lens replacement. They also make up a large proportion of patient symptoms at aftercare visits. Deposits fall into two general groups: (1) the general diffuse, denatured proteinaceous layer or areas seen on all types of hydrogel lens; and (2) white spots, possibly calcium, lipopolysaccharide, or a mixture of both. These often are localized in the lower half and presumably are exacerbated by an incomplete blink action (see Figures 19-9 and 19-10). Once formed, they maintain their inferior lens position by friction with the upper lid, much as in prism ballasting.

Deposits are worse in poor blinkers, dry-eyed patients, and possibly in those with loosely fitting Permalenses (Hodd 1976a) and tightly fitting Sauflon PW lenses (Hodd 1976b). Education in full blinking and the use of artificial tears, eye washes with normal saline, and in-eye cleaners such as Clerz, all help to a limited

Figure 19-9

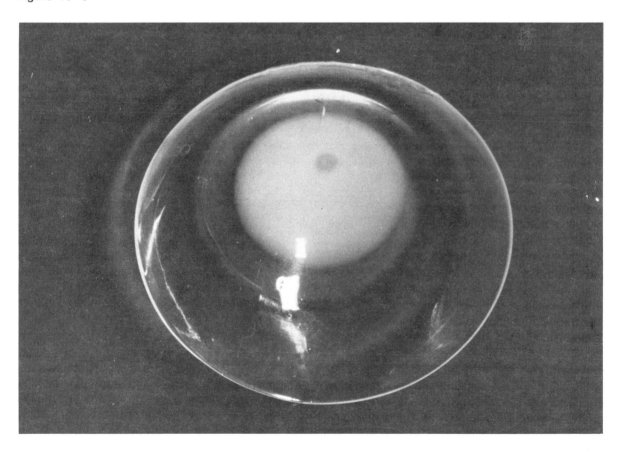

Opaque Central Area of Aphakic Permalens Repeatedly Inadvertently Boiled in Mirasol Preserved Storage Solution. The opacification is probably caused by a polymer in the solution.

Figure 19-10

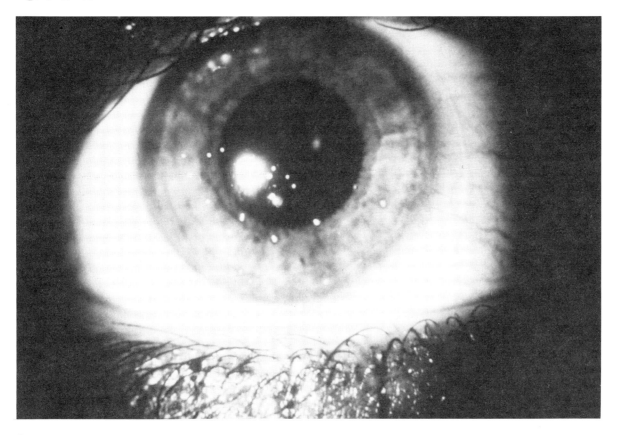

Calcium Deposits Localized in the Lower Half of an Extended Wear Lens

degree. Good lid margin hygiene with daily baby shampoo scrubs using cotton wool buds occasionally provides additional help.

Careful cleaning prior to fortnightly or monthly disinfection also will help avoid lens deposits. All normal surfactants may be used. Opticlean (Alcon/BP's Polyclens) can be used as a prophylactic in the prevention of major deposit formation. Enzyme cleaners such as papain (Allergan/Bausch & Lomb), pronase (Laboratoires Amisol's (Paris) Amiclair), or pancreatin (Alcon/BP) also may be used. Some protease enzymes may cause ocular irritation when used with lenses of higher water content. To prevent this, the tablet should be dissolved in saline, not distilled water. The subsequent shrinkage of the lens appears to prevent protease molecular entry into the lens surface. Cleaning and overnight soaking in a chemical storage solution is then essential both for lens disinfection and to restore isotonicity. The shorter contact times of the current effervescent papain tablets also reduce enzyme adsorption into the lens. Other "extra-strength" cleaners, such as Barnes-Hind's Soft-mate Weekly Cleaning Solution, may be used effectively.

Irritation. Assuming a correctly fitting lens, the two major causes of irritation are partial dehydration of the lens and lens deposits. Partial dehydration may be reduced by the use of artificial tears or in-eye cleaners such as Clerz, Blink-n-Clean, Adapettes, and so forth. Some dry-eyed patients are best changed to daily wear lenses and should then store their lenses in hypotonic saline. The saline initially should be diluted by 20 percent, and this figure then increased or decreased in 10 percent steps for optimal comfort to a maximum of 50 percent dilution. This artificially increases the water content of the lens and then slowly releases it onto the eye. Lens disinfection must be carried out either by a thermal method or by using the Softab chemical system (see *"Tear Film Disorders"* later in the chapter).

Some extended wear patients experience drying lenses at night, and actually are awakened by discomfort, redness, and irritation.

The probable cause of this problem is a borderline tear flow associated with primary nocturnal lagophthalmos or lagophthalmos secondary to ptosis or blepharoplasty. In mild cases a frequent application of artificial tears or a petroleum-based ointment at bedtime may alleviate the problem. Alcohol consumption also can cause a lens to dry out on the eye the next morning, because alcohol is an osmotic agent.

Red Eye Reaction. A red eye reaction can occur as diffuse keratoconjunctivitis, focal keratitis with sterile infiltrates, or keratouveitis. Frequently it occurs upon waking, and, although it can occur in both cosmetic and aphakic extended wear lenses, it is more likely to occur in the aphakic. Several causes have been postulated. One is that the lens tightens on the eye overnight, leading to the accumulation of metabolic waste and a drop in the tear pH. Another is that pathogens are trapped by mucous adhesion behind the lens, producing a conjunctivitis-like reaction. However, cultures of patients with red eye reactions often show negative results. Possibly the reaction is due to epithelial breakdown's being greater than regeneration because of anoxia, poor fitting, deposits, and so on. Red eye reactions often occur 1 to 2 days after the fortnightly or monthly disinfection cycle. Because of this, solution preservatives or cleaners have been blamed. Since the reaction is delayed and can occur with either no or minimal solution exposure, this theory has not been confirmed. A further possibility is the presence of bacterial endotoxins, that is, parts of the cell walls of gram negative organisms. Endotoxins are known to be able to precipitate inflammatory responses, and their presence would be likely to be increased by normal disinfection routines. Several causative mechanisms probably exist.

As has been mentioned, patients exhibiting a red eye also often show a very tightly fitting lens. The fitting previously may have been good and shown adequate movement. The apparent tightening may be due to dryness caused by nocturnal lagophthalmos or an acidic shift in the lens fluid. This could be caused by carbonic acid (from carbon dioxide buildup) or an accumulation of lactic acid. This would reduce the lens water content, steepen the fit, and trap potentially toxic epithelial waste under the lens. Using this theory, Keates (personal communication, 1980) found a significant reduction in the red eye/tight lens reaction by instructing patients to use an alkaline (pH 8 to 9) eye drop before sleep, during the night if possible, and again on awakening. Some patients also are helped by being refitted with materials that do not contain methacrylic acid, such as the Sauflon group, since these are lenses sensitive to parameter changes with reductions in pH and hence show less tightening effect under these circumstances.

When a patient presents with a red eye, the lens should be removed and the patient referred for hospital investigation. Cultures usually are taken and appropriate antibiotic therapy administered, if appropriate. However, in most cases the condition will heal spontaneously over 24 to 48 hours once the lens has been removed. The eye then should be observed for one week. The lens should be cleaned by strong oxidizing technique—for example, Liprofin (Alcon/BP)— or, if appropriate, a new lens refitted that is slightly flatter. Adequate movement of all aphakic extended wear lenses is essential.

Giant Papillary Conjunctivitis. Giant papillary conjunctivitis is seen only infrequently in extended wear patients. This might be considered evidence against the theory that the condition is caused by an immunologic reaction to denatured protein on the lens surface, since deposits are such a common problem in extended wear. However, the problem may be reduced in older patients because of their looser lids. Patients with giant papillary conjunctivitis have blurring, burning, and foreign body sensation, as well as perhaps a slight decrease in vision. The palpebral conjunctiva should always be examined when these symptoms are present.

Edema. Many patients comment on the mild blurring that edema produces when they first awaken during the first few weeks of wearing their lenses. This should disappear within half an hour and sometimes is helped by the administration of Clerz (which is mildly hypertonic) or the stronger Absorbonac 2 or 5 percent solution on waking.

If the edema persists for more than half an hour, the lens should be removed. Once normalcy has returned, a thinner lens or one of higher water content, a lens with a flatter fit, or both should be fitted. Sometimes edema occurs if fitting is carried out too soon after surgery. Waiting 2 to 3 months more will often help. If edema occurs after the lens has been successfully worn for some time, surface deterioration is implicated. The lens should be either laboratory cleaned or replaced. Periodic cleaners such as Liprofin or Monoclens (Contact Lens Manufacturing Co.) often help.

Vascularization. Neovascularization should not be mistaken for simple limbal vessel engorgement. However, lens wear should always be discontinued in such cases unless a reason for the condition can be determined. Often the lens is too tight; evidence may be the presence of edema, striae, and endothelial guttata. Vessels in or around surgical or suture scars may be ignored unless they progress beyond the scar lines. If a lens decenters, an exposure vascularization may occur. Vessels growing toward a corneal graft may precipitate donor rejection.

Diplopia and Asthenopia. Although diplopia and asthenopia are not frequent symptoms, the practitioner must be aware of their causes:

1. Intermittent or constant diplopia may be present if strabismus has occurred due to the prolonged occlusion effect of a long-term monocular cataract. If it is only occasional, it usually can be ignored. However, if it is more frequent or constant, orthoptic help or prismatic spectacles can be prescribed. In the latter case it is often possible to reduce the prism over a period of months.
2. Occasional vertical diplopia in the case of a monocular aphakic patient with good vision in the other eye can be caused by the lens' lagging low and inducing a prismatic effect. This problem is more likely to occur with hard lenses. Tightening the fit or increasing the overall lens diameter may help.
3. Asthenopic symptoms may be due to residual aniseikonia. This may be checked with an eikonometer, if one is available. Generally, the image size can be reduced by 6 to 8 percent (Enoch 1978) by overcorrecting the aphakic eye by +5.00 to +7.00D and then using a compensating negative spectacle lens (that is, an inverted Galilean telescope effect).
4. Asthenopic symptoms may occur in a patient involved in moderate or large amounts of intermediate vision. Normal bifocals are of little help. Trifocals may be used over the contact lenses, although it is simpler to correct the contact lens for intermediate vision and use conventional bifocals to compensate for optimal distance and near vision when required.

Hard and Gas-Permeable Contact Lenses

Hard or rigid lenses have several advantages over soft lenses for certain elderly patients. The development of gas-permeable materials has increased and added to these advantages, which include (1) better acuity, (2) better correction of astigmatism, (3) greater range of tints (for polymethylmethacrylate, or PMMA, lenses), (4) better tolerance in compromised corneas (for gas-permeable lenses), (5) ease of handling, (6) fewer deposit problems, and (7) reduced problems from the giant papillary conjunctivitis associated with soft lens wear.

Patient Selection

The younger range of elderly patients are often better suited for hard lenses, because this age group demands a higher acuity level. The ability to handle the lenses on a regular, daily basis is essential (although gas-permeable rigid lenses for extended wear are now becoming available) and the normal contraindications such as pathology, general health, and tear flow apply. Comfort is usually good in older patients because of loss of lid elasticity. However, a slightly reduced motivation compared with that of the younger age groups often will make patients initially opt for a soft lens unless the practitioner carefully explains all the advantages and disadvantages of each lens type.

Fitting Criteria

The general principle of fitting rigid lenses, of course, is to maintain full corneal integrity. This is done by providing as large an area of alignment between the lens and the cornea as possible and allowing normal tear flow between the lens and eye. The former prevents physical trauma, and the latter allows secondary oxygen supply via the tears and removal of cellular and other debris. Alternative fitting techniques are discussed in detail in the major undergraduate texts on contact lenses, but the following general principles normally are adopted in most cases.

The main base curve should be fitted to provide the maximum area of alignment between the lens and cornea. Therefore, the base curve normally is fitted on the flattest K reading in spherical or nearly spherical corneas. For astigmatic corneas, the base curve normally is approximated to one-third of the difference between flattest and steepest K readings. This compromise fitting is not as relevant with the more flexible gas-permeable lenses, since these lenses generally flex slightly on the eye. However, this is not necessarily true at the higher power range. A trial lens of the correct curve and approximately the correct power is very useful in such cases and allows keratometry to be performed over the lens while it is in the eye to ascertain the degree of lens flexure.

The keratometer typically measures the corneal curvature approximately 1.5 mm from the corneal apex. This gives a useful average corneal curvature and, hence, the base curve radius for lenses of the typical base curve diameter values of 6.0 to 7.0 mm. However, since the cornea flattens toward the limbus, then as base curve diameters increase beyond this, the average curvature over the area contacting the base curve will be slightly flatter. An approximate rule of thumb is that every 0.5 mm increase in base curve diameter requires a flattening in the base curve of 0.05 mm (0.25D). As the base curve diameter continues to increase, good alignment becomes increasingly difficult to achieve. This will be visible upon examination under ultraviolet light using sodium fluorescein. Therefore, a balance must be made between the optical requirements of, say, a large or displaced pupil and the physiological requirements of minimal zones of pressure at the corneal apex and base curve transition areas. Otherwise, tear fluid trapped in the midperiphery area of a large base curve zone will stagnate.

The peripheral curves of rigid lenses normally are fitted to give a gradual change from alignment of the base curve zone to minimal clearance at the lens edge. This allows the entrance of tears under the lens edge and prevents edge indentation as the lens moves to the flatter corneal periphery. Too tight an edge will cause physical discomfort and physiological trauma. A lens with flat edge curves will cause physical awareness and a lens that is overly mobile. Nevertheless, a large, flat-edge design sometimes is used to allow lens movement by the lids. Conversely, a steep lens with alignment of the main peripheral curve sometimes is used to aid lens centration and reduce too much mobility. Some examples for flattest K readings 7.25, 7.75, and 8.25 mm and overall diameters 8.80, 9.20, and 9.60 mm, respectively (Guillon, Lydon, and Sammons 1982), are given in Table 19–2 to show the base curve changes necessary as the base curve diameter is increased to give the same equivalent fitting and similar axial edge lift.

(See also Figure 19–11.) Thus, for a cornea with a flattest K reading of 7.25 mm, the base curve diameter of 7.40 mm typically will show a good alignment fit with a base curve radius of 7.25 mm (Example 1a). When the base curve diameter is increased to 7.80 mm on the same cornea, the base curve radius will need to be flattened to 7.30 mm to show the same fitting characteristics (Example 2a) because of the gradual flattening of the cornea from apex to periphery. For a base curve diameter of 8.20 mm, further flattening by the base curve radius to 7.35 mm will be necessary (Example 3a).

Lens Handling

As with soft lenses, it is helpful for patients inserting rigid lenses to use a well-illuminated concave mirror, at least initially. Hinged rims or reading spectacles with one lens and rim removed are also often helpful. Tinted lenses not only reduce photophobia in cases such as aphakia, but they also help a patient find a dropped lens.

Removal often presents a problem to the older patient because of lid flaccidity. The normal stare-pull-and-blink method frequently does not work. Although suction holders can be used, a technique that does not require artificial aids is always preferable. One useful method is shown in Figure 19–12. The opposite hand is brought over the forehead and the first or second finger directed in toward the nose. The same finger from the other hand is used for the lower lid. Gentle but firm pressure is applied to the lid margin and the lids stretched outward in an arc around the lens. As the lids come together, the lens should be ejected. The mistake made by many novice wearers is not to place the fingers on the very edge of the lids or to press the lids gently against the globe (Figure 19–13).

Rigid Aphakic Contact Lens Design

Single Curve Front Surface Lenses. Rigid aphakic lenses with a single curve front surface are useful for certain patients, especially those with a large or decentered pupil. The main problem is thickness (and hence weight) and upper lid action against the convex lens periphery, which tends to push the lens downward. Typically, a lens of 9.00 mm overall diameter and +15.00D power will have a center thickness

Table 19–2

Tricurve Corneal Lens Specifications and Resultant Axial Edge Lifts for Lenses of Overall Diameters 8.80, 9.20, and 9.60 mm to Give an Alignment Fit for Corneas of Flattest K Readings 7.25, 7.75, and 8.25 mm, Respectively

Lens Specifications	Axial Edge Lift (mm)	Overall Diameter (mm)
a. 7.25 / 7.95 / 10.00 7.40 8.20 8.80	0.106	
b. 7.75 / 8.55 / 11.00 7.40 8.20 8.80	0.099	8.80
c. 8.25 / 9.15 / 12.25 7.40 8.20 8.80	0.096	
a. 7.30 / 7.90 / 9.75 7.80 8.60 9.20	0.103	
b. 7.80 / 8.60 / 10.50 7.80 8.60 9.20	0.098	9.20
c. 8.30 / 9.20 / 11.50 7.80 8.60 9.20	0.093	
a. 7.35 / 7.95 / 9.50 8.20 9.00 9.60	0.108	
b. 7.85 / 8.45 / 10.50 8.20 9.00 9.60	0.098	9.60
c. 8.35 / 9.05 / 11.50 8.20 9.00 9.60	0.093	

Note: The slight reduction in axial edge lift at the end of the range of corneal radii is necessary to give the same fitting appearance.

Source: Adapted with permission from M. Guillon, D.P.M. Lydon, and W.A. Sammons. "Designing Rigid Gas Permeable Contact Lenses Using Edge Clearance Technique." *Journal of the British Contact Lens Association* 6, no. 1 (1982):24.

of 0.6 mm. The same lens reduced to 7.0 mm overall diameter has a center thickness of approximately 0.38 mm. Thus, as a general rule, such lenses must be fitted as small as possible commensurate with optical requirements. Generally, lenses work best on a well-centered pupil, average or steeper-than-average corneal curvature (since lenses center better), where the lower lid is such that it can provide some lens support, and where the lens is fitted with minimal edge clearance.

The main problems with such lenses are (1) the lenses' positioning low, remaining immobile, and thereby causing corneal edema; (2) flare if the lenses are fitted too small or positioned low; and (3) handling and locating problems with small lenses for the elderly aphakic.

Reduced Optic (Lenticular) Lenses. Cutting down the overall diameter of the front optic markedly reduces the center thickness and, hence, the lens mass. Not only will this improve lens centration, but it also will significantly improve the oxygen permeability of gas-permeable lenses. The diameter of the front optic cap is generally approximately 0.2 to 0.5 mm greater than the overall diameter because of the difficulty in producing a polish of good optical quality near the junction of the carrier. The junction thickness of a reduced optic lens normally is approximately 0.13 mm in PMMA lenses and sometimes slightly thicker in the more fragile gas-permeable materials. Depending on the lens's overall diameter and optic cap diameter, savings in lens thickness of between one-third and one-half are possible.

The design of the peripheral carrier portion is important. If the front carrier surface parallels the back surface, lens weight is kept to a minimum. However, the upper lid tends to bump the junction between central optic and carrier, pushing the lens downward. This design is satisfactory, however, when the lens is held up by resting on the lower lid.

If the upper lid covers part of the lens and is not too tight, a minus carrier reduced optic is best. The thicker edge is gripped by the lid and the lens held up. For such a design to perform adequately, the carrier portion must be at least 1.0 mm wide. Thus, for a typical front optic cap diameter of 7.0 to 7.5 mm diameter, the overall diameter must be 9.0 to 9.5 mm or greater. Since a lens of this design usually must ride under the upper lid to produce the desired effect, the necessity of a large diameter is not a disadvantage. Lenses of 10.0 to 10.5 mm overall diameter are not unusual and are becoming increasingly popular with the availability of gas-permeable materials.

Figure 19–11

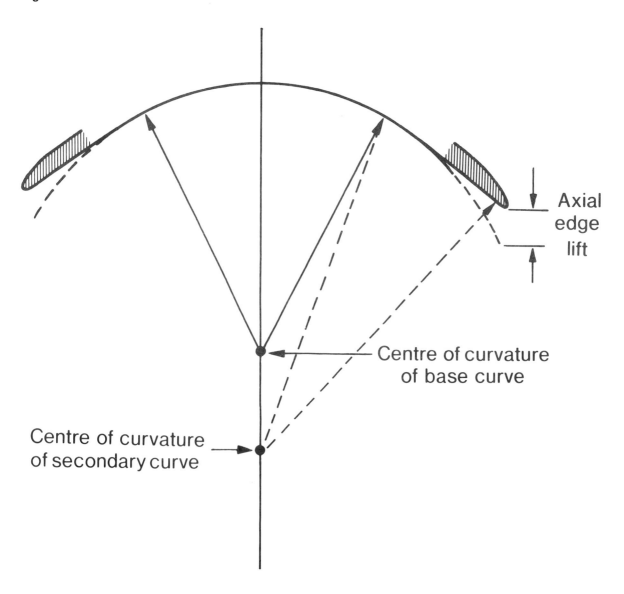

Axial edge lift

Centre of curvature of base curve

Centre of curvature of secondary curve

Cross Section of Axial Edge Lift (Edge Standoff) for a Bicurve Hard Lens.

Corneoscleral (Apex) Lenses. If persistent decentration is experienced with a conventional corneal lens design because of high corneal astigmatism, irregularity, or lid problems, a corneoscleral, or so-called apex, lens may offer stability where visual interference otherwise might be caused. The lens overall diameter is typically around 12.0 to 14.0 mm, with the edge resting just outside the limbus. This provides for a secure fit. However, there is a danger of inadequate lacrimal flow under the lens because of minimal lens movement. Take care to avoid a tightly fitting edge. One or more fenestrations may be necessary, even with gas-permeable materials. Keep the overall construction as thin as possible, and provide a reduced front optic. This larger lens often makes lens location and handling easier for elderly patients.

A base curve diameter of 8.0 to 8.5 mm typically is used in this lens design, so a base curve approximately 0.1 to 0.2 mm (0.50 to 1.00D) flatter than the flattest K reading is necessary to give corneal alignment over one-half to two-thirds of this relatively large base curve zone. The secondary curve is generally 0.6 to 0.7 (3.00 to 3.50D) flatter than the base curve, with still flatter, narrow edge bands near the lens edge to prevent edge indentation. The ideal fitting

Figure 19-12

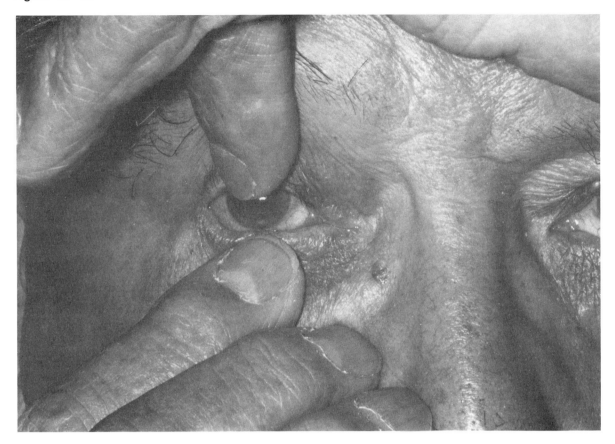

Correct Hard Lens Removal Technique

should give limbal clearance over three-quarters of the circumference, apical contact larger than 3 mm in diameter, and supporting intermediate peripheral zones of corneal alignment. The lens should sag downward by only 1 mm upon eye movement, with minimal horizontal slide. Nevertheless, corneal staining and distortion are common problems, so care must be taken both in patient selection and lens fitting.

Criteria for Selection of Lens Type and Material

Table 19-3 indicates the initial selection of lens type for typical situations and summarizes all the foregoing information. However, this information must be balanced against the fact that several conditions often occur simultaneously in one patient. In this situation, the fitter's expertise must be used to determine the optimal compromise. Also, new lens types and lens improvements continually widen the choice available to the practitioner, and borderline conditions further widen the choice.

Communication between Surgeon and Lens Fitter

Contact lenses for the elderly aphakic generally are not fitted until at least six to eight weeks after surgery. Fitting should not be attempted without the ophthalmologist's awareness and, preferably, instructions. Although most of the salient points can be determined by the fitter at the prefitting examination, it is often important to be aware of potential problems such as vitreous loss during surgery, a postoperative rise in intraocular pressure, current medication, and so on. During fitting, monitoring of the retina should be continued if the patient is not still seeing the surgeon. Look for the postoperative complications of retinal detachment and cystoid macular edema, and refer the patient back to the surgeon if any signs or symptoms of these or other abnormal conditions are detected. In certain pathological conditions or where there have been operative or postoperative complications, both fitter and surgeon must be in close communication and geographic proximity.

Figure 19-13

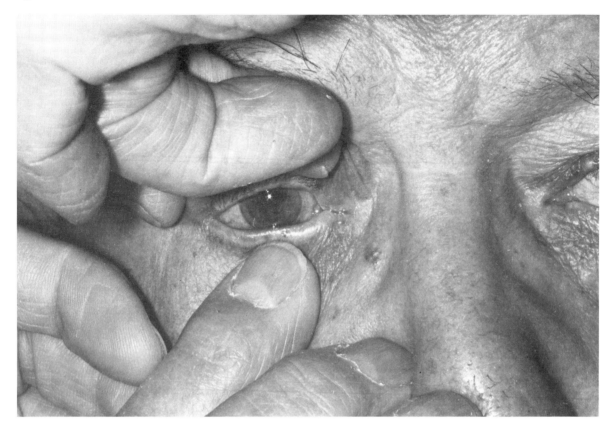

Incorrect Hard Lens Removal Technique. The fingers are not on the lid margin, and the pressure is being applied downward and upward, not inwards.

The choice of lens type generally is left to the fitter. In the case of extended wear lenses, however, the surgeon should be consulted. This insures the suitability of the eye for this lens type and also insures that the surgeon is aware of the lenses in case of emergency.

After the fitting and immediate postfitting aftercare, the fitter should inform the surgeon of the following:

1. The type of lens fitted and any related special advice.
2. The patient's wearing regimen.
3. Solutions and cleaners that have been recommended.
4. Acuity both with the lenses alone and with the lenses plus spectacle overcorrection, if appropriate.
5. Any abnormal observations so far.
6. The date of the next aftercare appointment and frequency of aftercare visits recommended.

Finally, the fitter should ask when the surgeon would next like to see the patient.

Therapeutic Contact Lenses

The use of therapeutic contact lenses—that is, lenses used for other than their refractive function—in the elderly population has increased in recent years. The general rate of success has increased as clinicians have become more aware of the uses and limitations of such lenses. In addition, the development of thin lenses of high water content, which have better oxygen transmission, has brought about the general availability of extended wear lenses. Both the nature of the conditions to be treated and the general state of the elderly patients dictates that extended wear lenses be used.

Many conditions managed with soft contact lenses can be corrected by surgery, and often surgery is the treatment of choice. However, surgery is not necessarily an option for elderly patients. In these situations soft contact lenses can be a salvation.

Therapeutic contact lenses have both benefits and limitations. They alter the general environment of the external eye, which may be beneficial or harmful, depending on the circum-

Table 19-3
Criteria for Selection of Material and Lens Type

Patient Characteristic	Extended Wear Soft	Daily Wear Soft	Gas-Permeable	Large Gas-Permeable	Silicone
Poor handling ability	✓				✓
High visual requirement			✓	✓	✓
Conjunctival bleb			✓		
Cataract sutures still in place	✓	✓			
Iridectomy or updrawn pupil		✓		✓	✓
Dry eye		✓ [a]			✓
Low acuity	✓				
Bifocal requirement		✓	✓		

[a]Use hypotonic saline for lens storage.

stances. Contact lenses can be used to splint an unstable epithelium, protect a vulnerable epithelium from the tear film and the eyelids, provide a regular anterior refracting surface, maintain the conjunctival fornices in the face of progressive fibrosis, and splint the cornea at times of corneolysis and threatened perforation. Contact lenses, however, reduce the availability of oxygen to the epithelium, and there is some suggestion that continuous wear brings about endothelial damage. In addition, contact lenses can damage the epithelium and provide a port of entry for microorganisms. The presence of the contact lens can affect the microbial flora of the eye, and a combination of factors could bring about infection. This is of particular concern in elderly patients, as their personal hygiene is not always optimal. Conditions in which these adverse effects may be produced are contraindications to the use of therapeutic lenses.

Splinting of Epithelium

In erosive diseases of the superficial cornea, the splinting influence of a contact lens often allows the epithelium to develop effective cellular adherence to underlying supporting structures. Erosive conditions include the recurrent erosion syndrome; superficial corneal dystrophies such as lattice, Meesemann's, and Reis-Bückler's; and various other, less common forms of dystrophic corneal disease.

It takes at least 6 weeks for effective hemidesomosomes to be formed and bridge the epithelium over the underlying basement membrane. In cases of recurrent epithelial breakdown, the use of a soft contact lens on a permanent wear basis for 6 weeks often will resolve a difficult problem to which there are few other solutions. The stabilization of the epithelium leads to increased patient comfort.

Protection of Unstable Epithelium

If the epithelium is unstable with edema, blebs, or ulceration, patients can suffer extreme pain. A common cause of epithelial disruption with pain is corneal edema, which usually results from endothelial failure. Dysfunction of the corneal endothelium may occur spontaneously as part of a dystrophic process such as the one that occurs in Fuchs' corneal dystrophy. Surgical trauma to the nonreplicating endothelium also can cause endothelial failure. This can occur after cataract extraction or with recurrent trauma from a mobile intraocular lens' coming into contact with the posterior corneal layer.

Fuchs' corneal dystrophy is now known to have its origin in the formation of guttata in the endothelium. The guttata themselves impair vision little or not at all, but they alter function of the endothelium as a barrier and may allow fluid to enter the cornea. As edema then progresses, bullae form; these may rupture, exposing the nerve endings and causing a red, irritated eye with a foreign body sensation. The cornea becomes progressively more opaque. Symptoms are often worse in the morning and in humid weather. The condition sometimes produces halos similar to those occurring in subacute glaucoma (Carden 1979). The condition is much more common in women than men.

The initial treatment consists of simple solutions and lubricants that use osmotic pressure to draw water from the cornea (for example, methylcellulose, glucose, hypertonic saline, and glycerin). Hydrogel lenses are helpful for patients who have advanced to the stage of bullous keratopathy. They relieve the discomfort by separating the painful bullae from the lids.

The lenses should be fitted for minimal movement, and large soft lenses of high water content give the best results. If K readings are not possible on the irregular surface, an approximation can be obtained from readings from the other eye. An actual reduction of the edema is more difficult to achieve, although Ruben and Wilson (1975) suggest compression of large areas of the cornea with a contact lens as a means of creating an anterior water barrier. The addition of 5 percent saline or methylcellulose every 1 to 2 hours produces an anterior surface hypertonicity; this causes a movement of fluid from the cornea and reduces the bullae. This also is aided by the greater rate of evaporation from the surface of a soft contact lens. The use of acetazolamide (Diamox) and similar diuretic drugs sometimes is helpful with or without the hypertonic saline solution therapy. The pupils are normally also kept dilated because of the concomitant iritis present in almost every case.

Partial or complete relief has been reported by about 80 percent of patients fitted (Gasset 1974). It is important that the lenses be worn 24 hours a day for long periods, as frequent removal may precipitate the formation of ulcers. Improvement in vision, however, is a little less predictable unless the condition is caught early (Mandell 1981). Dohlman and Hyndiuk (1972) report an increase in visual acuity in only about 20 percent of patients with advanced disease who were treated with hydrogel lenses.

Scleral lenses also occasionally are used as an alternative to soft lens therapy. Marriott (1981) states that these lenses should be fitted to obtain constant compression of the cornea over at least the central two-thirds of its area. A very close parallel fit is therefore necessary, and the lens must be as close to the cornea as possible without obliterating the tear flow. Good limbal clearance must be maintained at all times, and the fit will need modifying frequently as the disease passes through its various phases.

Although the condition sometimes improves to the point where lens wear can be discontinued, most patients become totally reliant on their lenses. In spite of this, the progress is sometimes not maintained. Also, the danger of secondary infection is always possible. Additionally, of course, extended wear lenses themselves reduce the amount of oxygen available to the cornea. This is particularly troublesome with aphakic bullous keratopathy from postsurgical endothelial damage, when the best visual result can be obtained from an extended wear aphakic soft lens. However, the performance of such lenses is usually inadequate, the edema of the cornea increases, and there is a tendency to induce corneal vascularization. A thin lens of high water content is the best solution to this difficult problem.

Ruben (1975) points out that because of the pain and discomfort associated with this condition, a contact lens always should be tried, but at least one-third of all patients may not be helped. Patients always should be referred to an ophthalmologist if there is any sign of secondary infection, if the pain persists, if the disease shows signs of progressing rapidly, or if neovascularization occurs. In a persistent or worsening condition, most surgeons will opt for a penetrating keratoplasty.

Protection from Eyelids
The health of the corneal epithelium is greatly affected by the tear film and the movement of the eyelid. It depends on the maintenance of normally situated lids that have a square posterior edge to maintain a regular covering of tears over the corneal epithelium. A disturbance of the posterior edge of the lid—either in position or in shape—can compromise the health of the anterior refracting surface of the cornea. Trichiasis is particularly troublesome in this situation; where it occurs, a contact lens can be used to protect the cornea from interference by the eyelids.

Most conditions of the eyelids that affect the cornea are best dealt with surgically. Entropion, ectropion, and trichiasis usually can be dealt with by minor surgery done under local anesthetic. Should this not be possible, a contact lens can be a very satisfactory alternative. If trichiasis is minimal, a soft lens alone will help prevent corneal damage and may reduce the causative blepharospasm by relieving the discomfort of the irritating lash. Although surgical correction or ablation are always preferable, fenestrated scleral lenses can be used for protection in more severe cases. In ectropion and lagophthalmos, where the cornea is unduly exposed, a scleral lens can keep the cornea moist.

Maintenance of Conjunctival Fornices
Mucosal scarring diseases in the elderly may obliterate the conjunctival fornices and cause severe ocular disease. This occurs in Sjögren syndrome, mucous membrane pemphigoid, and following chemical burns. In addition, where

attachment of the palpebral and bulbar conjunctivas occurs (symblepharon), normal blinking often is reduced. Secondary complications may result from exposure keratitis.

The condition frequently has been treated successfully with an annular ring cut from a scleral lens, although often the problem is one of ring ejection. Soft lenses with a flat radius and large overall size are also very effective. The soft lens must be large (15 to 20 mm) to prevent adhesions' forming or reforming (Westerhout 1981, 604). Also, because of the lens's large overall size, it must be made of an adequately gas-permeable material. A thin lens of low water content may wrinkle up in the eye, causing discomfort and reformation of the adhesions. Continuous use is obviously necessary, and local and systemic steroids often are given to discourage vascularization.

Ocular pemphigoid is an inflammatory disorder of the conjunctiva that in its chronic state, usually affects the elderly eye tissue and produces conjunctival scarring, ankyloblepharon, and symblepharon. The main task of the contact lens practitioner is to protect the cornea and keep it wet, especially if lid surgery is performed to overcome entropion. Although there is no proved association, some patients also are affected by rheumatoid arthritis. This may present difficulties if the patient is unable to handle lenses well.

Unfortunately, keeping the cornea wet is only a partial solution to the problem. Ruben and Wilson (1975) have pointed out that although devices such as spectacles with manual or electronic fluid injection are worthy of consideration, solutions without the necessary lipid or protein concentrations eventually will produce epithelial edema and necrosis. Therefore, no matter whether the contact lens used is hard or soft, the prognosis is poor, and the disease normally remains progressive and results in blindness.

Provision of a Regular Corneal Surface
In corneal scarring diseases, an irregular surface may preclude good vision. This usually can be overcome with an appropriate contact lens.

Tear Film Disorders
Generalized mucosal drying is a common problem in the elderly. Keratoconjunctivitis sicca is particularly common. Usually, it is mild and adequately controlled by tear film supplements and, occasionally, obliteration of the lacrimal outflow channels. With the reduction of the aqueous component of the tear film, there is a relative mucous excess. This may be troublesome in itself, as the mucous may adhere to the epithelium and create plaques or filaments.

Soft lenses with a high water content may be used in mild dry eye states, even though their use in this situation is limited. Although they can be used as a reservoir for the tear film, they do predispose patients to corneal infection. Patients with keratoconjunctivitis sicca have less protective lysozyme in their tear film and may have disturbances of the epithelium; the presence of contact lenses may predispose them to ocular infection. For this reason, the use of contact lenses in mild dry eye states is not generally encouraged. If mucous adherence is a problem, however, contact lenses are very helpful, as they can protect the epithelium from developing mucous tag and subsequent filament development. In this situation the concurrent use of artificial tears or 10 percent acetylcysteine and wetting agents is advised, and regular review is necessary.

Ocular dryness occurs at a variety of different levels and often where there is another indication for contact lens wear, for example, aphakia. The problem often is exacerbated by the high heat or air conditioning levels of nursing homes. In very mild cases, conventional hard and soft lens wear can be made more comfortable by the use of either isotonic or hypotonic artificial tears. These generally are used "on demand" in hard lens cases. A more definite routine must be decided upon for the soft lens wearer. As well as tear film's being deficient, tear film composition is also often abnormal in such cases, and these patients are prone to heavy deposit formation on soft lenses. This is particularly true for lenses of high water content, which usually are used in these cases for their higher fluid level reservoir.

Relief often is promoted in both mild and slightly more severe cases by switching the patient to a soft lens of medium or higher water content suitable for daily wear. The lens then is soaked in diluted saline overnight to artificially increase its fluid level. As has been discussed, this fluid then is slowly released onto the eye during the next wearing period. The saline dilution may be determined by experimentation for each patient and is typically between 10 and 50 percent. (The author generally starts patients at 20 percent.) Lens fitting does not seem to be affected, since the hypotonic saline counters the tightening effect on lens fitting of the patient's own hypertonic tears. The patient should use a thermal disinfection technique; the only chemical technique suitable for this method is the Softab system (Contact Lens Manufacturing).

In moderate cases the use of silicone lenses is often beneficial. Their advantages lie in the fact that, being nonhydrophilic, an osmotic gradient is not created across the lens by evaporation from the front surface. A tear film therefore is trapped between the lens and eye. Nevertheless, dry and hence tight lenses can occur with these lenses; possibly this is a result of water vapor, which, being gaseous, can still pass through the lens material. Tear supplements therefore may still be necessary.

In more severe cases, sealed scleral lenses must be used. To maintain a reasonable wearing time but not allow excess tear evaporation through a normal lens fenestration, an S-bend groove or channel can be cut into the superior and inferior haptic portions (McKay Taylor 1969). Pullum (1983) also has described the use of a limbal arcuate groove cut through the superior haptic portion; this again allows venting without excess tear fluid loss.

Corneal Splinting

If the integrity of the cornea is threatened by a destructive process, a soft contact lens can provide a protective splint until the process has been controlled or surgery is possible. Lenses are effective in cases of destructive corneal disease when inflammation is minimal. Perhaps the best example is keratolysis associated with rheumatoid arthritis. This slowly progressive condition can lead to perforation but has a tendency toward spontaneous arrest. No medical treatment is positively effective, and surgery is difficult. In this situation a continuous wear soft lens can protect the peripheral indolent ulcer as a bandage; it initially protects the area from the mechanical irritation of blinking and any environmental irritants, all or which may retard healing.

The ulcer margins should be cleaned of necrotic and hyperplastic tissue, under local anesthesia if necessary, before fitting is commenced. Regrowth of the epithelium under the bandage lens then usually occurs, and the cells sometimes use the back surface of the lens as a bridge across the crater (Liebowitz and Rosenthal 1971). The lens should not be removed for at least the first week, provided frequent slit lamp examination shows no abnormality, since this may damage the early regenerating tissue.

Contact lenses also are useful in cases of corneal perforation. Small perforations can be closed under contact lenses until healing occurs or surgery is performed. The lens closes off the flow of aqueous humor which helps small perforations to seal. Care must be taken, however, not to use contact lenses in destructive disease that is due to uncontrolled infection or in the presence of corneal infection and continuing inflammation. At these times the presence of a contact lens may make the disease worse.

Soft Contact Lenses as a Drug Delivery System

Because of the normal tear turnover and drainage system of the eye, absorption by the conjunctiva, impermeability of the cornea, and difficulty in maintaining contact with the cornea, less than 1 percent of topically administered drugs usually penetrate into the anterior chamber. Therefore, several researchers have investigated contact lenses as a means of improving this penetration and maintaining drug levels at a more constant value than the peak-and-trough situation normally existing when drugs are administered in conventional eyedrop form. The literature suggests that the effects of cycloplegics, pilocarpine, phenylephrine, idoxuridine, and possibly steroids and other water-soluble drugs of high molecular weight may be enhanced and prolonged by the use of hydrogel contact lens delivery systems (Robinson and Eriksen 1978, 265).

Soaking the lens in the medication seems to be more effective than simply wearing the lens and dropping the medication into the eye. Most researchers agree that within 1 to 2 hours of soaking, the lenses are at equilibrium with the drug solutions, although a little more may be taken up during continued soaking for 48 hours. Sterile, presoaked "therapeutic" lenses have been found to have a shelf life of 4 months if stored in a refrigerator (Hillman, Marsters, and Broad 1975). Generally, lower concentrations of the drug may be used than would need to be administered topically.

The uptake and release of the drug will depend largely upon the lens material, its water content, and the drug in question. In the case of pilocarpine, approximately 90 percent of the drug is released in the first 1 to 2 hours, and the remainder is slowly released over the rest of the waking hours. This may be useful in an acute attack, as 2 hours of intensive nursing therapy and drug administration may be saved. A supplementary effect may be maintained by administering further drops topically onto the lens in situ, by removing the lens for resoaking during the day, or by alternating with a presoaked reserve lens. In the case of herpes ulcers, it has been suggested that fenestrating the hydrogel lens over the site of the ulcer will allow direct supplementary topical therapy of idoxuridine; the lens is rotated manually to position the fenestration over the ulcer prior to drug administration. It would appear that in spite of most of the drug being released fairly quickly, intraocular pressure is controlled for as long as 23 hours after lens insertion (Podos, Becker, and Asseff 1972).

Generally a lens of higher water content will release its drug content quicker than a lens of lower water content. Thus, in the case of acute glaucoma, a presoaked lens of higher water content is the most appropriate, whereas a lens of lower water content is better for the chronic simple case.

In spite of the advantages already listed, contact lenses are not widely used as drug delivery systems. In some cases this is simply because of the availability of more modern, longer-acting drugs. However, it is largely because of the additional lens cost and patient management. Also, the drug release from contact lenses is not constant and therefore offers only a partial advantage over drops and ointments. The pulse-like drug release poses logistical problems for the patient: Should the patient remove the lens periodically and soak it in the medication, or will continuing topical medication be effective? Should the drug for lens soaking be preserved or unpreserved? If preserved, is it available in a form that will not bind to the hydrogel material? The lack of definite knowledge and known outcome usually encourages the ophthalmologist to adopt a more conventional approach. Nevertheless, if the patient is already a contact lens wearer, the possiblity of using the contact lens as a drug dispenser should not be forgotten.

Tonometry over Soft Contact Lenses

The need to monitor intraocular pressure continues, of course, after patients have begun wearing contact lenses. In certain cases this may be particularly important; for example, aphakic penetrating keratoplasty patients often have a marked rise in early postoperative intraocular pressure (Wood, West, and Kaufman 1972). These patients may be wearing bandage contact lenses for therapeutic purposes, and it may be inconvenient or not preferable to remove the lenses for routine measurement. A simple expedient in more normal eyes, of course, is to simply slide the lens onto the sclera, carry out routine tonometry, and then replace the lens. However, this normally involves the use of a topical anesthetic, which may reduce the adhesion of the epithelium to Bowman's membrane. Sliding the lens back onto the cornea could easily displace a segment of epithelium. In addition, the instillation into the conjunctival sac of a topical anesthetic, which is absorbed into the hydrophilic material, may maintain anesthesia for a prolonged period because of elution from the lens. For these reasons some clinicians have sought to ascertain the validity of tonometry carried out over the top of hydrogel lenses while it is in the eye.

Meyer, Stanifer, and Bobb (1978) compared intraocular pressure measurements with and without a Bausch & Lomb Plano T Bandage lens using a MacKay-Marg Electronic Applanation Tonometer. For normal eyes the measurement over the contact lens was approximately ±4.0 mm compared with what it was without the contact lens. This variation increased slightly in the grafted cases but was still felt to be useful as an indication of early glaucoma.

Draeger (1980) measured intraocular pressure by applanation tonometry both with and without plano and +12.00D lenses using a lens of 80 percent water content. The graphs in Figures 19–14 and 19–15 show his results. Although applanation tonometry may be carried out over a soft contact lens without using a fluorescing agent, the use of fluorescein of high molecular weight (for example, Fluorexon) will facilitate readings and prevent the absorption of normal fluorescein into the lens. Such information gives the clinician an approximate idea of the true intraocular pressure, although for accurate readings the lenses always should be removed.

Soft Contact Lenses
and Preserved Topical Solutions

Researchers have warned that the use of ocular medication in contact lens wearers (for example, glaucoma therapy or artificial tears in keratitis sicca) would either concentrate the drug or the

Figure 19-14

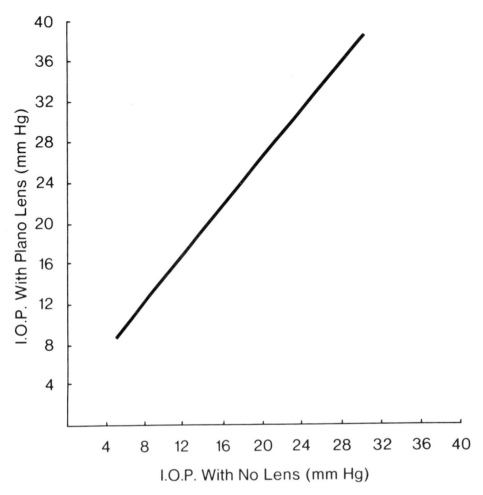

Conversion of Intraocular Pressure (I.O.P) Reading Obtained by Applanation Tonometry over a Plano Soft Contact Lens to a Reading without the Lens In Situ. Source: From J. Draeger. "Applanationstonometric auf Kontaklinsen mit hohem Wassergehalt Probleme, Ergebrisse und Korrekturfaktoren." *Klinische Monatsblatter fur Augenheilkunde* 176 (1980): 38.

preservative within the lens. In the author's experience, no discernible effects have been seen either due to drug or perservative concentration. Lemp (1978) showed that an artificial tear preserved with benżalkonium chloride and ethylenediamine tetraacetate (EDTA) instilled frequently into an eye wearing a bandage lens for keratoconjunctivitis sicca caused no discernible corneal toxicity or accumulation of the preservative according to spectrophotometric analysis. The one notable exception is epinephrine or its analogs, which should never be used because they cause marked lens discoloration (Miller, Brooks, and Mebilia 1976; Sugar 1977). There is also a report in the literature of soft lens discoloration related to the use of tetrahydrozoline (Kleist 1979).

The use of systemic medications should have

no adverse effect on the use of extended wear soft lenses, although drugs such as atropine and various tranquilizers that reduce tear secretion could precipitate lens intolerance in patients with only marginal tear flow. Systemic tetracycline use has been claimed to increase ocular sensitivity to thimerosal-preserved hydrogel solutions (Crook and Freeman 1982).

Certain locally administered medications that are inherently hypertonic, such as 10 percent sodium sulfacetamide or 8 percent pilocarpine hydrochloride, can cause soft lens dehydration, a change in lens fit, and temporary lens discomfort. Lenses of higher water content are more prone to producing this effect. Similar temporary lens intolerance and decreased visual acuity occurs when locally administered medications are buffered at pH values far from the ideal of

Figure 19-15

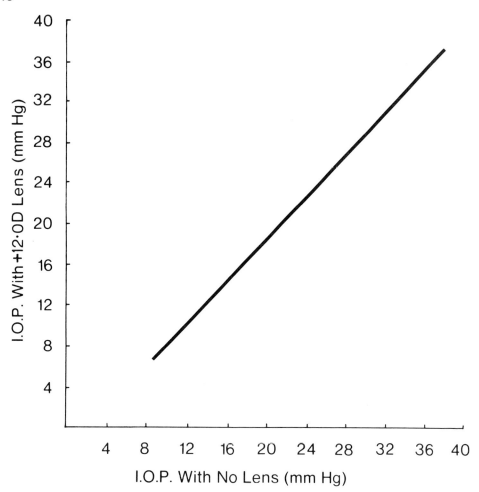

Conversion of Intraocular Pressure (I.O.P) Reading Obtained by Applanation Tonometry over +12.00D Soft Contact Lens of 80 Percent Water Content to a Reading without the Lens in Situ. Source: From J. Draeger. "Applanationstonometric auf Kontaklinsen mit hohem Wassergehalt Probleme, Ergebrisse und Korrekturfaktoren." *Klinische Monatsblatter fur Augenheilkunde* 176 (1980): 38.

7.4. An abnormally acidic pH promotes lens dehydration and steepening of some hydrophilic copolymeric lenses, particularly those with acidic functional groups in their matrices. Conversely, an alkaline pH promotes lens hydration and flattening.

References

Carden, R. G., "Optometric Management of Fuch's Endothelial Dystrophy." *American Journal of Optometry* 55 (1979): 642.

Crook, T. G., and J. J. Freeman. "Tetracyclines and Hypersensitivity to Thimerosal in Contact Lens Solutions." *American Journal of Optometry* 59, no. 10 (1982): 17.

Dohlman, C. H., and R. A. Hyndiuk. "Subclinical and Manifest Corneal Edema after Cataract Extraction." In *Symposium on the Cornea: Transactions of the New Orleans Academy of Ophthalmology*, eds. R. Castorviejo et al. St. Louis: Mosby, 1972, pp. 225–232.

Draeger, J. "Applanationstonometric auf Kontaklinsen mit hohen Wassergehalt. Probleme, Ergebrisse und Korrekturfaktoren." *Klinische Monatsblatter fur Augenheilkunde.* 176 (1980): 38.

El Hage, S. G. "Clinical Evaluation of the Presbycon Aspheric Contact Lens." *International Contact Lens Clinic* 3, no. 2 (1976): 65.

Enoch, J. M. "Restoration of Binocularity in Unilateral Aphakia by Nonsurgical Means." International Ophthalmology Clinics 18, no. 2 (1978): 273.

Fatt, I. "Changes in Dimensions of Soft Contact Lenses while on the Eye." *Optician* 185, no. 478 (1983): 11.

Gasset, A. R. "Correction of Bullous Keratopathy with Soft Contact Lenses." International Contact Lens Clinic 1, no. 1 (1974): 89.

Goldberg, J. B. *Biomicroscopy for Contact Lens Practice: Clinical Procedures.* 2nd ed. Chicago: Professional Press, 1984.

Goldberg, J. B. "A Comprehensive Method for Fitting Monocentric Crescent Bifocal Contact Lenses." *Optometric Weekly* 60 (1969): 24.

Guillon, M.; D. P. M. Lydon; and Sammons W. A. "Designing Rigid Gas Permeable Contact Lenses Using the Edge Clearance Technique." *Journal of the British Contact Lens Association* 6, no. 1 (1982): 19.

Hill, R. M., and L. G. Carney. " Extended Wear Systems." *Contact Lens Forum* 1, no. 6 (1976): 29–31.

Hillman, J. S.; J. B. Marsters; and A. Broad. "Pilocarpine Delivery by Hydrophilic Lens in the Management of Acute Glaucoma." *Transactions of the Ophthalmological Societies of the United Kingdom* 95 (1975): 79.

Hodd, N. F. " How to Fit Soft Lenses: 7." *Optician* 172, no. 4458 (1976): 12. a

Hodd, N. F. "How to Fit Soft Lenses: 8." *Optician* 172, no. 4462 (1976): 16. b

Holden, B. A. "Ocular Changes Associated with the Extended Wear of Contact Lenses." Paper presented at the 15th Contact Lens Congress, Aschattenburg, West Germany, March 1983.

Holden, B. A.; G. W. Mertz; and M. Guillon. "Corneal Swelling Response of the Aphakic Eye." *Investigative Ophthalmology and Visual Science* 19 (1980): 1394.

Holden, B. A., and S. G. Zantos, "Corneal Endothelium: Transient Changes with Atmospheric Anoxia." In *The Cornea in Health and Disease: Proceedings of the Sixth Congress of the European Society of Ophthalmologists.* London: Royal Society of Medicine, 1981, pp. 79–81.

Jurkus, J. "Bifocals Go Soft" *Review of Optometry* 120, no. 3 (1983): 46.

Kersley, H. J., and C. Kerr. "Aphakic Extended Wear: One Solution to the Problems that Occur." *Contact and Intraocular Lens Medical Journal* 7, no. 1 (1981): 57.

Kleist, F. "Prevention of Inorganic Deposits on Hydrophilic Contact Lenses." *International Contact Lens Clinic* 6, no. 3 (1979): 44.

Koetting, R. A., and C. E. Andrews. "The Relationship of Age, Keratometry, and Miscellaneous Physiological Factors in Hydrogel Lens Wear." *American Journal of Optometry* 56, no. 10 (1979): 642.

Lemp, M. A. "Bandage Lenses and the Use of Topical Solutions Containing Preservatives." *Annals of Ophthalmology* 10 (1978): 1319.

Mandell, R. B. *Contact Lens Practice: Hard and Flexible Lenses.* 3d. ed. Springfield, Ill.: Thomas, 1981.

Leibowitz, H. M., and P. Rosenthal. "Hydrophilic Contact Lenses in Corneal Disease: I. Superficial, Sterile, Indolent Ulcers." *Archives of Ophthalmology* 85 (1971): 163.

Marriott, P. "Impression Scleral Lens Fitting for Special and Pathological Conditions." In *Contact Lenses: A Textbook for Practitioner and Student*, Vol. 2, eds. J. Stone and A. J. Phillips. London: Butterworth, 1981, pp. 592–603.

McKay Taylor, C. "The S-Bend and Other Channelled Haptic Lenses." *Ophthalmic Optician* 9 (1969): 1256–1258.

Mertz, G. W., and B. A. Holden. "Guttate Endothelial Changes and Anterior Eye Inflammation." *British Journal of Ophthalmology* 65 (1981): 101.

Meyer, R. F.; R. M. Stanifer; and K. C. Bobb. "MacKay-Marg Tonometry over Therapeutic Soft Contact Lenses." *American Journal of Ophthalmology* 86 (1978): 19.

Miller, D.; S. M. Brooks; and E. Mebilia. "Andrenochrome Staining of Soft Contact Lenses." *Annals of Ophthalmology* 8, no. 1 (1976): 65.

Podos, S. M.; B. Becker; and C. Asseff. "Pilocarpine Therapy with Soft Contact Lenses." *American Journal of Ophthalmology* 73 (1972): 336.

Polse, K A., and R. B. Mandell. "Hyperbaric Oxygen Effect on Corneal Edema Caused by a Contact Lens." *American Journal of Optometry* 48, no. 3 (1971): 197.

Pullum, K. Paper presented at the British Contact Lens Society Clinical Conference, Harrogate, England, 1983.

Robinson, J. R., and S. P. Eriksen. "Drug Delivery from Soft Lens Materials." In *Soft Contact Lenses: Clinical and Applied Technology*, ed. M. Ruben. London: Baillière & Tindall, 1978.

Ruben, M. "Soft Contact Lens Treatment of Bullous Keratopathy." *Transactions of the Ophthalmological Societies of the United Kingdom* 95 (1975): 75.

Ruben, M. "The Factors Necessary for Constant Wearing of Contact Lenses." *Optician* 172, No. 4453 (1976):19.

Ruben, M. "Constant Wear versus Daily Wear." *Optician* 194, no. 4496 (1977): 7.

Ruben, M., and R. Wilson. "Cosmetic and Prosthetic Appliances." In *Contact Lens Practice: Visual, Therapeutic and Prosthetic*, ed. M. Ruben. London: Baillière & Tindell, 1975, pp. 343–352.

Sugar, J. "Andrenochrome Pigmentation of Hydrophilic Lenses." *International Contact Lens Clinic* 4 (1977): 35.

Vannas, A.; B. A. Holden; J. Makite; P. Ruusuvaara; and J. S. O'Donnell. "Specular Microscopy and Ultrastructure of Endothelial Blebs." *Investigative Ophthalmology and Visual Science* 18 suppl. (1979): 143.

Westerhout, D. "The Use of Soft Lenses in Ocular Pathology." In *Contact Lenses: A Textbook for Practitioner and Student*, Vol. 2, eds. J. Stone and A. J. Phillips. London: Butterworth, 1981.

Wood, T. O.; C. E. West; and H. E. Kaufman. "Control of Intraocular Pressure in Penetrating Keratoplasty." *American Journal of Ophthalmology* 74 (1972): 724.

Zantos, S. G., and B. A. Holden. "Guttate Endothelial Changes with Anterior Eye Inflammation." *British Journal of Ophthalmology* 65 (1981): 101.

Zantos, S. G.; B. A. Holden, and D. Pye. "Guide to Photography with the Nikon Photo-slit Lamp." *Australian Journal of Optometry* 63 (1980): 26.

Chapter 20

Vision Care in the Home and in Institutional Settings

John Anstice

As the human life span increases, the proportion of the population over 60 years old—including those who are bedridden because of disease or accident or are restricted in mobility—will become greater. It has been noted that as a group, older people have a greater need for vision care, as well as other professional services (Leslie and Greenberg 1974).

People who are housebound or unable to afford or arrange transport to the optometrist's office are likely to spend more of their time engaged in handiwork, reading, and watching television than they formerly did. Their spectacles may no longer satisfy their increased visual needs. For these people, the provision of vision care must be arranged for in their home or residential institution.

In spite of the difficulties involved in a home visit, it is usually a rewarding experience for the optometrist. Older people and their families usually appreciate the special nature of the vision care service.

An out-of-office examination is unlikely to be as satisfactory as a regular in-office examination, however, mainly because of the restrictions of available equipment and poor illumination control. Therefore, it is important to determine that no alternative to a house call can be arranged. As will be discussed, some aspects of office design and practice management can be implemented to allow some mobility-impaired people to visit the office, thereby reducing the number of house calls.

Previsit Management

The receptionist on an initial inquiry should explain that home visits are made by the optometrist only if it is impossible to transport the patient into the office. The receptionist should determine the reason why the inquirer considers the older person unable to visit the office and should explain, if necessary, the features that have been included in the office's design to help overcome mobility problems. It is usually more diplomatic for the receptionist to discuss the matter first with the practitioner and telephone the person back.

A ramp entrance always should be incorporated into a ground floor or cottage type of office design. Unrestricted access from the parking place to the door of a practice will enable a patient in a wheelchair to transfer from an automobile into the examiner's office with a minimum of effort. Office doors should be wide enough to accommodate a wheelchair, and there should be an unobstructed path from door to refracting room (New Zealand Optometrical Association 1970). In addition to people who rely on wheelchairs, many other older and cardiac patients will appreciate the ramp. An appointment should be made for these patients at a time when they can be examined without delay.

In many communities the public transportation system and some private welfare agencies provide buses equipped with ramps and elevators to make entry and exiting easy for those in wheelchairs and the less agile. People with limited mobility inquiring about home visits should be advised about special transport services (Figure 20–1).

By proper scheduling, appropriate office design, and discussion with the patient and family, most invalids and handicapped people can be examined more satisfactorily in the office. However, there remain some truly housebound individuals who must be visited at home if they are to receive professional vision care.

Advance preparation will reduce the time the

Figure 20-1

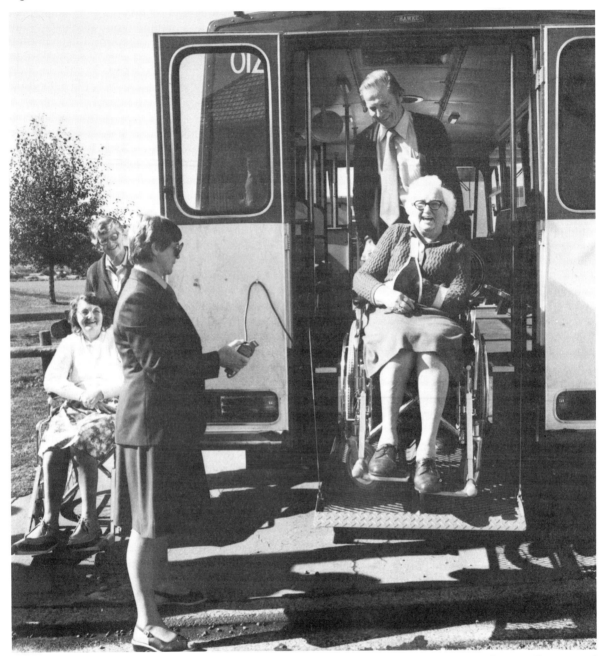

Public Transport Bus Equipped with Motorized Wheel Chair Lift for the Mobility Impaired. Source: Courtesy of the Christchurch Transport Board.

examiner is away from the office. A clinical record card should be filled out from information obtained by telephone, including the patient's name, address, age, and other similar data. The nature of the patient's infirmity, as well as his or her physician's name, visual needs, past history of visual care, and major symptoms, should be elicited. The exact location of the person's home and any special instructions for reaching

it also should be ascertained. The most convenient time of day for the examination should be determined to suit the patient's daily schedule. It often is helpful for a family member to be present to assist the optometrist in arranging furniture, moving the older person, and performing other chores.

The examiner or receptionist also should ascertain in advance from the patient or the patient's family whether suitable furniture is available. The following checklist will help in making arrangements:

1. *Testing distance.* The distance from the patient to where the chart can be suspended or propped up should be at least 3 m (10 feet).
2. *Table.* A bedside table for essential equipment is ideal, but even a chair can be used if that is all that is available.
3. *Electrical connections.* If instruments require electrical connections, plan the examination site nearby.
4. *Lamps.* Correct illumination is needed for near point testing and the visual acuity chart. If the needs are fully explained to family members, they usually can have suitable sources of illumination arranged in approximately the correct location.
5. *General illumination.* Although complete darkness is not necessary, it is useful to determine beforehand that there are adequate drapes or blinds to reduce illumination and thus enable retinoscopy and ophthalmoscopy to be carried out.

In general, the older person or his or her family should not have to provide equipment not customarily found around the house, but arranging the examination room as outlined can facilitate the examination. Similar arrangements apply to the examination of patients in institutions.

Equipment Necessary for Home Visits

Ideally for a home visit, the same range of equipment should be available as in the office. Ultimately, the decision about what equipment to take is a compromise between the clinical ideal of a full range of equipment and what can be conveniently carried.

Equipment can be divided into three parts. The first part forms a permanent kit of necessary but inexpensive items that can be assembled and ready for use at any time. The small cost of these items is justified by the convenience of having them packed and ready, even if only a small number of home visits are undertaken annually. The second part of the examiner's travelling kit is composed of those more expensive items normally kept in the refracting room. A list of these items should be kept with the permanent kit and checked off when the equipment is being assembled before a visit so that no essential equipment is left behind. The third part is a list that contains optional equipment. Since every examiner develops a personal routine including favored

tests, no one can draw up a "perfect" list.

Permanent Kit

Equipment to be kept as a permanent kit for house calls includes the following:

1. *Distance vision test charts.* A standard Snellen chart will be sufficient for most examinations. If an examiner relies heavily on an astigmatic chart, this also should be included. However, if a crossed cylinder usually is used to determine the astigmatic correction, a Snellen chart will be sufficient. If good illumination is provided at the patient's home, a simple cardboard or plastic chart will do the job adequately.
2. *Near point test cards.* A reduced Snellen chart or paragraphs of type and a card with a small, single object for phoria and duction testing will suffice. There also should be larger print cards for examining visually impaired people.
3. *Penlight and binocular loupe.* If a penlight is used infrequently, check the batteries before each visit. These instruments are used for the external eye examination, photostress recovery tests, and the investigation of pupillary reflexes.
4. *Millimeter PD rule.*
5. *Hatpin.* A hatpin can be used as a target for field testing by confrontation and for phoria and duction measurements. It also can be attached to a wall or curtain as a fixation point.
6. *Pen, pencil, or both.*
7. *Tape measure.* The bedridden patient often will read at an unusual distance. Hence, accurate measurement of the working distance is essential.
8. *Hand crossed cylinders.* Several hand crossed cylinders of different powers should be included.
9. *Occluder.* Hand-held and tie-on types of occluders should be included.
10. *Masking tape.* Masking tape is useful for mounting the Snellen chart on the wall, and for minor repairs to instruments, or for emergency spectacle repair.
11. *Extra bulbs and batteries for the retinoscope and ophthalmoscope.*
12. *Paper clips, thumb tacks, and bulldog clips.* Clips and tacks can be useful for mounting equipment or holding cards.
13. *Screwdriver and an assortment of screws for frames and temples.*

14. *Extension cord and electrical socket.* If the retinoscope and ophthalmoscope are electrically powered, it is wise to include the extension cord.

15. *Small packet of facial tissues.* Facial tissues are useful for cleaning lenses and spectacles and can be used as occluders when placed behind spectacles.

16. *Checklist of equipment.* A list of other equipment to be taken should be included.

This list is only a guide. When making up a kit, practitioners may think of extra items they wish to add. The important characteristics of the permanent kit are that it is inexpensive to assemble and not very extensive. Many traveling cases for trial lens sets have extra compartments that could hold most of the items of a permanent kit, and there is usually enough room above the tray of lenses to store the Snellen chart.

Equipment to Be Taken from the Office
The more complete the permanent kit, the less need there is to remember items to be taken from the refracting room. If a considerable number of home visits are made, many of these items also could be included in the permanent kit. The following list is only a guide, and individual examiners may wish to add to or omit from this list:

1. *Ophthalmoscope and retinoscope.* Include the transformer if necessary, and add it to the permanent kit checklist. It is desirable that a battery-powered ophthalmoscope and retinoscope be stored with the permanent kit so that the regular set need not be taken from the refracting room when a house call is made. Insure that the batteries are fresh.

2. *Trial lenses.* A complete set of trial lenses is necessary and should include Maddox rod, prisms, pinhole disc, and stenopaic slit.

3. *Clip-on lens holders, such as Halberg or Janelli clips.* Clip-on lens holders secure trial lenses in front of the patient's existing spectacles for overrefraction.

4. *Trial frame.* A good trial frame facilitates a trial case refraction. In addition to the conventional spectacle type of trial frame, a headband-mounted trial frame may be more comfortable for prolonged examination. Many practitioners find that a drop cell type of trial frame speeds up the refraction.

5. *Amsler grid.* This is a sensitive test of macular integrity and the central visual

fields.

6. *Opticianry tools.* Take a selection of pliers and file.

7. *Selection of sample frames.* It is wise to carry a sufficient number of frames to determine the correct fit. As the bedridden patient is not usually interested in fancy frames or fashions, the practitioner should need to take only a dozen or so on a visit.

8. *Bifocal segment height and monocular PD measuring devices.* If the optometrist relies on one of these, it should be taken, in addition to the PD rule, in the permanent kit.

9. *Patient's record card.* The record card will be partially filled out before the visit. Since this cannot be kept in the permanent kit, it is listed here as a reminder to include it.

Optional List
In addition to these items, a practitioner may wish to take other items of equipment on a home visit. Some of the following items should be included if the previsit information elicited from the patient indicates that they might be useful.

1. *Placido's disc.* If there is an indication that corneal problems are present, Placido's disc can indicate the integrity of the cornea and the presence of corneal irregularities.

2. *Hand-held lensometer.* Small battery-powered lensometers are now available; if sufficient home visits are made, the expense of buying one would be justified (Figure 20–2).

3. *Hand-held arc perimeter.*

4. *Tonometer.* Several portable tonometers are available, such as the Perkins, Tonomat, and EMT-20.

5. *Lens gauge and protractor.* These can be used for neutralizing spectacles in a patient's home.

6. *Lens bar.* This will facilitate retinoscopy and overrefraction.

7. *Prism bar.* Like a lens bar, a prism bar is more convenient than the loose prisms found in a trial set.

8. *Hand measuring prism.* A Risley prism, mounted on a handle and either with or without a Maddox rod, is useful for quickly determining phorias.

9. *Gooseneck or anglepoise lamp.* Such lamps will simplify the illuminating of test charts. However, if satisfactory lighting can be provided by the home to be visited, it will

Figure 20-2

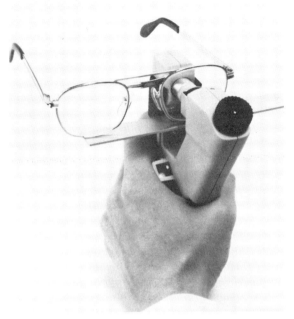

Small, Battery-powered Lensometer Suitable for Home Visits

Figure 20-3

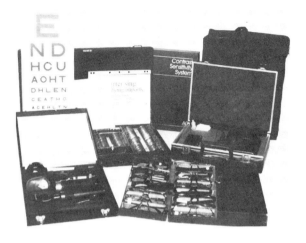

Equipment for Home Visits (Includes Tonometer and Contrast Sensitivity Test) Packs into Two Small Bags

Figure 20-4

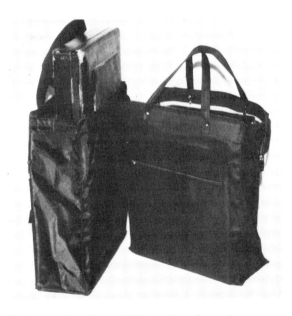

Equipment for Home Visits in Two Carry Bags

reduce the amount of equipment carried.

10. *Frame warmer.* If a frame warmer cannot be taken from the office, a hand-held hair dryer can be used for adjusting frames.

11. *Contrast sensitivity function test.* As a supplemental test of possible value, American Optical Corporation has produced a commercial version of the Arden grating test. This is an easily administered test for contrast sensitivity. As it is the size of a large book, it is portable enough to take on home visits (Figure 20–3).

12. *Color vision test.* In this age group, acquired color vision defects are important. The test used should include tests for blue-yellow disturbances. The D-15 test, the HRR, and City University color vision test include tests for this. It is important that proper illumination controls be provided for valid color vision testing.

As a general rule, the practitioner should limit the equipment taken on a visit to the minimum that will allow an accurate examination to be administered (Figure 20 – 4).

The Examination

When examining, it is wise to remember that most elderly people dislike the tendency for professionals to address them with patronizing

endearments such as "honey," "sweetheart," and "dear" instead of asking them how they prefer to be addressed or using terms such as "sir," "ma'am," or other forms of address that accord them dignity.

The key to a successful home examination is to solve the patient's problem with a minimum of time and strain on the patient (Hirsch and Wick 1960). A typical office examination should not be attempted, but the examiner's desire for precision and accuracy on all tests should be tempered by a knowledge of the patient's state of health. The examiner must judge which tests will yield useful information about the patient's problems. If a patient is complaining about difficulty reading, for example, it would be poor judgment to spend much time determining the axis of a quarter-diopter cylinder. Rather, the examiner should have determined quickly that the astigmatic correction was insignificant and corrected the error with spherical lenses.

Before the examination takes place, it is wise to have the prescription of the previous spectacles. If this was not obtained before the visit, the spectacles should be neutralized at this stage and the case history taken. Although some details will have been learned before the visit, there is no substitute for the information gained by the examiner's talking directly to the patient so that voice, inflections, facial expressions, and other mannerisms may be oberved. The case history and the prescription of the previous spectacles now will determine what tests are necessary.

The external eye examination, test of pupillary reflexes, ophthalmoscopy, and retinoscopy are carried out in the same manner as in the office. Field testing by confrontation, the use of a portable arc perimeter, or the Amsler grid for macular integrity should not be overlooked. If a patient already wears distance spectacles, the amount of change may be determined rapidly by performing retinoscopy over the spectacles.

If a patient can sit up, the distance subjective test is conducted using trial lenses, and the distance test chart is suspended at a suitable distance before the patient. If the patient cannot sit up and there is no active accommodation, the subjective examination can be conducted at the patient's reading distance. If spectacles are required, an allowance is made for the test distance in the prescription. Attention to proper lighting control is essential for an adequate refraction.

Table 20–1 gives the approximate lens power for level of visual acuity and thus a starting point for the distance refraction. When the best acuity has been found using spherical lenses, Table 20–2 gives an estimation of the cylindrical power required to correct any astigmatic error. With the estimated cylinder in place, the appropriate axis is found using the hand-held crossed cylinder, and the power then is refined. It should be noted that many elderly patients have a best visual acuity of less than 20/20 (6/6).

They usually give a more positive response in astigmatic testing if a crossed cylinder of at least $\pm0.50D$ is used, and it is useful to have one of $\pm1.00D$ if the patient finds it difficult to distinguish between the two choices of the $\pm0.50D$ cylinder in cases of reduced acuity. Brooks (1982) provides a good guide to full subjective trial frame refraction; however, care should be taken not to tire the patient by overtesting.

If the patient has a physical disability, the examiner should confine most of the examination to solving the patient's complaint. If a close facsimile of an office examination can be tolerated, that is desirable. However, if a person has difficulty in sitting for long and the main requirement is to read correspondence, for example, it is wise to concentrate on determining the reading prescription.

In determining a near point correction, the patient's reading requirements, best distance visual acuity, health condition, and present lenses frequently will suggest a suitable tentative prescription. This should be placed in a trial frame and refined with the patient's holding a near point card at the habitual reading position. The patient's reading distance should be noted. A person forced to remain in bed may find it more comfortable to read at distances other then those of people following a more active daily routine. A proper visual environment requires that bright illumination be provided over the shoulder and to one side of the better-seeing eye.

The extent of muscle testing to be performed is determined by the patient's signs and symptoms. Rapid tests of reasonable accuracy are all that is required for many people. The distance lateral phoria can be assessed rapidly using the cover test and a convenient small target such as a hatpin placed in a nearby curtain or a penlight held by a helper or placed on a table facing the patient. If loose prisms are used, accuracy of within 4Δ can be obtained. The vertical deviation can be determined easily using a Maddox rod placed in a trial frame and a 1Δ prism placed base down before the other eye. The patient is asked if the light is above or below the line. It should be seen above the line. The prism is now turned base up, and if there is no appreciable vertical phoria, the light will be seen below the line. Using these two simple questions only, the presence or absence of a vertical phoria in excess of 1Δ can be quickly established. If the phoria is greater than this, hand prisms of greater power are used to determine rapidly its amount

Table 20-1
Lens Power for Level Visual Acuity

Visual Acuity			Necessary Sphere (Diopters)
International	Snellen		
<0.50	20/400	(6/120)	±2.00
0.05-0.20	20/400-20/100	(6/120-6/30)	±1.00
0.21-0.50	20/100-20/40	(6/30-6/12)	±0.50
>0.50	20/40	(6/12)	±0.25

Source: C. W. Brooks. "A Systemic Method of Subjective Trial Frame Refraction." *Optometric Monthly* 73, no. 8 (1982): 437.

Table 20-2
Cylinder Estimation Table. Young people tend to obtain higher acuities than would be indicated for the amount of uncorrected astigmatism present.

Visual Acuity			Estimated Cylinder (Diopters)
International	Snellen		
1.00	20/20	(6/6)	0.00
0.70	20/30	(6/9)	0.50
0.50	20/40	(6/12)	1.00
0.35	20/60	(6/18)	1.50
0.25	20/80	(6/24)	2.00
0.20	20/100	(6/30)	2.50

Source: C. W. Brooks. "A Systemic Method of Subjective Trial Frame Refraction." *Optometric Monthly* 73, no. 8 (1982): 438.

and nature.

When testing the muscle balance at the reading position, remember that the positive fusional reserve is of greater diagnostic value than the near phoric position. The amount and type of phoria can be checked rapidly using the cover test, and the positive fusional reserves can be assessed rapidly using loose prisms of 6Δ or 8Δ. With the patient's fixating a small target, the hand prism is introduced in the base-in and then the base-out position. If, in each instance, the patient reports seeing only one target or seeing two that quickly merge together, it is safe to assume that the correction may be worn without the discomfort caused by a lateral muscle imbalance. However, if the patient sees double on one of these positions or if the two targets drift apart, the test should be repeated using prisms of smaller magnitude, and a prismatic element may be prescribed in the reading spectacles.

When testing muscle imbalance and fusional reserves, it is important to observe the patient's eyes carefully as the tests are conducted. Accurate measurements often can be obtained more easily by noting the speed and accuracy of eye movements rather than relying on a subjective response.

Additional Tests

Other tests that yield valuable information about a person's visual system can be carried out; they also can be used to monitor aspects of general health.

Contrast Sensitivity Function Testing

Contrast sensitivity function (CSF) testing gives a comprehensive picture of the functioning of a person's visual system. In contrast to visual acuity tests, which determine a person's ability to resolve fine targets at high contrast, CSF testing provides information on how well the individual perceives coarse and intermediate features in the environment. Studies show that CSF testing measures correlate well with patients' performance of daily tasks (Marron and Bailey 1982; Sekuler, Hutman, and Owsley 1980). American Optical produces a commercial version of Arden gratings for testing CSF (Arden 1978; Weatherhead 1980). This test is compact and easily administered, and it provides information useful in monitoring changes in the visual system that are caused by both ocular and systemic health conditions (Arden and Jacobson 1978; Arundale 1978; Laird 1978a; Marron and Bailey 1982).

Color Vision Testing

Color vision testing is another supplemental procedure that can be used to monitor changes in the visual system. If an older person has serious color deficiency, his or her environment should be arranged to take account of this fact. However, in this age group, acquired color vision defects are more important, as they can signal changes in a person's ocular or general health (Applegate, Adams, and Cavender 1979; Laird 1978b). Testing should include an investigation of the blue-yellow as well as red-green defects, so a test that incorporates this must be chosen. A quick screening test based on the Farnsworth F2 plate can be constructed easily and it has a high rate of correct diagnosis (Taylor 1975). It is important that color vision tests be presented under the correct lighting conditions (Chioran and Sheedy 1983), as well as monocularly, as the difference between the two eyes is an important diagnostic criterion.

Photostress Recovery Test

Although a full investigation of light and dark adaptation is beyond the scope of a typical home visit, a simple test that should give adequate clinical data can be carried out: the photostress recovery test (Glaser, et al. 1977; Lacey and Jacobs 1983; Severin, Tour, and Kershaw 1967). In this monocular test, the best visual acuity is measured, and a bright light then is shone into the eye for 10 seconds. The time taken for the visual acuity to return to its original level is measured. A recovery time of more than 50 seconds is considered abnormal. The test is repeated with the other eye; if there is a difference in recovery time of more than 20 seconds between the two eyes, further investigation should be undertaken.

Field Testing

Field testing of both the peripheral and central fields can be important for some patients. Early detection of defects at the macula is important in older people, and this is most conveniently done with the Amsler grid. A simple hand-held arc perimeter or testing by confrontation usually will give adequate information about the peripheral fields.

Institutional Care

When an older person is examined at home, the examiner deals with that person and his or her family. However, when the older person is living in an institution, the person is seen in conjunction with the institution's staff. This means a team approach should be followed, and additional information can be obtained from the medical records and the medical and nursing staff. Most elderly people in institutions are multihandicapped; they often have hearing and mobility defects as well as visual problems. Chapter 16 of this book discusses the importance of the visual environment of institutions.

The examiner should consult with the institution's staff about the best time to carry out a visual examination; the increased use of psychotropic medication with elderly people means that the examination should be scheduled to achieve maximum responsiveness. The examiner should be aware of the visual side effects of these drugs and alert to the importance of periodic review of drug type and dosage. The staff with prior notice often can assist the examination procedure by transferring the patient into a suitable environment and being present as part of the care team.

Spectacle Dispensing

The case history will determine what form the spectacle prescription will take. Whether to use multifocal lenses, bifocals, two pairs of spectacles, or reading lenses will be determined largely by the patient's needs, general health, range of mobility, and physical environment.

In prescribing for older people with limited mobility, the lens design should be chosen to deal with their primary need or needs so that if necessary, head movement can be kept to a minimum. Because many may need a higher-than-normal reading addition, single vision lenses are often more practical than bifocals. Similarly, a bedridden person may find the greater field of view of single vision distance spectacles easier for viewing television or looking about a room.

If the person requires an aphakic correction, particular attention must be given to lens design to minimize weight, lens thickness, and lens aberrations (Chapter 17 contains a full discussion on aphakia). Moving about with a bifocal correction may be a problem for elderly aphakics with mobility problems. In these cases, a single vision correction can be fitted close to the face for distance vision and pushed down the nose for reading.

The practitioner also should keep in mind that spectacles may not be the best solution to a person's visual problem, and magnifiers may offer the best solution. For those with unsteady hands, a neck-suspended magnifier could be of real benefit. In intermediate powers, it can be used for sewing, knitting, writing, eating, and other activities in which the hands are otherwise occupied.

In addition to optical aids, a range of nonoptical aids can help elderly people maintain their independence. The practitioner should be aware of the range of aids available from agencies like the New York Lighthouse and the American Foundation for the Blind. Simple aids that can be included as part of a traveling kit include felt-tip pens and heavy, lined writing paper, enlarged numerical telephone dials, check-signing guides, and examples of large print books. Talking Books are an efficient alternative to high-magnification lenses for extended "reading," and their source in the community should be known to the examiner.

If it appears that the patient will be able to visit the office within a few months, the best course of action could be to prescribe a pair of temporary spectacles that will solve the immediate problem. These should be replaced by a more accurately determined prescription when the person is able to visit the office.

The selection of the type of frame and the adjustments necessary for a comfortable fit will be done in much the same manner as in the office. Because older people have fragile skin, lens weight and the use of plastic materials always should be considered. Frames should be selected that distribute weight evenly and comfortably on the nose (see Chapter 18).

The person's posture while reading in bed, the illumination, and the possibility of supplying a reading stand or table all should be considered. A stable and easily adjustable bookstand/knee table can be made by attaching a tray to a small beanbag, which stays stable on an uneven surface. Adequate illumination must be provided where the person does the most reading, and the examiner should not hesitate to recommend the type of lamp, bulb power, and position of the lamp in the room that will give the best visual environment (Cole 1974; Lovie-Kitchen, Bowman, and Farmer 1983). These recommendations should be reinforced by involving a family or staff member in the discussion. The placement of the bed in relation to windows or the television set also may be suggested.

Older people and their families should be told about the nature of the lenses being recommended; what they can expect to see with them; and, possibly more important, what not to expect and any limitations and side effects that may be experienced.

The method of delivery and adjustment of the spectacles is determined by the nature of the prescription and the patient's circumstances. If the patient's home is some distance from the office and one of the sample frames can be used, that frame can be adjusted at the time of the examination visit and the lens inserted later without altering the adjustment. The spectacles then can be mailed to the patient or collected by a family member. If the patient lives close to the office and the spectacles will require adjustment to give optimum performance, it is better for the examiner to deliver them and adjust them on the patient. If adjustments are made at home, a portable frame warmer or hair dryer, a file, and pliers are all the equipment necessary. If the spectacles have been mailed, the examiner should telephone the patient's family after a few days to determine if there are any problems with the new spectacles.

The optometrist should keep in mind specialized devices such as recumbent spectacles, the use of yoked prisms, nonstandard bifocal segment positions, and minus addition bifocals when dealing with patients with limited mobility. Although these may not be prescribed often, a person with restricted mobility may greatly appreciate the wider range of vision these devices offer.

Financial and Legal Questions

Since eye care practitioners make only a limited number of house calls, frequently they are in doubt as to the proper fee to charge. The fee, of course, will have to be determined by the individual, but some factors should be kept in mind in arriving at an appropriate fee. In many localities, physicians in general practice have a set fee for mileage in making calls some distance from the office to compensate for automobile expenses and for the time away from productive work while traveling to and from the patient's home. In addition, the time required to prepare for a house call must be considered. In an efficient office this should not be great, but a house call does take more time than a regular office examination. The fee is calculated simply from the regular examination fee, plus a charge for the extra time involved in the home visit, plus a charge for the mileage.

Each state in the United States administers Medicaid separately, and each professional should be aware of the current services provided locally. Other countries provide different payment mechanisms within their health care services. Local and national professional organizations should be contacted for up-to-date information about any third-party payment available.

Although it is not a legal requirement, it is a courtesy, as well as a potential help, to consult the attending physician before visiting a patient undergoing treatment. As well as providing valuable medical information, the physician may advise against a visit at a particular time because of the patient's medical condition. A physician could be justifiably concerned at not being consulted and then discovering that a patient had been subjected to a procedure that may do general harm. Consulting the patient's physician is particularly important when the patient is hospitalized. The patient's physician also should be informed of the results of the examination.

References

Applegate, R. A., A. J. Adams, and J. C. Cavender. "Early Visual Function Loss in Senile Macular Degeneration." Paper presented at the annual meeting of the Association of Research on Vision and Ophthalmology, April 30 –May 4, 1979, Sarasota, Fla. (ARVO Abstracts, 1979, p. 254.): and in suppl. to *Investigative Ophthalmology and Visual Science, April 1979.*

Arden, G. B. "The Importance of Measuring Contrast Sensitivity in Cases of Visual Disturbance." *British Journal of Ophthalmology* 62 (1978): 198–209.

Arden, G. B., and J. J. Jacobson. "A Simple Grating Test for Contrast Sensitivity: Preliminary Results Indicate Value in Screening for Glaucoma." *Investigative Ophthalmology and Visual Science* 17 (1978): 23–32.

Arundale, K. "An Investigation into the Variation of Human Contrast Sensitivity with Age and Ocular Pathology." *British Journal of Ophthalmology* 62 (1978): 213–215.

Brooks, C. W. "A Systematic Method of Subjective Trial Frame Refraction." *Optometric Monthly* 73, no. 8 (1982): 433–438.

Chorian, G. M., and J. E. Sheedy. "Pseudoisochromatic Plate Design: Macbeth or Tungsten Illumination?" *American Journal of Optometry and Physiological Optics* 60 (1983): 204–215.

Cole, B. L. "Prescribing Light for the Aging Patient." *Australian Journal of Optometry* 57 (1974): 207–214.

Glaser, J. S., P. J. Savino, K. D. Sumers, S. A. McDonald, and R. W. Knighton. "The Photostress Recovery Test in the Clinical Assessment of Visual Function." American Journal of Ophthalmology 83 (1977): 255–260.

Hirsch, M. J., and R. E. Wick, eds. *Vision of the Aging Patient.* Philadelphia: Chilton, 1960.

Lacey, J. A., and R. J. Jacobs. "The Macular Photostress Test." *Australian Journal of Optometry* 66, no. 4 (1983): 147–150.

Laird, I. K."Contrast Sensitivity and Clinical Developments." *Transactions of the 48th Annual Conference* (New Zealand Optometrical Association), 1978, 101–105. (a)

Laird, I. K. "The Use of Colour Vision Tests in Screening for Acquired Defects." *Archives of the New Zealand Optometric Association* 6 (1978): 9–14. (b)

Leslie, W. J., and D. A. Greenberg. "A Survey and Proposal Concerning Visual Care at the Nursing Home Level." *Journal of the American Optometric Association* 45 (1974): 461–466.

Lovie-Kitchen, J. E., K. J. Bowman, and E. J. Farmer. "Technical Note: Domestic Lighting Requirements for the Elderly." *Australian Journal of Optometry* 66 (1983): 93–97.

Marron, J. A., and I. L. Bailey. "Visual Factors and Orientation Mobility Performance." American Journal of Optometry and Physiological Optics 59 (1982): 413–426.

New Zealand Optometrical Association. *Design of Optometric Premises.* Wellington: New Zealand Optometrical Association, 1970.

Sekuler, R., L. P. Hutman, and C. J. Owsley. "Human Aging and Spatial Vision." *Science* 209 (1980): 1255–1256.

Severin, S., R. Tour, and R. Kershaw. "Macular Function and the Photostress Test: 1." *Archives of Ophthalmology* 77 (1967): 2–7.

Taylor, W. O. G. "Constructing Your Own PIC Test." *British Journal of Physiological Optics* 31 (1975): 22–24.

Weatherhead, R. G. "Use of the Arden Grating Test for Screening." *British Journal of Ophthalmology* 66 (1980): 591–596.

Chapter 21

Functional Therapy in the Rehabilitation of Elderly Patients

Bruce C. Wick

Vision is a complex synkinesis of biochemistry, neural structures, physiology, and learning. The relationships are complex and often not well understood. Aging causes major changes in visual performance, and, as is true in youth, specific deficits frequently do not account for overall performance decrements. A loss of visual sensory and motor abilities impairs performance of all perceptual tasks. The decline of visual abilities with age is a fact of mature life and ranges from severe deterioration to minor reductions in visual function.

Perception of the environment through vision requires that the visual system be able to effectively gather information. Generally, people do not experience severe visual acuity impairment with increasing age (Weymouth 1960); however most suffer from decreases in oculomotor function. Losses of accommodative ability (presbyopia), field of vision, and eye movement speed and accuracy can cause profound difficulties in binocular information gathering and processing.

These losses often can be remedied by selective rehabilitative techniques. Although perceptual aspects of vision care are very important, these aspects will be dealt with only partially. This chapter will discuss the functional rehabilitation of vision problems with emphasis on motor aspects of binocular vision for patients with normal static visual acuity.

Oculomotor Functions

A thorough understanding of the basis and development of normal oculomotor function

My thanks to my father, Dr. Ralph E. Wick, for his help and support in all my writing and especially this chapter. He was free with his comments and suggestions, as usual.

is necessary before any rehabilitation can begin. Equally important is an understanding of the changing normals of age that occur in all individuals. For example, losses in vergence ability and changes in tonic vergence accompany presbyopia and the normal aging process. (Chapter 10 of this book discusses normal changes in visual function with aging.) Rehabilitative techniques are used when normal aging changes cause individuals to depart from required abilities to perform adequately.

Vergence Eye Movements

The diagnosis and rehabilitation of oculomotor system dysfunction requires understanding pursuit, saccadic, and vergence eye movements (Schor and Ciuffreda 1983). Vergence eye movements generally are considered to consist of four components: tonic, accommodative, disparity (fusional), and proximal (Maddox 1893). In the diagnosis and treatment of visual motor problems, vergence magnitudes are related to one another using various criteria to evaluate whether symptoms are likely to be caused by the findings present.

Components of the total vergence response depend on age and show specific decrements as time passes. There are especially dramatic decreases in accommodative function and a corresponding loss in accommodative vergence and, subsequently, near convergence ability (Sheedy and Saladin 1975). In light of other decrements in motor and sensory ocular ability with age, it is not surprising that disparity vergence ability also decreases with age.

Diagnosis of Oculomotor Dysfunctions

The proper diagnosis of visual problems of the aged is facilitated by taking a thorough, careful history. The value of a complete, accurate history increases with the patient's age. Ocular disease, systemic disease, side effects of medication, and accidental injury all have increased incidence. Patients usually have two or three main visual problems they want solved. Careful listening by the examiner combined with well-directed questions and a systematic approach to obtaining pertinent information will improve the chances of an accurate history. Pertinent visual complaints often are obscured by rambling, and sometimes incoherent, details. The history can be conveniently divided into two parts: general and visual.

General and Visual History
A general history should be taken prior to any examination, and it frequently indicates many tests that should be performed. Often an accompanying member of the family can (or needs to) be consulted, as an aged patient may overlook key points of the history. In these instances the family can be of great help, as well as prevent exasperation to the patient.

Visual history taking should be continued throughout the examination. A fixed sequence of questions can be useful, but information volunteered by the patient during the examination often has the greatest value (Wick 1960). Information gathered during the examination may lead to other areas that need to be explored and indicate ancillary tests needed for accurate diagnosis of the visual problem.

Determining the patient's occupation and hobbies is of utmost importance for prescriptive purposes, including working distances, times, lighting conditions, and occupational requirements. Frequently, the aged are unaware that different types of lenses are needed or available for various visual tasks. Thus, in spite of a careful history, many visual requirements may be neglected because the patient is unaware of the visual requirements of specific tasks.

Specific questions related to binocular problems should be asked: When do symptoms occur? When do they start? How long do they last? What relieves the symptoms? With what tasks do they occur? and Is there any diplopia? When the patient complains of newly acquired diplopia, there is usually a paretic or restrictive etiology involving oculomotor pathology. However, patients frequently confuse double vision with distorted or blurred vision, so it is important to be sure that diplopia truly exists.

The following are nonpathological causes of diplopia:
1. Strabismus/heterophoria.
   a. *Fusional disturbances.* Intermittent diplopia may be associated with uncompensated heterophoria and comitant heterotropias with inadequate suppression.
   b. *Postoperative diplopia.* This is a complication of strabismus surgery that may persist for years. It frequently follows cosmetic operations on older patients.
   c. *Onset of comitant strabismus.* Diplopia is experienced briefly at the onset of a comitant deviation before suppression begins. These patients are typically young children who rarely describe their symptoms accurately.
   d. *Uncompensated congenital palsy.* In patients with congenital muscle palsies who have maintained single binocular vision by appropriate head posturing and fusional mechanisms, a breakdown in fusional ability may result in sudden diplopia. This occurs in particular with congenital superior oblique palsies in which fusional resources are weakened (for example, following a long illness). A review of old photographs will reveal a head tilt that has been maintained throughout life.
   e. *Sudden onset comitant strabismus.* Although almost all comitant strabismus develops insidiously, occasionally a comitant deviation appears suddenly and is accompanied by annoying diplopia. This is most common in patients with high heterophorias who have undergone an artificial interruption of binocular vision for several days (for instance, with unilateral patching for ocular injuries). When the patch is removed, fusion cannot be maintained, and there is constant diplopia. Although some cases resolve spontaneously, most require treatment in the form of prisms, lenses, or visual training.
   f. *A and V patterns.* In these complex forms of horizontal strabismus, the deviation varies with vertical gaze. For example, in A exotropia, the exotropia increases on downgaze. Such patients frequently experience diplopia, especially with reading and other near tasks.
   g. *Brown's superior oblique tendon sheath syndrome.* This condition involves a

congenital superior oblique sheath defect that mechanically limits the eye's ability to elevate from an adducted position. Diplopia is noticed on upgaze.

2. *Physiological diplopia.* Many patients are alarmed by a sudden awareness of normal physiological diplopia experienced for objects off the singleness horopter.

3. *Anomalous prismatic effect of spectacles.* This occurs with poorly adjusted glasses, errors in spectacle fabrication involving the inclusion of unwanted prism, omission of previously worn prism, or the need for slab-off prism in anisometropia.

After it has been determined that diplopia does exist, a routine history is augmented with questions related to: the duration of diplopia, its first occurrence, the location of diplopic images, and the frequency and course of their occurrence.

Tests and Measurements

Comitant Deviations. Once an accurate initial history has been completed, tests are done to thoroughly evaluate binocular function. Ocular health is evaluated (through fundus evaluation, biomicroscope examination, tonometry, visual field testing, the Amsler grid, and testing pupillary reflexes) to be sure that ocular, neurological, or systemic disease is not causing the reported signs or symptoms. The analysis of binocular dysfunction on the aged is described in this section.

A thorough refraction, including tests of binocular and monocular visual acuity, should be performed. Monocular refraction under binocular conditions helps stabilize fusion and visual acuity. (American Optical vectographic slides or Turville's distance testing combined with the Borish or other binocular tests for near vision are recommended.) Fusional difficulties may cause binocular acuity to be less than the acuity of the better eye.

Obviously, plus additions are needed for the aged to maintain clear vision at near due to loss of accommodative ability. Proper history taking will help determine the best choice of near addition power and form (bifocal, trifocal, reading, or any other). Many tests can determine the addition. Excellent theoretical (Morgan 1960) and test (Borish 1970) descriptions are available. The basic premise is to prescibe the addition so that one-half of the accommodative amplitude is kept in reserve, or so that the desired working distance is in the central part of the range of clear vision through the addition.

Heterophoria and binocular vision are evaluated at distance and near. Near evaluations are done through any plus addition indicated by refractive findings. Lateral heterophoria can be measured by various methods: objective and subjective cover tests, Maddox rod–flash and nonflash, and von Graeffe's technique–flash and nonflash (Hirsch and Bing 1948). Tests in the natural environment are frequently superior to those made through the phoropter. A properly performed cover test for assessment of phoria magnitude, as well as quality of fusional recovery, can be useful (Morgan 1960). The cover test consists of two parts: the unilateral cover test (to detect strabismus) and the alternate cover test (to measure the angle of heterophoria or strabismus).

To perform the unilateral cover test, do the following:

1. Direct the patient to fixate a small, detailed target.

2. Closely observe one eye (the limbus may be used as a guide), and simultaneously occlude the other eye.

3. Note the direction and estimate the amount of movement required of the eye to fixate the target.

4. Immediately uncover the eye.

5. Repeat, if necessary.

6. Bring the occluder beneath the eyes to the opposite side. (*Be sure* the patient uses alternate fixation.)

If fixation is central for each eye and there is no movement of either eye upon covering the opposite eye, there is heterophoria. Strabismus is indicated if there is movement of one eye upon covering the other. The test should be repeated in different fields of gaze to analyze noncomitancy. For aged patients, the near cover test is done through any plus addition required.

To perform the alternate cover test, do the following:

1. Occlude one eye, and direct the patient to fixate a small target with the unoccluded eye.

2. Direct your gaze to the cover at a point where you assume the temporal limbus to be.

3. Quickly move the occluder to the fixating eye. Do not allow your gaze to follow the occluder.

4. Note the direction and estimate the amount of movement required of the uncovered eye to fixate the target. Movement of the eye with the occluder signifies an exodeviation, and

movement opposite to the occluder indicates an esodeviation

5. Return the occluder to the original position before the eye.
6. Between the occluder and the eye, orient a loose prism or prisms of sufficient power to neutralize the movement just seen.
7. Repeat the test, changing the power of the prism or prisms until just-perceptible movements of opposite direction are observed.
8. The midpoint of this pair of prism values represents the angle phoria or tropia.

The test is done in different fields of gaze to analyze noncomitancy. Occasionally, the alternate cover test will reveal a larger angle than did the unilateral cover test in the presence of strabismus. Such measurements are often evidence of unharmonious anomalous correspondence, although for exotropic patients (especially those with pseudodivergence excess), a properly performed (prolonged) near cover test will reveal more exodeviation than will just short, rapid occlusion.

Vertical heterophoria may be measured at distance and near by Maddox rods, a cover test, and prism dissociation. When a vertical heterophoria is present in an aged patient, comitancy should be carefully evaluated. Fixation disparity tests probably are the most accurate techniques for prism prescription. Fixation disparity measures have the added advantage that they can be conducted in all fields of gaze under more natural binocular viewing conditions.

Disparity (fusional) vergence ranges are measured using loose or rotary prisms in free space and through the phoropter at distance and near. Because loose prisms are presented in discrete steps, they give good indications of the patient's fusional recovery ability. Measuring vergence ranges using rotary prisms through the phoropter frequently can be eliminated from the test sequence if forced vergence fixation disparity curves are measured at distance and near.

For determining lateral phorias, forced vergence fixation disparity curves are plotted at distance and near. Prism to reduce fixation disparity to zero is measured in all positions of gaze. Actual fixation disparity is only measured by instruments specifically designed for the task, for example, the Disparometer, and Woolf near card (Schor and Narayon 1982). Most clinical tests (Mallett Distance and Near Fixation Disparity Tests, as well as Bernell lanterns) measure the prism to reduce fixation disparity to

zero—the associated phoria. Forced vergence fixation disparity curves (Disparometer and Wolff near card) are valuable for the analysis of binocular vision (Sheedy and Saladin 1977). Figure 21–1 shows typical distance and near forced vergence fixation disparity curves for a symptomatic presbyopic subject with poor control of a near lateral phoria.

Figure 21–1

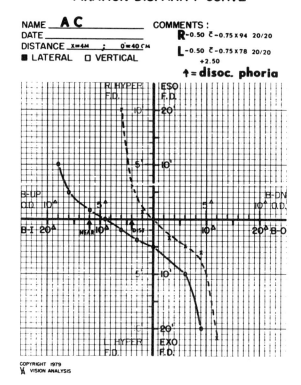

Fixation Disparity Curves Measured at Distance (x) and Near (o) on Patient with Symptomatic Near Exophoria. There is a near exofixation disparity of 5′, and nearly 10Δ base-in is required to reduce the fixation disparity to zero. Source: Graph reprinted with permission from James E. Sheedy, University of California, Berkeley.

Flat curves indicate better compensation for the phoria than do steep curves. For symptomatic patients, prism can be prescribed to approximately center the curve about the y-axis, or the center of symmetry (Schor 1983). The associated phoria measurement (prism to reduce fixation disparity to zero) generally gives smaller prism prescriptions for symptomatic patients with steep curves than do other criteria for prescribing prisms, and the prescription found usually gives adequate relief of symptoms (Sheedy 1980).

When a lateral and a vertical fixation disparity exist simultaneously, the vertical fixation disparity should be corrected first. Then the horizontal fixation disparity curves should be measured. Correcting the vertical fixation disparity often will normalize (flatten) the slope found in horizontal fixation disparity curve measurement (Wick and London 1984).

Vision therapy can be prescribed to improve binocularity and modify the curve shape. For the elderly patient, vision therapy progress can be followed using forced vergence fixation disparity curves. These curves generally flatten with successful therapy, just as do those of younger patients. After therapy, a small fixation disparity generally remains when the actual fixation disparity is measured (Schor 1983).

Arriving at the prism prescription for a vertical phoria frequently requires maximum clinical judgment. Various techniques have been recommended for prescription design, including equating vergence ranges, flip prism techniques (Eskridge 1961), and fixation disparity tests (Morgan 1949). Tests that measure prism to reduce vertical fixation disparities to zero (measured clinically by American Optical vectographic slides, Turville's infinity balance, the Mallett distance and near unit, and the Borish near card) generally give vertical prism prescriptions that reduce symptoms. Nearly all patients can appreciate a difference of 0.5Δ on vertical fixation disparity tests (Morgan 1949).

Vertical prism should not be prescribed for all vertical fixation disparities—only when it gives improved visual performance (less suppression, increased fusion ranges, and flatter lateral forced vergence fixation disparity curves) and reduced symptoms. Generally, a reduction of vertical misalignment to zero under binocular viewing conditions (prism to reduce fixation disparity to zero) gives the most accurate prism prescriptions.

Stereopsis should be measured at distance and near. The stereoscopic threshold is relatively constant up to ages 45 to 50. After age 50, stereopsis declines gradually with increasing age (Pitts 1982). However, there are large variations in individuals, and "normal" stereopsis may be found even in the extremely aged.

Finally, the near point of convergence should be measured. In youth the near point of convergence ranges from 1 to 4 cm from the spectacle plane (Cooper and Duckman 1978). With the onset of presbyopia, there is decrease of about 1 cm per decade, so by age 70 the normal convergence near point is 3 to 7 cm from the spectacle plane. Debility, systemic medication, and changes in binocular status can cause dramatic individual decrements.

Heterophoria, convergence, and binocular vision should be examined without the patient's wearing glasses if he or she does not normally wear them and with glasses (correct or not) if the patient does wear them. To evaluate the effects of lens prescriptions, and prism prescriptions, or both, the examination is repeated with the best possible correction and appropriate prescription modification.

Noncomitant Deviations. Deviations that vary significantly (greater than 5Δ) when the eyes are directed into various fields of gaze are noncomitant (Griffin 1976). These deviations also increase when an eye with one or more paretic muscles fixates; the secondary deviation is larger than the primary. Diagnosis is facilitated by taking a case history and performing tests to measure the amount and extent of diplopia, fusion, and noncomitancy. Noncomitant deviations are characterized by the following:
1. A limitation of monocular motility.
2. A change in magnitude of the deviation in various fields of gaze.
3. A change in diplopia with various fields of gaze.
4. An increase in the angle of deviation when the eye with the paretic muscle fixates.

Identification of the affected muscles begins with observation. The examiner looks for gross deviations in alignment, signs of lid abnormality, or an unusual head turn or tilt. Patients who have noncomitant deviations often adopt distinctive head positions to compensate for diplopia. Table 21–1 shows head positions adopted in noncomtancy and the extraocular muscles affected.

Noncomitancy generally is caused by three conditions:
1. Trauma, including head and orbital trauma.
2. Neurological disorders (disorders of gaze and muscle palsies caused by dysfunctions of cranial nerves III, IV, and VI).
3. Muscle disorders, including orbital tumors and pseudotumors, which compromise muscle action; thyroid disease; and myesthenia gravis.

Tests to detect the affected muscle in noncomitancy must take into account that restrictive syndromes (thyroid disease and blow-out

Table 21–1
Abnormal Head Posture
and Affected Extraocular Muscle

Face Position			Muscle Affected
Turn	Chin Position	Tilt	
R	None	None	RLR
L	None	None	RMR
L	Down	L	RSO
L	Up	R	RLO
R	Up	L	RSR
R	Down	R	RLR
L	None	None	LLR
R	None	None	LMR
R	Down	R	LSO
R	Up	L	LLO
L	Up	R	LSR
L	Down	L	LLR

fractures) affect eye alignment differently than nerve or muscle dysfunctions (myesthenia gravis and cranial nerve dysfunction cause muscle palsy). In restrictive syndromes diplopia is caused by mechanical resistance to movement of the eye, and diplopia is most noticeable during attempted movements *opposite* the field of action of the involved muscle or muscles. With nerve dysfunctions the deviation increases on attempted gaze into the field of action of the muscle. Recent paretic involvements are charac-

terized by: (1) a larger secondary than primary deviation and (2) a sudden onset of symptoms such as diplopia, blurring, and head tilt or turn.

The diagnostic field of action of each extraocular muscle is shown in Table 21–2. To properly diagnose noncomitancy, the examiner must evaluate the deviation in the primary position, in each of the six positions of gaze, and with each eye fixating. Evaluation is done monocularly and binocularly. This will allow determination of the affected muscles. Some tests used for evaluation are the alternate cover test, the Hess-Lancaster screen, and the Maddox rod.

A shortcut method to isolate a single cyclovertical muscle in recent noncomitancy is the Parks (1958) three-step method, which consists of various measurements of ocular alignment. It is not appropriate for lateral muscle palsies or when more than one muscle is affected. Determining which eye has the hyper component in primary position; in which field of gaze the hyper component increases; and, finally, whether the hyper increases on right or left head tilt allows differentiation of the affected muscle (Table 21–3).

Two tests are especially helpful for evaluating noncomitancy and subsequently monitoring therapy progress (Cohen and Soden 1981). Using a projective or arc perimeter or tangent screen, measure the following:

1. Monocular field: how far the patient can

Table 21–2
Extraocular Muscles and Their Fields of Action

Right Eye				Left Eye	
Gaze Direction	Muscle			Gaze Direction	Muscle
R	RLR			L	LLR
L	RMR			R	LMR
L, down	RSO			R, down	LSO
L, up	RLO			R, up	LLO
R, up	RSR			L, up	LSR
R, down	RLR			L, down	LLR
Rotational separation	LLO			RIO	Rotational separation
Vertical separation	{ LSR { RIO			RSR } LIO }	Vertical separation
Patient's left	{ LLR { RMR	Primary position		RLR } LMR }	Patient's right
Vertical separation	{ LIR { RSO			RIR } LSO }	Vertical separation
Rotational separation	LSO			RSO	Rotational separation

Table 21−3
Three-Step Method for Determining Cyclovertical Muscle

Paretic Muscle	Hyper Eye in Primary Position	Hyper Greater on Gaze	Hyper Greater on Head Tilt
LIO	R	R	R
RIR	R	R	L
RSO	R	L	R
LSR	R	L	L
RSR	L	R	R
LSO	L	R	L
LIR	L	L	R
RIO	L	L	L

foveally fixate (follow) a target as it moves along the perimeter surface. This is measured in degrees.

2. Binocular field: to what extent the patient can bifoveally fixate (follow) a target along the perimeter surface before diplopia or suppression occurs. This is measured in degrees. Anaglyphic or Polaroid techniques help diplopia awareness. Frequently there is an area of suppression or confusion before diplopia is noticed. Figure 21−2 shows possible diplopia fields for a right lateral rectus paresis.

During and after optometric rehabilitation, these tests are used to monitor therapy by checking whether the monocular fixation field has expanded. The extent of the binocular field before diplopia awareness also should increase. This allows objective assessment of therapy progress.

Pupillary and visual field studies should be done when diagnosing any noncomitancy (see Chapter 12 for more complete description). When pupillary function is affected, tumors or aneurysms are suspected. Etiology is not determined in every noncomitancy, however.

Rehabilitation of Oculomotor Dysfunctions

In geriatrics it has long been recognized that the object of treatment is to restore function maximally based on the normal for the age of the patient and the condition present. This may seem obvious to the experienced clinician; however, attempts to restore function beyond normals for the age, visual condition, and individual patient will only result in frustration for both practitioner and patient. This may explain the reluctance of many optometrists to engage in the rehabilitation of visual dysfunctions of aged patients.

After an accurate history and diagnosis have been obtained, lens management, prism management, or both are used to improve binocularity maximally. Decisions about lens prescription types (bifocals, single vision reading, and so on) generally are made based on a case history of working conditions rather than any possible subsequent binocular therapy. The patient is reevaluated after 2 weeks to 1 month. If the patient still shows evidence of decreased binocular function (for example, macular suppression, decreased amplitude of fusion, fixation disparity, or decreased stereopsis) and symptoms persist, vision therapy is indicated if the patient can be properly motivated. Home vision therapy is generally sufficient for the rehabilitation of elderly patients' binocular dysfunctions, especially exodeviations. Occasionally, the management of esodeviations will need to incorporate office-based therapy.

Comitant Deviations

Binocular rehabilitation attempts to develop efficient, comfortable, well-sustained binocular vision using prisms, lenses, vision therapy, or a combination of these techniques. Motor and peripheral sensory fusion are generally already present. The rehabilitative therapies discussed in this chapter will be limited to lateral deviations. Although vertical heterophorias can be treated with vision therapy techniques, the processes needed are somewhat more complicated. Furthermore, experience indicates that vision therapy techniques for vertical deviations are usually less successful in reducing symptoms of aged patients than vertical prism prescriptions.

Vision therapy is designed to maximally enhance stereopsis, version and saccadic ability, and vergence ranges. It is indicated at any age—

Figure 21–2

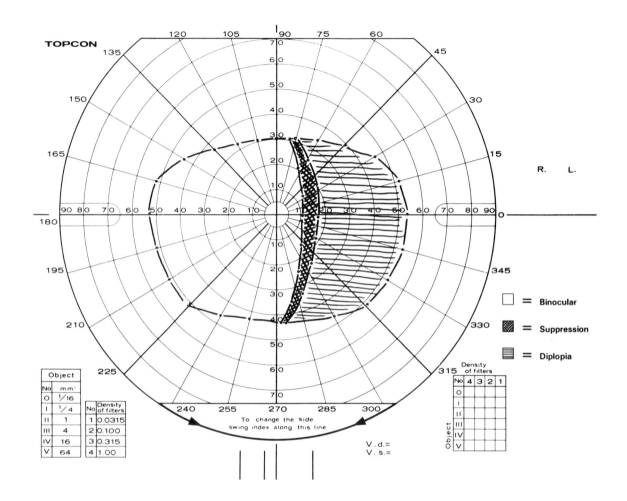

Possible Diplopia Fields for Right Lateral Rectus Paresis

even into the 90s—when symptoms exist and binocular findings are abnormal. When there are age-related decreases in monocular skills (pursuit and saccadic ability), a short period of monocular training may be needed (one to two weeks at most). Rehabilitation for the aged proceeds faster when binocular therapy accompanies monocular therapy and is emphasized exclusively after monocular skills are essentially equal.

Occasionally, elderly patients have problems with even very small heterophorias. Central suppression, reduced vergence ranges, poor version and saccadic ability, and reduced stereopsis influence the extent of these problems. Rehabilitative therapy using appropriate lens and prism corrections is done when these "general skills" problems exist.

Rehabilitative Management of Exophoria.
The overall goals in the rehabilitation of exophoria in the elderly patient follow:
1. Sustained compensation for the exodeviation using increased convergence ability.
2. Comfortable binocular vision for needed visual tasks.

Refractive management is usually less successful than vision therapy management for exophoria. Obviously, overminusing is inappropriate for presbyopic patients, and base-in prism can actually increase the exodeviation because of prism adaptation (Carter 1965). Vision therapy is generally sufficient without modification of the refractive correction. However, base-in prism can be useful when vision therapy is not possible.

The following are vision therapy goals for the

elderly patient with exophoria:

1. Increase voluntary fusional convergence maximally (break points).
2. Enhance jump vergences (recovery points).
3. Establish central and foveal sensory fusion in free space at the ortho position.
4. Enhance stereopsis.
5. Develop reflex vergences.

The following lists give typical rehabilitative vision therapy procedures for symptomatic near and distance exophoria. Procedures are listed in the order usually prescribed for home therapy. All procedures are not used for all patients. Aged patients with symptomatic exophoria at distance and near are managed using rehabilitative vision therapy techniques from all four lists. Therapy for both distance and near exophoria is grouped into two parts: vergence training and antisuppression/stereopsis training. Home therapy is prescribed from each category, and the level of difficulty is increased with improved binocular responses.

Vergence Training for Near Exophoria:

1. *Pencil push-ups.* A detailed target is moved from arm's length closer until fusion is lost. This technique is sometimes combined with lights, anaglyphs, or both for antisuppression training.
2. *Colored circles (Mast/Keystone).* These provide a flat fusion convergence demand and can be modified for antisuppression training simultaneously.
3. *Aperture-rule trainer.* Using a single aperture, positive fusional vergence training is done using antisuppression and stereoscopic targets. This is often combined with a distance target for jump vergence training.
4. *Eccentric circles.* Using these circles with stereopsis demand, fusion training is done by crossing the eyes to develop convergence ability. This technique can be combined with two targets for jump vergence training.
5. *Near point chiastopic fusion.* This develops convergent fusion using two ordinary objects (often with antisuppression cues) such as coins, thumbs, buttons, and so on.
6. *Anaglyphic reading.* Using a Polaroid or anaglyphic grid of bars and spaces, combined with appropriate glasses, antisuppression training is done. This technique can be combined with lenses or prisms for simultaneous vergence training (Gibson 1955).
7. *Mirror stereoscope.* A Wheatstone-type stereoscope using two mirrors for dissocia-

tion and shaped in the form of a W, using various targets, can train vergence ranges of 40Δ base in to 50Δ base out.

8. *Brock's Posture Board.* Using anaglyphs and lights on a Plexiglas board near antisuppression tests can be done. The technique can be combined with lenses and prisms.
9. *Three-eye mirror method.* A circle is drawn on a mirror. The patient converges and fuses his or her eyes to see one eye fused in the center and two eyes on the outside – all inside the circle. This technique can be combined with a letter on the mirror for jump vergence training.
10. *Combinations.* All these techniques can be combined to increase vergence demand, reduce suppression, and enhance stereopsis.

Antisuppression/Stereopsis Training for Near Exophoria:

1. *Polachrome Orthoptic Trainer.* Vectograms or tranaglyphs (Bernell Corporation) and appropriate spectacles are used in antisuppression and convergence therapy (Vodnoy 1970).
2. *Pola-mirror push-ups.* The patient looks at his or her eyes in a mirror while wearing Polaroid glasses. Any "blacking out" of one lens (suppression) is noted (Griffin and Lee 1970). The mirror is moved closer and farther away.
3. *Eccentric Circles.*
4. *Anaglyphic reading.*
5. *Brock's Posture Board.*
6. *Aperture-rule trainer.*
7. *Orthofusor, base-out kit (Bausch & Lomb).* The Polaroid kit is used to improve positive fusional vergence and give antisuppression and stereoacuity training.
8. *Bar reading (custom-made).* A septum is placed between the reading task and the patient to dissociate one eye from the other. Suppression is noted when words are missing. This technique can be combined with lenses and prisms for vergence training.
9. *Combinations.* All these techniques can be combined to increase vergence demand, reduce suppression, and enhance stereopsis.

Vergence Training for Distance Exophoria:

1. *Voluntary convergence.* In training willful crossing of the eyes, visual stimuli sometimes are used. Patients are to become aware of the feeling in their eyes as they converge.
2. *Ductions and versions.* Some improvement of saccadic and version ability is often helpful. A swinging Marsden ball can train pursuit movements. Any two targets can be

used for saccadic training.

3. *Pencil push-aways.* A detailed fixation target is held close and gradually moved farther away. Sometimes anaglyphs and a light are used.

4. *Hand-held Brewster's stereoscope.* This is a refracting stereoscope with a septum. Using any of the hundreds of stereograms available, vergence and antisuppression training are done. Vergence demand is varied by changing the target separation or fixation distance (tromboning).

5. *Prism demand flippers.* Using prisms in a lens holder, vergence demand is changed in discrete steps. This technique can be combined with antisuppression exercises (anaglyphs or Polaroid glasses) for powerful training of vergence and fusion ability.

6. *Chiastopic fusion at far.* Two pictures with suppression cues give a fusion demand. Near chiastopic fusion usually must be learned first.

7. *Risley prism for pursuit.* This variable prism, which can be used to increase vergence demand, may need to be combined with antisuppression exercises.

8. *Polachrome orthoptic trainer.* Vectograms or tranaglyphs (Bernell Corporation) and appropriate spectacles are used in antisuppression and convergence therapy (Vodnoy 1970).

9. *Vis-à-vis walkaways.* Both examiner and patient wear Polaroid glasses. The patient is to tell of any blacking out of one of the examiner's eyes. This also can be done with a mirror by the patient alone (Griffin 1976).

10. *Combinations.* All these techniques can be combined to increase vergence demand, reduce suppression, and enhance stereopsis.

Antisuppression Stereopsis Training for Distance Exophoria:

1. *Peripheral stereopsis.* Using large stereoscopic targets (Root rings or Brock's rings), stereopsis responses are elicited peripherally. The patient works to increase the distance from the test so that the test, as well as subsequent stereopsis demand, becomes more central.

2. *Television trainer.* An anaglyphic or Polaroid attachment for the television is available. When appropriate spectacles are worn, suppression is noted when part of the picture turns black. This technique can be combined with prisms or lenses for simultaneous vergence training.

3. *Brock string techniques.* A string is held from a distant target to the nose. The patient sees two strings crossing at the visual axes' crossing point. Beads can be put on the string to increase diplopia awareness, and anaglyphs can help eliminate suppression.

4. *Pola-mirror training with afterimages.* A mirror and Polaroid lenses are combined with afterimages. The goal is to see crossed afterimages and both eyes (no suppression).

5. *Pola-mirror training with two mirrors.* This is the same technique as in Item 4, but this one uses two mirrors so that fixation distances can be altered to increase or decrease vergence demand and fusion difficulty. It also can be combined with afterimages.

6. *Chiastopic fusion at far.*

7. *Hand-held Brewster's stereoscope.*

8. *Prism bar for saccadic vergences.* Prism bars increase vergence demand in discrete, rapid steps. They often are combined with antisuppression exercises. Prism bars can be custom-made for each patient to give maximal training (Wick 1974).

9. *Combinations.* All these techniques can be combined to increase vergence demand, reduce suppression, and enhance stereopsis.

When home therapy is appropriate, detailed instruction sheets can help insure patient compliance. Figure 21–3 shows a typical instruction sheet for home therapy using push-up convergence. Other sheets can and should be prepared for each rehabilitative technique, and examples will be given throughout the chapter.

As with young patients, the primary therapeutic consideration in treating exophoria in the elderly is the patient's ability to compensate for the deviation (an ability that has large individual variations). Because of normal reductions in overall vergence ability in the elderly, the magnitude of the deviation is important to the final outcome. Rehabilitative vision therapy alone is generally sufficient for the treatment of exophoria. Frequently, a vertical and lateral heterophoria coexist, and it is occasionally difficult to decide whether it is necessary to correct the vertical phoria. When the vertical phoria is not corrected and initial lateral vergence training is unsuccessful, vertical prism correction frequently is needed to reduce symptoms and insure the success of lateral therapy.

Some older patients complete all the rehabilitative therapy techniques with little symptomatic relief. These patients require a decrease

Figure 21-3

These exercises will develop the coordination and focusing ability of your eyes when you are looking at near objects and when you look from far to near objects. You will know you are doing the exercise or exercises correctly when you can fuse the two sets of circles into one circle, with a smaller circle inside that stands out or falls away.

Exercise a total of _____ minutes each day. After you can accomplish Procedure 1, add one new procedure each week as you do the exercises. In the beginning you may experience some discomfort such as headaches and eyestrain, so you may have to limit the exercises to a few minutes. As your ability improves, your discomfort will disappear, and the exercise time can be increased. Remember that exercising 15 minutes daily is better than exercising 2 hours once a week! It would be best if you did this exercise at _(insert times)_ ,and _____ each day. Try to establish a routine so that you always do the exercises at the same time each day.

Procedure 1: Hold the two cards together with the *A*'s overlapping. Hold a pencil centered between the circles. Look at the top of the lead, and observe the circles on either side without looking directly at them. Slowly move the pencil toward your nose (always looking at the lead and keeping it centered) until you see *Four* large circles, or more than two. Continue moving your pencil. Observe the center large circles approaching each other until you see them overlap (superimpose). You then will see *Three* large circles with the center one under the pencil. The center large circle will have a smaller circle inside it that appears to be behind the large circle. If the center circle looks even with the large circle, you are not using one of your eyes (suppresion).

Note: If you find that only one eye is being used, then in order to use both eyes, do the following:
1. Blink your eyes rapidly.
2. Cover one eye, and then quickly remove the cover.

Next, try to clear the letters. While you continue to maintain the fused circles and depth (one circle behind the other), concentrate on holding the letters clear.

Correct Response: When Procedure 1 is done correctly, you should see three large circles. The center one should be *clear* and composed of two circles—one behind the other.

Note: This exercise also can be done with the *B*'s overlapping. These are the correct responses:
1. When the *A*'s overlap, the center circle should appear behind the large circle.
2. When the *B*'s overlap, the center circle should appear ahead of the larger circle.

If you cannot see the depth or see it as the reverse of the previous description, you are doing the exercise incorrectly and need to try again.

Procedure 2: Repeat Procedure 1, but without the aid of the pencil. When you can easily fuse the circle without the pencil, begin moving the cards apart. Keep moving them farther apart until the center circle blurs and then breaks into two. Repeat the exercise _____ times, trying to get the cards farther apart each time.

Procedure 3: Look to a detailed distant (more than 10 feet away) object, and make it clear. Then look to the cards and fuse the circles, making the center clear and single and noticing the depth. Repeat this until you can easily look from a distant object to the cards and fuse them when they are separated by 12 inches or more. No pencil is to be used in this exercise. Remember to clear the distant object, then look to the cards and fuse and clear the circles. Move the circles farther apart each time.

Procedure 4: Place the cards against a wall at a distance of about 5 to 6 feet. The cards should be 5 to 6 inches apart. Fuse them in the same manner you have been using for near. When you can fuse and clear the cards easily at this distance, begin moving them farther apart each time.

Procedure 5: When you can fuse the cards (at 5 to 6 feet away) when they are about 2 feet apart, begin alternating your fixation from the fused cards at a distance to a detailed near object. Repeat this until you can easily look from the fused cards to the near object, making each clear before you look to the next one.

Procedure 6: Fuse the cards at a distance of 5 to 6 feet with the cards approximately 12 inches apart. Walk toward the cards (keeping them fused) as close as you can until they get blurry or split into two. Repeat this, trying to walk closer each time before the center circle breaks into two. Always try to maintain the correct response: The cards should be clear, and you should see the depth.

Patient Instructions: Home Vision Therapy—Free Fusion Rings (Convergence) in overall convergence demand for comfortable, efficient binocularity. Vergence demand can be reduced with base-in prisms or surgery when the deviation is large enough at all distances. After the deviation has been reduced with prism or surgery, some patients need further vision therapy to eliminate persistent conditions such as foveal suppression and fixation disparity or to develop fine stereopsis.

Rehabilitative Management of Esophoria.
The overall goals in the rehabilitative management of esophoria are the following:
1. Enhance compensation of the esodeviation through increased divergence.
2. Provide comfortable binocular vision for needed visual tasks.
Prescription modification is more helpful for esodeviations than for exodeviations and may be successful in relieving symptoms without vision therapy or with minimized therapy time. Patients with a distance esophoria frequently are helped by base-out prism. Vision therapy then is done if needed to enhance sensory fusion and give the patient the most comfortable clear binocular vision possible.

The following are vision therapy goals in the management of esophoria:
1. Extend fusional convergence maximally.
2. Enhance awareness of stereopsis.
3. Exercise the present ability to achieve sensory fusion (especially peripheral fusion) in as many varied instruments as are available in office.
4. Increase fusional divergence (break points) by teaching "relaxation" of the eyes through mental effort.
5. Enhance jump vergence ability (recovery points).
6. Establish central and foveal sensory fusion at the angle of deviation (a) using instruments and (b) not using instruments.
7. Develop reflex vergences.
Rehabilitative therapy procedures for esophoria attempt to increase disparity (fusional) divergence involuntarily as a response to increased sensory fusion (stereopsis) demands. Sensory fusion is maintained by adding stereopsis to flat fusion skills. Fusional divergence is stimulated reflexly by increased demand. Because of the absence of accommodation (compensated by plus additions for clear vision at near), there are seldom symptomatic near esophorias.

The home rehabilitative therapy sequence for distance esophoria follows:
Vergence Training for Distance Esophoria:
1. *Ductions and versions.* Some improvement of saccadic and version ability is often helpful. A swinging Marsden ball can train pursuit movements. Any two targets can be used for saccadic training.
2. *Pencil pushaways.* A detailed fixation target is held close and gradually moved farther away. Sometimes anaglyphs and a light are used.
3. *Eccentric circles.* Using these circles with stereopsis demand, fusion training is done by turning the eyes out to develop divergence ability. This technique can combine with two targets for jump vergence training.
4. *Prism demand flippers.* Using prisms in a lens holder, vergence demand is changed in discrete steps. This technique can be combined with antisuppression exercises (anaglyphs or Polaroid glasses) for powerful training of vergence and fusion ability.
5. *Brock string techniques.* A string is held from a distant target to the nose. The patient sees two strings crossing at the visual axes' crossing point. Beads can be put on the string to increase diplopia awareness, and anaglyphs can help to eliminate suppression.
6. *Combinations.* All these techniques can be combined to increase vergence demand, reduce suppression, and enhance stereopsis.
Antisuppression Stereopsis Training for Distance Esophoria:
1. *Prism demand flippers.*
2. *Hole-in-hand game.* The patient looks through a tube with one eye while holding a hand in front of the other eye. The patient strives to see both the hand and an object in the field of view through the "tube-hole" in the hand.
3. *Hand-held Brewster's stereoscopes.* This is a refracting stereoscope with a septum. Using any of the hundreds of stereograms available, vergence and antisuppression training are done. Vergence demand is varied by changing the target separation or fixation distance (tromboning).
4. *Brock string techniques.*
5. *Polachrome orthoptic trainers.* Vectograms or tranaglyphs (Bernell Corporation) and appropriate spectacles are used in antisuppression and convergence therapy (Vodnoy 1970).
6. *Flannel board training.* Red, green, and

yellow pieces are made to put on a piece of black flannel. Using anaglyphic glasses, antisuppression exercises can be done. This technique is often combined with lenses and prisms and distance anaglyphic targets.

7. *Worth dot lights.* Four lights—one red, two green, and one white—are arranged in a diamond pattern. They are used with anaglyphs and moved nearer and farther as a good antisuppression technique. This technique can be combined with lenses and prisms for simultaneous vergence training.

8. *Bagolini's striated lenses.* These lenses with fine striations cause a visible streak when the patient looks at a light. Any suppression is noted when one line or part of a line disappears (Winter 1971). This technique can be combined with lenses and prisms for vergence training.

9. *Combinations.* All these techniques can be combined to increase vergence demand, reduce suppression, and enhance stereopsis.

Figure 21–4 shows a typical home therapy instruction sheet for an esophoria rehabilitation technique.

Rehabilitative Management of Central Suppression and Fixation Disparity. When aged patients have reduced visual skills and binocular instabilities, fixation disparity, foveal and macular suppression, or both are frequently found. Goals in rehabilitation include the following:

1. Eliminate central suppression.
2. Establish bifoveal fixation.
3. Develop fine stereo-acuity.

Refractive management includes modification of the refractive correction using prism. Prescriptions are designed using forced vergence fixation disparity curves (see Figure 21–1). Prism is prescribed to reduced fixation disparity to zero (associated phoria) when steep curves are present. Prism is prescribed to center the flat portion more approximately on the y-axis (center of symmetry) when flat forced vergence fixation disparity curves are measured. Careful refractive management can reduce the need for rehabilitative therapy, enhance therapy success, or both.

Successful rehabilitative therapy of central suppression and fixation disparity requires targets that are small and detailed enough to necessitate bifoveal fixation and enhance central sensory fusion. Using stereoscopic targets rather than flat fusion targets will aid motor processes

and thus maintain bifoveal fixation. The techniques used are "finishing off" procedures for heterophorias with reduced visual skills. Whenever possible, targets should be chosen that have (1) binocular contours, (2) foveal-sized suppression targets, and (3) fine stereopsis stimulation.

Typical home rehabilitative therapy procedures for fixation disparity and central suppression follow:

Vergence Training for Central Suppression and Fixation Disparity:

1. *Polachrome orthoptic trainer.* Vectograms or tranaglyphs (Bernell Corporation) and appropriate spectacles are used in antisuppression and convergence therapy (Vodnoy 1970).

2. *Biopter cards, E series.* These are targets with antisuppression cues for use in Brewster-type stereoscopes. They are combined with changeable vergence demand in the stereoscope (tromboning).

3. *Spache binocular reading.* These are targets with antisuppression cues for use in Brewster-type stereoscopes. They are combined with changeable vergence demand in the stereoscope (tromboning).

4. *MKM binocular reading cards.* These are targets with antisuppression cues for use in Brewster-type stereoscopes. They are combined with changeable vergence demand in the stereoscope (tromboning).

5. *Combinations.* All these techniques can be combined to increase vergence demand, reduce suppression, and enhance stereopsis.

Antisuppression/Stereopsis Training for Central Suppression and Fixation Disparity:

1. *Cheiroscopic tracing.* Using a cheiroscope, targets are traced, colored or filled in. Training can be enhanced by having the patient close his or her eyes and then reopen them, striving to see all lines and colors previously drawn.

2. *Projectopter.* Tranaglyphs or vectograms (Bernell Corporation) are projected on a screen for distance antisuppression and vergence training.

3. *Titmus stereo slides.* Slides are used to enhance stereopsis. Vergence ability is altered using prisms and lenses.

4. *American Optical vectographic adult slide.* A projected polarized slide is used to monitor fixation disparity and suppression as prisms and lenses change vergence demand.

5. *Mallet Distance and Near Fixation Disparity Test Unit.* These fixation disparity tests are

used with Polaroid glasses. Lenses and prisms can be used to train vergence while reducing fixation disparity and suppression.

6. *Combinations.* All these techniques can be combined to increase vergence demand, reduce suppression and enhance stereopsis. A home therapy training sheet is shown in Figure 21–5 for a typical antisuppression training technique.

A different prism correction frequently is indicated for aged patients for distance and near. Bifocals can be prescribed with cement-on or press-on prism segments. It is often better to provide bifocals for occasional reading only. For prolonged reading, a single vision reading correction incorporating the proper near addition and indicated prism correction is frequently the best and most comfortable rehabilitation possible.

Noncomitant Deviations

Management of the noncomitant deviation depends on whether it is of recent onset or is long-standing. Noncomitancy of recent onset requires accurate, immediate diagnosis and referral to the appropriate medical practitioner –usually an internist, ophthalmologist, neuro-ophthalmologist, or neurologist. The optometrist plays a significant role in diagnosis, directing the patient to the proper specialist, and judging the urgency of the situation. When the necessary medical care has been completed (and sometimes while it continues), functional aspects of the paretic noncomitant deviation are managed optometrically by fusion maintainance programs and ocular calisthenics to help prevent secondary contracture. These programs involve careful use of lenses, prisms, and occlusion.

When an extraocular muscle becomes paretic, its antagonist acts unopposed; an eye turn results from weakness of the paretic muscle and subsequent overreaction by the antagonist. Long-standing action by an unopposed muscle can lead to a slow contracture of that muscle. Contracture is thought to be caused by atrophy and hyalinization. When contracture occurs— even when the cause of the noncomitancy is muscle paresis–contracture frequently occurs over a long time course (months or years). The paresis frequently lessens, the deviation becomes more equal, and a residual deviation remains. This is known as the "spread of comitancy." Optometric intervention can help prevent and relieve the problems of noncomitancy (diplopia, spatial localization problems, and contracture).

When diplopia is a significant problem, prism and occlusion often can restore fusion or eliminate the diplopic image. Occlusion will always eliminate diplopia. However, this technique must be used cautiously, as spatial localization is impaired when an eye muscle is paretic. When critical or dangerous tasks are done (for example, driving, cooking, or dangerous work), the eye with the paretic muscle should be occluded.

Sector occlusion on a spectacle lens can help prevent diplopia when fusion exists in certain fields of gaze (Figure 21–6). Alternate occlusion can help give both eyes as much action into the paretic field of gaze as possible.

Occlusion must be done in a manner consistent with attempts to prevent muscle contracture secondary to the paresis. Although it is doubtful whether any method of preventing secondary contracture is fully effective, preventive methods are important to try, and they can only help. The following optical techniques attempt to prevent contracture:

1. Conjugate prisms (bases in the same direction) may be worn. Both prisms are placed so that the eyes are forced to look in the direction of the field of the paretic muscle. This stimulates the paretic muscle and relaxes its antagonist.
2. A prism can be worn before the eye without the paretic muscle to force that eye into the field of gaze of the paretic muscle. This again attempts to relax the antagonist muscle and stimulate the paretic one.

Nonoptical methods of secondary contracture prevention are also possible. Medical techniques include anesthetic injection into the antagonist muscle, early recession surgery of the antagonist before contracture can develop, or both (O'Connor 1943).

Optometric techniques for the prevention of secondary contracture are primarily designed to force the paretic eye toward the field of action of the affected muscle. Monocular therapy is designed for each eye while the other is occluded. The sound eye exercises in the field of action of the paretic muscle to relax the antagonist muscle and stimulate the paretic one. To exercise the eye with the paretic muscle, systematized programs requiring accurate fixations farther and farther into the field of action of the paretic muscle are employed.

The following techniques can be used for monocular calisthenic therapy when there is a muscle paresis:

Figure 21-4

These exercises will develop good binocular vision while your eyes are diverging (turning outward) as if looking at distant objects. You will know you are using both eyes correctly in each procedure when the pictures viewed are seen as one, they are seen clearly, parts of the targets seen by each eye alone are present simultaneously, and depth is seen in certain cards.

Exercise a total of _____ minutes each day, and increase the number of procedures in each session as you can do them. In the beginning you might experience discomfort such as headaches and eyestrain, so that you may have to limit the exercises to a few minutes. As you ability improves, your discomfort will disappear, and the exercise time can be increased. Remember that exercising 15 minutes daily is better than exercising 2 hours once a week! It would be best if you did this exercise at _(insert times)_, and _____ each day. Try to establish a routine so that you always do the exercises at the same time each day.

Procedure 1: Place the instrument on a table at a comfortable height, with light falling evenly on the target cards. The double-aperture slider is placed at the position marked 1 or 2 on the front ruler. The target cards should be placed at the 0 position on the back ruler. The AP1 and AP2 cards are the targets for this procedure. To see the targets through the double aperture, place the tip of your nose against the end of the front ruler. If you are wearing a bifocal, tip you head back slightly, and place your lower lip against the ruler. Concentrate and actively try to fuse the targets at all times. Do not be discouraged if you are unsuccessful at first. Repeated efforts at looking at the targets and attempting fusion will lead to success.

Look through the double aperture at card AP1 (later, follow the same procedure with AP2). Close your left eye, and your right eye will see only one box with a black cross. Close your right eye, and your left eye will see only one box with a black ball. The ball is seen only by the left eye, and the cross is seen only by the right eye. If necessary to achieve this, move the aperture slider toward or away from you. Your eyes are now in this position:

The right eye sees the target on the right side of the card.

The left eye sees the target on the left side of the card.

Look with both eyes, and make the two targets into one target.

Correct Response: When you have made the two targets into one (fusion), you will see this:

One box with the cross and ball are seen simultaneously.

Note: If either the cross or the ball is seen alone, it means that although both your eyes are open, the visual information from one of your eyes is not being received (suppression). The result is that of closing one eye. One of your goals in this exercise is to become aware of the information from both eyes and unify it into one visual percept (sensory function). To do so, follow these steps:

1. Cover and uncover one eye, exposing both targets for brief periods while attempting fusion.
2. Blink your eyes rapidly, looking for fusion between blinks.

If you see two boxes instead of one, the visual information is being received, but your eyes are not aimed correctly. Your second goal is to diverge your eyes correctly so that sensory fusion can take place. To do so, look over the aperture slide across the room at a target. You should feel your eyes going outward. As you keep your eyes in an outward position, just notice the targets in the foreground. Now direct your attention to the targets. You should see them as one, and as you concentrate, the fused picture should clear. Repeat this procedure until you can maintain *one fused clear* target.

Patient Instructions: Home Vision Therapy—Double Aperture Rule Trainer

Figure 21-4 continued

Ask yourself these questions as you do each exercise, and be sure to tell the answers to your doctor when he evaluates your progress:
1. Can I feel both eyes moving when I look at the targets?
2. Can I see one fused target? If so, slowly or rapidly?
3. Is the target *clear*?
4. Do the suppression checks (the parts in the picture seen by only one eye) ever disappear?
5. Does the exercise get easier as I do it more often?

Procedure 2: Look from a distant target to the target card _____ times. Then look at the small letters on the aperture slide. Alternately, look at the three places (the distance target, the target card, and the small letters on the aperture slide) _____ times.

Correct Response: Your goals are smooth, accurate, and comfortable eye movements when looking at the targets together with fast fusion and no suppression. Each target you look at should be *clear*. It is very important that each target be clear before you look at the next one.

Procedure 3: Alternately fixate as in Procedure 2; in addition, pull your eyes in (converge) until the red and green circles (on the upper corner of the slide) are seen as one. Be sure to notice the suppression checks.
You should now be looking alternately at the following:
1. At the card.
2. At the small letters below the center bar between the aperture.
3. At a distance.
4. At the red and green circles (at the upper corners of the slide), making them into one.

Correct Responses: Your goals are smooth, accurate, and comfortable eye movements when looking at the targets, together with fast fusion and no suppression. The fused target always should be clear before you look at the next target.

Procedure 4: Look at cards AP3 to AP7, always moving the aperture slides to the position marked on the card. Fuse the targets, keeping the suppression checks (the circle and cross) present both on the soldier and at the larger circles. When you look at the large circles, note whether the inner circle looks behind or in front of the outer circle (depth perception). Close one eye, and see if the soldier or circles change in appearance. (Do they look flat or less real?) Then alternately fixate from distance, to the small letters, to the read and green circles, to the target card, and so forth as in Procedure 3.

Correct Responses: Your goals are smooth, accurate, and comfortable eye movements when looking at the targets, together with fast fusion and no suppression. The fused target should always be clear and seen with depth.

Procedure 5: Look at cards AP8 to AP12, always moving the aperture slider to the position marked on the card. Fuse the targets, keeping the suppression checks (the *X* and *Y*) present simultaneously. Be sure to be aware of the depth in the fused pictures, noting the relative position of all objects. Close one eye, and note the flattening of the pictures as compared with what is seen by both eyes. When you can fuse and clear the fused target, alternate fixations as in Procedures 3 and 4.

Correct Responses: Your goals are smooth, accurate, and comfortable eye movements when looking at the targets, together with fast fusion and no suppression. The fused target always should be clear and seen with depth.

Figure 21–5

These exercises will develop simultaneous perception from your two eyes when you are looking at a distance. You will know you are using both eyes when you can see the television clearly through both parts of the therapy device. Remember, your task is to see the whole television picture through both parts of the device at once.

Exercise a total of _____ minutes each day, and increase the number of procedures in each session as you can do them. In the beginning, one part of the television may be dark, or you may experience some discomfort; therefore, you may have to limit the exercises to a few minutes. As your ability improves, your discomfort will disappear, and the exercise time can be increased. Remember that exercising 15 minutes daily is better than exercising 2 hours once a week! It would be best if you did this exercise at _(insert times)_, and _____ each day. Try to establish a routine so that you always do the exercises at the same time each day.

Procedure 1: Attach the therapy device to the television set vertically with the suction cups:

If the device is red and green, put the red part on top. It is very important that the device be vertical; otherwise, the therapy may be ineffective. Put on the special glasses provided by the doctor. If the glasses are red and green, put the red lens over your right eye. If the glasses are not red and green, be very careful to watch the television with your head straight upright. Turn on the television, sit _____ feet away from it, and watch it.

Correct Response: Looking at the television, you will see the television through both parts of the therapy device at the same time.

Note: During this exercise, if one part of the therapy device is black (cannot be seen through), the visual information from one of your eyes is not being received (suppression). The result is like closing one eye. If first one part of the device is black and then the other is black, it is similar to alternately closing one eye and then the other. The visual information is still being received only from one eye at a time. Your goal in these exercises is to become aware of the visual information from both eyes simultaneously.

If you find that only one eye is being used (suppression), do the following to use both eyes:
   1. Blink your eyes rapidly, looking for the other eye's image between blinks.
   2. Cover one eye; then quickly remove the cover.
   3. Turn the room lights down or out.
   4. Do any or all of the above in combination.

Ask yourself these questions, and be sure to tell your answers to the doctor evaluating your progress:
   1. Does one part of the television therapy device ever go black? If so, when and how often?
   2. Does the black part of the therapy device jump from top to bottom and back?
   3. If both parts of the device are easy to see through, is the picture on the television clear or blurry?
   4. Does the exercise get easier as I do it more often?

Procedure 2: Repeat Procedure 1 at a different distance (about _____ feet). Always try to maintain the correct response: clear, easy viewing through both parts of the therapy device at the same time.

Procedure 3: As Procedure 2 becomes easy for you, move (closer) (farther) and continue trying to maintain the correct response.

Patient Instructions: Home Vision Therapy—Television Trainer

Figure 21-6

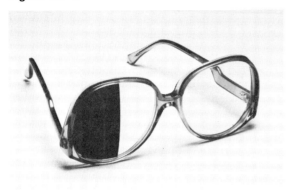

Spectacles with Temporal Occlusion

Sound Eye Fixing (gaze direction in field of action of paretic muscle):

1. *Watching television or related activity.* This is done with the eyes directed in the field of action of the paretic muscle.
2. *Walking.* This is done with the eyes directed toward the field of action of the paretic muscle.
3. *Balancing exercises.* These are done with the eyes directed toward the field of action of the paretic muscle.
4. *Tracing exercises.* Targets are traced toward the field of action of the paretic muscle.
5. *Prism ductions: large prism changes.* Prism vergence is done in large steps toward the field of action of the paretic muscle. The patient tries to maintain fixation farther each time.

Paretic Eye Fixing (gaze direction toward action of paretic muscle):

1. *Tracking a suspended moving ball.* The patient attempts to track a Marsden ball farther and farther into the field of action of the paretic muscle.
2. *Tracing exercises.*
3. *Batting or ringing a moving, suspended ball.* The patient attempts to keep a circular ring around a swinging Marsden ball as it swings toward the field of action of the paretic muscle.
4. *Prism ductions: small prism changes.* Prism vergence is done in small steps toward the field of action of the paretic muscle. The patient tries to maintain fixation farther each time.
5. *Repeating Step 4 while walking.*
6. *Rotating pegboard.* The patient tries to put golf tees in a rotating perforated disk. Gradually the disk is moved toward the field of action of the paretic muscle.

Fusion should be maintained as much as possible in all cases of noncomitancy. Sensory fusion usually was present before noncomitancy developed, so this type of training may not be needed in all fields of gaze.

Prism may be needed to restore fusion in the primary position. Sector prisms in Fresnel form can be used to give increasing fusion ability in the field of the paretic muscle. Prism power is determined empirically, and varying prism power can be used if noncomitancy is severe. Prism for fusion does not prevent secondary contracture.

Expansions of motor fusion ranges are indicated in practically all cases of muscle paresis. Motor fusion training is designed to give maximal fusion ability.

Vision therapy goals for patients with muscle paresis follow:

1. Maximally expand voluntary motor fusion ranges in the field of gaze *opposite* the paresis.
2. Develop reflex vergence in the primary position.
3. Expand fusional vergence training into the field of action of the paretic muscle.

Rehabilitative therapy is done in the manner indicated for the type of phoria present (see the section on therapy for comitant deviations). Therapy is similar for recent or long-standing noncomitant deviations. The progress of the therapy should be monitored according to the monocular field of view and binocular diplopia fields, which should increase as fusion and eye movement ability improve.

Prognosis

Vision therapy is an effective procedure that can improve binocularity in presbyopic patients. These patients are able to learn therapy procedures easily and often carry them out more faithfully than do younger patients. Thus, the tradition of reserving vision therapy primarily for children or young adults is not justified. Problems such as blurred vision, tired eyes, or headaches after reading that are associated with binocular problems can be helped for most patients of any age.

To establish the prognosis for success of vision therapy in the elderly, Wick (1977) studied records of presbyopic subjects (n = 161) who had undergone vision therapy for convergence problems (n = 134) or general skills problems (n = 27). The age range was 45 to 89. Patients all had normal acuity for their age. After appropriate refractive management, vision therapy was prescribed as needed. When vision therapy was needed, exophoric patients generally were successful with 6 weeks of therapy, and esophoric patients were successful in 6 to 8 weeks. Elderly patients generally carried out therapy procedures well, and home therapy was satisfactory for the majority. The conclusion of the study was that for binocular vision problems in the elderly that are treated with appropriate prism correction and vision therapy, symptoms are eliminated and test findings are restored to normal for the age and physical condition of the patient 92 percent (148 of 161) of the time. When the elimination of symptoms was the primary criteria, the success rate for therapy was 97 percent (156 of 161).

Approximately one-half of the patients who needed vision therapy remained asymptomatic after therapy was discontinued. In a 3-month follow-up to the study on vision therapy for patients with presbyopia, 47.8 percent (77 of 161) needed some additional therapy to remain asymptomatic. Generally, patients over age 70 needed to continue with a maintainance therapy program (68.8 percent, or 22 of 32). These patients needed to continue minimal home therapy weekly or biweekly, with yearly examinations to assess visual function (Wick 1977).

For elderly patients, just as for younger patients, exophoria responds better than esophoria to vision therapy alone. Vision therapy is generally the only necessary treatment for exodeviations. Esophoria, in contrast, often requires base-out prism management combined with vision therapy. Even when therapy causes symptoms to disappear, the magnitude of the heterophoria usually does not change. Patients more than 20Δ exophoric and 15Δ esophoric may have symptoms remaining after therapy. Surgery can provide additional relief for selected cases.

Elderly patients who develop noncomitancy frequently have partial or complete recovery of paretic muscle function. The recovery of muscle function depends on the nerve innervation, the muscle involved, and the cause of the noncomitancy (Rucker 1958). Overall rates of recovery of paretic muscle function based on the involved nerve are: 48.3 percent for the third nerve, 53.5 percent for the fourth nerve, and 49.6 percent for the sixth nerve. When the cause of noncomitancy is vascular, the chance of muscle function recovery is approximately 70 percent. Usually recovery is within 3 to 6 months. After that time, recovery of paretic muscle function is unlikely (Hugonnier and Hugonnier 1969). When contracture does not occur or can be prevented by functional therapy and muscle function recovers, normal binocularity is restored.

The prognosis for comfortable binocular visual function in noncomitancy using the best medical management combined with appropriate optometric intervention (lenses, prisms, patching, and vision therapy) is probably 70 to 80 percent. Visual function may not be "normal," but the patient should be comfortable with minimal diplopia.

Sensory Adaptation Training

Monocularity
Elderly people frequently become monocular because of disease or accident. They need advice in adapting to this condition. For example, when monocularity comes suddenly, there is a loss of depth judgment, particularly for distances within arm's reach. Teaching the patient to touch a plate to the table or a teapot spout to the cup will save much embarrassment and help prevent accidents. A description of monocular cues to depth – for example, size constancy, overlap, and perspective – and of proper head motion for increased parallax will help facilitate safer driving and parking.

Perceptual Rehabilitation
Declines in visual function with age can be attributed to a reduced ability to gather data (reduced saccades, version and vergence ability, visual acuity, and so on) and to a reduced ability to process the data gathered. Optometrists interested in the ability of children to process data gathered through vision and other senses have worked, through various types of visual/perceptual training, to increase abilities in this area.

Visual processing in the elderly significantly decreases when more complex processing tasks are attempted (Craik 1977) because of an age-related slowing of the rate of information processing (Welford 1964), different allocation of the resources that control visual function, or both (Hoyer and Plude 1980). Perceptual function in the aged can be evaluated by the following techniques:

- Copy forms (adult variety) and an additional three-dimensional form.
- Motor free visual perception test.

- Reading test.
- Pegboard test.
- Jordan right-left test.
- Identification test using objects and pictures.

Optometric visual perceptual therapy is used to enhance attention span, form discrimination, and auditory and visual memory in children. Similar procedures can be used to improve visual perceptual function in the aged. A sequenced therapy program using sensory-motor interaction enhances basic visual perceptual skills for the aged, as well as for children.

Aphakic Rehabilitation

Patients with cataracts already have experienced visual function decrease and often are apprehensive about the prospects of life without sight. The optometrist can provide much assurance about the outcomes of surgery. Working closely with the ophthalmic surgeon will enable the optometrist to advise the patient about what to expect from aphakia or pseudophakia. A careful explanation of the adaptation to and correction options in aphakia and the necessary spectacle correction (at least for near) in pseudophakia will help alleviate the fear and apprehension patients experience. Unfortunately, this necessary assurance sometimes is neglected in referrals back and forth between optometrist and surgeon.

Vision correction after surgery for cataracts presents some unique rehabilitative problems. First, visual acuity must be restored through the use of intraocular lens implants, contact lenses, or aphakic spectacle lenses, and each presents specific problems. Frequently, the patient must learn a new way of seeing because of that correction. Finally, convergence demand is increased by the surgery itself, especially for patients who do not have intraocular lens implants.

Aphakic spectacle lenses generally require the most comprehensive rehabilitative techniques. From a purely optical standpoint, an aphakic spectacle lens causes serious adaptive problems. The lenses magnify what is seen by over 25 percent, so objects appear larger and closer than they really are. Aphakic corrections significantly impair initial judgment of depth. The spherical aberration of high plus lenses causes pincushion distortion—lines seem to curve inward—and movement of the eyes behind a fixed spectacle lens causes objects to swim.

The highly magnified central visual field of aphakic spectacle lenses overlap a portion of the peripheral field and produce a characteristic ring scotoma. The stronger a lens in plus power, the worse the problem is. At intermediate distances (10 to 2 feet), the scotoma causes problems that are not easily overcome. Objects (people, chairs, and so on) pop in and out of the blind area, and patients see things they cannot turn their eyes to look at, bump into objects, and have trouble negotiating their environment. Visual field limitations of aphakic spectacle lenses are best solved by contact lens correction.

Coordinating hand and eye movements also becomes difficult when aphakic spectacles are first worn, so coordination for near tasks frequently is impaired. Small wooden puzzles, building block figures, and jigsaw puzzles can be used to help patients redevelop the spacial judgment needed for daily tasks. Aphakic adaptation therapy sessions attempt to redevelop the depth judgment and head and eye movements necessary for accurate hand/eye coordination.

Convergence Requirements. Convergence requirements are altered by cataract surgery. Removal of the crystalline lens of the eye shifts the normal visual angle temporalward by 2 to 3 degrees per eye. This shift causes an induced exophoria of 10 to 12Δ for distance and near, which must be overcome by fusional (disparity) vergence reserves. Postsurgically induced exophoria combined with the usually receded near point of convergence in the aged can cause binocular problems that interfere with the aphakic patient's ability to read comfortably or for very long.

Convergence demands of binocular aphakic spectacle correction are affected by the following:
1. Phoria (preexisting phoria combined with altered convergence demands that are due to the change in the visual angle resulting from lens removal).
2. Interpupillary distance.
3. Spectacle lens vertex distance.
4. Correcting lens strength (both distance and bifocal additions).

Convergence requirements increase slightly with each diopter of distance lens power increase (provided the vertex adjustment, near additions, and interpupillary distance remain constant). This amounts to approximately 1Δ of increased convergence demand for each diopter of distance correction. Increasing the bifocal addition causes dramatic increases in convergence demand.

Near work must be held closer to be clear, and the combined power of the distance lens and the bifocal increases vergence demand still more. Each diopter of increased bifocal addition power increases convergence demand about 12Δ. Each 2 mm increase in interpupillary distance increases convergence demands about 1Δ. Greater vertex distances increase convergence demand about 1Δ per millimeter of increase.

Increased bifocal addition power is the most significant cause of increased vergence demand with aphakic spectacle correction. In general, prescribing the closest spectacle lens vertex distance and the weakest addition possible will minimize problems of increased convergence demand with initial aphakic correction. Aphakic patients who need strong (+14.00 to +15.50D) or very strong (greater than +15.50D) spectacle lens corrections with wide interpupillary distances have very large demands on near convergence and are best corrected with contact lenses, especially when high (above +2.50D) near additions are needed.

Increased convergence demands with the spectacle correction of aphakia are treated with the rehabilitative therapy techniques previously described for near exophoria. These can be combined with puzzle tasks to enhance spacial awareness simultaneously. Rehabilitative therapy is generally successful in developing the convergence ability necessary for near tasks. Occasionally, prism segments or near reading corrections with base-in prisms are required for comfortable sustained near vision.

Difficulties in adapting to aphakic spectacle lenses are largely solved by contact lenses or pseudophakic correction. These corrections eliminate many of the size differences and spectacle lens distortions of aphakic spectacle lenses, thus causing significantly fewer adaptive problems. Increased convergence requirements after cataract surgery, however, are not eliminated by contact lens correction. Convergence therapy is still needed by many of these patients to obtain the best binocularity at near. Increased convergence requirements are reduced after intraocular lens implants, and convergence therapy is needed less frequently.

Intraocular Lens Implants. Intraocular lens implants after cataract surgery are becoming the rule rather than the exception. This solves the problem of spectacle adaptation for cataract patients but can cause new problems when sur-

gery initially is on only one eye: aniseikonia and anisometropia. The problem of aniseikonia also exists when contact lenses are used to correct monocular aphakia. Spectacle lens overcorrections, which are needed for clear vision at near, can be designed to minimize the problems of aniseikonia and anisometropia.

Aniseikonia and Anisometropia. Aniseikonia is a relative difference in the size, the shape, or both the size and shape of the ocular images. Clinically significant aniseikonia is aniseikonia that is greater than 0.75 percent associated with symptoms related to the use of the eyes (headaches, asthenopia, and spacial distortions) and that is not relieved by accurate refractive or motility correction (Bannon 1965).

Intraocular lens implants and contact lenses to correct the refractive error after cataract surgery reduce aniseikonia to a minimum in unilateral aphakia. Aniseikonia is not usually considered in spectacle overcorrection of unilateral pseudophakic patients. Lens correction is always needed—even if just a near addition—for clear near vision. After a lens implant there is an average ocular image size difference from 1.52 to 2.17 percent for various anterior chamber lenses (Choyce 1961; Troutman 1962). The image of the eye without the implant generally requires magnification. Contact lens correction of unilateral aphakia leaves approximately a 6 percent image size difference between the two eyes. A 2 to 6 percent image size difference still can cause symptoms.

The rehabilitation of aniseikonia after a unilateral lens implant or monocular contact lens correction of aphakia uses iseikonic lenses. Lens corrections are designed to equalize magnification as much as possible for the two eyes. Lenses are modified by making a thicker, steeper base curve lens for the eye requiring the magnification. If necessary, the opposite lens can be made thinner with a flatter base curve. Complete lens design techniques are available (Wick 1973).

Increasing anisometropia during cataract development and after unilateral implants can also lead to binocular vision problems. This rapidly developed anisometropia causes prismatic differences in all fields of gaze, but it especially causes problems upon downgaze. Rehabilitation uses lens corrections for reading only or slab-off prism when bifocal lenses are used. The amount of slab-off prism to be prescribed can be measured using fixation disparity tests. In general, the amount measured by fixation disparity can be prescribed and is almost always less than the amount expected based on calculated prismatic differences between the two lenses. When contact lens corrections are used for unilateral aphakic correction, the contact lens is prescribed so that there is isometropic (equal) spectacle lens overcorrection. In this way, the problem of anisometropia and slab-off prism can be avoided with contact lens correction.

Visual Field Defects

Visual field evaluations provide a functional assessment of the location, extent, and quality of the area of best vision (Bailey 1978). The location, density, size, and number of scotomas are significant in determining the visual care of the patient (Jose and Ferraro 1983). Recent field losses may be caused by life- or vision-threatening conditions, and patients with them should be referred to appropriate medical practitioners.

When central visual field defects affect visual acuity or patient fixation, the patient is best served by comprehensive low-vision evaluation. Some patients have binocular peripheral field loss. Careful analysis using the tangent screen, arc perimeter, and Amsler grid is indicated for optimal evaluation. When complex field loss (multiple scotomas, ring scotomas, peripheral islands of vision, and so on) is present, a low-vision evaluation should be done.

Partial monocular field loss is usually not a large problem, because the intact field of the other eye compensates adequately. Occasionally, in the presence of a high phoria, partial monocular field loss will cause fusion difficulty. Vergence training and prism corrections are indicated for these patients to give the best possible fusion ability and minimize diplopia.

When binocular congruous field loss is present, techniques such as partial mirrors, mirrors, or prisms can increase the patient's awareness of objects located in the blind area. Bilateral conjugate prisms (with bases in the same direction) will enable the patient to become more aware of objects in the scotomatous area. Although prism does not expand the visual field, without it the patient must make large head or eye movements toward the blind area to detect objects. Prism allows the use of small scanning eye movements to locate objects in the peripheral field. With the prism in place, the apparent position of objects is displaced toward the primary visual direction; they are then easier for the patient to

locate. Usually, visual acuity must be essentially normal for prism field enhancement; patients with reduced acuity need appropriate low-vision care.

A binocular mirror system also can be used for field defect rehabilitation (Goodlaw 1982). Semitransparent mirrors with a 30 percent reflectant coating on the ocular surface are used to allow use of the remaining nasal fields, and temporal fields are seen by reflection. However, the two fields are seen simultaneously, and the mirror device is somewhat cumbersome. Generally, prisms are cosmetically superior and probably easier to adapt to.

Monocular mirrors can expand peripheral awareness by blocking out the seeing field of one eye and projecting a superimposed field of the lost area. The mirror allows the user to monitor major changes occurring in the blind field. Images seen in the mirror move rapidly with head movement and are reversed. The patient must learn to suppress the mirror image for many tasks and only use it when needed. Large eye movements, hand movements, or both are needed to look at an object in the blind field. The success rate with mirrors is not very high (Bailey 1982) because of nausea or disorientation from the moving reversed mirror image.

Prism rehabilitation of visual field defects uses Fresnel prisms put on one sector of each spectacle lens. Prism power is chosen based on the lateral excursion of the patient's habitual eye movements. Larger eye movements allow prisms to be placed farther from the line of sight and lower powers to be used. Prism powers from 10 to 30Δ can be used, depending on the scanning area and the patient response. Initial prism power may have to be reduced as the patient's scanning ability improves.

Prisms are placed on the lenses where they will not interfere with primary gaze and normal eye movements. The patient should not be aware of the prisms during normal eye movements and should need to make only small scanning movements into the prisms to see objects in the blind field. Prisms usually are placed 1 mm or more away from the primary position of gaze (Jose and Smith 1976; Weiss 1972). They are placed on one lens at a time by occluding one eye and having the patient make eye movements into the blind field with the other eye while the prism is positioned. The leading edge of the prism is moved until the patient is just aware of the prism location. This procedure then is repeated for the other eye, and finally binocular adjustment is done so that both lines of sight simultaneously meet the prism edges. Generally, prisms must be used binocularly. When monocular prisms are used, patients may experience confusion when their gaze first encounters the prism and diplopia when looking further into the prism.

The necessity of using prisms is based on the location of the field loss. Right hemianopsias cause reading problems, because the patient has difficulty knowing where the next word is and often loses the line. Typoscopes, margin markers in books and reading slits help the patient improve tracking ability. Occasionally a patient is assisted by learning to read from right to left on an inverted book or by holding the book sideways and reading from the top down, thus avoiding reading into the scotomous areas. Rehabilitative techniques will assist patients in learning these techniques when they are necessary.

Left hemianopsias cause fewer problems. Reading ability (right saccades) is generally not impaired, but patients tend to lose their place on returning to the next line. A marker (a finger or other object placed at the start of the next line) usually solves the problem. Superior field losses cause some problems. Because vertical (upward) scanning is difficult, base-up conjugate prism (with bases in the same direction) seems to be superior when prisms are required (Jose and Ferrero 1983). Inferior field losses cause mobility problems and reading confusion when the patient tries to find the next line or scan a picture. Prism scanning aids are less successful than improving mobility with head movement, cane travel training, or both (Jose and Ferrero 1983).

Careful instruction and training can be valuable in the rehabilitation of visual field defects. Patients must be told that scanning eye movements into the prisms may cause initial confusion and that objects, usually invisible, will appear suddenly in front of them. Images are displaced from their actual position by an amount that depends on the distance of the object seen.

Visual and perceptual rehabilitative therapy can improve judgment of object distance and location. The patient is seated, and objects are brought from the blind field into the seeing field at various distances and speeds (a swinging Marsden ball and ring work well). The patient is trained to judge correct responses by "ringing" the ball as it moves. As improvement is shown, the same and more complex tasks are repeated

while the patient stands or walks. When mobility is substantially impaired, referral for mobility training can often greatly benefit the patient.

Patient Education, Monitoring, and Selection

The availability of the most expert techniques and the finest instrumentation do not insure the success of therapy. The patient must be educated to understand alternative therapy (lenses or prisms, vision therapy, or both), along with the scope and magnitude of the problem. Unless the patient can be properly motivated and fully understands the need for and the technique of the treatment being used, management will not succeed. Literature describing lens corrections, vision therapy, heterophoria, stroke, and so on is valuable in explaining therapy and reinforcing patient cooperation. The following are psychologically sound techniques of greatly increasing patient cooperation with therapy:

1. It is best to work well within the patient's limitations in order to give a feeling of success at each session.
2. Emphasis on positive results is preferable to a detailed explanation of any dire results that could occur if the therapy is not completed.
3. Rehabilitative vision therapy, like any other health routine, must be done regularly. Help the patient set a time of day that insures the therapy's completion. Instructions to do therapy techniques 15 minutes each day at 9 in the morning, noon, and 6 in the evening are superior to simple instructions to do these techniques 45 minutes every day.
4. Written instructions often are helpful. A daily checklist showing results also can be used in more difficult cases. Routine instruction sheets can be prepared for the patient to reinforce a careful, friendly, personal explanation by the doctor. A typical home therapy instruction sheet is shown in Figure 21–7.

Monitoring rehabilitative therapy is easy if the reasons for the therapy are kept in mind. It is important to question the patient about any decrease in symptoms, the amount of time spent in therapy, and the understanding of techniques. Therapy progress can be monitored objectively by repeating appropriate tests. Vergence ranges, the convergence near point, suppression tests, and forced vergence fixation disparity curves generally can be repeated as appropriate. As therapy progresses, vergence ranges expand, the near point of convergence improves, and suppres-

Figure 21-7
Your specific problems determine the frequency and type of vision therapy (orthoptics) needed to establish a good visual system. Doing orthoptics at the times prescribed is important if learning is to occur, and doing the orthoptics actively and with maximum concentration is equally important if progress is to be made. Remember, your cooperation and efforts at home will largely determine your success.

The following orthoptic program is designed to develop the visual skills needed for comfort and efficiency. When you can do these visual tasks correctly, you will possess visual abilities transferable to your everday seeing needs.

Exercise 1
1. Starting with Procedure ____, practice _____ times per day for _____ minutes.
2. When you are able to do all the procedures correctly, limit the exercise to Procedure ____, and practice _____ times per _____ for _____ minutes.

Exercise 2:
1. Starting with Procedure ____, practice _____ times per day for _____ minutes.
2. When you are able to do all the procedures correctly, limit the exercise to Procedure ____, and practice _____ times per _____ for _____ minutes.

Exercise 3:
1. Starting with Procedure ____, practice _____ times per day at _____, _____, and _____ for _____ minutes.

2. When you are able to do all the procedures correctly, limit the exercise to Procedure ____, and practice _____ times per day at _(insert times)_, and _____ for _____ minutes.

Patient Instructions for Home Vision Therapy

---

sion lessens. Forced vergence fixation disparity curves are especially helpful for monitoring near binocularity improvement of presbyopic patients. As binocularity improves, curves generally flatten; this indicates better compensation over a larger range of vergence changes.

Patients should be selected on an individual basis. Nearly all elderly patients can have some relief of symptoms related to faulty binocular vision when appropriate medical care is combined with subsequent optometric rehabilitative therapy as needed. Rehabilitative therapy consists of lenses and prisms combined with vision therapy to improve vergence ranges, eliminate suppression, reduce adverse adaptations after stroke, and improve motility in muscle weakness or restrictive syndromes.

When the patient is mentally capable of understanding instructions, therapy is generally successful in alleviating or reducing symptoms. As with all physical therapy, however, some patients are unwilling or unable to comply. These patients should be managed with lens or prism modification of the spectacle correction to give maximal symptom relief. Occasionally, patients have progressive problems that therapy can help only minimally. These patients need continued medical monitoring to be sure the condition is controlled maximally. Optometric rehabilitative therapy can be done concurrently to give the best possible relief of symptoms.

References

Bailey, I. L. "Visual Field Measurement in Low Vision." *Optometric Monthly* 69 (1978): 697–701.

Bailey, I. L. "Mirrors for Visual Field Defects." *Optometric Monthly* 73 (1982): 202–206.

Bannon, R. E. *Clinical Manual on Aniseikonia.* Buffalo, N.Y.: American Optical Co., 1965.

Borish, I. *Clinical Refraction.* 3rd ed. Chicago: Professional Press, 1970.

Carter, D. B. "Fixation Disparity and Heterophoria Following Prolonged Wearing of Prism." *American Journal of Optometry and Archives of American Academy of Optometry* 42 (1965): 144–152.

Choyce, D. P. "All-Acrylic Anterior Chamber Implants in Ophthalmic Surgery." *Lancet* 2 (July 22, 1961): 165–171.

Cohen, A. H., and R. Soden. "An Optometric Approach to the Rehabilitation of the Stroke Patient." *Journal of the American Optometric Association* 52 (1981): 795–800.

Cooper, J., and R. Duckman "Convergence Insufficiency: Incidence, Diagnosis, and Treatment." *Journal of the American Optometric Association* 49 (1978): 673–680.

Craik, F. I. M. "Age Differences in Human Memory." In *Handbook of the Psychology of Aging,* eds. J. E. Birren and K. W. Shaie. New York: Van Nostrand, 1977.

Eskridge, J. B. "Flip Prism Test for Vertical Phoria." *American Journal of Optometry and Archives of American Academy of Optometry* 38 (1961): 415–419.

Gibson, H. *Textbook of Orthoptics.* London: Hatton, 1955.

Goodlaw, E. "Rehabilitating a Patient with Bitemporal Hemianopia." *American Journal of Optometry and Physiological Optics* 59 (1982): 677–679.

Griffin, J. R. *Binocular Anomalies: Procedures for Vision Therapy.* Chicago: Professional Press, 1976.

Griffin, J. R., and J. M. Lee. "The Polaroid Mirror Method," *Optometric Weekly* 61, no. 40 (1970): 29.

Hamasaki, D.; J. Ong; E. Marg. "The Amplitude of Accommodation in Presbyopia." *American Journal of Optometry and Archives of American Academy of Optometry.* 33 (1956): 3–14.

Hirsch, M. J.; M. Alpern; H. L. Schultz. "The Variation of Phoria with Age." *American Journal of Optometry and Archives of American Academy of Optometry.* 25 (1948): 11.

Hirsch, M. J., and L. Bing. "The Effect of Testing Method on Values Obtained for Phorias at Forty Centimeters." *American Journal of Optometry and Archives of American Academy of Optometry* 25 (1948): 407–416.

Hofstetter, H. W. "A Comparison of Duane's and Donder's Tables of the Amplitude of Accommodation." *American Journal of Optometry and Archives of American Academy of Optometry* 21 (1944): 345–363.

Hofstetter, H. W. "A Longitudinal Study of Amplitude Changes in Presbyopia." *American Journal of Optometry and Archives of American Academy of Optometry* 42 (1965): 3–8.

Hoyer, W. J., and D. J. Plude. "Attentional and Perceptual Processes in the Study of Cognitive Aging." In *Aging in the 1980's: Psychological Issues,* ed. L. W. Poon. Washington, D.C.: American Psychological Association, 1980.

Hugonnier, R. and S. Hugonnier. *Strabismus, Heterophoria, Ocular Motor Paralysis.* Ed. and trans. Veronneau-Troutman. St. Louis: Mosby, 1969.

Jose, R. T., and J. Ferraro. "Functional Interpretation of the Visual Fields of Low Vision Patients." *Journal of the American Optometric Association* 54 (1983): 885–893.

Jose, R. T., and A. J. Smith. "Increasing Peripheral Field Awareness with Fresnel Prisms." *Optical Journal and Review of Optometry* 113 (1976): 33–37.

Maddox, E. E. *The Clinical Use of Prisms and the Decentering of Lenses.* Bristol, England: John Wright & Sons, 1893.

Morgan, M. W. "The Turville Infinity Binocular Balance Test." *American Journal of Optometry and Archives of American Academy of Optometry* 26 (1949): 231–239.

Morgan, M. W. "Accommodative Changes in Presbyopia and Their Correction." In *Vision of the Aging Patient,* eds. M. J. Hirsch and R. E. Wick. Philadelphia: Chilton, 1960, pp. 83–112.

O'Connor, R., "Contracture in Ocular-Muscle Paralysis." *American Journal of Ophthalmology* 26 (1943): 69.

Parks, M. M. "Isolated Cyclovertical Muscle Palsy." *Archives of Ophthalmology* 60 (1958):1027–1035.

Pitts, D. G. "The Effects of Aging on Selected Visual Functions: Dark Adaptation, Visual Acuity, Stereopsis, and Brightness Contrast." In *Aging and Human Visual Function,* eds. R. Sekuler, D. Kline, and K. Dismukes. New York: Alan R. Liss, 1982, pp. 131–159.

Rucker, C. W. "Paralysis of Third, Fourth, and Sixth Cranial Nerves." *American Journal of Ophthalmology* 46 (1958): 787.

Schor, C. "Analysis of Tonic and Accommodative Vergence Disorders of Binocular Vision." *American Journal of Optometry and Physiological Optics* 60 (1983): 1–14.

Schor, C. and K. J. Ciuffreda. *Vergence Eye Movements: Basic Clinical Aspects.* Boston: Butterworths, 1983.

Schor, C. and V. Narayan. "Graphical Analysis of Prism Adaptation, Convergence Accommodation and Accommodative Vergence." *American Journal of Optometry and Physiological Optics* 59 (1982): 774–784.

Sheedy, J. E. "Actual Measurement of Fixation Disparity and Its Use in Diagnosis and Treatment." *Journal of the American Optometric Association.* 51 (1980): 1079–1084.

Sheedy, J. E., and J. J. Saladin. "Exophoria at Near in Presbyopia." *American Journal of Optometry and Physiological Optics* 52 (1975): 474–481.

Sheedy, J. E., and J. J. Saladin. "Phoria, Vergence and Fixation Disparity in Oculomotor Problems." *American Journal of Optometry and Physiological Optics* 54 (1977): 474–478.

Troutman, R. C. "Artiphakia and Aniseikonia," *Transactions of the American Ophthalmological Society* 60 (1962): 590–658.

Vodnoy, B. E. *The Practice of Orthoptics and Related Topics.* 4th ed. South Bend, Ind · Bernell Corp., 1970.

Weiss, N. J. "An Application of Cemented Prisms with Severe Field Loss." *American Journal of Optometry and Physiological Optics* 49 (1972): 261–264.

Welford, A. T. "Experimental Psychology in the Study of Aging." *British Medical Bulletin* 20 (1964): 65–69.

Weymouth, F. W. "Effect of Age on Visual Acuity." In *Vision of the Aging Patient,* eds. M. J. Hirsch and R. E. Wick. Philadelphia: Chilton, 1960, pp. 37–62.

Wick, B. "Iseikonic Considerations for Today's Eyewear." *American Journal of Optometry and Archives of American Academy of Optometry* 50 (1973): 952–967.

Wick, B. "A Fresnel Prism Bar for Home Visual Therapy." *American Journal of Optometry and Archives of American Academy of Optometry* 51 (1974): 576–578.

Wick, B. "Vision Therapy for Presbyopes." *American Journal of Optometry and Physiological Optics* 54 (1977): 244–247.

Wick B., and R. London. "Effect of Vertical Fixation Disparity Correction on the Horizontal Forced Vergence Fixation Disparity Curve." *American Journal of Optometry and Physiological Optics.* Forthcoming.

Wick, R. E. "Management of the Aging Patient in Optometric Practice." In *Vision of the Aging Patient,* eds. M. J. Hirsch and R. E. Wick. Philadelphia: Chilton, 1960, pp. 214–240.

Winter, J. "Striated Lenses and Filters in Strabismus." *Optometric Weekly* (June 10, 1971): 531–534.

Chapter 22

Care of the Visually Impaired Elderly Patient

Alfred A. Rosenbloom, Jr.

Between 1970 and 1980 the U.S. population aged 60 and over grew by about 18 percent, while the total population expanded by only 9 percent. According to the 1980 census information, life expectancy at birth is now over 73 years of age, and people living to age 65 can expect to live for an average of 16 more years (National Council on the Aging 1982).

Today's greater life expectancy is accompanied by a higher incidence of ocular and degenerative disorders. According to Kirchner and Peterson (1979), nearly 25 percent of the elderly population, or over 6 million U.S. citizens, have some form of visual impairment. Statistical projection to the year 2000 suggests that the 1977 National Council for Health Statistics (NCHS) survey population of severely visually impaired individuals over age 65 will double (Kirchner 1985). The vast majority of these individuals can be helped with a comprehensive low-vision care program and appropriately prescribed low-vision aids.

There are also demographic and psychosocial dimensions to the burgeoning population of elderly people. Women and nonwhites have the highest incidence of severe visual disabilities. Furthermore, approximately two-thirds of visually impaired older people have at least one other impairment, such as orthopedic impediments, paralysis, or hearing loss. Older people in the United States are demanding that more attention be paid to the quality and comprehensiveness of their health care. Serving these needs is truly a continuing challenge. This chapter considers four aspects of the problem: I. Contemporary aspects of low-vision and aging as frames of reference; II. Effective optometric care for the elderly; III. Essential clinical skills and understandings; IV. New directions in elderly patient care.

I. Contemporary Aspects of Low-Vision Care

The Elderly in Western Society

In the future health care providers will serve a greatly increased number of people in the 70- to 90-year age range. Recent data show that approximately 21 percent of the U.S. population is 55 or over; 15 percent is 60 or over, and 12 percent is 65 or over (45 million, 33 million, and 24 million people, respectively). The number of people over age 65 is growing at twice the rate of the general population. People in this age group represent one of every eight U.S. citizens and head one of every five households. Those over 75 are in the fastest growing group of all.

Contrary to popular opinion, the majority of older people in the United States live independent lives (Population Resource Center 1981):

- Only 5 percent over age 65 are institutionalized.
- Nearly three-quarters aged 65 to 74 are home owners.
- In the 65 to 74 age group, 62.6 percent are living with a spouse; 24 percent live alone, and most of these are women.
- One-half of all women over 75 live alone.
- Two-thirds of all households are headed by people over age 55.

In other developed countries the elderly population makes up an even larger proportion of the whole.

The incidence of visual impairment increases markedly among the elderly. Robbins' (1981) survey of patients examined at the Low Vision Clinic, Kooyong, Melbourne, Australia, indicated that patients aged 80 or more make up about 35 percent of the patient population. Within this group, those aged 80 to 89 years represent the modal group, a distribution that closely follows that given by Sorsby (1972) for the United Kingdom and for Wales alone. This finding has particular clinical relevance, since in the aging U.S. population two-thirds of the low-vision population is already over the age of 60.

Aging

Aging describes physiological and related changes in a person's life from maturity to death, including adjustment to the total environment. It is a continuous and highly individualized process, especially in the area of health. Each person adjusts to old age differently. The optometrist's role is to understand the effects of aging in dealing with vision rehabilitation.

The impact of vision loss is rarely felt in isolation from the other losses associated with growing older. No two people experience visual loss or the changing self-perceptions associated with aging in the same way. The impact of visual impairment, however, is felt more keenly because of other problems associated with aging (for example, physical and physiological changes; economic limitations; loss of social independence; and altered roles in the family, work place, and community) (Weg 1982).

The Jarvik (1975) longitudinal study of a random sample of elderly people suggests that those who engage in cognitive, emotive, and physical activities on a regular basis throughout adulthood age more successfully than those who are relatively inactive. Activities of later life, rather than those of earlier years, are primarily related to successful aging.

The goal of optometrists in relation to elderly patients with impaired vision, therefore, is to help them live happy and useful lives and enjoy self-sufficiency, emotional independence, and satisfactory social interactions. Too often the practitioner's goals are aimed at physical well-being, and social and psychological aspects are not given the emphasis they deserve.

II. Effective Optometric Care for the Elderly

The optometrist should adhere to five key principles for geriatric patient care, regardless of the nature of the patient's disease, disability, or impairment:

1. Distinguish *aging* from *disease*.
2. See the patient as a *whole person* focusing on health status, ability, psychosocial well-being, and socioeconomic needs.
3. Use a *team approach;* employ support resources from the family; community ser-

vices; health care and rehabilitation; social service counseling; and occupational therapy, including environmental support services.
4. Emphasize the *goals* of geriatric patient care. These include prevention, preservation, restoration, and maintenance leading to the enrichment of quality of life.
5. Improve the patient's *quality of life* by facilitating independence and goal-directed activity.

Effective optometric service involves the art and science of patient care. Patients have become discontent, critical, and hostile as the art of health care gradually becomes separated from the science of health care (Remen 1980). They are increasingly disenchanted with a specialized high technology health care system that frequently treats "health problems" rather than human needs (Grayson, Nugent, and Oken 1977; McKay 1980). The practitioner must view patients as individuals with special needs and abilities. To overlook this diminishes the doctor-patient relationship.

Since health problems in the elderly tend to be complex, effective communication between patient and health provider is essential. Indeed, older adults share with everyone the dual needs for self-importance and social acceptance. Physical limitations often cause older adults to feel isolated. Deficits in hearing and vision may interfere directly with communication. The optometrist should understand the psychological stress that accompanies aging, including loneliness, a sense of uselessness, and anxiety over increasing dependency and impending death.

The care of elderly patients should be effective, humane, and tailored to the limitations and priorities of each individual. In addition to obtaining information essential to a correct diagnosis and treatment plan, the optometrist should assess the cognitive and psychological states of elderly patients, their ability to carry out activities of daily living, and their socioeconomic needs. The practitioner must be sensitive to the patient's psychological set; the patient's expressed and perceived needs; the collection of clinical data; and an agreed-upon plan of action paced to the individual's needs, understanding, and motivation.

Psychological and Functional Effects of Low Vision

Ocular and degenerative disorders tend to increase in incidence and severity among elderly persons. For a complete discussion of these changes, see Chapters 9 and 11.

Many "normal" aging changes are exacerbated for the low-vision patient (Lederer 1982). To understand the visual performance characteristics of low-vision patients, it is necessary to differentiate between optical and neural effects (Lubinas 1980). For example, a patient with an optically reduced visual loss resulting from irregularities in the refractive surfaces or media usually suffers from a degradation of the visual image. This deficit results from excessive intra ocular scatter, which causes lower visual acuity and reduced contrast sensitivity. This patient has greater difficulty with resolution tasks, and as the angular extent of scatter broadens, resolution capacity and performance suffer.

In some patients visual acuity may remain unaffected, but contrast sensitivity of all objects within the visual field is diminished. Marron and Bailey (1982) showed that loss of contrast sensitivity and loss of visual field were approximately equally important contributions to impaired mobility because of decreased vision. They also showed that visual acuity was a relatively poor predictor of mobility performance. Research results by Cunningham and Johnston (1980) suggest that the detection of low-contrast objects (such as steps, pavement, and textures) is critical for pedestrian mobility. Jos Verbaken (personal correspondence 1982), of the Department of Optometry, University of Melbourne, measured the contrast threshold for a luminous edge profile using a photographic plate technique in 349 consecutive clinic patients with normal acuity. The data showed that the edge contrast threshold is constant between the ages of 5 and 49 and declines steadily thereafter. For the 80 to 89 age group, the contrast threshold was twice as great as in the younger age group.

With increased intraocular scatter and absorption of light by the media, higher than normal luminance levels are necessary. If the individual's environment includes poorly designed light fittings, dimly lit passageways, shadows surrounding objects, and impairments such as disability glare, performance difficulties are increased.

Regardless of their etiologies, losses involving structures within the neural pathway are most commonly expressed as visual field defects. Central field losses typically affect low-vision patients with a reduction in visual acuity. These losses may be complicated by metamorphopsia, poor tolerance to variation in luminance, dependence on high luminance levels, lowered contrast sensitivity, and poor mobility despite an intact peripheral visual field. The size and extent of scotomas limit sensitivity of the retina, as only objects of sufficient size, illuminance, or contrast will be recognized within these areas. If these scotomas are numerous, the correct localization and subsequent evaluation of visual information may become so difficult that some patients, despite relatively good visual acuity, are unable to read with any efficiency even when using magnification. This effect may be likened to the crowding phenomenon, in which letters can be seen but not interpreted by some amblyopic patients.

Although not as common as central field losses, peripheral field losses are important within the low-vision population. Mobility and the ability to detect environmental hazards are hindered when poor dark adaptation makes patients dependent on high light levels. The fact that older people require higher levels of illumination to meet their visual needs is well established, but frequently overlooked. The role of the practitioner in the assessment of the response of older patients to illumination levels and the appropriate standards for domestic lighting are described by Lovie-Kitchin and Bowman (1985) and Merz (1982).

Psychological Set

In addition to physical conditions and aging changes, a patient's performance is influenced by the attitude of the practitioner. Sinick (1976) notes that professional personnel in service settings may fail to realize the presence of prejudice despite their commitment to a professional service role. In so doing, they may become condescending, overprotective, and insensitive to the basic needs of elderly people. Members of the rehabilitation team must confront their own attitudes toward visually impaired people to render the most effective services.

In caring for the elderly, professionals must make very clear that an elderly person's well-being is as important as that of younger individuals. A reduced life span is no basis for making compromises in the scope or quality of health care services.

A recent World Health Organization (1981) meeting noted that the identification of the elderly as the most vulnerable group for visual impairment has important implications for health planning. A number of reasons explain why the elderly may be relatively neglected in the provision of services:

- They accept the gradual loss of vision and fail to seek appropriate help.
- A number of elderly patients cannot effectively communicate their needs and may be reluctant to seek professional help.
- Elderly patients are assumed to be less readily rehabilitated than more youthful patients.
- Professionals may believe they are examining patients too late in the disease process to permit optimal treatment and prevent disability.

Barraga and Morris (1980) report that many elderly patients resist learning to see because they fear their inability to live up to visual expectations, fear becoming more independent and possibly losing the care and emotional support of family and friends, and lack a desire to invest extra time and effort in the process. These authors also suggest that motivation may decline because patients do not understand that low-vision aids only improve blurred or distorted visual images rather than provide or restore vision. Elderly patients also often do not understand that visual performance may vary from day to day. Other patients have high expectations and unbridled hopes. Mehr (1974, 49) notes: "Before prescribing, the patient must be ready and eager for help, *not* seeking restoration of his former vision without limitations. For the patient playing "yes, but" or preferring dependency to increased visual abilities, a program of masterful inactivity is preferable to an expensive aid." In making a decision about an appropriate therapeutic plan for the low-vision patient, the optometrist must consider the psychosocial factors influencing the patient's readiness.

The visually impaired person may face inadequacy in all daily activities, such as dressing, grooming, personal hygiene, eating, telling time, caring for clothes and personal effects—virtually every facet of daily life. He or she may need to relearn many routines. Social insecurities and communication difficulties are experienced, independence may be reduced, and self-esteem affected.

Thus, the cognitive and psychological states of elderly patients, their ability to perform daily activities, and their socioeconomic frameworks should be clinically assessed. The services available to assist patients in maintaining their independence should be established. To the extent that the practitioner can develop understandings about, and sensitivities to, the realities of being and growing old, he or she will enhance the quality of the interpersonal relationship with the patient.

III. Essential Clinical Skills and Understandings

Five aspects of providing optometric care for the aged visually impaired person include the case history interview, low-vision examination and functional assessment, therapeutic approaches (appropriate low-vision designs and accessory aids), low-vision patient management, and patient education and compliance.

Case History Interview

The success of the rehabilitation process depends on the quality and scope of the case history. The history for elderly patients should establish their specific needs or desires, their ability to adapt to new situations, their motivation to learn new visual habits, and their understanding of the uses and limitations of the visual aids. If an elderly patient lives with sighted family members, efforts may be directed toward finding aids that allow participation in normal family activities (for example, television, card playing, sewing, and games). If the patient lives alone, more attention may be focused on functional tasks, such as reading mail and identifying labels on medicine bottles and canned goods (Rosenbloom 1982). Other important case history information includes ocular and health history, visual capabilities at distance and near, illumination requirements, life-style history, present and previous interests, travel abilities, education and reading interests, vocational and avocational activities and goals, and familiarity with rehabilitation services.

The patient should be the primary source of information in gathering the case history; if doubt arises as to accuracy, other sources such as family or friends should be consulted. To compile a complete case history, multiple sessions may be needed to minimize patient fatigue.

Key questions for the case history interview include the following:

- What is the duration of the visual impairment?
- What is the ophthalmologic diagnosis, treatment, and prognosis?

- What is the state of the patient's general health?
- What drugs or medications are being taken, and for what purposes?
- Do any other health or psychosocial factors impair the patient's life-style?
- What is the patient's present level of visual functioning?
- Are there preferred light levels? Is there sensitivity to glare?
- What are the patient's principal vocational, recreational, and daily living activities?
- Are orientation and mobility impaired? Can the patient travel independently and successfully?
- What are the patient's primary visual needs and expectations?
- Is reading an important activity? If so, reading of what type and purpose?
- Are any aids or appliances being used?
- What is the patient's life-style? Is he or she living with others or alone?
- Is there psychological readiness and motivation for visual rehabilitation?

This information is useful not only for in-office questioning by the practitioner, but also in a pre-examination interview by telephone or by a low-vision assistant in the office.

Low-Vision Examination and Functional Assessment

Flexibility and readiness to alter standard procedures are necessary to secure the most accurate and reliable findings. The visual examination must be adapted to the special needs and requirements of the patient. Environmental setting, test distance (usually 10 feet or less), and surrounding illumination are important considerations. Use of the trial frame (including clips for overrefraction), trial lenses, and printed test charts add accuracy, flexibility, and improved patient control. Bailey and Lovie–Kitchin (1976) note that the examiner may wish to predict how much change in working distance, dioptric power of an addition, or magnification is required to enable the patient to read a certain size print; they recommend using a chart with unrelated words arranged in a logarithmic size progression.

Much of the examination procedure follows a conventional pattern: determination of visual acuities at far and at near; internal and external ocular health examination; tonometry and slit lamp biomicroscopy; ophthalmometry; determi-

nation of central and peripheral visual fields, including use of the Amsler grid; and distance and near point subjective testing with low-vision and accessory aids suited to the needs and capabilities of the patient.

Functional assessment requires a full understanding of the patient's needs and the complex interaction of factors that influence the perceptual response. These factors include the acuity level required for tasks at various working distances; luminance; figure-ground and contrast differences; and contour interaction relationships involving size and style of type, spacing, and print quality. It is important to realize that magnification alone may not improve function in terms of daily activities, orientation, and mobility in the environment. Visual performance is poorly correlated with visual acuity. Accurate refractive technique is of utmost importance, as is the prescription of proper light levels for the patient's various environments. The goal of the low-vision practitioner should be to improve function by whatever means to enhance quality of life for the patient.

When possible, previously acquired skills must be reactivated by the practitioner's continuing encouragement, guidance, patience, and empathy. Techniques for achieving accurate clinical findings and their evaluation are described in Chapter 14.

Therapeutic Approaches (Appropriate Low-Vision Designs and Accessory Aids)

Low-vision aids most valuable to elderly patients include hand and stand magnifiers, compact telescopic systems for spot checking, high plus reading additions in bifocal or single vision designs, microscopic types of reading lenses, closed-circuit television systems, and various nonoptical or accessory aids.

Which aid or aids to prescribe depends not only on the optometric evaluation derived from the case history and examination findings, but also on the evaluation and interpretation of the functional field of vision. According to Faye (1984), the visual field is the single most important factor affecting visual function. Faye identifies three types of field defects that can influence the practitioner's decision on therapeutic correction: no demonstrable field loss, functional field loss involving retinal disease marked by central or paracentral scotomas, and peripheral field loss.

No Demonstrable Field Loss. Typically, patients with no demonstrable field loss complain of blurred vision or an image poorly resolved centrally, haze, or a sensation of glare. The evaluation of visual performance depends on the type and size of test objects, contrast, illumination levels, pupil size, and figure-ground interaction.

Therapeutic approaches to a blurred or poorly resolved image include telescopic devices, which help some patients retain their ability to read street, bus, and directional signs and avoid obstructions in travel. For such short-term spotting tasks, hand-held monocular telescopes from 2.5 to 10× are available.

Stand magnifiers are often used by patients with hand tremors, by those with aphakia where added magnification for reading is needed, and as a supplemental correction for the occasional reading of small print.

Most informational display signs can be identified with 20/70 vision under suitable illumination. Patients with diffusely blurred vision need telescopes with good light-gathering properties—often a prism monocular with the largest field. For reading, high addition spectacles, hand or stand magnifiers, or telemicroscopes should be prescribed according to near reading acuity.

Functional Field Loss Involving Retinal Disease Marked by Central or Paracentral Scotomas. Faye (1976, 217) notes the common denominators of macular disease to be visible pathology by ophthalmoscopy, central or paracentral field defects of varying density, decreased central acuity, and central scotoma. Peripheral field functions remain relatively normal. Visual complaints vary from lack of clear vision, recognition of faces, and disappearance of parts of words, to search difficulties in travel vision.

The specific design of the low-vision aid depends on the patient's level of visual acuity, preference and adaptability, and requirements for daily living. In descending order of frequency, the aids commonly prescribed for elderly patients are single vision or bifocal spectacles, hand and stand magnifiers (2 to 9× power), hand-held and spectacle-mounted telescopes (2.5 to 8×), telemicroscopic units, and closed-circuit television. Stand magnifiers are often used by patients with hand tremors, by those with aphakia where added magnification combined with the bifocal power is needed for reading and as a supplemental correction for the occasional reading of small print.

Peripheral Field Loss. The most potentially disabling form of functional vision impairment is peripheral field loss. Magnification may not help those with peripheral field loss, and many patients adopt techniques in traveling and reading that prove more effective than low-vision aids. The practitioner must also differentiate between overall contraction of the visual field and sector or hemianopic losses.

Patients with irregular scotomatous patterns often have unpredictable near vision responses. They may identify isolated letters more easily than words, and they may use eccentric viewing and angling of reading materials. An accurate assessment and interpretation of the central and peripheral visual fields should be performed before low-vision aids or a rehabilitation program is considered.

High addition spectacles may be ineffective as low-vision aids because of the close distance they impose. Telemicroscopes alleviate the working distance difficulties, but the field of vision becomes small. Patients should participate in selecting the best compromise.

Low-powered hand and stand magnifiers can increase the working distance and allow the patient to adapt to a preferred image size. Patients with small central or paracentral fields may prefer closed-circuit television because of the flexible reading distance and the improved ease and speed in reading, as well as the illumination and contrast controls. Accessory aids for mobility and orientation should be considered. Light control is especially important.

For patients with sector or hemianopic field defects, trials should be conducted with prisms of varying power and position. Mirrors have been used with some success by patients with homonymous hemianopias. Prisms also can enhance mobility and scanning, but their success with the elderly tends to be limited. With elderly people the success rate with all these techniques is relatively low and depends on patient motivation and adaptability. Adaptive training by the orientation and mobility specialist is most desirable.

Accessory or Nonoptical Aids. Accessory or nonoptical aids take many forms. These include large-print materials, matte black cardboard reading slits (typoscopes) to improve contrast, reading stands, adequate illumination, fiber-tipped pens, and visors to control light intensity and glare. Talking Books should be recommended where there are limited or unsuccessful trials with optical aids; this is especially appropriate if reading is an important part of a patient's life-style. Other technological advances include text-to-speech synthesizers, large-print computers, and image intensifiers.

Accessory or nonoptical aids should be considered to reduce glare and heighten contrast and illumination. Patients can control outdoor glare by wearing hats with wide brims; visors that attach to the eyeglass frame; and absorptive lenses that reduce ultraviolet and infrared radiation as do NOIR and Corning photochromic lenses.

Disability glare presents a special challenge in the diagnosis and management of the elderly patient. Robert Jacobs and Nasoha Saabin (personal correspondence 1982) of the Department of Optometry, University of Melbourne, indicate that elderly patients with cortical cataracts are so sensitive to disability glare that many are housebound at night. Contrast threshold or contrast sensitivity functions of these patients can be essentially normal in low photopic luminance (about 30 footcandles), but thresholds for high and medium spatial frequency targets are drastically reduced in the presence of any bright glare source. Because these patients often have 20/20 acuity, their problems can be overlooked by the examiner who does not specifically ask about night vision or glare problems during the case history. These patients can be helped with advice on lighting design to reduce luminance levels and restore contrast. Also generally recommended are clear antireflective coatings, side and sun shields, and a cardboard reading mask of the appropriate length and width (typoscope) to reduce glare from the surrounding field and improve contrast. Large-print materials, marking pens, heavily lined writing paper, and reading lamps and stands are a few of the many available aids.

The use of nonoptical or accessory aids is especially important because contrast sensitivity is generally lessened in low-vision patients. Cullinin (1978) identifies the importance and effects of poor lighting control: "Among those surveyed who had recently been seen at specialist's clinic, over 60% apparently saw worse at home than they did at the time of examination." Poor lighting in the home is virtually a universal problem.

A loan system for aids that allows a patient to become accustomed gradually to the effects of greater magnification may be appropriate.

This process requires reassessment, supervision, and counseling on a continuing basis as frustrations and new needs emerge. The loan program is sometimes more important than the low-vision aid itself.

Home visits by the assistant or allied professional should be considered. Questions about patient compliance and problems of illumination and contrast in the home can often be resolved by on-site assessment. Hazards such as loose mats and worn electrical fixtures can be detected and remedied.

Various patterns of reinforcement or encouragement are needed to keep the patient's enthusiasm and motivation high. Adaptive training should be flexible and emphasize the most effective use of residual vision. Since comprehensive low-vision care is time consuming, help from an understanding, experienced low-vision assistant is desirable. This frees the professional examiner for procedures necessitating special skills and knowledge.

Low-Vision Patient Management

The management of adaptive problems in the low-vision patient requires more than the prescription of aids. Proper management frequently requires painstaking instruction and supervised training to create and sustain motivation for visual tasks along with the use of training materials and activities chosen according to the patient's interests.

Barraga and Morris (1980) offer some helpful thoughts:

- Focus on how the remaining vision can be used effectively.
- Teach the individual to rely on visual memory for the performance of tasks.
- Assist the patient in making interpretations and decisions (based on visual imagery) using less immediate visual information.
- Emphasize visual tasks previously performed by the individual or those chosen for learning.
- Remember that adaptation to less efficient functioning is slow and far more difficult than learning to perform tasks for the first time.
- Use different patterns of reinforcement to keep enthusiasm and motivation high. Work with the entire family.

Depending on the clinical setting and the needs of the patient, the practitioner should make appropriate referrals. In some cases multidisciplinary care is unnecessary; in others, however, services should be coordinated. Where the services of several specialists are required, one member of the team must take responsibility for identifying needs and coordinating services. Establishing constructive relationships with the health care and social service agencies is essential. Because of changing social and family structures, the elderly patient must often seek other support systems. Social service agencies, senior citizen support groups, and religious and service organizations are available in the community for health care and social support (Jacobs 1984). The practitioner should furnish the patient and the patient's family with a list of resources in the community that will provide needed services. Periodic follow-up increases the patient's compliance and success.

The optometrist must be able to look behind the traditional stereotypes and focus on the special needs of each individual. These needs include independence and individuality, physical health and mobility, self-respect, dignity, and privacy. Good health and mobility, in turn, depend on the satisfaction of diverse subsidiary needs such as adequate services to compensate for loss of vision and hearing; a proper nutritional standard; adequate dental care; the maintenance of personal and household standards of cleanliness; and quality, accessible health service (Brearley 1978).

All professionals and paraprofessionals involved in the care of the elderly low-vision patient should assist in the process of rehabilitation, which can be thought of as a transition from dependence to independence, and finally to interdependence. This transition can be typified by some commonly encountered phrases. The statement "Of course, I can't read; you will have to do it for me" typifies dependence. Independence can be expressed by "I will try to read this myself" but this also can be a stubborn and self-defeating experience leading to "This print is just too small. No, you can't help me—I didn't want to read it anyway." Ideally, independence should lead to the ultimate state of interdependence: "I can read this section, but these words are too difficult. Could you help me, please?" This state of rehabilitation recognizes abilities and limitations and graciously requests and accepts assistance. This process requires time, and the patient will fluctuate between stages. The optometrist should seek an understanding of the

patient's present state.

Patient Education and Compliance

For the elderly patient unaccustomed to, or overwhelmed by, the diversified maze of the health care system, the optometrist can develop a trusting relationship of support and encouragement. In contrast to the traditional model of health care, low-vision rehabilitation should be oriented to the person rather than the disease. Such an approach establishes an ongoing, personal relationship with the patient. At the same time that this humanistic approach to health care is rightly desirable for the general population, it is critical for the elderly and will greatly enhance the patient compliance essential for successful low-vision rehabilitation.

There are few studies of patient compliance in optometry and medicine that specifically concern the elderly. Libow and Sherman (1981) found that for elderly patients who had medication prescribed, 50 percent deviated from the prescribed regimen, and 70 percent did not comprehend the regimen. Errors in medication and self-medication have accounted for 25 to 95 percent of the noncompliance problem (Gabriel, Gagnon, and Bryon 1977). Compliance difficulties are increased for the elderly for a variety of reasons. Explanations are given too rapidly or poorly, and written instructions are lacking. Environmental hazards such as weather conditions, transportation, or fear of crime deter patients from keeping appointments. Patients have trouble receiving or retaining instructions due to visual and hearing problems, or from loss of short-term memory. They are sometimes unable to open child-resistant medication containers and are confused about regimens with multiple medications (Ernst 1981).

In a study using experimental and control groups, Talkington (1978) found that four factors significantly increased patient compliance (from 53 to 73 percent):

1. Good rapport and communication between the patient and health provider.
2. Effective interaction whereby the patient's concerns were understood and expectations were met.
3. Patient understanding of the health problem, causes, treatment regimen, expected outcome of treatment, and consequences of noncompliance.
4. Patient participation in planning the treatment regimen, including the identification,

analysis, and solution of problems that might interfere with compliance.

The practitioner must stress that directions for medication dosages must be followed exactly. Some elderly believe that if one drop or one pill will help, then double the requirement will be doubly beneficial.

The optometrist must explain the low-vision aid or aids (their purpose, use, and limitations); the adaptive training program and its goals; environmental variables, especially lighting; and the importance of continuing follow-up. Informational reinforcement can consist of handouts, demonstrations, discussions, and audiovisual aids; handouts are especially useful as a continuing reminder. Vivian and Robertson (1980; cited in Glazer-Waldman, 1983, 249) developed guidelines for patient education that consider word choice, sentence length, and typography to maximize patient comprehension. They also suggest testing the education materials on a sample population before putting them into general use.

The optometrist must pace the instructions according to the learning ability of the patient. The response rate and reaction time of the elderly are slower, but not because of lack of motivation. Rushing the elderly patient may result in frustration and reduced motivation. Fear of failure, frustration, and confusion can be reduced by simplifying the environment and the tasks demanded of the elderly person. Presentation of material both in amount and content should be planned so that it reduces the patient's potential for failure and increases his opportunity for success.

The optometrist must realize that every low-vision problem is unique, and that individual differences increase with age. A slowing of motor functioning is not automatically equated with decreased learning ability; when older people can pace their own learning, studies show no significant age-related differences in ability. Diversity, rather than homogeneity, is the norm.

To ensure patient participation, the practitioner must provide sufficient opportunity for practice, repetition, and feedback about performance. Adaptive training must emphasize positive reinforcement for correct responses or procedures and re-training for incorrect ones. Evaluation involves assessment of the patient's progress at periodic intervals. An elderly person's sense of security, control, and orientation to the environment can be heightened with a set schedule of appointments at similar times, as well as the use of methods such as telephone inquiries or letter questionnaires. In all cases, rehabilitative success depends on the practitioner's ability to work together with the patient to realize attainable goals.

IV. New Directions in Elderly Patient Care

The focus for the future must be toward *research* and *development*. There is a need for greater scope and depth in basic and applied research on aging. Relevant topics range from basic biological knowledge to the design of better health care delivery systems, including diagnostic and therapeutic approaches to visual-perceptual problems of aging people.

Today, emerging findings from reliable clinical studies make research in low vision care of the elderly an exciting field of inquiry. New technological developments and the broader approach to patient management through involvement of allied health professionals adds to the research mandate to expand the boundaries of knowledge about health, disease, and sensory impairment during old age. The ultimate goal is optimum care of visually impaired elderly persons. This can be achieved by a synthesis of information from studies of normal aging and studies of disease in the elderly, yielding a data base that allows quantification of and differentiation between the effects attributed to age and those attributed to disease.

Assessment of Visual Performance

There is a need for greater research into visual performance. Topics include perceptual problems and adaptations; focusing, landmark spotting, and pursuit fixations involving movements of head, eyes, and body; adaptation to changing environmental conditions; optimal light levels indoors and outdoors; color cues; and figure-ground relationships.

Research should continue in the various conditions that cause loss of vision to allow the development of new procedures for alleviating their effects.

Studies of aging people who maintain good vision in spite of debilitating disease are also needed. Such studies might identify factors that offer preventive approaches to selected ocular diseases.

New techniques in the assessment of visual performance are needed, with improved correlation between clinical measurements of visual function and visual skills related to a person's life-style. This entails new instruments capable of measuring visual functions to understand the visual processes involved in everyday living.

There needs to be a greater understanding of the activity levels and interests of the elderly and their implications to behavior patterns of those with impaired vision. Such knowledge would enable the low-vision team to set realistic goals for rehabilitation.

The process by which elderly patients relearn skills necessary for the successful use of residual vision is poorly understood, and soundly based techniques must be developed for extensive re-adaptation. This involves perceptual relearning, the use of eccentric fixation, and methods of expanding the functional field of view.

The outcome of these and related studies may result in the development of a battery of tests used by the practitioner to create a profile of visual function for each visually impaired patient. A multidisciplinary approach would be necessary to consider the patient's overall ability to perform common visually related tasks in everyday life. This data could then be used to predict life-style improvements with the use of specific low-vision aids.

Therapeutic Approaches

New low-vision aids must be designed for wider application, versatility, and patient acceptance. The technical challenge is to optimize optical design parameters in order to combine magnification with distortion-free fields of view.

New accessory aids are required for varied levels of patient disabilities and handicaps. These may involve microprocessor technology, speech synthesis and recognition, and artificial intelligence. Closed-circuit television or similar display systems should be highly portable and gain additional technical features as supporting technology develops. Efforts should continue toward integrating large-character displays with computer and word-processing systems.

Lighting techniques must be examined in relation to intensity, spectral characteristics, heat properties, contrast, and the type of luminaires in various environments. Further objective and subjective evaluation is necessary to determine optimal lighting according to a person's near visual acuity, working distance, ocular disease type, and reading position to enhance patient comfort and visual efficiency.

Approaches to the Delivery of Low Vision Patient Care

Another major focus must be on the education and preparation of the health professional for the delivery of care to elderly visually impaired people. Since there is a positive correlation between knowledge and attitudes, professional educators should consider planning strategies to impart knowledge about the aging process and about the health care and social problems of the elderly early in school curricula. Training in gerontology should be undertaken at both professional school and the postgraduate levels (Rosenbloom 1982). A health care professional who understands the social, psychological, and economic aspects of aging can prevent exacerbations of illness, achieve patient cooperation with treatment programs, and interact more effectively with patients and their families.

A needs assessment study should be undertaken to determine the number and types of professionals needed to adequately serve the growing population of older blind and visually impaired people

Various alternative models of low-vision care delivery should be developed. Such models should delineate the total needs of the patient. The integration of the practitioner into a team is a necessary part of this planning; the nature of the interaction will depend on the health care delivery mode—be it clinic, private or group practice, hospital, or domiciliary patient care.

Pioneer and current rehabilitation programs for the elderly blind and visually impaired should be analyzed and their relative merits evaluated in terms of basic concepts, standards, and principles. Innovative approaches, such as mobile units to provide low-vision care for the rural elderly, represent another health care delivery need of increasing significance.

Multidisciplinary teamwork is especially important when caring for elderly patients. Delegates at the World Health Organization (1981) conference in Copenhagen emphasized the value of developing one or more comprehensive multidisciplinary centers that encompass patient care, planning, interdisciplinary research, and personnel training. These centers would be responsible for ameliorating the disability (but not necessarily prevent the disease), as well as for diagnosis, treatment, and rehabilitation. They should be staffed by specialists in the basic clinical, social, and public health sciences, bioengineering, and other technical disciplines.

In agency service, a need exists for in-service training of new staff to ensure a comprehensive approach to patient care. The actions of the low-vision team must dovetail the programs of care to ensure successful rehabilitation. Feedback from patients is needed to evaluate the quality and adequacy of the services offered, for the most important member of any team is the low-vision patient.

A delivery system should be developed that is economically viable; disseminates new information and techniques; trains appropriate personnel; and provides grass roots care, specialized assessment, and ongoing support structures. Vision care should be continually evaluated at both the patient and the clinic levels to ensure cost-effective and relevant service delivery. This assumes that goals and objectives have been considered carefully and are realistic, given the limits of resources in personnel and money. Finally, patient care within the community should avoid unnecessary duplication.

Professional services for the low-vision patient have progressed a long way in the last 30 years since the first low-vision clinic was opened in the United States, and they still have a long way to go. New research, advanced technology, and multidisciplinary expertise will enhance our ability to meet important human needs.

The optometrist must realize that every low-vision patient is different and unique. There is not only technical expertise in rendering effective low vision rehabilitation but also a personal and humane component. Perhaps the optometrist's greatest service lies in encouraging the visually impaired older person to become independent in every way possible and to learn as quickly as is practical the new skills needed to be once again a contributing member of society. The extent to which this is possible depends significantly on the optometrist's ability to help foster the patient's aspirations, self-confidence, and potential to realize attainable goals. It is a challenge worthy of our best efforts.

References

Bailey, I., and J. Lovie-Kitchin. "New Design Principles for Visual Acuity Letter Charts." *American Journal of Optometry and Physiological Optics.* 53 (1976): 740.

Barraga, N., and J. Morris. *Program to Develop Efficiency in Visual Functioning.* Louisville: American Printing House for the Blind, 1980.

Brearley, P. "Aging and Social Work." In *The Social Challenge of Aging,* ed. D. Hobman. London: Croom Helm, 1978, p. 180.

Cullinin, T. "Low Vision in Elderly People: Light for Low Vision." Proceedings of a Symposium. London: University College, April 1978.

Cunningham, P., and A. Johnston. "Edge Detection: A New Test of Visual Function." Paper presented at the ANZAAS Jubilee Conference, Adelaide, Australia, May 1980.

Ernst, N., ed. *Pharmaceutical Interventions and the Aged.* Dallas: University of Texas Health Science Center, 1981.

Faye, E. *Clinical Low Vision.* Boston: Little, Brown, 1976.

Faye, E. "The Effect of the Eye Condition on Functional Vision." In *Clinical Low Vision,* 2d ed., ed. E. Faye. Boston: Little, Brown, 1984, pp. 172–189.

Gabriel, M.; J. Gagnon; and C. Bryon. "Improving Patient Compliance through the Use of a Daily Drug Reminder Chart." *American Journal of Public Health* 67 (1977): 968.

Glazer-Waldman, H. "Patient Education." In *The Aged Patient: A Sourcebook for the Allied Health Professional,* eds. N. Ernst and H. Glazer-Waldman. Chicago: Year Book Medical, 1983, chap. 14.

Grayson, M; C. Nugent; and S. Oken. "A Systematic and Comprehensive Approach to Teaching and Evaluating Interpersonal Skills." *Journal of Medical Education* 52 (1977): 906–913.

Hobman, D., ed. "The Social Challenge of Aging." In *Aging and Social Work.* London: Croom Helm, 1978, p. 181.

Jacobs, P. "The Older Visually Impaired Person: A Vital Link in the Family and the Community." *Journal of Visual Impairment and Blindness* 78, no. 4 (1984): 154–162.

Jarvik, L. "Thoughts on the Psychobiology of Aging." *American Psychologist,* May 1975, 578.

Kirchner, C. and R. Peterson. "The Latest Data on Visual Disability from NCHS." *Journal of Visual Impairment and Blindness* 74 (1980): 42–44.

Kirchner, C. and R. Peterson. "The Latest Data on Visual Disability from NCHS." *Journal of Visual Impairment and Blindness* 73, no. 4 (1979): 151–153.

Kirchner, C. *Data on Blindness and Visual Impairment in the U. S.* New York: American Foundation for the Blind, 1985.

Lederer, J. "Geriatric Optometry." *Australian Journal of Optometry* 65, no. 4 (1982): 141–143.

Libow, L, and F. Sherman. *The Core of Geriatric Medicine.* St. Louis: Mosby, 1981.

Lovie-Kitchin, J.; K. Bowman; and E. Farmer. "Technical Note: Domestic Lighting Requirements for the Elderly." *Australian Journal of Optometry* 66 (1983): 93–97.

Lovie-Kitchin, J., and K. Bowman. *Senile Macular Degeneration: Management and Rehabilitation.* Woburn, Mass.: Butterworth, 1985.

Lubinas, J. "Understanding the Low Vision Patient." *Australian Journal of Optometry* 63, no. 5 (1980): 227–231.

Marron, A., and I. Bailey. "Visual Factors and Orientation-Mobility Performance." *American Journal of Optometry and Physiological Optics* 59, no. 5 (1982): 413–426.

McKay, S. "Wholistic Health Care: Challenge to Health Providers." *Journal of Allied Health* 9 (1980): 194–201.

Mehr, E. "Psychological Factors in Low Vision Care." In *A Guide to the Care of Low Vision Patients,* ed. J. Newman. St. Louis: American Optometric Association, 1974, p. 49.

Merz, B. "Lighting in Homes: A Study of Quantity and Quality." *Lighting in Australia* 2, no. 4 (1982): 26–28.

National Council on the Aging. *Aging in North America: Projection and Policies.* Washington, DC: National Council on the Aging, 1982.

Padula, W. "Low Vision Related to Function and Service Delivery for the Elderly." *Aging and Human Visual Function,* eds. R. Sekuler, et al. New York: Allan R. Liss, 1982, p. 315.

Population Resource Center, *Technology Adaptation and the Aging.* New York: Population Resource Center, 1981.

Remen, N. *The Human Patient.* New York: Doubleday, 1980.

Robbins, H. "Low Vision Care for the Over 80s." *Australian Journal of Optometry* 64, no. 6 (1981): 243–251.

Rosenbloom, A. "Care of the Elderly People with Low Vision." *Journal of Visual Impairment and Blindness* 76, no. 6 (1982): 209–212.

Rosenbloom, A. "Optometry and Gerontology." *Optometric Monthly* 73, no. 3 (1982): 143–144.

Sinick, D. "Counseling Older Persons: Career Change and Retirement." *Vocational Guidance Quarterly* 25, no. 1 (1976): 18–24.

Sorsby, A. *The Incidence and Causes of Blindness in England and Wales 1963–1968.* Reports on Public Health and Medical Subjects no. 128. London: Her Majesty's Stationery Office, 1972.

Talkington, D. "Maximizing Patient Compliance by Shaping Attitudes of Self-Directed Health Care." *Journal of Family Practice* 6 (1978): 591–595.

Vivian, A., and E. Robertson. "Readability of Patient Education Materials." *Clinical Therapy* 3 (1980): 129–136.

Weg, R. "The Image and Reality of 'Old': Time for a Change." *Journal of the American Optometric Association* 53, no. 1 (1982): 26–27.

World Health Organization. *The Use of Residual Vision by Visually Disabled Persons: Report on a WHO Meeting.* Euro Reports and Studies No. 41. Geneva: WHO, 1981.

American Foundation for th Blind, 1984.

Sekuler, R., D. Kline, and K. Dismukes. *Aging and Human Visual Function.* New York: Allan R. Liss, 1982.

Simonson, W. *Medications and the Elderly: A Guide for Promoting Proper Use.* Rockville, Md.: Aspen Systems, 1984.

Sloan, L. *Reading Aids for the Partially Sighted.* Baltimore: Williams and Wilkins, 1977.

Steinberg, F. U., ed. *Care of the Geriatric Patient.* 6th ed. St. Louis: Mosby, 1983.

Weale, R. A. *The Aging Eye.* London: H. K. Lewis, 1963.

Weale, R. A. *A Biography of the Eye: Development, Growth, Age.* London: H. K. Lewis, 1982.

Suggested Readings

Atchley, R. C. *Aging: Continuity and Change.* Belmont, Calif.: Wadsworth Publishing, 1983.

Conrad, K. A., and R. Bressler. *Drug Therapy for the Elderly.* St. Louis: Mosby, 1982.

Covington, T. R., and J. Walker. *Current Geriatric Therapy.* Philadelphia: Saunders, 1984.

Ernst, N. S., and H. R. Glazer-Waldman. *The Aged Patient: A Sourcebook for the Allied Health Professional.* Chicago: Year Book Medical, 1983.

Genensky, S. M.; S. H. Berry; T. H. Bikson; and T. K. Bikson. "Visual Environmental Adaptation Problems of the Partially Sighted: Final Report." HEW RSA Grant 14-P-57997, 1979. Santa Monica, Calif.: Center for Partially Sighted, Santa Monica Hospital Center, 1979.

Mehr, E. B., and A. N. Freid. *Low Vision Care.* Chicago: Professional Press, 1975.

Morgan, M. W. *The Optics of Ophthalmic Lenses.* Chicago: Professional Press, 1978.

O'Hara-Devereaux, M.; L. H. Andrus; and C. D. Scott, eds. *Eldercare: A Practical Guide to Clinical Geriatrics.* New York: Grune and Stratton, 1981.

Rosenbloom, A. A. "Low Vision." In *Principles and Practice of Ophthalmology,* eds. G. Peyman, D. Sanders, and M. Goldberg. Philadelphia: Saunders, 1980, pp. 241–277.

Ross, M. A. *Fitness for the Aging Adult with Visual Impairment: An Exercise and Resource Manual.* New York:

Chapter 23

Low-Vision Care in a Clinical Setting

Samuel M. Genensky
Steven H. Zarit

Definition of Terms

To insure good communication and a clear understanding of terms, the authors have carefully defined the visual groupings or subsets referred to in this chapter. No claim is made as to the merit of these definitions relative to alternatives offered by other researchers. However, these definitions are rational, self-consistent, and operational:

Fully sighted. People are fully sighted if they are not visually impaired.

Functionally blind. People are functionally blind if they are either totally blind or if they have, at most, light projection.

Legally blind. People are legally blind if the best-corrected visual acuity in their better eye does not exceed 20/200 or if the maximum diameter of their visual field does not exceed 20 degrees, even though the best-corrected visual acuity in their better eye exceeds 20/200.

Light perception. People have light perception if, with their better eye, they can only see light but are unable to determine the direction from which it is coming.

Light projection. People have light projection if, with their better eye, they can only see light and can determine the direction from which it is coming.

Partially sighted. People are partially sighted if the best-corrected visual acuity in their better eye does not exceed 20/70 but is better than light projection, or if the maximum diameter of their visual field does not exceed 30 degrees, even though the best-corrected visual acuity in their better eye exceeds 20/70.

Partially sighted and legally blind. People are partially sighted and legally blind if they are legally blind but not functionally blind.

Partially sighted and not legally blind. People are partially sighted and not legally blind if they are visually impaired but not legally blind.

Totally blind. People are totally blind if they cannot visually detect light with either eye.

Visual enhancement devices. Various visual aids permit partially sighted people to perform tasks that otherwise would be beyond their visual capability or that they could handle only with great difficulty. Examples of visual enhancement devices are telescopic spectacles that permit partially sighted people to view objects at a distance, microscopic spectacles that allow them to view objects at very close range, and closed circuit television systems that permit them to read ordinary ink-printed material, write with a pen or pencil, and carry on other tasks that require precise eye-hand coordination.

Visual enhancement techniques. Visual enhancement techniques may or may not involve the use of visual aids, but they permit partially sighted people to handle one or more tasks using their residual vision (for example, pouring dark-colored liquids into light-colored glasses in order to be able to distinguish more clearly the surface of the liquids in the glasses and hence avoid underfilling or overfilling those containers).

Visual substitution devices. Visual substitution devices call for the use of one or more senses other than sight (for example, talking watches or calculators, or the Opticon, a device that employs an electro-optical probe to scan printed material letter by letter and presents a raised image of each scanned letter to an index finger resting on a cradle or in a slot).

Visual substitution techniques. Visual substitution techniques require the use of one or more senses other than sight (for example, the nonvisual procedures that are needed to properly use a cane or dial a telephone without viewing the dial).

Visually impaired. People are visually impaired if they are either functionally blind or partially sighted.

The Population

Since this book is primarily concerned with older people, the reader undoubtedly will be interested in the population breakdown for individuals who are at least 65 years old. Table 23–1 gives estimates of the partially sighted, partially sighted but not legally blind, legally blind, legally blind but not functionally blind, and functionally blind populations in the United States for 1980. It also shows estimates of the age distribution for each of these populations.

These estimates were made by first using (1) information obtained by the National Institute for Neurological Diseases and Blindness (NINDB) and by its successor, the National Eye Institute (NEI), in the course of a 1962–1971 population data collection and analysis study known as the Model Reporting Area (MRA) study and (2) estimates of the 1970 legally blind, as well as partially sighted and not legally blind, populations made by a committee of the National Academies of Sciences and Engineering. Subsequently, the change in age distribution that occurred in the United States population from 1966 to 1980 was accounted for.

From Table 23–1 we see that 1,044,500, or 53.7

percent, of the partially sighted population is estimated to be at least 65 years old. Likewise, 837,200, or 53.7 percent, of the partially sighted but not legally blind population is in that age range; 263,200, or 51.7 percent, of the legally blind population; 207,200, or 53.7 percent, of the legally blind but not functionally blind population; and 56,000, or 45.5 percent, of the functionally blind population.

There is a very large difference between the number of people at least 65 years old who are legally blind but not functionally blind and those who are functionally blind. This difference can be explained in part by the fact that, with the exception of diabetic retinopathy, the other three major causes of severe visual loss among older people rarely lead to functional blindness either because of the inherent nature of the ocular pathology or because surgical and medical techniques exist that in most cases either check the progession toward functional blindness or, with the help of appropriate visual aids, nearly restore lost eyesight.

Common Visual Disorders in the Older Population

An erroneous myth prevails that individuals who are both partially sighted and legally blind should learn vision substitution methods and techniques to cope with daily needs, because eventually most of them will become totally blind or will at best be left with only light perception or light projection. Fortunately, as the

Table 23–1
Summary of National Data on Various Components of the Visually Impaired Population, 1980

Age	PS	PS-LB	LB	LB-FB	FB
0–4	5,500	4,400	1,800	1,100	700
5–19	123,800	99,300	37,500	24,600	12,900
20–44	328,500	263,300	89,700	65,200	24,500
45–64	444,000	355,900	117,200	88,100	29,100
65–74	338,900	271,600	87,400	67,200	20,200
75–84	371,400	297,700	93,100	73,700	19,400
85 +	334,200	267,900	82,700	66,300	16,400
Total	1,946,300	1,560,100	509,400	386,200	123,200

Note: PS = partially sighted; PS-LB = partially sighted but not legally blind; LB = legally blind; LB-FB = legally blind but not functionally blind; and FB = functionally blind.

previous section pointed out, medical evidence clearly indicates that most people who are both partially sighted and legally blind will continue to retain vision that is better than functional blindness throughout the remainder of their lives and hence, in most cases, will continue to benefit from visual enhancement techniques and devices. A recent study (Genensky 1978) has shown that even under the most pessimistic assumptions concerning the visual future of people who are both partially sighted and legally blind, a partially sighted child aged 5 would have less than 12 chances in 100 of becoming functionally blind before age 65. If the data were available to permit the use of more realistic assumptions, it is probable that the chances of the child's becoming functionally blind over the 60-year span would turn out to be less than 5 in 100. The probability of an older partially sighted and legally blind individual's losing total sight is very likely greater than that for a child, but it is still small enough not to invalidate the assertion previously made concerning the likelihood of a partially sighted person's becoming functionally blind.

The four most commonly encountered visual pathologies that afflict older people are macular degeneration, diabetic retinopathy, glaucoma, and cataracts. They account for more than 75 percent of severe visual impairment among older people in the United States. For a description of these eye diseases, see Chapter 11. This section concerns these four major causes of visual loss as they bear on the visual care of the low-vision patient.

Macular Degeneration. Macular degeneration patients tend to respond well, visually speaking, to a variety of visual aids that can help them see details up close, as well as far away. As is the case with other partially sighted people, the acceptance of visual aids depends heavily upon patient motivation, self-image, and the presence or absence of other sensory disorders and/or physical or mental disorders.

Diabetic Retinopathy. There are two major forms of diabetic retinopathy: *background retinopathy* and *proliferative retinopathy*. All retinopathy begins as background retinopathy, and most patients do not develop the proliferative type. People with proliferative retinopathy make up between 3 and 10 percent of all diabetics. Individuals with proliferative retinopathy often

encounter large, sometimes reversible fluctuations in the quality of their eyesight. One day they may be seeing well enough to drive a car or at least take a walk by themselves, and the next day they may be functionally blind (sometimes temporarily and sometimes permanently). Although individuals with proliferative retinopathy usually retain valuable eyesight over many years, some individuals suffer significant non-reversible losses rather suddenly. Vision care professionals should help these people use all their remaining eyesight as long as they have it. However, such people also should be advised to acquaint themselves with various visual substitution techniques and devices so that should they become irreversibly functionally blind, they will have useful information about what can be done for them and what they can do for themselves.

Partially because of the potential effects of diabetes itself and partly because of the fluctuations in vision, people with diabetic retinopathy, as well as members of their immediate families, frequently benefit from counseling. In addition, diabetics often find participation in patient support groups very beneficial.

Glaucoma. Glaucoma patients frequently have difficulty seeing at night and are bothered by glare during both the day and night. Impairment of night vision usually is due to partial loss of rod, or peripheral, vision. Furthermore, in the early stages of the disease, many people with glaucoma have good central vision, even though an examination of their visual fields indicates that they have substantial scotomas in an annular or partially annular region about the macula.

Cataracts. Some ophthalmologists hesitate to remove a cataract if the patient is severely visually impaired by way of macular degeneration in the affected eye, even if the patient has no other ocular diseases. They argue that (1) the removal of the cataract will not restore the patient's vision; (2) the patient will very likely remain legally blind; and, hence, (3) cataract surgery is contraindicated. We believe that this argument is sometimes fallacious. For example, in some instances the cataract is very dense and either pervades a large portion of the lens or obscures a critical portion of it. If this is the case and if the patient has no other ocular or systemic disorders that make surgery inadvisable, it appears reasonable to seriously consider removing the cataractous lens. New low-vision techniques and visual aids frequently will permit the patient who has undergone successful cataract surgery and who has macular degeneration to advance from functional blindness to partial sightedness and to make better use of the remaining eyesight.

Philosophy of Low-Vision Care at The Center for the Partially Sighted

One example of a low-vision care facility providing comprehensive rehabilitation services is The Center for the Partially Sighted in Santa Monica, California. The Center, established in 1978, has demonstrated that it is possible to provide partially sighted people of all ages with a set of services that are tailored to meet their special needs and that permit them to use all their remaining sensory capabilities, including their residual vision, to gain, regain, or maintain their visual independence.

At The Center, the needs of each patient are assessed, and a determination is made as to which of the following services might prove beneficial to the patient: low-vision optometric care; psychological counseling; orientation and mobility instruction; and direction to educational, vocational, social, and recreational services not offered at The Center. All services are given on an out-patient basis. Every attempt is made to help patients understand the difference between partial sightedness and functional blindness; the value of residual vision and how that vision can be used to perform tasks that are important to the patient; how all sensory capabilities, including residual vision, can be used to enter, reenter, or remain within the framework of fully sighted society. This program provides partially sighted people with visual aids and teaches independent living skills that can reduce their medium- and long-range dependence on scarce tax dollars.

Low-Vision Optometric Care

A low-vision optometric examination differs from a general ophthalmological examination in that it concentrates on determining what patients can do with their remaining eyesight rather than on determining the nature and extent of patients' ocular pathologies and how best to treat them medically or surgically.

Low-vision optometric examinations should be designed to determine the patients' functional visual capability. Based on the results of these examinations and information gleaned from

patients concerning their objectives and significant vision-related environmental problems, optometrists should determine which visual aids, if any, will help the patients perform one or more of these problematic tasks with comparative ease. Before purchasing these aids, patients should be encouraged to borrow and work with one or more appropriate loaner aids. A loaner program permits patients to try the aids in their home or work environments and enables them to make more informed decisions about which aids to purchase for long-term use. Patients should be trained in the use of the aids, including the loaner aids, before they take them home. Thorough training is essential for patients to use visual aids effectively and avoid the aids' being relegated to the bureau drawer.

About four to six months after the initial low-vision examination, a follow-up visit should be made to patients at their home or work place by, for example, a case coordinator, social worker, or orientation and mobility instructor. These visits enable staff members to determine how the patients are getting on with the aids prescribed for their use and to ascertain whether a recheck or additional visual aids training is necessary. At this time, these professionals also can look for inexpensive modifications that would make the visited environment safer or more visually comfortable.

Psychological Aspects of Aging and Low Vision

To successfully work with older patients with low vision, the clinician needs technical skills, such as those for the measurement of remaining vision or prescribing appropriate visual aids. However, the difference between a good or poor outcome will depend on the interactions between the patient and clinician. Under the best of circumstances patients can be difficult, but especially following the loss of vision they may be irritable, contrary, or distractible, or they may not even hear what the clinician has to say. Some patients will not accept the clinician's conclusions about their condition, or they may reject the visual aids or other assistance offered. In the face of all evidence, they even may maintain that all they need is a new pair of glasses to correct for the vision loss.

Many older people approach low-vision services enthusiastically and learn to use aids quickly and effectively. However, some present complex problems in psychosocial adaptation, even when their vision loss is not severe. On the one hand, clinicians who expect that patients will be rational or will do what is best for them will be continually frustrated in low-vision work. On the other hand, there are effective ways of interacting with many difficult patients to increase their positive response to optometric services. Just as the eye care specialist relies on the scientific foundations of practice, there are appropriate procedures for managing interactions, the practitioner can increase the numbers of people who can benefit from low-vision optometric services.

To work effectively with older patients, optometrists experienced in low-vision practice must be able to evaluate the possible causes of a poor response to services and what remedies can be tried. One potential cause is the effects of aging on behavioral capacity to respond. A second area, which applies to patients of any age, involves problems in compliance with treatment. These two areas will be reviewed, and the program of psychological services at The Center for the Partially Sighted, which has been developed to address these concerns, will be described.

Psychological Changes with Age

The most central question in dealing with older patients is the extent to which aging can be expected to interfere with successful adaptation to a vision loss. The predominant belief is that aging is associated with decline, and there are certainly people who have suffered irreversible physical and mental declines that interfere with their response to low-vision services. However, the course of aging is highly variable. Some older people function at or near levels typical of the young, whereas others experience only mild, relatively benign psychological changes. Major decrements in functioning typically result from illnesses rather than aging per se. Nonetheless, many people confuse the effects of age and illness and view all older people as having major psychological impairments.

An example of the way old age and disease are confused is senile dementia. Senility involving severe decrements of memory and personality is considered by many people to be synonymous with old age. However, only 5 to 7 percent of people over age 65 have the type of progressive mental deterioration that could properly be termed *senile*. Furthermore, senile dementia is brought about by degenerative diseases of the brain, the most common being Alzheimer's dis-

ease and multiinfarct dementia (see Chapter 5). Just as older people are more prone to other chronic and degenerative conditions, the prevalence of dementia increases at advanced ages, but it is not a universal part of the aging process.

Individuals with senile dementia will be recognizable by their extreme forgetfulness. The dementia patient literally may be unable to remember from one minute to the next. This is different from the average older person, who— like anyone else—will forget occasionally. A person who is anxious or depressed may be more distractible, and it is important not to mistake his or her forgetfulness for the more permanent, persistent type found in dementia.

Working with dementia patients usually involves enlisting the cooperation of family members or other people involved in their care. Because of their extreme forgetfulness, the patients need to be reminded to follow any procedures the clinician might recommend. Furthermore, problems they have with reading may involve comprehension as well as vision. Although the gains dementia patients can make from low-vision services are small, it is worthwhile at least to evaluate their response to visual aids.

In the absense of the catastrophic decrements caused by an illness creating dementia, the psychological changes associated with aging are relatively mild. Some practical suggestions can help the practitioner adjust for age-related differences in three areas of functioning: (1) learning and memory, (2) cautiousness, and (3) hearing. The older person generally will need more time to learn new information, especially when it is novel or unusual. When information is given at too fast a pace, learning can be seriously disrupted. Distractions also may interfere with learning to a greater extent for older people than for younger ones. Problems in learning often are magnified by hearing and vision losses. Once information is learned, however, the older person will remember effectively—perhaps as well as when younger (Botwinick 1978; Craik 1977). Steps the clinician can take to enhance learning include pacing the presentation of information or instructions more slowly, cutting down distractions, and writing or typing instructions so the patient can review them later.

Another dimension of behavior with practical relevance is cautiousness. In general, older people have been found to make more cautious responses in a number of situations. For instance, they are less likely to guess when taking tests, even when they are fairly sure they know the answer (Botwinick 1978). This reluctance to guess carries over to other situations. In an auditory examination, for example, older people failed to report hearing tones that were faint but had previously been determined to be within their range of hearing (Rees and Botwinick 1971). As a result, they gave the impression of having far more hearing loss than was actually present. Cautiousness may have a similar effect on the vision examination. Encouraging older patients to guess can overcome this inhibition.

Hearing loss is fairly common among older people and may be a major reason for communication problems (Corso 1977). The hearing-impaired person can, at times, be mistaken as senile or confused, although with proper methods of communication the effects of the hearing loss can be minimized. Some ways of working with patients with hearing loss include speaking slowly, distinctly, and in complete sentences; using a room with good acoustics; and eliminating background noises. It is not necessary to shout to be heard. Although many hearing-impaired people are helped by hearing aids, others have conditions that cannot be corrected, or the benefits of the aids are outweighed by the discomfort caused by the ways sounds are reproduced ("How to Buy a Hearing Aid" 1976).

Perhaps the most important factor that emerges from studies of normal aging is that older people as a group are more variable or different from one another than are younger people. On any given test of abilities, some older people will score as well as the young, whereas others will do more poorly (Schonfield 1974). Even for reaction time, where the most consistent differences between old and young have been reported, some older people can respond as fast as younger individuals; for others, the slowing is minimal. It is therefore difficult to make predictions about the "average" older person. More so than at any other age, averages are misleading. One older person will have difficulty with memory, another will be rigid, and still another will be lively, flexible, and have a good memory.

A major implication for working with older patients is to evaluate each person individually and not make assumptions based on chronological age. People's current behaviors and attitudes can be understood in the context of values and habits they had in the past, as well as their current circumstances. Rather than look upon an elder as someone for whom nothing can be done, the vision care practitioner can consider the role vision has played in the person's life and how that individual has adapted to change in the past. Although adaptation may be slower than for younger patients, the practitioner who takes time with older people will obtain good results.

Common Problems in Adaptation and Compliance

The aging person who has experienced recent losses in vision represents a major challenge for the vision care practitioner. As with any major life stress, adaptation to visual loss is a difficult process. Often the person's emotional reaction will be intense or self-defeating and will interfere with appropriate adaptational responses. The key to a successful outcome is for the clinician to understand that the patient's emotional response is an integrated part of the eye problem and has to be dealt with as part of the rehabilitative process. By understanding the basis of self-defeating or irrational behaviors, clinicians can assist patients to make better choices about visual aids and other low-vision assistance.

Many older patients have a poor initial response to low-vision aids. They may reject them without trying them, use them briefly and then give up, or use the aids in ways that do not produce maximum benefit. Perhaps as many as one of every two older patients has a poor first response to low-vision aids.

These patients often are described as "unmotivated." The vision care specialist may believe that if only the patient wanted to get help, the response to treatment would be adequate. However, lack of motivation is too general a concept for understanding patients. A few patients derive benefits from their vision loss, such as having someone take care of them or being eligible for disability, and they are not interested in increasing their own independence. Most partially sighted people, however, truly want to use their vision again. Furthermore, patients who are difficult or noncompliant rarely believe they are the cause of the problem. Instead, they regard the treatment as inadequate for their condition. Even when patients are aware they are noncompliant, they may not be able to understand why.

The low-vision specialist must identify the specific reasons for noncompliance for a given patient. This means gathering information from several sources, including the patient's verbal reports about the eye problems and observations of how the patient uses visual aids. Possible reasons for noncompliance include the patients' beliefs about their visual condition and about the use of visual aids, as well as behavioral problems that prevent adequate adaptation to visual aids. Once the basis of noncompliance has been identified, interventions can be made to improve the response to treatment. Such interventions may involve testing self-defeating beliefs, involving patients in managing their own problems better, and breaking down complex visual tasks such as reading into a series of simpler steps. These interventions have been found useful for dealing with a variety of emotional problems (Beck et al. 1979; Lewinsohn et al. 1978; Meichenbaum 1977). Several common problems and ways of managing them will be described.

One of the most straightforward and frustrating obstacles to compliance is when patients believe that what they need is a new, stronger pair of spectacles, and they do not understand why the optometrist has shown them more cumbersome devices such as magnifiers or telescopes. When they first come to a low-vision service, patients have varying degrees of information about their condition. Some may not understand what their condition means for visual functioning. Although the low-vision specialist can give a careful explanation and answer the patient's questions, that does not always mean the patient will understand.

When a patient does not respond to a brief explanation, it is important to go into more detail. The clinician can discuss why new glasses would not correct the condition—for example, stating that glasses correct for errors in refraction, whereas the patient's condition involves damage to the retina. Using the analogy that the eye is like a camera sometimes helps. It should then be determined if the patient believes the explanation. If so, the patient then can be encouraged to try visual aids again, with the instruction of finding out if there is anything that makes even a small difference. By emphasizing to the patient the importance of determining if there is a "small difference," the clinician guards against creating other unrealistic expectations, such as being able to see as well as in the past. However, if patients do not respond to these efforts to explain the nature of the vision problem or continue to insist that they just want a new pair of glasses, they can be

encouraged to continue their search. However, it must be stressed that these patients are welcome to come back if they decide to try the other aids available. For some patients, keeping open the possibility of returning at a later date may be the best that can be done.

A related belief that interferes with adjustment is that it is too embarrassing or demeaning to use visual aids. Some patients think the aids will call too much attention to them or will cause others to pity them or think of them as strange. Through questioning a patient, the specific reason why aids are embarrassing and the situations in which the patient would be uncomfortable can be determined. It sometimes may be sufficient to explain that most partially sighted persons are a bit ill at ease when they first use their aids. They generally find that other people respect them rather than pity them. One patient, for example, said he initially would not use his aid (a hand-held telescope for distance viewing), but he subsequently found that when he did use it in social situations, it provided a helpful way to initiate conversations with strangers. He evaluated the change in his attitude this way: life had handed him a lemon (his visual problem), but he was trying to turn it into lemonade. Sometimes giving patients examples such as this one helps, but occasionally the best tactic is to introduce them to other partially sighted people who are using aids. Hearing firsthand from someone who has a similar problem that the gains from using aids far outweigh any minor embarrassments can make the most difference.

Other beliefs that interfere with compliance involve pessimism and hopelessness about what the aids can do. Some patients believe they cannot be happy unless the aids restore their vision to what it used to be. Using what Beck et al. (1979) call "all-or-nothing" thinking, these patients maintain there is no reason to use low-vision aids, because their vision is not totally restored. They will make statements such as "It's not the same" or "It's just no good," and they will actively frustrate efforts by the clinician to determine how much use they potentially might get from a given aid. They also may be disturbed by some aspects of how they see with the aid. For instance, some patients complain about the reduced visual field they have when using magnifiers. Others complain about how they have to use the aids; for example, a reading position might be too awkward or uncomfortable, or they may have to read more slowly than in the past.

There are several ways in which patients can be helped to question these pessimistic attitudes. First, the clinician can explain to them that it takes time to get used to an aid. Improvement is gradual and does not occur all at once. This is particularly the case with someone who maintains that the aids are too awkward or uncomfortable or who reports reading too slowly or tiring too easily. The clinician also can ask patients about other situations in which they faced changes to determine how they generally adapt to new circumstances. One woman who did not like the way she had to read with microscopic spectacles remembered that she did not like Talking Books when she first received them but now uses them all the time. Once she gave this example, she was able to understand that she often responds negatively to changes. At that point, she was able to accept the microscopic spectacles that were being suggested to her.

A particularly difficult type of patient is the "help rejector." This person says "Help me," but then refuses anything that is offered. The help rejector maintains that nothing makes a difference, even when objective testing of visual functioning with aids indicates differently. Once someone with this negative belief has been identified, the clinician needs to present the aids in a paradoxical way, for example: "This is an aid that helps a lot of people, but I am not sure you can use it. Tell me if it makes any difference." This approach upsets the patient's usual negative response. Another strategy is to ask the patient what amount or percent of improvement he or she would consider significant. Many people with all-or-nothing thinking will scale down their expectations when forced to be more specific. The extent to which aids can help them fulfill their expectations then can be discussed.

With some oppositional and negative patients, the best approach is to give them a choice between different visual aids. They may not always choose the aid that gives them the most benefit, but their choice will reflect other, intangible factors, such as which aid fits best into their life-style.

One final reason for a poor response to low-vision aids is a patient's never having been a good reader. Adequate magnification of print is possible, but the patient cannot put together the simplest words or sentences. These patients differ from those with just negative expectations in that their reading skills are just not adequate

to meet the increased challenge of reading with magnification. An approach using the method of "successive approximations" may be beneficial to these patients (Rimm and Masters 1978). Successive approximations involves breaking a task down into small, manageable components. A person can master a skill by starting at a very simple level and gradually increasing the complexity level. Most of the problem with poor readers appears to be in figuring out individual words quickly. To build up this ability, they can begin with simple words or pairs of words. When their speed begins to pick up, they can move to sentences and, eventually, to printed material. The goals often can be modest, since patients' goals may involve reading a label or letter, not a complicated text.

Psychological Services for Low-Vision Patients

A viable psychology program should have five components: assessment, individual and family psychotherapy, patient groups, consultation, and peer counselors. Assessments should be made when patients are referred by an optometrist or by other health and/or rehabilitation professionals as paraprofessionals. The assessment seeks to determine if the person has a significant psychological problem interfering with rehabilitation and what type of intervention would be best. Depending on the assessment, the patient may be referred for individual or family psychotherapy, he or she could be recommended to a patient support group, or there could be a consultation between the psychologist and other clinical personnel on better ways of interacting with the patient.

People judged to be in need of psychotherapy are those manifesting severe adjustment reactions. Some examples are severely depressed, anxious, angry, or worried individuals or those having pronounced interpersonal difficulties. In many instances, the problems preceded the vision loss but may have been exacerbated by it. Individual or family therapy that may be time limited should be offered, or, if the patient lives too far away to travel in regularly for assistance, referrals should be made to mental health professionals in their own communities.

When the symptoms of distress are not severe or if a person is socially isolated, a patient group often is useful. Such a group should emphasize the exchange of information among patients and developing positive self-images. Much of the benefit will come from observing and learning from the successes of other patients. For instance, people may observe others using visual aids successfully or learn strategies for compensating for their visual loss, such as how they might identify people in a social situation. Finding out they are not alone in having a vision problem is often very helpful in itself to older patients.

A consultation with the optometric staff should occur for each patient who is referred for psychological assessment. The consultation should involve conveying the findings of the assessment and working out strategies for interacting with the patient. Many of the referrals will involve patients who do not have prominent psychiatric symptoms such as depression or anxiety, but whose attitudes or behaviors interfere with successful adaptation, as described earlier. In collaboration with the low-vision staff, the psychologist will use the findings of the assessment to formulate new approaches for working with the patient in question.

Because of the benefits patients can derive from talking to someone else with a similar vision problem, a peer group counseling program is recommended. Volunteers for this program might be former patients who have gone through a special training program in communications skills. Their role might be to greet new patients and answer any questions they might have while waiting for their examination. They should not respond to technical questions about vision; they should tell the patient to ask the low-vision specialist these questions. Instead, they should talk about the different services available and how they have been able to adjust to their vision problem. New patients will frequently welcome the opportunity to ask questions of a peer and will be often surprised and pleased to meet someone else with a vision problem.

Summary
Although aging has some effects on mental processing, most older people have the capacity to adapt to changes, including learning to use visual aids. Many patients, however, make a poor initial response to low-vision aids. The clinician's task is to identify the reasons for this poor response and give the patient information that counters the negative beliefs. Patients' compliance and understanding can be increased considerably by working with them in this way.

Environmental Adaptation
As can be gleaned from the prior sections of this chapter, we believe that comprehensive low-vision care is much more than a low-vision examination, the prescription of visual aids as a result of such an examination, and training in the proper use of those aids. The chapter has demonstrated the relevance of competent psychological counseling to comprehensive low-vision care. This section will discuss orientation and mobility; home visits; and information that can and should be conveyed to the older partially sighted patient during those visits, as well as at comprehensive centers.

Orientation and Mobility
In general, emphasis should be placed on teaching patients how to move about safely and independently using visual enhancement techniques (that is, all their remaining sensory capabilities, including their residual vision, augmented when necessary with appropriate visual aids). Thus, patients should be taught, for example, how to use a monocular, binoculars, or telescopic spectacles to perform distance tasks such as determining the status of a traffic signal, the number or name of a bus, the name of a street, a street address or office number, or a name on an office door in a public building. However, the mere acquisition of a monocular or other distance-viewing device does not guarantee that it will be used or used properly. Patients need training in the use of the aids, and the training preferably should take place daily in a context in which the patient can be expected to use the aids.

There are circumstances in which some partially sighted people should be encouraged to carry and display a cane, even though visual parameters such as best-corrected distance visual acuity and size and shape of visual fields would not indicate a need for such an aid. For example, people who have both macular degeneration *and* very slow reaction rates to visual and other sensory information should be encouraged to carry and display a cane when moving on a crowded street or passing through automobile traffic in order to inform others that they have a visual problem.

Some partially sighted people should be taught to use a cane properly to move from place to place. For example, people who have very restricted visual fields, regardless of what their best-corrected visual acuities might be, should be encouraged to obtain thorough training in the proper use of a cane. This follows from the fact that these people cannot visually comprehend enough of a complicated traffic situation fast enough to avoid being injured or perhaps being the cause of injury to others. Many people with retinitis pigmentosa or with advanced glaucoma fall into this category. Partially sighted people who experience fluctuations in vision that at times leave them functionally blind (as is sometimes the case among people having very advanced cases of diabetic retinopathy) also need instruction on how to use a cane properly during periods in which they are effectively functionally blind.

Home Visits
With patient permission, follow-up visits should be made to the homes or work sites of older patients to ascertain how they are getting on with the visual aids prescribed for them. The follow-up visits could be made, for example, by case coordinators, social workers, or orientation and mobility instructors. These professionals should be able to help patients learn to work with aids when necessary. However, if it is apparent that the patient needs assistance and training that requires more skill or time than the visiting staff member can give, the patient should be encouraged to return for additional training from a low-vision technician or optometrist. Patients also should be encouraged to return for additional help when a negative change in visual status is reported, and they should be referred to the pyschologist when the staff member detects possible patient need for individual, group, or family counseling. During the visits to patients' homes, staff members should also look for opportunities to make suggestions to the patient that, if heeded, would make the visited environment safer and more visually comfortable (Genensky 1979, 1980, 1981; Genensky et al 1979).

Important and Useful Information for the Partially Sighted
What follows illustrates the kinds of information and advice that teacher counselors of the blind and rehabilitation counselors of the blind should give to their partially sighted clients, whether they are or are not legally blind. General information about services available to the visually impaired is useful. For example, local services may include special transportation services or discounted taxi fares, and state services may include identification cards available from the state department of motor vehicles, which are similar in appearance to drivers' licenses and which can be used for identification or check-cashing purposes.

Probably the best-known national program is the Talking Book Program. For people who enjoy reading and who cannot read long articles or books for long enough periods of time or rapidly enough to make it practical, the Library of Congress provides a service that may prove useful. The Talking Book Program provides free recordings or tape cassettes of a large number of current and classical books and periodicals for the benefit of visually impaired people, as well as other handicapped people who are not able to read printed material. The Talking Book Program provides record players and tape recorders for use with its records and tapes, and it also services this equipment—all at no charge to the user. Talking Books and Talking Book machines (record players and tape recorders) are distributed by the Library of Congress through a system of regional and branch libraries. Although this program is admirable and has enriched the lives of tens of thousands of legally blind and physically handicapped people for over 40 years, the selection of materials available is limited. Thus, it would appear that the partially sighted person who is a serious reader and who can use visual aids for reading will also want to use the aids to maintain reading independence and avoid curtailing the selection of reading material.

In addition to the information already described, patients should receive specific advice concerning things they should or should not do to make their adaptation to partial sight smoother and perhaps more efficient. Table 23–2 gives specific examples illustrating the scope, degree, or kind of advice and information that most partially sighted older people might benefit from having.

A comprehensive program of supportive rehabilitative services is essential to achieve success with selected low-vision patients. It is strongly recommended that vision care specialists who do not have such supportive services available through their own offices or clinics seek them in their communities for those patients who might benefit.

Table 23-2
Aids to Daily Living Guidelines for the Partially Sighted

1. Keep all room doors totally open or totally closed to minimize the dangers of inadvertently walking into the vertical edge of a door.
2. Use dishes and glasses that contrast in color with the tablecloth or table (that is, white or light dishes on a dark cloth or table, or dark dishes on a light cloth or table). When pouring liquids, pour dark liquids into light cups or mugs and light liquids into dark cups or mugs. For example, pour coffee into a white cup and milk into a dark mug. This use of the color-contrast technique will allow you to avoid underfilling as well as overfilling the container.
3. Tack down or otherwise inhibit the motion of a scatter rug. This will reduce the possibility of falling because of rug slippage.
4. Avoid placing lamps and other sources of artificial light in places or positions that result in people's having to look at bare lightbulbs or at reflections of those bulbs coming from reflectors that may be associated with them. Bare lightbulbs or light coming from such reflectors can be annoying even to fully sighted persons. For many partially sighted people it can be physically painful or blinding in the sense that other objects in the visual field that otherwise would be visible are fully or nearly completely obscured by the light generated by the bulbs or off the reflectors.
5. When reading or writing, make sure the lighting sources illuminate the printed word or the writing paper and not the eyes of the person trying to read or write.
6. Arrange clothing according to color or put clothes together in matching sets. In the former case, for example, clearly labeled dividers can be placed on clothes racks to distinguish one color set from another. Many partially sighted people have good color vision, but many others have difficulty distinguishing among low- or medium-saturation colors, especially in the presence of incandescent lighting.
7. Use brightly colored reflecting tape to mark dial settings on stoves, washers, dryers, and other appliances to indicate critical settings. Partially sighted people frequently have great difficulty reading these dials and need this additional visual boost.
8. Do not reach across burners on a gas or electric stove. Partially sighted people often have difficulty determining visually whether or not a gas burner is lit or an electric element is heated, particularly when the color or gray value of the flame or heated coil is not in high contrast with the color or gray value of the portion of the stove immediately adjacent to it. For safety's sake, try to confine cooking to the gas burners or electric elements closest to the front of the stove. By doing this, there will be less chance of inadvertently reaching across a lit burner or hot electrical element.
9. Avoid the use of glass-top coffee tables or other low glass-top furniture to prevent severe leg bruises caused by bumping into the virtually invisible glass.
10. Clearly mark sliding glass doors with colorful decals or other clearly visible markings to reduce the chance of serious injury from glass door-human collision.
11. Mark the leading edge of all interior and exterior steps with a stripe of paint or a strip of nonskid material that runs the width of the step. The stripe should be 5 cm wide on both the runner and the riser and have a color and gray value that stands out in high contrast to the color and gray value of the rest of the step. (A coating of clear resin mixed with clear transparent aggregate protects painted stripes and provides some traction.) Steps marked in this way can be seen by at least 95 percent of all partially sighted people. Furthermore, marking steps in this way is also useful to fully sighted older people, many of whom have a great fear of falling or tripping on stairs (Genesky 1979, 1980, 1981).
12. Place knives, forks, and other sharp objects with their points downward in drainers and dishwasher silverware baskets. This will avoid the problem of your inadvertently grasping the blade of a knife or the pointed end of the prongs of a fork.
13. *Never move your face close to an object to view it more clearly until you have carefully and cautiously checked with your hands whether it has any pointed or sharp edges that could injure your eyes. Similarly, never*

move an object close to your face to see it more clearly until you have inspected it with your hands.

14. If a steel needle or a common pin is missing and its approximate location is known, a small, strong magnet can be used to "sweep" the area and find the missing needle or pin. If the sharp object is in the area and the magnet is close enough to the surface — say, about 1 to 3 cm — the needle or pin will be attracted to the magnet. To determine that the needle or pin has in fact been picked up by the magnet, move your fingers carefully over or near the magnet. *Never bring the magnet close to your eyes:* if the needle or pin is present, it could cause serious injury.

15. When sweeping or washing a floor or vacuuming a rug, mentally divide the floor or rug into squares or other convenient shapes enclosing about 9 or 16 square feet. First, thoroughly sweep (wash, or vacuum) a square in one corner of the room; then do the same to the square to the immediate right (or left) of it and to each successive square in the row until you reach the end of the row. Follow the same procedure across each row, and continue doing this until the last row has been completed. In this way if you cannot see the dirt or dust on the floor or rug, you still can be reasonably sure you did a good job of cleaning. A still better procedure requires that the successive squares overlap somewhat with their closest neighbors.

16. Carefully order the paper money in your wallet or billfold either in increasing or decreasing order of value. For those who still would have difficulty telling one bill from another even with any visual aid they carry about with them, a money-folding convention used by the totally blind may prove useful. The convention calls for leaving one-dollar bills unfolded, five-dollar bills folded in half lengthwise, ten-dollar bills folded in half widthwise, and twenty-dollar bills folded in half widthwise and then folded in half again widthwise. You also may find it convenient to separate bills of various denominations from one another by ordinary paperclips. Thus, the one-dollar bills are all clipped together, the five-dollar bills are all clipped together, and so on, and the clipped bills are arranged in the billfold either in increasing or decreasing order. Imaginative use of the paperclips would make it possible to differentiate the various denominations from one another without having to see them visually. For example, a single paperclip at the longest side of the bills indicates that they are ones, a single paper clip at the shorter side of the bills indicates that they are fives, two paper clips at the long side of the bills indicates that they are tens, and so on.

17. If you have trouble seeing the numbers on a telephone dial, try using a special enlarged telephone dial cover that has enlarged numbers and letters. You also may be able to learn to dial strictly by touch. For many people, this is not hard to do with a bit of practice. For example, placing the nonthumb fingers of the right hand in the first four holes of the dial immediately tells you where the numbers *1, 2, 3,* and *4* are located and that the number *5* is below and slightly to the left of your index finger. Placing the same fingers in the last four holes of the dial immediately tells you where the numbers *7, 8, 9* and *0* are located and that the number *6* is above and slightly to the left of your index finger. Using this finger map, the right index finger can be trained to dial as rapidly as you please. For many individuals, "dialing" via push buttons is much easier than dialing via the circular dial. With the right hand, the index finger can be placed on the button labeled *1,* the big finger on the button labeled *2,* and the ring finger on the button labeled *3.* The same fingers on the second row of the push buttons cover *4, 5,* and *6,* respectively, and on the third row they cover *7, 8,* and *9,* respectively. On the fourth row they cover the asterisk, the *0,* and the number sign, respectively. For those who prefer to use the push button telephone with a display of enlarged numbers and letters, a plastic cover having these properties is also available.

18. To avoid losing contact with friends, for example, on the street or at a large gathering, ask those friends to say hello to you and tell you their names when they see you. Explain to them that because of your impaired vision, you are no longer able to recognize them, even if they are standing very close. We have found that by doing this, both partially sighted people and their

friends are put at ease. The former no longer wonder who passed by, who is approaching them, or who is standing in front of them, and the latter are no longer at a loss as to how to cope with their friend's visual impairment in this regard. Furthermore, friends tend to respect people who have accepted their partial sightedness and have, as it were, taken command of their visual loss. Thus, both parties are more at ease. As a result, they frequently find it easier to talk to one another about the visual problem and, perhaps, further ease any tension that might still exist because of the reduction in vision.

19. When it is necessary to approach the entrance of a bus and ask the driver a question such as the number of the bus, it is best to also let the driver know that you cannot see well. For example, say to the driver, "Excuse me. I don't see very well. Could you please tell me if this is number *38?*" By doing this, you alert the driver to the existence of your visual problem and hence reduce the chance of responses like "Can't you read?" or "You blind or something?" Both of these responses are uncalled for, but the driver is human and, like the rest of us, is subject to making "dumb statements." This same technique would be helpful in asking people for directions or assistance in determining the name of a street or number of a building. It is best to help others help you and in so doing avoid confrontations.

20. Do not let your ego or vanity interfere with using your vision and your visual aids. Experience has shown that fully sighted people soon get used to the use of visual aids, and they accept their presence and use as perfectly normal. In addition, they frequently develop a greater admiration and respect for you because you accept your visual status; use the aid; and, as a consequence, participate more effectively in fully sighted society. Also, as noted in Item 18, when you use your aids, you put your fully sighted friends and family at ease. You ease the anxiety they sometimes experience because they want to help you and do not know what to do.

References

Beck, A., D. Rush, D. Shaw, and G. Emery. *Cognitive Therapy of Depression.* New York: Guilford Press, 1979.

Botwinick, J. *Aging and Behavior.* 2nd ed. New York: Springer Publishing, 1978.

Corso, J. F. "Auditory Perception and Communication." In *Handbook of the Psychology of Aging,* eds. J. E. Birren and K. W. Schaie. New York: Van Nostrand Reinhold, 1977.

Craik, F. I. M. "Age Differences in Human Memory." In *Handbook of the Psychology of Aging,* eds. J. E. Birren and K. W. Schaie. New York: Van Nostrand Reinhold, 1977.

Genensky, S. M. "Data Concerning the Partially Sighted and the Functionally Blind." *Journal of Visual Impairment and Blindness* 72, no. 5 (1978): 177–180.

Genesky, S. M. "Architectural Barriers to Partially Sighted Persons." *Report* (National Center for a Barrier Free Environment) 5, no. 2 (1979): 8.

Genensky, S. M. "Architectural Barriers to the Partially Sighted—And Solutions." *Architectural Record,* May 1980, 65–67.

Genensky, S. M. "Design Sensitivity and the Partially Sighted." *Building Operation Management,* June 1981, 50–54.

Genensky, S. M., S. H. Berry, T. H. Bikson, and T. K. Bikson. *Visual Environmental Adaptation Problems of the Partially Sighted: Final Report* (CPS-100-HEW). Santa Monica, CA: Santa Monica Hospital Medical Center, Center for the Partially Sighted, January 1979.

"How to Buy a Hearing Aid." *Consumer Reports* 41 (1976): 345–351.

Lewinsohn, P. M., R. F. Munoz, M. A. Youngren, and A. M. Zeiss. *Control Your Depression.* Englewood Cliffs, N. J.: Prentice-Hall, 1978.

Meichenbaum, D. *Cognitive-Behavior Modification.* New York: Plenum, 1977.

Rees, J., and J. Botwinick. "Detection and Decision Factors in Auditory Behavior of the Elderly." *Journal of Gerontology* 26 (1971): 133–136.

Rimm, D. C., and J. C. Masters. *Behavior Therapy: Techniques and Empirical Findings.* 2d ed. New York: Academic Press, 1978.

Schonfield, D. "Translations in Gerontology—From Lab to Life: Utilizing Information." *American Psychologist* 29 (1974): 796–801.

Suggested Readings

"Argon Laser Photocoagulation for Senile Macular Degeneration." *Archives of Ophthalmology* 100 (June 1982): 912–918.

Bernstein, C. "Altering SMD Victims in Time." *Sight-saving: Journal for Blindness Prevention* 51, no. 2 (1982): 16–20.

Birren, J. E., and J. Botwinick. "Age Differences in Finger, Jaw, and Foot Reaction Time to Auditory Stimuli." *Journal of Gerontology* 10 (1955): 429–432.

Botwinick, J. "Intellectual Abilities." In *Handbook of the Psychology of Aging,* eds. J. E. Birren and K. W. Schaie. New York: Van Nostrand Reinhold, 1977.

Chown, S. M. "Age and the Rigidities." *Journal of Gerontology* 16 (1961): 353–362.

Coughlin, W. R., and A. Patz. "Diabetic Retinopathy." *Diabetes Forecast,* 1978.

Hassinger, M. J., J. M. Zarit, and S. H. Zarit. "A Comparison of Clinical Characteristics of Multi-infarct and Alzheimer's Dementia Patients." Paper presented at the meetings of the Western Psychological Association, Sacramento, 1982.

National Institutes of Health, U. S. Department of Health, Education, and Welfare, *Model Reporting Area for Blindness Statistics.* Washington, D. C.: U. S. Government Printing Office, 1962–1970.

NIA Task Force. "Senility Reconsidered." *Journal of the American Medical Association* 244, no. 3 (1980): 259–263.

Rosenbloom, A. A. "Care of Elderly People with Low Vision" *Journal of Visual Impairment and Blindness,* June 1982, 209–212.

Schaie, K. W. and G. Labouvie-Vief. "Generational versus Ontogenetic Components of Change in Adult Cognitive Behavior: A Fourteen Year Cross-Sequential Study." *Developmental Psychology* 10 (1974): 305–320.

"SMD: Clearing up the Picture." *Eye Care Digest* 1, no. 1 (1982): 4.

Zarit, S. H. *Aging and Mental Disorders.* New York: Free Press, 1980.

Zarit, S. H. "Affective Correlates of Self-reports about Memory of Older People." *International Journal of Behavioral Geriatrics* 1 (1982): 25–34.

Zarit, S. H., and J. M. Zarit. "Families under Stress." *Psychotherapy: Theory, Research and Practice.* 19 (1982), 461–471.

Chapter 24

The Need for Innovation: Services and Programs for Vision-impaired Older People

Lorraine G. Hiatt

Goals for Developing Program for Older People

An estimated 1,334,000 seriously vision-impaired older people in the United States live at home, yet very few of these people's lives are touched by services that help them live independently despite their vision losses (American Foundation for the Blind 1981).

Occasional reports have described local projects to compensate for vision losses, but too many people are needlessly giving up interests and curtailing routines because they (1) do not understand their vision needs, (2) have no information on what can be done to work around or compensate for vision losses, or (3) presume that these losses are to be expected with old age. There are strong indications that older people with vision losses are more likely to become candidates for costly, restrictive institutional care (Kirchner and Peterson 1980).

Vision care specialists could make an outstanding contribution to the future of a community's aging by working toward the development of a continuum of vision care services for older people. Their efforts would serve as a model, and they would need to be documented so that others could learn. Innovation in vision care for older people often involves efforts to disseminate information on available services—services offered by vision care professionals, as well as those offered by other agencies or individuals—that would be beneficial to an older person with limited vision.

What can be done to respond to these needs? Participants in the 1981 Mini-Conference on Vision and Aging for the White House articulated some fairly succinct goals (*Vision and Aging* 1981).

1. To allow older people to live at home and do the following:
   a. Seek services from a community source, including (1) generic agencies or those providing a variety of services to people for reasons other than vision impairments; and (2) categorical sources, such as centers specifically serving the needs of people who are partially sighted, elderly, or blind.
   b. Receive services, if necessary, at home (in people's own houses or in community spaces associated with apartment residences).
2. To provide services, as necessary, to people in institutions so that they can be aided along with everyone else (rather than being segregated, as a result of their vision impairments, into separate facilities or programs solely on the basis of their being vision impaired), as well as to provide special training and services related to vision impairments.

The purpose of this chapter is to present a continuum of services that ideally should be available to older people in each community, and then to describe two special areas of interest to vision care professionals: self-help groups and better utilization of the physical environment.

Worth the Effort

Several excellent reviews of the literature on the sensory functioning of older people have appeared in the past few years (Birren 1964; Flood 1979; Fozard et al. 1977; Fozard and Popkin 1978; Koncelik 1979; Ordy and Brizzee

1979; Pastalan 1979). The common theme of studies both grand and humble is that it is worth the effort to maximize residual vision or compensate for vision losses of people from midlife through old age.

Starting with Evaluation

Something needs to be done about the nearly 75 percent of those over age 75 who experience vision changes that are neither adequately assessed nor generally amenable to treatment (Fozard et al. 1977). A good place to start is to participate in ongoing evaluation programs. Chapter 20 of this book describes some specific evaluation procedures. The objective of participating in community organizations involved in services to older people is to offer convenient, ongoing programs of vision care and education. Some leadership groups in aging have sponsored health fairs, mobile units, and educational programs that could serve as a forum for high-quality vision care services.

Nationally, there is no system or required policy of vision and hearing evaluation of older people (American Foundation for the Blind 1981). Furthermore, there have been too few interest groups advocating such evaluations. It is difficult for one professional to spark communitywide commitments to vision evaluations; it is not as difficult for organizations to collaboratively generate an interest in vision care.

In some states, communities, and institutions, the adequate evaluation of the vision of older people is stymied by medical directors, private physicians, or other gatekeepers who fail to recognize the significance of such evaluations (Leslie and Greenberg 1974; Miller 1974; Newman 1977; Rosenbloom 1974; Sartoris 1975; Snyder, Pyrek, and Smith 1976; Woodruff and Pack 1980). Gatekeepers are more easily persuaded by numbers—by the political clout that comes from group efforts.

It is difficult to interest individual older people and sponsors of senior centers or other groups in services for visually impaired consumers without having some system for vision evaluation. Moreover, sometimes vision evaluations have been superficial, and information has not been used to develop priorities and services. Nothing is more frustrating for the older person than learning of a condition and not being able to do anything about it. For this reason, it would be helpful for vision care professionals to work with the leaders of various community-based ser-

vices for older people to develop follow-up beyond refraction or medical procedures. The American Foundation for the Blind in the 1980s found that few organizations in the field of aging had ever heard of the term *low-vision services*, for example. Nor did they have the slightest idea as professionals that something could be done to maximize residual vision skills.

Vision care professionals also need to listen to consumers and professionals as they develop a package of vision evaluations. For example, a community that has a driver retraining program for older people may want to emphasize certain aspects of an evaluation. A community interested in working with memory-impaired individuals needs to know if there are professionals who are comfortable screening forgetful clients. The more functionally based the vision examination procedures become—that is, the more they relate to the daily lives and routines of older people—the easier it may be to generate clients. The person who no longer reads is less likely to take a vision examination that relates only to print legibility.

Not only are functionally based assessments likely to create a demand for increased technology, environmental design, and self-help techniques; the converse also may hold true. As consumers become more aware of aging, more assertive through self-help group experiences, and more widely exposed to the possibilities for optical aids, they are likely to request clinicians to provide information pertinent to their own lifestyles and activities.

At least three gaps must be filled before adequate vision evaluation will be widely implemented for older people:

1. Eye care professionals now have inadequate information on which to base and develop functional assessments for older people. Professionals in vision care need to develop a better understanding of how older people really spend their time. Generalizations about older people have become an impediment to good service. Sometimes older people have given up doing things because they do not know that professionals can help them pursue activities. Not only should assessments include information on how the eye functions; they need to tap into how the people function and what they would like to do.

2. Practicing professionals need to have access to education on new techniques of vision

evaluation. Through continuing education, professionals need to be trained on methods of conducting functional assessments, as well as on techniques for speaking to older people and their families about the meaning of their findings.

3. Eye care professionals have inadequately conceptualized the environment in which the evaluation of vision occurs (Fozard 1980). An emerging design issue in assessment relates to the topic of ecologically valid or realistic assessments (Cullinan 1979, 1980a, 1980b; Hiatt 1981a; Sekuler and Hutman 1980; Willems 1977). Measurements of the vision abilities of older people often are performed in well-lit and acoustically controlled offices that do not reproduce the features of the everyday world. In the near future, two types of evaluations are necessary; those that give controlled measures of vision and hearing and those that indicate performance in actual settings.

Basic Services and Implications for Vision Care Specialists

Several types of services are required by visually impaired individuals, according to the data collected by those providing such programs. These include the following:

1. Referral to appropriate vision care professionals.
2. Low-vision evaluation and services.
3. Referral to rehabilitation agencies.
4. Training in mobility indoors and outdoors, basic daily living skills, reading and writing communication skills, and information on and instruction in reading alternatives (large print books, Talking Books, or the use of magnification and lighting aids).
5. Recreation.
6. Transportation.
7. Counseling regarding chronic depression or coping with losses.
8. Driver refresher course (as feasible).
9. Information specific to vision impairment, as well as other services and programs (including payment procedures).
10. Demonstration on consumer aids and appliances.
11. Assistance in employment and work force participation.
12. Access to peer groups or to other older people who are coping with similar vision problems.

Few communities have this full range of services in place. However, many have more services than the vision care professional may be aware of. In the United States, to learn about what is available, the vision care professional must meet with active community groups interested in aging; such groups may be discovered by contacting the area agency on aging, the director of the nearest senior citizens center, or the state office on aging. Ideally, a representative of the local optometric or vision care professionals group should serve as a regular member and liaison with the leadership of community aging organizations.

Service Developments and Aging People

Three particularly significant developments in services include (1) a greater recognition that older people benefit from training, (2) an emphasis on the maximization of residual skills (low-vision services), and (3) the growth in self-help groups and techniques.

Low vision services are particularly interesting to gerontologists. The notion of maximizing capabilities or eliciting untapped potential of older people is considered innovative. Despite the overwhelming literature suggesting that older people's talents are underutilized, gerontologists (and older people) have had few examples of services that truly help them overcome their disabilities.

Prototypical Innovations

This section offers two approaches for optimizing vision:

1. Self-help programs, where *self-help* refers to efforts in which older people play a significant, decisive role (either individually or in groups) in dealing with the effects of chronic or acute visual impairments.
2. Environmental design, where the *environment* refers to the world from the skin to the walls and beyond, including the characteristics and arrangement of physical features, as well as the interactive effects they create.

Environmental design and self-help would be additions to the continuum of vision care. They may be considered innovative, because they are seldom practiced. These two concepts are particularly appropriate, because they offer solutions for people whose vision cannot be fully corrected. They are challenging, because they use professionals in new ways.

What Do Self-Help and Environmental Design Have to Do with Vision Care?

Vision (and hearing) changes typically bring about the first functional changes experienced in late adulthood. Self-help programs offer a method whereby older people can exchange experiences and practical advice regarding how to cope with diminished capabilities. Self-help is valuable because it (1) respects the dignity and value of older peoples' experiences; (2) is most likely to touch on priorities, because the topics are generated by participants rather than professionals; and (3) should not be costly. Techniques for more prudently using the environment and technology to cope with and compensate for unremediable vision losses can be effectively taught using self-help programs (Hiatt et al. 1982).

For the older person, the environment is no innocent bystander in daily life; features of the environment actually may contribute to visual handicaps (Cullinan 1978a, 1978b, 1980b; Hiatt 1980a; Silver et al. 1978; Snyder, Pyrek, and Smith 1976). Cullinan's research of British older people at home and in institutions indicates that poor light may hasten the rate of retinal deterioration.

Environmental design can be an appealing, nonthreatening intervention that shifts the focus from dysfunctions of humans to the failings of environments as it unites professionals, families, and older adults in problem solving.

Learning More about Self-Help

One goal for aging services in the area of low vision is the creation of services that make judicious use of each professional's time while making sure that the technology or optical aids do not overshadow training or teaching. Self-help groups offer a technique for dealing with older people's reluctance to seek services (Moen 1978).

Group meetings also afford opportunities for peer training on the very practical aspects of adapting to the use of optical aids or other aspects of a low-vision life-style. Professionals often have been charged with the responsibility for this type of education on a one-to-one basis. This becomes expensive and frustrating, and it is inconsistent with the literature on how older people learn and the importance of integrating their own expertise into the training and teaching process (Balts and Schaie 1974; Okun 1977).

The vision care professional plays three primary roles in a self-help program:

1. In the evaluation of vision, the vision care professional can provide a *referral,* suggesting that the older person take part in a group and even offering information on where and how to contact one (Gartner and Riessman 1979).

2. The professional may help through *sponsorship.* Research on self-help has suggested that older people have more faith in self-help when the groups are sponsored by professionals. The vision care professional may do this through involvement with either vision care associations or associations involved with aging (Hiatt et al. 1982; Winer 1981).

3. The professional may serve as a *resource,* offering credible information and publications, as well as coming to speak when invited by the participants (Dory 1979; Lieberman and Borman 1979; Winer 1981).

Self-help programs are no substitute for rehabilitation services or specialized design, but they may be a viable means for increasing the direct participation of older people in self-assessment, stimulating the assertiveness necessary to cope in social contexts, and formulating practical solutions to everday tasks and environments (Butler et al. 1979–1980; Elderly Hearing Impaired People 1981; Hiatt et al. 1982).

Both the self-help group experience and the idea of using features of the environment to help compensate for losses may be usefully generalized to other imminent functional changes associated with aging (Fozard 1981; Fozard and Popkin 1978; Marsh 1980). For example, once a person learns to cope with vision and hearing loss, it may be easier to deal with forgetfulness, arthritis, and psychosocial issues such as grieving or depression.

Self-help books and programs abound. However, successful programs for older people are fairly recent. More information can be obtained from Butler et al. (1979–1980); Dory (1979); Gartner and Reissman (1979); Hiatt et al. (1982); Lieberman and Borman (1979).

Using Environmental Design

The environment, available 24 hours a day, can be a resource or a detriment to visually impaired people (Fozard 1981; Fozard and Popkin 1978; Hiatt 1981a; Willems 1977). Attention needs to be directed to households (Dickman 1983; Hale 1979; Hiatt 1983), institutions (Hiatt 1978, 1980b; Koncelik 1979), and community and commercial facilities (Braf 1974; Genensky 1980; Wardell 1980). Literature on the use of design to compensate for visual losses typically refers to the following topics.

Arrangement. Placing tasks in orderly formats, improving body positioning in relation to work, and encouraging the use of arrangement to overcome sight losses all seem to improve visibility for persons with partial vision (Dickman 1983; Markle 1977; Yeadon and Grayson 1979).

Reducing Distractions. Background noise, which is confusing to older people, can be reduced in homes and clinical settings to improve the visual skills of older people (Elderly Hearing Impaired People 1981; Hiatt 1978). Background noise may come from industrial sources and machines, from music or television, and from conversations.

Maximizing Textural Information. Using contours, pressure variations, and texture where visual information is insufficient are among the ways to improve textural inputs for the older person (Hiatt 1980c). With minimal training, the older person often can use texture to identify key features (Kimbrough, Heubner, and Lowry 1976; Sicurella 1977; Welsh and Blasch 1980).

Increasing Lighting While Decreasing Glare. As people grow older, they probably will rely on magnification for at least some close work visual tasks. The greater the magnification, the greater the need for additional lighting. Whereas many of the preceding recommendations on environmental design can be accomplished with available information, the topic of lighting requires substantially more research with respect to older people (Fozard 1981). Standards have not been developed, and techniques for adapting information to home lighting are scarce (Hiatt et al. 1982).

Lighting levels in households and institutions are typically inadequate for the visual needs of older people (Cullinan, 1980a, 1980b; Hiatt 1981b; Lefitt 1980; Silver et al. 1978). Improvements usually involve increasing lighting levels, especially by directing light directly on tasks (Blackwell and Blackwell 1971; Duncan et al. 1977; Fozard et al. 1977; Koncelik 1979). For examples of how to increase lighting, see Dickman (1983); Hiatt (1978, 1980a); Hughes and Neer (1981); Nuckolls (1976).

Older people often require formal instruction on their need for increased lighting. They may resist using lights because of strongly held convictions about conserving energy costs (Cullinan 1980a, 1980b; Hiatt et al. 1982; Lefitt 1980). Older consumers should be advised about the uses of artificial lighting, such as reducing fatigue by using full-spectrum fluorescent lighting sources (Hughes and Neer 1981). Older people also need information on using nonglare lighting, minimizing reflection, "flashing," and shiny surfaces (Hughes and Neer 1981).

The environments in which older people live and function should be designed with an overall, even lighting, that avoids abrupt changes from high to low levels of illumination (Hiatt 1978; Hughes and Neer 1981; Koncelik 1979; Nuckolls 1976; Welsh and Blasch 1980). Similarly, elderly consumers need insights on minimizing shadows that can result in confusing environmental patterns and problems with mobility and steadiness in walking (Koncelik 1979; Nuckolls 1976).

Older consumers typically need to be instructed on how to avoid direct and indirect glare by minimizing excessively bright or unshielded lighting sources, by properly placing light sources so that bulbs are nonintrusive, and by minimizing reflections and shiny surfaces (Dickman 1983; Hiatt 1978; Hughes and Neer 1981; Nuckolls 1976; Welsh and Blasch 1980). Older people can be encouraged to use lighting (and color) to meaningfully call attention to important features of the environment (Dickman 1983; Fozard 1981; Hiatt 1980b; Hughes and Neer 1981; Nuckolls 1976; Sicurella 1977).

Contrast. Contrast can be creatively used to differentiate edges, that is, contrast in terms of color, texture, or both (Dickman 1983; Hiatt 1983; Hiatt et al. 1982). For example, if the focal object and background are two to three values different from each other, they will be more easily "read" or seen by people with low vision (Blackwell and Blackwell 1971; Dickman 1983; Hiatt 1981b; Sicurella 1977). At times, the older consumer needs to minimize contrast that creates optical illusions of objects or surface changes, such as patterns on a floor (Blackwell and Blackwell 1971; Dickman 1983; Hiatt 1978, 1980a; Sicurella 1977).

Eye/Muscle Resting Techniques. Older people can be taught techniques for both using and relaxing their eyes, as well as alleviating facial muscle strain. Exercises to strengthen residual visual capacities can be provided (Hiatt et al. 1982). Eye-resting techniques are helpful in teaching people that they can read under appropriate lighting and that they can relieve tension without giving up close work activities.

Size. People may need specific ideas on how to increase the size of focal objects, as determined by a low-vision evaluation (Rosenbloom 1974); techniques may include magnification, larger-size consumer products or labeling, or similar technical product changes (Dickman 1983; Hiatt et al. 1982).

Color. The eye care professional can help distinguish between trivial and meaningful notions about the benefits of color. It is highly unlikely that one color will make all people rested or excited. No data suggest that all older people function well with certain wall colors. Color coding often is not effective as a wayfinding technique for many older people who need more concrete, less abstract information about their whereabouts and route (Hiatt 1980b, 1981b).

Older people may see and name colors differently, because the eye's lens tends to yellow during old age, and the ability to differentiate among similarly light tones (pastel colors) or dark shades (black, brown, and navy) diminishes. Data do indicate that as people age, they are able to distinguish between greens, blues, and violets (Fozard et al. 1977; Hiatt 1981b). Almost any color can be made more visible by improving lighting, using it on a highly contrasting surface, and using full-spectrum light sources (Hiatt 1981b; Hiatt et al. 1982; Hughes and Neer 1981).

Alternative Technologies and Senses. Older people in general have not been adequately introduced to technologies or products that might assist them in daily activities despite their vision losses (American Foundation for the Blind 1983; Hale 1979). Independence in daily living might be increased if people were encouraged to take fuller advantage of mobility aids and communication devices as well as optical aids (Hale 1979; Hiatt 1981a; Mellor 1981; Rosenbloom 1974).

Sensory Retraining Based on Environmental Features. Sensory retraining involves learning to identify sounds for orientation and mobility; using tactile, kinesthetic, and thermal changes; learning techniques for estimating size, weight, distance, and time; and training in the identification of odors (Barns, Sack and Shore 1973; Kimbrough, Heubner and Lowry 1976). It also may include training for reduced peripheral vision and for orientation or wayfinding (Blasch and Hiatt 1983; Hiatt 1980b). The American Foundation for the Blind maintains a directory of services that offer training to partially sighted, as well as blind persons. Directories issued since 1983 indicate whether the training is specifically geared toward older people.

Specific Instruction in Prevention of Falls and Other Accidents. The three most common places for accidents that involve older people are the bathroom, next to the bed, and in transitional spaces (between rooms and halls, and indoors to outside; Maguire 1971). Training on accident prevention at home and while driving is too seldom offered for older people (Daubs 1973; Overstall 1980; Waller 1978).

Print Legibility. Several studies have added to our understanding of the print legibility requirements of older people (Badar 1980; Ralph 1982; Vanderplas and Vanderplas 1980; Yelland 1980). For printed matter, type styles with serifs are more legible than sans serif styles. Type sizes larger than 12 points do not seem to increase legibility or reading speed. Line width, the amount of white space available, and the simplicity of the background are factors of print legibility that are often overlooked. Just as reflective floors may contribute to disabilities of orientation (Hiatt 1978; Waller 1978), shiny paper may reduce legibility and produce reading discomforts (Ralph 1982; Yelland 1980).

The vision care professional's role with regard to environmental design may range from simply making people aware of the environment by talking about it, to offering consumers and other professionals publications or information on the topic, to serving on committees that make settings more visually accessible. Vision care professionals are also needed as consultants in industry, technology, and design to develop and market more appropriate amenities for older people.

Why Hasn't More Been Done, Sooner?

The lack of transportation and funding mechanisms all too often have discouraged sensory-impaired individuals away from community-based services and enticed them into institutions. Sometimes community services are too fragmented or seem difficult to contact, especially for people who have trouble reading a telephone book or telephoning.

The environment often is taken for granted. People in midlife are accustomed to thinking of themselves as independent of their surroundings; when things are not to their liking, they change them, ignore them, or leave. Older people may be less mobile and more vulnerable to features of the environment. Sometimes habits keep people from changing lighting or doing things new ways. At other times, they just fail to think beyond the loss of vision itself. Professionals who value the environment may well pass along this sensitivity to their clients.

Sometimes older people and their families have not demanded services because they do not believe improvements are possible. Professionals may have similar misconceptions regarding the values of prevention and rehabilitation of older vision-impaired people. Some would argue that professionals have poor incentives for bringing vision services to older people (Kane and Kane 1978). By contrast, pharmacologic interventions have been well financed and too widely adopted (Green 1978).

People, organizations, and communities respond well to models, or examples. More innovative vision evaluation and services will require the following:

1. A systematic effort to disseminate information on what is available, what does work, and how to go about doing it.
2. Information on what programs cost, in dollars and professional time.
3. Cooperation with agencies outside the field of vision care.
4. Truly new ideas (uses of computers in retraining or technology enhancements in lighting, vision, or mobility, for example).

Summary

Although research has amply documented the potential for using a variety of services, technologies, and environmental design techniques in overcoming vision losses in old age, older people are inadequately receiving the benefits of this information. This chapter offers a variety of

reasons for the gaps between knowledge and practice; paramount may be the lack of information that something can be done.

Vision care professionals can assume many worthwhile roles at this time. We need technological improvements to aid evaluation, as well as community liaisons to work with existing programs and older people. We also need spokespeople to convey ideas and information through a variety of sources so that we raise the expectations of older people and of our peers among vision care professionals.

References

American Foundation for the Blind. *Products for People with Vision Problems.* New York: American Foundation for the Blind, 1983.

Bader, J. E. "The Legibility of Print and the Indexing of Printed Reference Materials Intended for Use by Older People." Ph.D. diss. University of California, San Francisco, 1980.

Baltes, P. B., and K. W. Schaie. " The Myth of Twilight Years." *Psychology Today* 7, no. 10 (1974) 35–40.

Barns, E.; A. Sack; and H. Shore. "Guidelines to Treatment Approaches." *Gerontologist* 13 (1973) 513–527.

Birren, J. E. *The Psychology of Aging.* Englewood Cliffs, N.J.: Prentice-Hall, 1964.

Blackwell, O. M., and H. R. Blackwell. "IERE Reports: Visual Performance Data for 156 Normal Observers of Various Ages." *Journal of the Illuminating Engineering Society* 1 (1971) 2–13.

Blasch, B. and L. G. Hiatt. *Orientation and Wayfinding.* Washington D.C.: U.S. Architectural and Transportation Barriers Compliance Board, 1983.

Braf, P. G. *The Physical Environment and the Visually Impaired.* Bromma, Sweden: ICTA Information Centre, 1974 FACK, S-161 03.

Butler, R. N.; J. S. Gertman: D. L. Oberlander; and L. Schindler. "Self-Help, Self-Care, and the Elderly." *International Journal of Aging and Human Development* 10, no. 1 (1979–1980) 95–107.

Cullinan, T. R. "Epidemiology of Visual Disability." *Transactions of the Ophthalmological Societies, United Kingdom* 98 (1978):267–269. (a)

Cullinan, T. R. "Visually Disabled People at Home." *New Beacon* 63, no. 743 (1978): 57–59. (b)

Cullinan, T. R. "Studies of Visually Disabled People in the Community." *Regional Review* 63 (Spring 1979): 21–25.

Cullinan, T. R. "Low Vision in Elderly People." In *Light for Low Vision,* ed. R. Greenhalgh. Proceedings of a symposium. London: University College, 1980, pp. 65–70. (a)

Cullinan, T. R. "Visual Disability and Home Lighting." *International Journal of Rehabilitation Research* 3, no. 3 (1980): 406–407. (b)

Daubs, J. G. "Visual Factors in the Epidemiology of Falls by the Elderly." *Journal of the American Optometric Association* 44 (1973): 733–736.

Dickman, I. R. *Making Life more Liveable.* New York: American Foundation for the Blind, 1983.

Dory, F. *Building Self-Help Groups among Older Persons: A Training Curriculum to Prepare Organizers.* New York: Center for Advanced Study in Education, Graduate Center, City University of New York, 1979.

Duncan, J.; C. Gish; M.E. Mulholland and A. Townsend. *Environmental Modifications for the Visually Impaired: A Handbook.* New York: American Foundation for the Blind, 1977.

Elderly Hearing Impaired People. *Report on a Mini–White House Conference on Aging.* Washington, D.C.: U.S. Government Printing Office, 1981.

Flood, J. T. "Special Problems of the Aged Deaf Person." *Journal of Rehabilitation of the Deaf* 12, no. 4 (1979): 34–35.

Fozard, J. L. "The Time for Remembering." In *Aging in the 1980s,* ed. L. Poon. Washington, D.C.: Amercian Psychological Association, 1980, pp. 273–287.

Fozard, J. L. "Person-Environment Relationships in Adulthood: Implications for Human Factors Engineering." *Human Factors* 23, no. 1 (1981): 7–28.

Fozard, J. L., and S. J. Popkin. "Optimizing Adult Development: Ends and Means of an Applied Psychology of Aging." *American Psychologist* 33 (1978): 975–989.

Fozard, J. L.; E. Wolf; B. Bell; R. A. McFarland, and S. Podolsky. "Visual Perception and Communication." In *Handbook of the Psychology of Aging,* eds. J. E. Birren and K. W. Schaie. New York: Van Nostrand, 1977, pp. 497–534.

Gartner, A., and F. Reissman. *Self-Help in the Human Services.* San Francisco: Jossey-Bass, 1979.

Genensky, S. "Architectural Barriers to the Partially Sighted –And Solutions." *Architectural Record* 167, no. 5 (1980): 65, 67.

Green, G. "The Politics of Psychoactive Drug Use in Old Age." *Gerontologist* 18, no. 6 (1978):523–530.

Hale, G. *The Sourcebook for the Disabled.* New York: Bantam, 1979.

Hiatt, L. G. "Architecture for the Aged: Design for Living." *Inland Architect* 23 (1978): 6–17.

Hiatt, L. G. "Disorientation Is More Than a State of Mind." *Nursing Homes* 29, no. 4 (1980): 30–36. (a)

Hiatt, L. G. "Is Poor Light Dimming the Sight of Nursing Home Patients? Implications for Vision Screening and Care." *Nursing Homes* 29, no. 5 (1980):32–41. (b)

Hiatt, L. G. "Touchy about Touching?" *Nursing Homes* 29, no. 6 (1980): 42–46.

Hiatt, L. G. "Aging and Disability." In *America's Retirement Population: Prospects, Planning and Policy,* eds. N. McClosky and E. Borgotta. Beverly Hills, Calif.: Sage, 1981, pp. 133–152. (a)

Hiatt, L. G. "Color and Care: The Selection and Use of Colors in Environments for Older People." *Nursing Homes* 30, no. 3 (1981): 18–22. (b)

Hiatt L. G. "Environmental Design and the Frail Older Person at Home." *Pride Institute of Long-Term Home Health Care* 2, no. 1 (1983): 13–22.

Hiatt L.G.; R. Brieff; J. Horwitz; and C. McQueen. *What Are Friends For? Self-Help Groups for Older Persons With Sensory Loss: The U.S.E. Program.* New York: American Foundation for the Blind, 1982.

Hughes, P. C., and R. M. Neer "Lighting for the Elderly: A Psychobiological Approach to Lighting." *Human Factors* 23, no.1 (1980): 65–86.

Kane, R., and R. Kane. " Care of the Aged: Old problems in Need of New Solutions." *Science* 200 (1978): 913–919.

Kimbrough, J. A.; K. Heubner; and L. Lowry. *Sensory Training: A Curriculum Guide.* Professional Series 2. Pittsburgh: Greater Pittsburgh Guild for the Blind, 1976.

Kirchner, C., and R. Peterson. "Multiple Impairments among Non-Institutionalized Blind and Visually Impaired Persons." *Journal of Visual Impairment and Blindness* 74 (1980): 42–44.

Koncelik, J. A. " Human Factors and Environmental Design for the Aging: Physiological Change and Sensory Loss as Design Criteria." In *Environmental Context of Aging,* eds. T. O. Byerts, S. C. Howell and L. A. Pastalan. New York: Garland, 1979, pp. 107–118.

Lefitt, J. "Lighting for the Elderly: An Optician's View." In *Light for Low Vision,* ed. R. Greenhalgh. Proceedings of a symposium, University College, London, April 1978; Hove, Sussex, 1980, pp. 55–61.

Leslie, W. J., and D. A. Greenberg. "A Survey and Proposal Concerning Visual Care at the Nursing Home Level." *Journal of the American Optometric Association* 45 (1974): 461–466.

Lieberman, M. A., and L. D. Borman, eds. *Self-Help Groups for Coping with Crisis.* San Francisco: Jossey-Bass, 1979.

Markle, R. J. *Household Arts: A Curriculum Guide.* Professional Series 3. Pittsburgh: Greater Pittsburgh Guild for the Blind, 1977.

Marsh, G. R. "Perceptual Changes with Age." In *Handbook of Geriatric Psychiatry,* eds. E. W. Busse and D. G. Blazer. New York: Van Nostrand, 1980, pp. 147–168.

McGuire, M. "Preventive Measures to Minimize Accidents among the Elderly." *Occupational Health Nursing* 19 (1971): 13–16.

Mellor, M. *Aids for the 80s: What They Are and What They Do.* New York: American Foundation for the Blind, 1981.

Miller, D. "Vision Screening and Hearing in the Elderly." *Eye, Ear, Nose and Throat Monthly* 53 (1974): 128–133.

Moen, E. "The Reluctance of the Elderly to Seek Help." *Social Problems* 25 no. 3 (1978): 293–303.

Newman, B. Y. "Vision Care in Nursing Homes." *California Optometrist* 3, no. 9 (1977).

Nuckolls, J. L. *Interior Lighting for Environmental Designers.* New York: Wiley, 1976.

Okun, M. A. "Implications of Geropsychological Research on Instruction of Older Adults." *Adult Education* 27, no. 3 (1977): 139–155.

Ordy, J. M., and K. R. Brizzee, eds. *Sensory Systems and Communication in the Elderly.* New York: Raven, 1979.

Overstall, P. W. "Prevention of Falls in the Elderly." *Journal of the American Geriatric Society* 28, no. 11 (1980): 481–484.

Pastalan, L. A. "Sensory Changes and Environmental Behavior." In *Environmental Context of Aging,* eds. T. O Byerts, S. C. Howell and L. A. Pastalan. New York: Garland, 1979, pp. 118–126.

Ralph, J. B. "Guidelines for Printing Published Materials for Our Aging Population." *Journal of the American Optometric Association* 53, no. 1 (1982): 43–50.

Rosenbloom, A. A. "Prognostic Factors in the Visual Rehabilitation of Aging Patients." *New Outlook for the Blind* 64, no. 3 (1974): 124–127.

Sartoris, R. "Eye Care in Nursing Homes." *Minnesota Optometrist* 1975: 6.

Sekuler, R., and L. Hutman. "Spatial Vision and Aging: 1. Contrast Sensitivity." *Journal of Gerontology* 35, no. 5 (1980): 692–699.

Sicurella, V. "Color Contrast as an Aid for Visually Impaired Persons." *Journal of Visual Impairment and Blindness* 71 (1977): 252–257.

Silver, J. H.; E. S. Gould; D. Irvine; and T. R. Cullinan. "Visual Acuity at Home and in Eye Clinics." *Transactions of the Ophthalmological Societies of the United Kingdom* 98, part 2 (1978) 252–257.

Snyder, L; J. Pyrek; and K. Smith. "Vision and Mental Function." *Gerontologist* 16, no. 3 (1976): 491–495.

Vanderplas, J. M., and J. H. Vanderplas. "Some Factors Affecting Legibility of Printed Materials for Older Adults." *Perceptual and Motor Skills* 50 (1980): 923–932.

Vision and Aging. Report of the Mini-Conference on Vision and Aging prepared for the 1981 White House Conference on Aging. Washington, D.C.: U.S. Government Printing Office, 1981. (Also available from the American Foundation for the Blind, New York City.)

Waller, J. "Falls among the Elderly: Human Environmental Factors. *Accident Analysis and Prevention* 10 (1978): 21–33.

Wardell, K. T. "Environmental Modifications." In *Orientation and Mobility,* eds. R. L. Welsh and B. Blasch. New York: American Foundation for the Blind, 1980, pp. 477–525.

Welsh, R. L., and B. B. Blasch, eds. *Foundations of Orientation and Mobility.* New York: American Foundation for the Blind, 1980.

Willems, E. P. "Behavioral Ecology." In *Perspectives on Environment and Behavior: Theory, Research and Applications,* ed. D. Stokols. New York: Plenum, 1977, pp. 39–68.

Winer, M. A. "Method for Setting Up a Self-Help Support Network for People with Progressive Eye Disease." *Braille Forum* 29, no. 10 (1981): 22–27.

Woodruff, M. E., and G. Pack. "A Survey of the Prevalence of Vision Defects and Ocular Anomalies in 43 Ontario Residential and Nursing Homes." *Canadian Journal of Public Health* 71 (1980): 413–423.

Yeadon, A., and D. Grayson. *Living with Impaired Vision: An Introduction.* New York: American Foundation for the Blind, 1979.

Yelland, M. "Large Print Difficulties." In *Light for Low Vision,* Proceedings of a symposium, London: University College, 1980, pp. 47–54.

Contributing Authors

Karen Altergott, Ph.D., is assistant professor of family studies, Purdue University, West Lafayette. Altergott's research and publications are on aging and the family, social networks, and social policy. She has received fellowships from the National Institute on Aging and the National Institute on Mental Health and currently helps administer predoctoral and postdoctoral training programs in social gerontology.

John Anstice, Dip. Opt., M.Sc., received his optometric training at the Auckland University School of Optometry and his M.Sc. degree in psychology from the University of Canterbury (New Zealand). He is in private optometric practice with an emphasis on orthoptics and contact lenses. Anstice has lectured and published in these areas and was the 1983 recipient of the New Zealand Contact Lens Society's Allergan Travel Award.

Jeanne E. Bader, Ph.D., is director of the Center for Gerontology at the University of Oregon. She has held previous positions at the Hubert H. Humphrey Institute of Public Affairs (University of Minnesota), the Graduate School of Public Policy (University of California, Berkeley), and the Philadelphia Geriatric Center.

Ian L. Bailey, O.D., M.S., F.B.O.A.(H.D.), is an associate professor and director of the Low Vision Center of the School of Optometry, University of California, Berkeley. He is a Diplomate in Low Vision of the American Academy of Optometry. Most of Bailey's research and publications deal with low vision and clinical optics. He was elected a life governor of the Association for the Blind, Melbourne, Australia, in recognition of his contribution to the establishment of the Kooyong Low Vision Clinic.

Susan Bettis, Ph.D., is associate professor of psychology and nursing and chair of the humanities department at the Linfield Good Samaritan School of Nursing in Portland, Oregon. Prior to this position she was an assistant professor of gerontology at the University of Oregon's Center for Gerontology.

David M. Cockburn, O.A.M., M.Sc. Optom., is senior academic associate in the Department of Optometry, University of Melbourne; chair of the board of administration, National Vision Research Institute of Australia; and chair of the board of continuing education, Victorian College of Optometry. Besides teaching and research interests centered on ocular manifestations of systemic disease, he conducts a private optometry practice.

Daniel F. Detzner, Ph.D., is associate professor, social and behavioral sciences, and coordinator of the Aging Studies Program at the University of Minnesota. His research interests include cross-cultural gerontology, stereotyping, and life review. Service activities include workshops, in-service training, and conferences for people involved in direct service roles with the elderly.

Jay M. Enoch, Ph.D., is professor of physiological optics and optometry and dean, School of Optometry, University of California, Berkeley. He also is professor of physiological optics in ophthalmology at the School of Medicine, University of California, San Francisco. Enoch has dedicated a lifelong career to visual science research and vision needs, including studies on retinal receptor optics and function; experimental perimetry; studies of infant vision; contact lens fitting in complex cases; and assessment of vision through dense opacities such as cataracts, leukomas, and hemorrhages.

Eleanor E. Faye, M.D., F.A.C.S., is the ophthalmological director of the New York Lighthouse Low Vision Service and attending surgeon at Manhattan Eye, Ear and Throat Hospital. She holds an honorary doctor of humane letters degree from Illinois College of Optometry, and the Honor Award and Senior Honor Award from the American Academy of Ophthalmology for her contribution to the education of ophthalmologists and optometrists in low vision. She is the author of numerous textbooks and articles on low vision.

Samuel M. Genensky, Ph.D., F.A.A.O., is executive director of The Center for the Partially Sighted in Santa Monica, California. Genensky's research on electro-optical aids led to the production of the first practical closed-circuit television systems for the partially sighted. His research on behalf of the partially sighted population also includes multicamera, multimonitor two-way video communications systems; visual environmental adaptation problems; and solutions to environmental and architectural barriers. He is a recipient of the Paul Yarwood Award and of an honorary doctor of humane letters degree from the Illinois College of Optometry.

Lorraine G. Hiatt, Ph.D., is an environmental psychologist/gerontologist who consults nationally from her base in New York City. For 15 years she has conducted research, lectured, and written on optimizing the sensory and mental functioning of elderly people through programs and design. From 1979 to 1982 she was national consultant on aging for the American Foundation for the Blind. Hiatt is currently an associate of the Center for Human Environments at the City University of New York.

Jule Griebrok Jose, O.D., Ph.D., is an associate professor of optometry and physiological optics at the University of Houston College of Optometry, where she also lectures in ocular pharmacology. Her primary research interest is in the area of cataracts, particularly ultraviolet- and photosensitizer-induced anomalies in the lens. From her research Jose developed the hypothesis that senile cataracts may develop as a consequence of DNA damage in the lens.

David D. Michaels, M.S., O.D., M.D., is clini-

cal professor of ophthalmology at UCLA School of Medicine and chair of the Department of Ophthalmology at San Pedro Peninsula Hospital. His widely recognized text *Visual Optics and Refraction* is now in its third edition.

Meredith W. Morgan, O.D., Ph.D., is professor emeritus and former dean of the School of Optometry, University of California, Berkeley. Morgan's primary interest is binocular vision and clinical optometry. His contributions to optometry and visual science have been recognized by the Apollo Award of the American Optometric Association, the Prentice Medal of the American Academy of Optometry, and the Berkeley Citation from the University of California.

Marion Nestle, Ph.D., is associate dean, School of Medicine; lecturer in family and community medicine; and director of the John Tung–American Cancer Society Clinical Nutrition Education Center at the University of California (San Francisco) School of Medicine. She is the author of *Nutrition in Clinical Practice,* a text for health professions students and practitioners.

Anthony J. Phillips, M. Phil., F.B.C.O., F.B.O.A. (H.D.), is head of the Contact Lens Unit, Department of Ophthalmology, Flinders Medical Centre, Adelaide, South Australia. He is also in general optometric practice specializing largely in contact lenses. Phillips is co-editor with Janet Stone of *Contact Lenses: A Textbook for Practitioner and Student* and has written numerous papers on contact lenses, optometric politics, practice management, visual aspects of night driving, and ocular anatomy.

David Pickwell, M.Sc., F.B.C.O., F.B.O.A. (H.D.), D. Orth., is professor of optometry, University of Bradford, Great Britain; and president of the International Optometry and Optical League. His primary interest is binocular vision, and he is author of a clinical book for optometrists, *Binocular Vision Anomalies.* Pickwell was awarded the Owen Aves Medal (1974) and the Walter Green Prize (1979) for contributions to research and teaching in binocular vision.

Albert L. Pierce, optician, is presently assistant professor and chief of the ophthalmic division at the University of Alabama at Birmingham School of Optometry. Prior to this position he was director of the ophthalmic dispensary and lecturer at the University of California (Berkeley) School of Optometry.

J. Randall Pitman, O.D., B.A., B.S., received his B.A. degree (Phi Beta Kappa) from the University of Idaho in 1980. Subsequent work at Pacific University College of Optometry led to a B.S. degree in 1981 and an O.D. degree in 1984. Pitman is currently in private practice in St. Maries, Idaho.

Derek M. Prinsley, M.D., F.R.C.P., F.R.A.C.P., F.R.S.H., is the professor of geriatric medicine, University of Melbourne, and director of the National Research Institute of Gerontology and Geriatric Medicine at Mount Royal Hospital in Australia. Prinsley is a member of the WHO Expert Advisory Panel on Health of Elderly Persons and has contributed extensively to the literature in gerontology.

Robert Rosenberg, O.D., is professor and chair of the Department of Vision Sciences at the State University of New York College of Optometry; consultant to the New York Lighthouse Low Vision Service; and former chair of the ANSI Subcommittee Z80.9 on Low Vision Aids. He was the founding chief of the Low Vision Clinic, University Optometric Center, State University of New York. Rosenberg is the author of several papers on low vision in geriatrics, as well as contributor to optometric public health and low-vision textbooks.

Alfred A. Rosenbloom, Jr., O.D., D.O.S., M.A., is an educator and administrator whose primary academic and research interests are in the fields of low vision, optometric gerontology, and clinical optometry. He serves as the Illinois College of Optometry's first Distinguished Professor of Optometry. For 25 years Rosenbloom served as dean and then president of the Illinois College of Optometry. Since 1956 he also has been an optometric consultant to the Chicago Lighthouse for the Blind. He is a Diplomate in Low Vision of the American Academy of Optometry. Rosenbloom is contributing author to six textbooks, as well as a writer in the fields of optometry, visual rehabilitation, and education.

E. Richard Tennant, O.D., D.O.S., is professor emeritus of the Illinois College of Optometry, where he served as chair of the Department of Physical Science. His primary teaching and research interests are in the fields of geometrical and physical optics. He has lectured on many clinical topics, including aphakia, binocular refraction, and ophthalmic optics.

C. Edwin Vaughan, Ph.D., is currently professor of sociology and director of the Center for the Study of Aging, University of Missouri, Columbia. He has a personal interest in problems of the blind and partially sighted. Vaughan is doing research and administering programs related to the needs of impaired older people.

Bruce C. Wick, O.D., has been in private practice for 13 years in Rapid City, South Dakota. He is currently an Associate Professor of Optometry at the College of Optometry, University of Houston. Wick's primary interests are binocular vision and aniseikonia. He is a Diplomate in Binocular Vision and Perception of the American Academy of Optometry and has served on the review board of the *Journal of the American Optometric Association* and the editorial council of the *American Journal of Optometry and Physiological Optics*.

Robert L. Yolton, O.D., Ph.D., received B.A., M.A., and Ph.D. degrees in psychology from the University of Wisconsin, California State University at Sacramento, and the University of Texas at Austin, respectively. His O.D. degree was granted by the New England College of Optometry in 1975. He is currently an associate professor at Pacific University College of Optometry, teaching psychophysiology of vision. Yolton's research interests include electrodiagnostic techniques, biofeedback, and the effects of visual anomalies on human physiology.

Steven H. Zarit, Ph.D., is associate professor of gerontology and psychology, Andrus Gerontology Center, University of Southern California, Los Angeles. Zarit's primary interests are in the adaptation of older people to chronic disabilities, including vision impairment and memory loss. He was director of psychological services at The Center for the Partially Sighted in Santa Monica, California, from 1979 to 1983. Zarit is the author of several articles and books on mental health problems in later life.

Index

Page numbers in *italics* refer to tables or figures.

DATE DUE